W0043757

Ultrasonography in Ophthalmology

Documenta Ophthalmologica
Proceedings Series volume 29

Editor H.E. Henkes

Dr W. Junk Publishers   The Hague — Boston — London 1981

Ultrasonography in Ophthalmology

Proceedings of the 8th SIDUO Congress

Edited by J. M. Thijssen and A. M. Verbeek

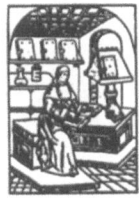

Dr W. Junk Publishers   The Hague — Boston — London 1981

Distributors:

for the United States and Canada

Kluwer Boston, Inc.
190 Old Derby Street
Hingham, MA 02043
USA

for all other countries

Kluwer Academic Publishers Group
Distribution Center
P.O. Box 322
3300 AH Dordrecht
The Netherlands

Library of Congress Cataloging in Publication Data

Ultrasonography in Ophthalmology. Proceedings of the 8th SIDUO Congress:
  Nijmegen, Netherlands

  (Documenta Ophthalmologica Proceedings series; v. 29)
  Bibliography
1. Ophthalmology–Congresses. 2. Eye–Diseases and defects–Congresses.
3. Adnexa oculi–Diseases–Congresses. I. Thijssen, J.M. II. Verbeek, A.M.
III. Title. IV. Series.
RE11.S55   1980   617.7   81-14271
                                        AACR2

ISBN-13: 978-94-009-8661-9   e-ISBN-13: 978-94-009-8659-6
DOI: 10.1007/978-94-009-8659-6

Cover design: Max Velthuijs

Copyright © 1981 Dr W. Junk Publishers, The Hague.

Softcover reprint of the hardcover 1st edition 1981

All rights reserved. No part of this publication may be reproduced, stored in a retrieval system, or transmitted in any form or by any means, mechanical, photocopying, recording, or otherwise, without the prior written permission of the publishers.

Dr W. Junk Publishers, P.O. Box 13713, 2501 ES The Hague, The Netherlands.

TABLE OF CONTENTS

PART ONE: THE EYE

1. Vitreous pathology

V

2. Intraocular tumours

3. Oculometry, lensimplantation

4. Miscellaneous

PART TWO: THE ORBIT

1. Orbital tumours

2. Optic nerve, muscles

3. Miscellaneous

PART THREE: NEW TECHNIQUES

1. Tissue characterization

2. Equipment

OPENING OF SIDUO 8
BY PROFESSOR AUGUST F. DEUTMAN,
HONORARY PRESIDENT OF THE SYMPOSIUM

Ladies and Gentlemen:

I am very happy and honoured having been asked to open this VIIIth meeting of the SIDUO. We are proud to have been chosen as the meeting place of this important congress.

Echography has developed into both an art and a science, and has conquered a very important place in modern ophthalmology. I would specifically like to mention oculometry because of lens implantation and the diagnostic examinations in vitreous opacities, ocular tumours and orbital lesions.

We are very honoured, indeed, that one of the foremost pioneers of ultrasound in ophthalmology, Gil Baum (New York), is here. Furthermore I would like to welcome specifically the great forerunners in echography, Karl Ossoinig (Iowa) and Jackson Coleman (New York). Four years ago in Lausanne, both, together with Dr. Oksala from Finland, received the prestigious Wacker award from the Jules Gonin Club, stressing the clinical importance of their pioneering work. When they received this award the whole ophthalmic echography world was honoured.

We are especially pleased to see Karl Ossoinig of the '3rd Viennese Eye Clinic (Dritte Wiener Augenklinik)' here in Iowa City, because he often helped our staff-members, Thijssen and Verbeek, set up a first class diagnostic unit. It is unquestionable that both A- and B-scan techniques have found an important place and beautifully complement one another, A-scan for oculometry and tissue differentiation and B-scan for the more exact localization of pathological processes. Together with computerized tomography, the diagnostic possibilities in ophthalmology have improved tremendously. Except for its well-known use in the fragmentation of lenses, therapeutic use of ultrasound still has to find a place.

I would also like to welcome the President of the International Council of Ophthalmology, Professor François, who is as active as ever and by his presence gives this meeting extra stature.

I wish this meeting the success it deserves and hope that this meeting will stimulate many researchers to develop ultrasound in ophthalmology into an even more important science.

Dr. Thijssen and Dr. Verbeek, I know how hard you both worked to organize this meeting and, therefore, I wish you all the success you deserve. Herewith I declare the VIIIth SIDUO Congress to be opened.

WELCOME BY PROFESSOR F. DAEMEN,
DEAN OF THE MEDICAL SCHOOL

Societas Internationalis pro Diagnostica Ultrasonica in Ophthalmologia: Symposium Octavum

It is indeed a great pleasure for me to welcome all of you on behalf of the board of the Medical School of the University of Nijmegen. We highly appreciate that you have come from many countries in Europe, and from as far as Egypt, Lebanon, United States, Argentina and Japan.

Myself being engaged in basic eye research, the biochemistry of photo-reception, I feel somewhat envious of your discipline: ultrasound in ophthalmology. Not only is it immediately clear to everybody that results in your field are applicable in patient care, or at least diagnosis, but the technique that you have developed, and are developing further, is very elegant and without any hint of harmful side-effects. Therefore, I may assume that you are spared the well-known troubles to have to prove the relevancy of your work and, hence, finding funds for your research cannot possibly be a problem.

In addition, your Society has an impressive Latin name. However, upon its foundation Latin was no longer the language of scientists and physicians, at least here in Europe. So why Latin? Of course I pass indignantly along the possibility of dog Latin. I suppose it has to do with a true international atmosphere and it suggests that you all are combining in your person and work modern skills with classic cultural values.

Anyhow, I am sure that the Organizing Committee from our Department of Ophthalmology, chaired by Dr. Han Thijssen, has carefully prepared the scientific and the social program. The presence of an honorary president like Professor August Deutman can only add to your confidence in this matter. Thus, you have every reason to expect a successful Eighth Symposium of your Society.

You certainly have my best wishes.

Symposium Octavum, Floreat

WELCOME BY DR. J.M. THIJSSEN,
PRESIDENT OF THE SYMPOSIUM

I am very happy to welcome you all, on behalf of the Organizing Committee, and personally. It is great to host so many friends in our city of Nijmegen.

I had some philosophies before the start of the organization of this Symposium. To be more specific, I wanted to make this Meeting as attractive as possible to young ophthalmologists, and even to residents. We have worked this out, as you may have noticed, by announcing the Symposium twice in one year to 1000 training Hospitals in Europe. We have held a special training course yesterday afternoon, and we have asked four prominent ophthalmologists to present lectures which are introductory in a broad clinical sense to the main topics of the Symposium.

This is all you know already, but we also have added a few other things which you yourself may make highly successful by your full cooperation and enthusiasm. We have created a Discussion Room on this floor, to the left of the Secretariat, where we expect the speakers of every morning or afternoon session to stay during the scheduled Discussion time and to be so open minded to give the other participants the opportunity to reopen the discussion on their Presentation. At the same time, during this Discussion time we will ask a few people who have brought with them one of these splendid Posters, to be available for discussion in front of their own Poster. This will be announced every day at the end of the Sessions.

Another hint I would like to give you is that we have a very extensive commercial exhibition, which is not only located here on the first floor, but also on the ground floor, and to make it more attractive to go downstairs we have foreseen a second coffee stand downstairs as well.

We received a few letters from people who were not able to come and liked to send you their regards, they are: Prof. Douglas Gordon, from London, Prof. S. Tane from Kawasaki, Prof. A Oksala, Turku, Dr. M. Wainstock from Detroit and Dr. H. Hughes from Sydney.

Ladies and Gentlemen, on behalf of the Organizing Committe may I wish you a very interesting, fruitful and enjoyable Symposium.

WELCOMING ADDRESS BY KARL C. OSSOINIG, M.D., PRESIDENT OF SIDUO, 1975–1980

Professor Deutman, Doctor Thijssen, Ladies and Gentlemen:

It is with great pleasure that I welcome you, both members and guests of SIDUO, to our eighth Congress. I am particularly pleased to greet our honorary members present, Professor Jules François, Professor Gilbert Baum and Professor Hermann Gernet. The large number of participants (nearly 150) present at this Congress is a new record for SIDUO meetings, and clearly shows the great popularity of our hosts, and of the famous university and beautiful city of Nijmegen. It is convincing evidence as well of the growing strength of our society.

I know that we all are very grateful to our hosts, the Honorary President of this Congress, Professor August Deutman, and the President of the Congress, Doctor Han Thijssen. Professor Deutman, an internationally renowned ophthalmologist, the head of the Eye Department of the Catholic University of Nijmegen, and an old frield of SIDUO, has contributed greatly to insure the success of this Congress. We are particularly grateful to Doctor Thijssen, who, as one of the pioneers in ophthalmic echography, and through his unique energy and skills, and his great scientific and administrative expertise, has succeeded, with the help of his organizing committee, in presenting us with a scientific and social program which is outstanding in every way. I am confident that we all will thoroughly enjoy this excellent program, as it will widen and deepen our understanding and knowledge of ophthalmic echography, and will provide the stimulus for further developments in this exciting medical field. And, equally important, this meeting will surely strengthen SIDUO's international ties, and all of our personal contacts and friendships.

ECHOGRAPHY AND VITREOUS SURGERY

Introductory lecture

AUGUST F. DEUTMAN, M.D.

(Nijmegen, The Netherlands)

Echography has developed into an important examination technique for the ophthalmic surgeon, particularly in patients with vitreous abnormalities. A-scan techniques are very important for biometry in the implantation of intraocular lenses and for tissue differentiation, whereas B-scan techniques are quite helpful in outlining pathological structures in, around and behind the globe. Especially since the development of vitreous surgery by Machemer and associates (1971) examination techniques of the vitreous have become increasingly important. Combination of A- and B-scan techniques is necessary to get maximal and optimal information about the morphology in the eye. Additional electro-ophthalmological testing methods have shown to be equally important to give information about the functional state of the eye.

Electro-retinography (ERG) and electro-oculography (EOG) can give one information about the functional state of the attached retina, while visually evoked cortical potentials (VECP) can give information about the macula, the papillomacular bundle, the optic nerve and its connections to the occipital cortex. We have to stress here that the ERG is not helpful in detached retinas since a detached retina, even if the retina itself is potentially quite good, will generally not respond. Moreover, the expected visual acuity after vitreous surgery cannot be predicted by ERG examinations; in this respect the VECP offers better possibilities.

A relatively good VECP with a poor ERG may indicate an attached posterior pole of the retina and a detached retinal periphery as we have seen in a few cases. In very dense vitreous haemorrhages an extra bright flash ERG may be necessary to elicit an ERG-response (Fuller *et al.* 1975).

For the vitreous surgeon a combination of ultrasound and electro-ophthalmological testing methods is very helpful, even though relatively simple tests like lightprojection (for the retinal periphery) and entoptic phenomena and gross colour vision (for the posterior pole of the eye) can give him important information. In massive periretinal proliferation (MPP) the far retinal periphery may still be attached and lightprojection may still be good. Even so, more extensive testing is important.

The most frequent indications of vitreous surgery in clinical practice are traumas and complications of diabetic retinopathy. In perforating ocular injuries with vitreous haemorrhage, trans pars plana vitrectomy (TPPV) has to be performed in most cases between one and two weeks after the primary wound closure, ideally some ten days after the injury. After two weeks there may already be tractional retinal detachment and hypotony, making recovery of the eye almost impossible. Hypotonic eyes with cyclitic membranes are very difficult to analyse with echography and sometimes a detached retina will not be detected embedded as it is in fibrovascular proliferations.

Echography can help us very well in detecting a beginning retinal detachment thus indicating the necessity of vitreous surgery. However, even when echography shows that a retina is attached one should not be lured into expecting too much, nor into conservatism, because frequently later on a retinal detachment may occur and a MPP-type of detachment may happen overnight, as we have seen in several cases. In addition to echography and electro-ophthalmological testing, monitoring of the ocular tension is very important. Increasing hypotony usually indicates the formation of cyclitic membranes that pull on the ciliary body and ultimately may detach the retina. Simple removal of the cycliting membrane by TPPV will save the eye in such cases.

When B-scan echography shows a triangle-shaped retinal detachment (Fuller *et al.* 1977), the prognosis for successful vitrectomy is rather poor and injection of intraocular silicone oil with drainage of subretinal fluid should be performed. We developed a microscopical technique for the injection of silicone oil with the help of parts of the Ocutome system (Deutman *et al.* 1980).

When there is no triangle shaped detachment echography is also helpful in outlining the detachment so that the surgeon knows beforehand where the infusion line should be brought into place and where he can expect to encounter a detached retina. Results of vitreous surgery in diabetic retinopathy have improved considerably with the use of the Medical Workshop 45°-angled vitreous scissors and Steve Charles's flute needle principle. Peeling of preretinal membranes may lead to iatrogenic tractional retinal detachment and iatrogenic retinal holes whereas cutting with scissors may severe these membranes without endangering the retina too much. The automated vitreous scissors that are available now make this type of surgery even more safe to perform. Use of bipolar cautery and intraocular photo-coagulation probes have further improved the ultimate results by cutting down the amount of bleeding and neovascular glaucoma. In order to decrease the amount of postoperative neovascular glaucoma in complicated diabetic retinopathy it seems, at this stage, best to leave the lens in the eye at the time of vitrectomy. If the lens is densely cataractous it should be removed first. Then if the vitreous does not clear afterwards, a trans pars plana vitrectomy can be performed a few months later.

Detachment of the posterior vitreous with ensuing haemorrhage from retinal vessels is an equally important indication for echography. Retinal detachment may occur immediately, days, or even weeks after such a posterior vitreous detachment. Echography therefore has to be repeated at regular intervals to examine the condition of the vitreoretinal relationships.

In choroidal tumors or in Junius-Kuhnt senile macular degeneration complicated by secondary vitreous haemorrhage, echography is indispensable for rendering a good diagnosis. The presence of endophthalmitis is also a good indication for the use of echography since the extension of the vitreous absces can then be monitored. If the retina is still free of the suppurative process, vitreous surgery with infusion of antibiotics may be considered, particularly when the ERG responses are still fairly good.

A developmental abnormality, such as the so-called persistent hyperplastic primary vitreous (PHPV), can be examined and diagnosed quite well with the help of echography techniques and successful TPPV surgery is often possible in PHPV. In retrolental fibroplasia (RLF) echography is equally helpful, differentiating retinoblastoma, Coats' disease, PHPV and the like. Vitreous surgery however is generally less successful in RLF than in PHPV.

In this short introductory paper I have indicated the importance of ultrasound in the evaluation of patients who are candidates for vitreous surgery. There is no doubt that improved techniques such as the use of computer analysis will make echography an even more important diagnostic technique in ophthalmology in the near future.

REFERENCES

Machemer, R., Buettner, H. & Norton, E.W.D. et al. Vitrectomy: a pars plana approach. Ophthalmology (Rochester) 75: 813 (1971).

Deutman, A.E., Eijkenboom, G.J.M. & Fanuriakis, C. A microsurgical method for the injection of intraocular silicone oil. Int. Ophthalmol. 2: 63 (1980).

Fuller, D.G., Knighton, R.W. & Machemer, R. Bright flash electroretinography for the evaluation of eyes with opaque vitreous Am. J. Ophthalmol. 80: 214 (1975).

Fuller, D.G. Laqua, H. & Machemer, R. Ultrasonographic diagnosis of massive periretinal ration in eyes with opaque media (triangular retinal detachment) Am. J. Ophthalmol. 83: 460 (1977).

Author's Address:
Dept. of Ophthalmology
University of Nijmegen
6500 HB Nijmegen
The Netherlands

ULTRASONOGRAPHIC CHARACTERISTICS OF OPERABLE MASSIVE PERIRETINAL PROLIFERATION

H. HAYASHI, K. OSHIMA, N. NAKAMA & Y. NISHIMURA

(Fukuoka, Japan)

INTRODUCTION

Massive periretinal proliferation (MPP) is a miserable condition in retinal detachment. Unfortunately, visual prognosis is still poor in the cases with MPP despite vitrectomy, preretinal membrane peeling and intraocular injection of gas, or silicone oil injection (Machemer & Laqua 1978, Okun & Arrivas 1969). In eyes with opaque media, identification of associated retinal detachment is important for effective vitrectomy. In particular, knowledge of the presence of associated MPP is essential for preoperative assessment of the visual prognosis. Ultrasonography is a most useful method for visualising the structure of an opaque eye.

Fuller and Machemer described the B-mode ultrasonographic characteristic of advanced MPP as triangular retinal detachment (Fuller & Machemer 1977).

Since we have begun to take a therapeutic approach to MPP with the aid of modern vitrectomy techniques, the eyes with MPP were also carefully examined ophthalmoscopically and ultrasonographically. Although many eyes with MPP showed typical triangular configuration as has been described previously, a considerable number of cases showing other configurations on B-scan tomographic section were observed.

We then studied a series of eyes with MPP for establishing the ultra-sonographic characteristics of MPP other than 'triangular retinal detachment', and for evaluating the usefulness of ultrasonographic characteristics for the assessment of operative prognosis.

MATERIALS AND METHOD

Total 48 eyes with MPP were examined over the past one year and nine months at the Ultrasonography Clinic, Department of Ophthalmology, Fukuoka University. Forty of the all eyes did not have the history of previous vitreous surgery. Other eight eyes had received vitreous surgery before ultrasonic examination. In this postvitrectomy group, previous vitrectomy had been performed for MPP in five eyes in which the retina had detached following the vitrectomy, and for other vitreous pathology in three eyes. Of all 48 eyes, 42 had clear media and six had opaque media. In the clear media group, MPP had been confirmed with ophthalmoscopy before the

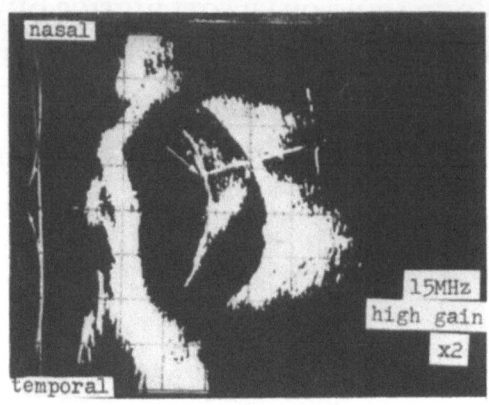

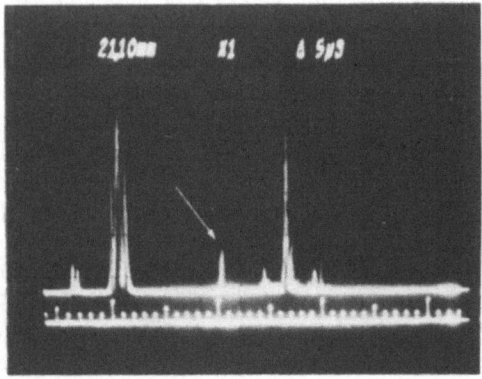

Fig. 1. The ultrasonographic finding of a triangular retinal detachment. Note the equatorial bridging membrane adhered with peripheral retina and bridge in the vitreous cavity.

ultrasonic examination. In the six eyes with opaque media, MPP was confirmed during the vitrectomy in one eye, after cataract extraction in two eyes and after spontaneous regression of vitreous hemorrhage in three eyes.

Twenty-nine eyes were treated by means of vitrectomy coupled with preretinal membrane peeling, intraocular injection of SF6 (40%) gas and buckling procedure. Fourteen eyes were not operated upon since the patients had severe systemic disorders or refused operation.

Ultrasonic examination was perforemed with the commercially available Sonometrics Ophthalmoscan 200 Model A- and B-scan equipment. The eyes were scanned under a water bath as previously described (Coleman *et al.* 1969). We used a 15 MHz focused transducer in a high sensitivity setting. Compound B-scan was made primarily in the horizontal plane, and photographs were taken with a Polaroid camera. The Bronson-Turner Ophthalmic B-scan contact B-scanner (Bronson & Turner 1973) was used simultaneously for observing the movements of intraocular structures during and after voluntary ocular movement.

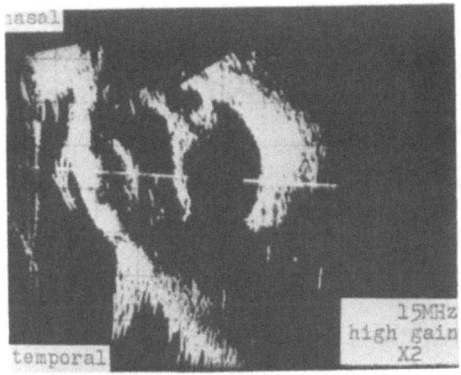

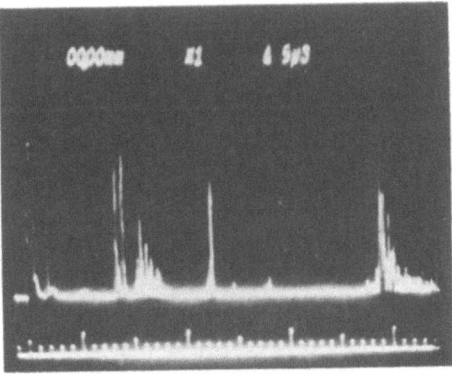

Fig. 2. A T-sign retinal detachment on ultrasonography. The two leaves of the retina have become to adherent and present T formation on the B-scan ultrasonography.

RESULTS

Ultrasonographic characteristics of MPP. Of 40 eyes with MPP which did not receive vitrectomy before examination, 18 showed typical triangular con-figuration as described by Fuller on B-scan ultrasonography (Fig. 1). Ophthalmoscopically, all 18 eyes showed advanced MPP and the presence of a circumferential equatorial bridging membrane was identified in most cases.

The other 22 eyes in this group did not show the proliferating membrane uniting both leaves of the highly detached retina in the anterior vitreous cavity at the base of the intraocular triangle. In seven of these 22 eyes B-scan ultrasonography revealed a structure similar in shape to the letter 'T' or 'Y' in the globe (Fig. 2). As seen with the 'T' shape, one leaf bridged both sides of the ora serrata, and another leaf originating from the optic disc connected at the midline of the former one. This T-sign was found in eyes which showed a closed funnel appearance ophthalmoscopically. Two eyes with T-sign were

7

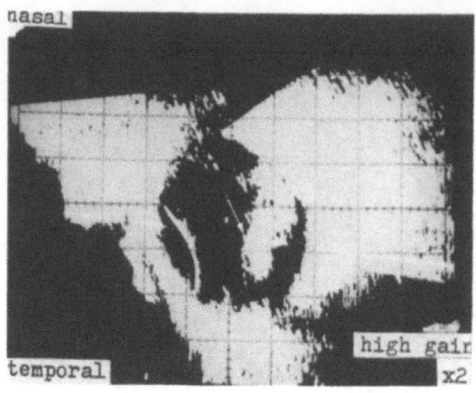

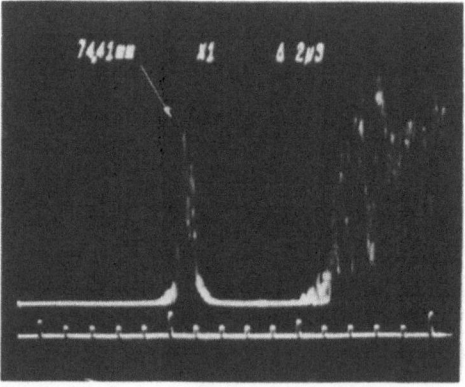

Fig. 3. The detached retina showed irregulary thickened appearance. Equatorial bridging membrane was not seen.

operated on and it was found that the two leaves of the detached retina had adhered posteriorly as a stalk connecting with the optic disc. Nine eyes showed irregular thickening or folding of the retina on B-scan ultrasonography. Usually, thickened retina was found in one or two quadrants of whole retina on which a star figure fold or irregular fold of the retina was found with ophthalmoscopy (Fig. 3). In the remaining six eyes, marked differences from uncomplicated rhegmatogenous retinal detachment without MPP were difficult to find on B-scan ultrasonography. Only the sign of bending of the detached retina, in which the detached retina appears to extend from the optic disc into the vitreous cavity after making an angle of some degrees and then becomes parallel to the posterior ocular wall, was found in some cases (Fig. 4).

Eight eyes with a history of previous vitrectomy did not show triangular configuration. Thickening of the retina was identified in four eyes by B-scan ultrasonography, no remarkable sign being found in the other four eyes. All

8

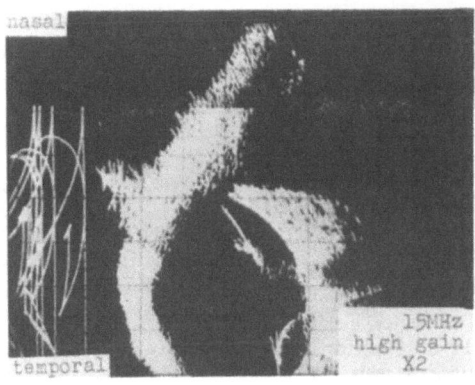

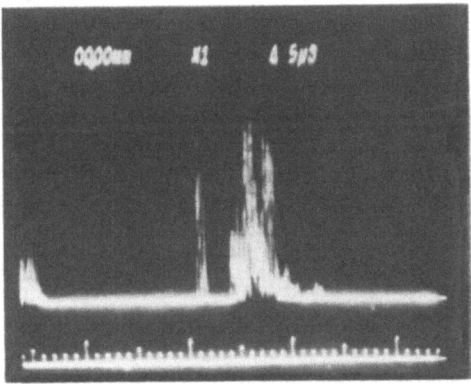

Fig. 4. The detached retina showed bending in the vitreous cavity. The presence of traction was suggested.

findings are shown in Table 1. In all 48 eyes, the detached retina was immobile on dinamic scan.

Ultrasonographic findings and surgical results. Of 29 eyes operated on, ten had the retina attached. In nine eyes, the retina had remained flat six months after operation. The follow-up time was less than six months in one eye. This result might be influenced by additional problems for evaluating surgery of

Table 1. Ultrasonographic findings from eyes with MPP.

	Number of eyes (%)	
Ultrasonographic finding	Previtrectomy group	Postvitrectomy group
Triangular retinal detachment	18/40 (45%)	0/8 (0%)
T-sign retinal detachment	7/40 (18%)	0/8 (0%)
Irregular thickening of retina	9/40 (23%)	4/8 (50%)
Others (Bending of retina etc.)	6/40 (15%)	4/8 (50%)
Total	40/40	8/8

Table 2. Surgical success rate in relation to different ultrasonographic findings.

Ultrasonographic finding	Success rate (%)
Triangular retinal detachment	6/13 (46%)
T-sign retinal detachment	0/2 (0%)
Irregular thickening of retina	3/8 (37%)
Others (Bending of retina etc.)	1/6 (17%)
Total	10/29 (34%)

*This series includes the patients who suffered from MPP after perforating ocular injury or in combination with giant tears.

MPP since this series included the patients that suffered from MPP after perforating ocular injury or in combination with giant tear. The surgical success rate in relation to preoperative findings with ultrasonography is shown in Table 2. It appeared that a similar prognosis for retinal reattachment was obtained regardless of preoperative ultrasonographic finding. Although the retina had not reattached in two eyes with the preoperative ultrasonographic finding of T-sign, no definite conclusions could be drawn because of their insufficient numbers and one of the two eyes was associated giant tear.

DISCUSSION

Massive periretinal proliferation (MPP) has been recognized as a proliferative membrane-forming disease in which metaplastic pigment epithelial cells and glial cells grow to form membranes along available surfaces, such as retina and vitreous. Contraction of intravitreal membrane causes equatorial circumferential fold and/or irregular fold of the detached retina, and preretinal and subretinal membrane cause irregular retinal folding and/or fixed fold (Laqua & Machemer 1975, Machemer & Laqua 1975, Machemer et al. 1978, Machemer 1978) (Fig. 5). When the proliferations occur simultaneously and extensively, the retina is pulled anteriorly, and a typical morning glory appearance of end-stage MPP is formed (Laqua & Machemer 1975).

In end-stage MPP, intravitreal membrane which is attached to the peripheral retina and bridges the vitreous cavity is a typical features (Fig. 5). And the presence of this equatorial bridging membrane associated with retinal detachment on B-scan ultrasonic tomogram is thought to be pathognomic for advanced MPP (Fuller & Machemer 1977). Twenty-two of 40 eyes of the previtrectomy group revealed this triangular configuration in this series. On the other hand, the equatorial bridging membrane was not observed in all eight eyes of the postvitrectomy group in which the vitreous was removed almost completely. This explains the role of the vitreous as a scaffold of this bridging membrane. In extremely severe MPP the detached retinal segments were pulled together with adhesion to one another. The T shape of the detached retina should reveal this change. Triangular retinal

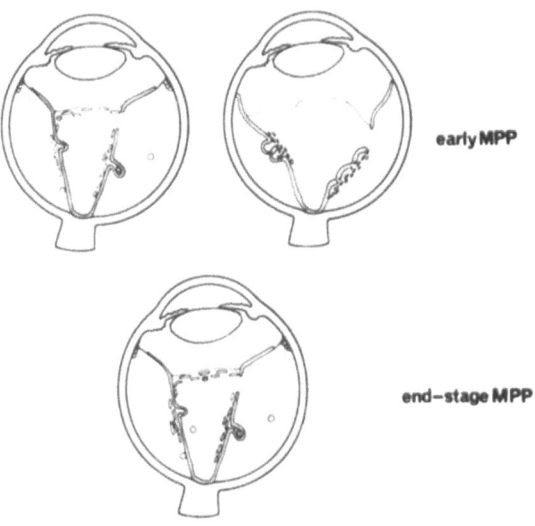

early MPP

end-stage MPP

(Machemer, R., Br.J.Ophthalmol., 1978, 62, 740)

Fig. 5. Schematic drawing of the development of MPP.
top right: Pre- and subretinal membranes contract and throw the retina into the fold in early MPP.
top left: Proliferating membrane along the posterior vitreous surface is shortend, pulling the retina centrally, and causes circumferential fold.
bottom: Both intravitreal and periretinal proliferations occurred extensively, intravitreal membrane become dens.

detachment with acoustically full triangle also has been known as the sign of this extreme situation, though, the triangle often becomes full when proliferating tissue fills its inner space. T-sign seems a more adequate expression.

The clinicopathological studies revealed remarkable variability of the clinical pictures depending upon the varying degree and extent of the proliferation in early MPP. Fixed retinal fold is the most obvious sign in the clinical pictures (Laqua & Machemer 1975). Pre- and subretinal proliferation may cause the fixed fold regardless of the degree of intravitreal proliferations as shown in Fig. 5. This explains the sign of thickened retina without equatorial bridging membrane as indicative of early MPP. Similarly, ultrasonographic sign of bending of the retina seems to represent the circumferential retinal fold in early MPP in which intravitreal proliferation is still not so dense. Additionally, retinal immobility suggests the presence of contracting force on the retina, as previously described (McLeod, *et al.* 1977). We believe that the irregular thickening and bending of the retina supplemented with retinal immobility are good guides for the indentification of MPP.

No marked differences among the operative success rates in relation to various ultrasonographic figures appeared. It seems quite similar to that the preoperative severity of MPP does not influence the final outcome (Machemer & Laqua 1978). And it appeared that the importance of detecting the early MPP since it will have similar operative prognosis to severe case.

SUMMARY

Forty-eight eyes with massive periretinal proliferation were examined with ultrasonography. In addition to the triangular retinal detachment T-sign was indicative of severe MPP. And irregular thickening and bending of the retina were observed on ultrasonography in eyes with MPP. The detached retina was immobile in all eyes. Preoperative ultrasonographic findings did not prove the value on the assessment of operative prognosis.

REFERENCES

Bronson, N.R. & Turner, F.T. A simple B-scan ultrasonoscope. Arch. Ophthalmol. 90: 237 (1973).

Coleman, D.J., Koning, W.F. & Katz L.: A Hand-Operated ultrasound scan system for ophthalmic evaluation, Am. J. Ophthalmol. 68: 258 (1969).

Fuller. D.G., Laqua, H. & Machemer, R. Ultrasonographic diagnosis of massive periretinal proliferation in eyes with opaque media (triangular retinal detachment). Am. J. Ophthalmol. 83: 460 (1977).

Laqua, H. & Machemer, R. Glial cell proliferation in retinal detachment (massive periretinal proliferation). Am. J. Ophthalmol. 80: 1 (1975).

Laqua, H. & Machemer R. Clinical-pathological correlation in Massive periretinal proliferation. Am. J. Ophthalmol. 80: 912 (1975).

Machemer, R. & Laqua, H. Pigment epithelial proliferation in retinal detachment (massive periretinal proliferation). Am. J. Ophthalmol. 80: 1 (1975).

Machemer, R. & Laqua, H. A logical approach to the treatment of massive periretinal proliferation. Ophthalmology 85: 584 (1978).

Machemer, R. Van Horn, D. & Aaberg, T.M. Pigment epithelial proliferation in human retinal detachment with massive periretinal proliferation,

Machemer, R. Pathogenesis and classification of massive periretinal proliferation. Br. J. Ophthalmol. 62: 737 (1978).

McLeod, D., Restori, M. & Wright, J.E. Rapid B-scanning of the vitreous. Br. J. Ophthalmol. 61: 437 (1977).

Okun, E. & Arrivas P.N. Therapy of retinal detachment complicated by massive periretinal fibroplasia (long term follow-up of patients treated with intravitreal liquid silicone). Transactions of New Orleans Academy of Ophthalmology. St. Louis: C.V. Mosby Co. (1969) p. 278

Authors' Address:
Dept. of Ophthalmology
34, Narakuma, Nishiku
Fukuoka University
Fukuoka 814-01, Japan

ULTRASONIC DIAGNOSIS
OF MASSIVE PERIRETINAL PROLIFERATION

S. TAKEUCHI

(Tokyo, Japan)

INTRODUCTION

Massive periretinal proliferation (MPP) is one of the serious complications of retinal detachment. Total retinal detachment with advanced MPP has so far been regarded as inoperable. However, the number of successful operations is increasing due to development of vitreous surgery. In the case of advanced MPP, there are many cases in which detailed findings on the fundus cannot be obtained because of complicated cataract and vitreous opacity. Ultrasonic diagnosis is the most useful method for examination of such cases, and it not only enables diagnosis of complications of retinal detachment but also progressive stages of MPP. The author examined 20 eyes with advanced MPP by means of A- and B-scan, in order to establish ultrasonic characteristics of MPP.

MATERIALS AND METHOD

All 20 eyes with advanced MPP were cases of rhegmatogenous retinal detachment which had no traumatic or secondary retinal detachment. According to Machemer's classification (Machemer 1978), all cases were stage IV. Regarding the equipments used, General ZD-251 was used for A- and B-scan and General ZD-252 for contact B-scan. A 10 MHz unfocused transducer was used for A-scan and a 10 MHz focused transducer for B-scan. With A-scan, vitreous opacity, degeneration and mobility of retinal detachment were examined and quantitative echography was also performed according to Ossoing *et al.* (1971). As a control, quantitative echography was also performed on 30 eyes with uncomplicated rhegmatogenous retinal detachment without MPP. With contact B-scan, retinal mobility was mainly examined, and the whole picture of retinal detachment was displayed by a water bath method.

RESULTS

With A-scan, various spikes showing degeneration and opacity of the vitreous body of all 20 cases were recognized, and retinal mobility was found to be

Table 1. ΔdB values obtained wtih quantitative echography from retinal detachment with MPP and retinal detachment without MPP.

ΔdB value	6	9	12	15	18	21	Total
Retinal detachment with MPP	2	1	3	3	1	0	10
Retinal detachment without MPP	0	0	3	8	12	7	30

ΔDB = difference between sensitivity of detached retina and sclera.
T = 4.637**
**·········P < 0.01

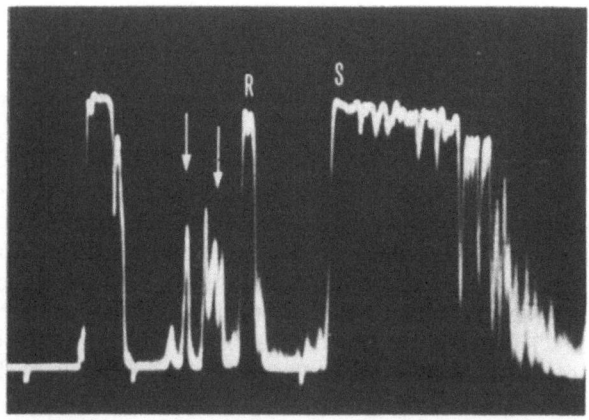

Fig. 1. A-scan echogram of retinal detachment with advanced MPP showing various spikes of the vitreous. R = retinal spike S = scleral spike arrow = vitreous spike

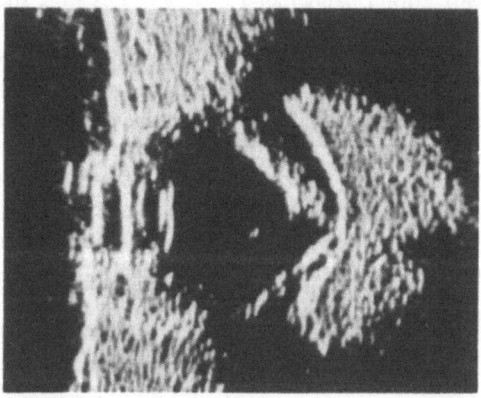

Fig. 2. B-scan ultrasonogram of total retinal detachment with advanced MPP. Temporal retina is thickened by proliferative membrane.

reduced (Fig. 1). As a result of quantitative echography, detached retina with MPP showed higher reflectivity than detached retina without MPP and a significant difference was also recognized statistically (Table 1). With B-scan retinal mobility was more clearly observed and showed that retinal mobility with MPP decreased remarkably. Furthermore, retina with proliferative membrane was found to be thickened and shruken (Fig. 2, 3). In total retinal detachment with advanced MPP, facing retinas approached each other and bridging membrane was formed. In such cases, a triangular configuration was seen ultrasonographically (Fig. 4). In the event of further advance, this bridging membrane shrank further and peripheral retina was gradually pulled toward the axis of the eye (Fig. 5). Consequently, facing retinas came into contact with one another and a T-shaped configuration was formed (Fig. 6).

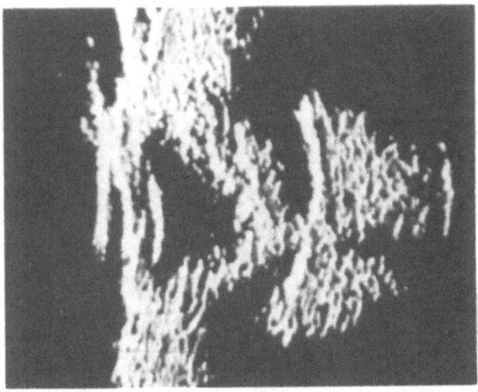

Fig. 3. B-scan ultrasonogram of total retinal detachment with advanced MPP showing extremely thickened and organized retina.

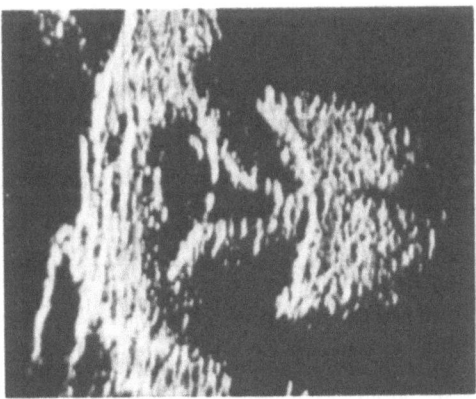

Fig. 4. B-scan ultrasonogram of acoustically empty triangular retinal detachment. Bridging membrane pulls the peripheral retina toward the axis of the eye.

15

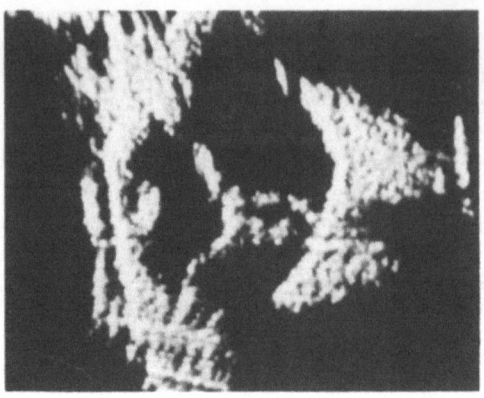

Fig. 5. B-scan ultrasonogram of total retinal detachment of advanced MPP. With further constriction of bridging membrane the anterior retinas come into contact with one another.

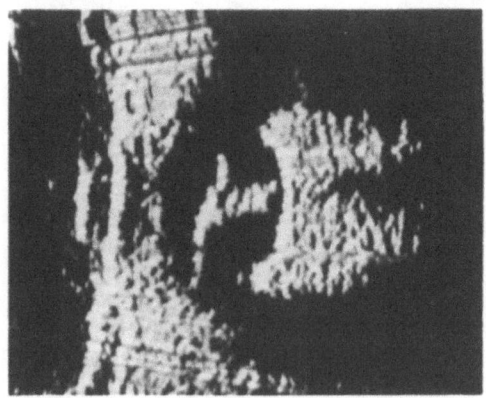

Fig. 6. B-scan ultrasonogram of T-shaped configuration. Posterior facing retina also come into contact with one another in the final stage.

DISCUSSION

MPP results from proliferation of retinal pigment epithelium and retinal glial cells, and fibrous metaplasia. Proliferative membrane causes retinal fold and also causes vitreous membrane to shrink. Machemer clinically classified MPP into 4 stages, and stated that in stages I & II, opacities of the vitreous body and subretinal space were mainly recognized and in stages III & IV, proliferative membrane was formed.

In the present study by A-scan on such cases, various spikes were detected in the vitreous cavity in all cases. However, these spikes are not peculiar to retinal detachment with MPP. In the cases of uncomplicated rhegmatogenous retinal detachment with retinal tear or of advanced age, abnormal spikes were

Table 2. Relationship between vitreous spikes and type of retinal break.

Break's type	equatrial tear		equatrial hole		macular hole		intermediate tear		oral dialysis	
vitreous spikes age, years	+	−	+	−	+	−	+	−	+	−
10−19	0	0	0	4	0	0	0	0	0	1
20−20	2	0	3	14	0	0	1	0	1	1
30−39	3	0	3	5	0	0	0	0	0	0
40−49	5	1	2	2	0	0	0	0	0	1
50−59	12	1	1	1	2	0	0	0	0	0
60−69	20	2	1	1	2	0	1	0	0	0
70−79	4	0	0	1	0	0	0	0	0	0
Total	46	4	10	28	4	0	2	0	1	3

very likely to be detected in the vitreous cavity (Table 2). Moreover, Oksala (1977) also stated that abnormal spikes were detected in the vitreous cavity in all 32 cases of eyes with retinal detachment.

However, the present study revealed that in the case with the spikes of the vitreous body is high and multiple, proliferative membrane is liable to be formed. At an advanced stage of MPP, it is observed that retina ophthalmoscopically becomes rigid and immobile, the same being observed with A- and B-scan. In quantitative echography, detached retina with MPP shows higher reflectivity than detached retina without MPP. It is often experienced that a strong return echo from the retina is received, which is considered to be due to an increase of reflectivity of retina with proliferative membrane. Sawada (Sawada *et al.* 1979) stated in his experimental and clinical study that eyes with detached retina with proliferation showed higher reflectivity which agrees with our result.

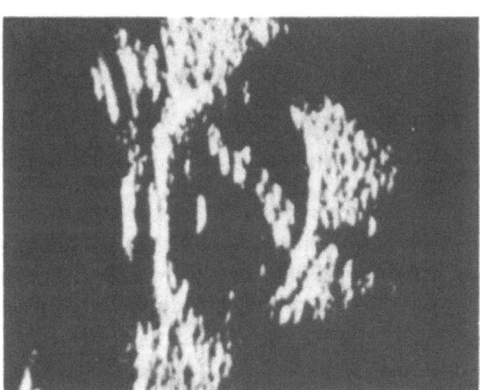

Fig. 7. B-scan ultrasonogram of pre-phthisical eye showing choroidal thickening, shortening of axial length and posterior out line of sclera.

17

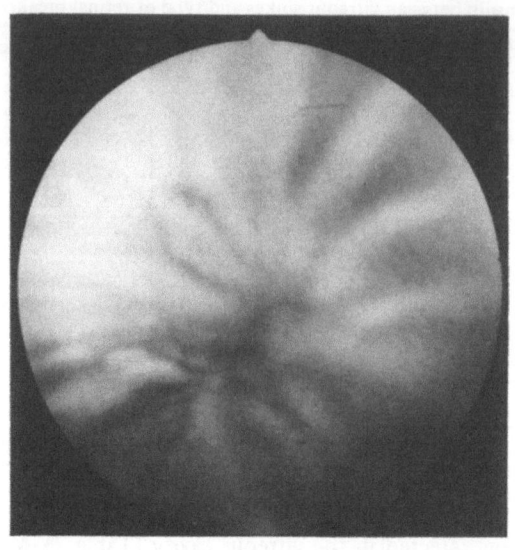

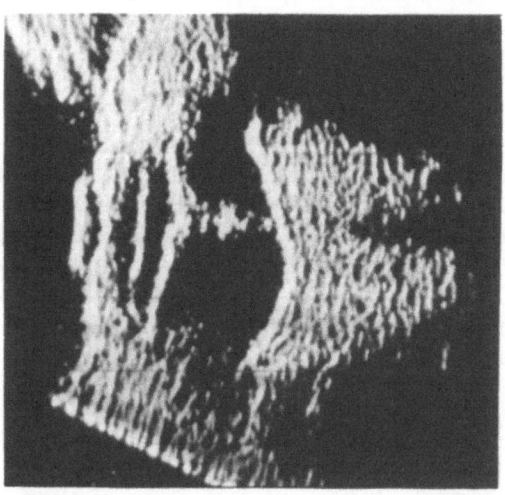

Fig. 8. Preoperative appearance of total retinal detachment with final stage MPP. Optic disc is not visualized and B-scan ultrasonogram shows T-shaped configuration.

With B-scan, it is observed that detached retina becomes thickened and shruken due to proliferative membrane. Coleman *et al*. (1977) stated that a freshly detached retina appeared as a thin white line, equal in length to the sclera from ora to ora. In a long-standing detachment, the retina was thickened and overall length often shorter, a chord being formed from optic disc to ora serrata. This type of detachment, however, seems to be complicated with MPP and the present study demonstrated even in long-standing retinal detachments, without MPP, thin atrophic detached retina appears as a thin shrunken line with B-scan.

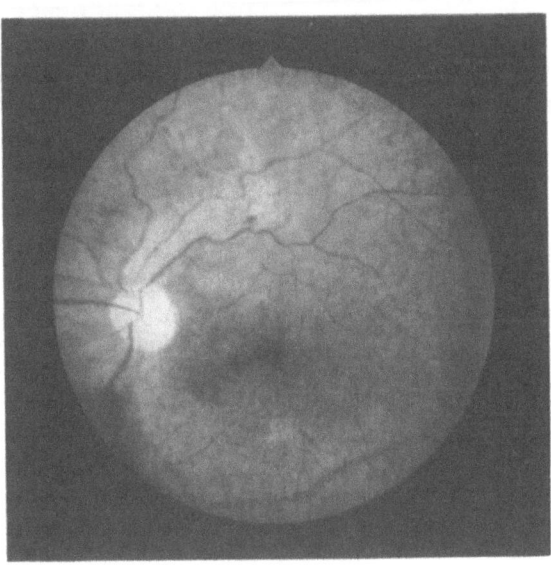

Fig. 9. Postoperative appearance of Fig. 8 case, retina is reattached completely by means of vitrectomy, membrane peeling and intravitreal gas injection.

Fuller (Fuller *et al.* 1977) called total retinal detachment with advanced MPP as a triangular retinal detachment and reported that bridging membranes were composed of condensed, newly formed collagen and proliferating metaplastic epithelial cells.

When shrinkage of this bridging membrane increases, retinal detachment is considered to finally result in a T-shaped formation. The present study revealed that ultrasonographic characteristics of retinal detachment with MPP are as follows: multiple and high amplitude spikes of vitreous body, in advanced stage, high reflectivity of detached retina, thickened and shrunken retina and reduction of retinal mobility. In final stage, bridging membranes are formed, thus forming triangular and T-shaped configurations.

Accordingly, it is clear that the respective stages of MPP can be accurately diagnosed by means of ultrasonic diagnosis. Moreover, this is also effective for detecting chroidal thickening and shortening of the axial length, which is a sign of phthisic globe (Fig. 7).

Fuller also stated that surgical prognosis for triangular retinal detachment was still poor even by means of modern vitrectomy techniques. However, successful cases of operation on advanced MPP are increasing because of technique such as vitrectomy, membrane peeling and intravitreal gas or silicone oil injections (Fig. 8, 9).

Therefore, operation is possible even in such cases with triangular and T-shaped configurations, and cases which are considered to be inoperable are limited to those with highly organized retina.

Our findings indicate that preoperative ultrasonic diagnosis not only enables diagnosis of the progressive stages of MPP but is also indispensable in determining the operability, estimation of difficulty of surgery and planning of surgical procedures. Preoperative ultrasonography also contributes to the safety of vitreous surgery.

SUMMARY

With A-scan, eyes with MPP exhibit various spikes in the vitreous cavity and higher retinal reflectivity than retina without MPP. With B-scan, the retina thickens and shrinks because of proliferative membrane, and its mobility is weakened. In the case of total retinal detachment with advanced MPP, facing retinas approach each other and then bridging membrane with a triangular configuration is formed. When bridging membrane further shrinks, facing retinas come into contact with one another, resulting in a T-shaped formation. With the development of vitreous surgery, it is possible to operate even on advanced MPP which shows triangular or T-shaped configurations and only cases with highly organized retina are considered inoperable.

REFERENCES

Bronson, N.R. Contact B-scan Ultrasonography. Am. J. Ophthalmol. 77: 181 (1974).

Coleman, D.J., Lizzi, F.L. & Jack R.L. Ultrasonography of the Eye and Orbit. Philadelphia: Lea & Febiger (1977).

Fuller, D.G., Laqua, H. & Machemer, R. Ultrasonographic diagnosis of massive periretinal proliferation in eyes with opaque media (Triangular retinal detachment). Am. J. Ophthalmol. 83: 460 (1977).

Machemer, R. Pathogenesis and classification of massive periretinal proliferation. Brit. J. Ophthalmol. 62: 737 (1978).

Machemer, R. & Laquq, H. A logical approach to the treatment of massive periretinal proliferation. Ophthalmology. 85: 584 (1978).

Oksala, A. Ultrasonic-findings in the vitreous space in patient with detachment of the retina. Albrecht. V. Graetes. Arch. Ophthalmol. 202: 197 (1977).

Ossoinig, K.C., Frazier, S.L., Watzke, R.C. & Diamond, J.G. Combined A-scan and B-scan echography as a diagnostic aid for vitreoretinal surgery. In: New and controversial aspect of the vitreoretinal surgery. (McPherson, ed.) St. Louis: C.V. Mosby (1977) p. 106.

Sawada, A., Inahara, M., Masuyama, Y. & Baba, Y. Significance of quantitative echography in membrane-like structures in the vitreous. Acta Soc. Ophthalmol. Jpn. 83: 1434 (1979).

Takeuchi, S., Kato, S., Ota, Y. & Minoda, M. Significance of ultrasonic diagnosis prior to vitreous surgery. Jap. J. Clin. Ophthalmol. 33: 967 (1979).

Author's Address:
Dept. of Ophthalmology
Tokyo Kosei-Nenkin Hospital, 23 Tsukudo-cho Shinjuku-ku
Tokyo, Japan

RAPID B-SCANNING IN DIABETIC EYE DISEASE

D. MCLEOD & M. RESTORI

(*London, United Kingdom*)

One of the commonest indications for ultrasonic assessement of the posterior segment is diabetic eye disease in which vitreous haemorrhage or cataract precludes ophthalmoscopic visualisation of the fundus (Fig. 1a). The vitreoretinal interrelationships in eyes with proliferative retinopathy are often complicated and, notwithstanding the excellent topographic data obtained from B-scanning (Fig. 1b), interpretation of the findings may be difficult (Fig. 1c). Correct interpretation depends to a considerable extent on detailed knowledge of the pathogenesis and pathological anatomy of proliferative retinopathy and its sequelae. Despite the potential complexity of this subject, however, the underlying principles can be clearly defined. We propose to illustrate these principles by means of examples from some of the several hundred diabetic cases examined in the Ultrasound Department of Moorfields Eye Hospital in the last six years.

Our system comprises a focussed 10 MHz transducer scanning rapidly in a linear fashion to produce real-time B-scan sections with good tonal quality. We generally examine the eye in the horizontal plane by consecutive serial scanning, though oblique or vertical sections may be obtained as necessary.

There are eight basic principles to be considered when discussing the pathogenesis of severe proliferative diabetic retinopathy:

1. *Vasoproliferation occurs in association with, and probably as a response to, ischaemia of the inner retina.* The ischaemia principally affects the peripheral rather than the central retina, and the new vessels tend to grow at the optic disc and at the junction of ischaemic and non-ischaemic retina. Characteristically, epiretinal proliferation commences nasal to the disc and along the major temporal vascular arcades i.e. posterior to the equator. The newly-formed membranes comprise both blood vessels and fibrous tissue, and the foci of proliferation may be isolated or may coalesce. In eyes in which the membranes are very thick, they can be identified by ultrasound (Fig. 2a).

2. *Fibrovascular tissue only proliferates in the most cortical part of the vitreous gel (epiretinal fibrovascular tissue – flat new vessels) or, after vitreous detachment, along the posterior hyaloid interface in continuity with epiretinal neovascularisation (preretinal fibrovascular tissue – forward new vessels).* Fibrovascular tissue does not grow into the central part of the

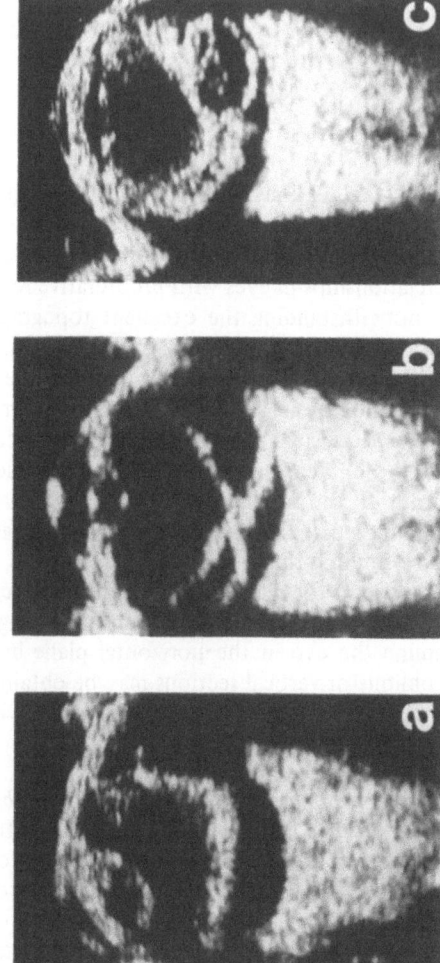

Fig. 1. Horizontal B-scan Sections
(a) Ochre membrane (eye deviated left)
(b) Traction retinal detachment
(c) Traction detachment & vitreous haemorrhage

22

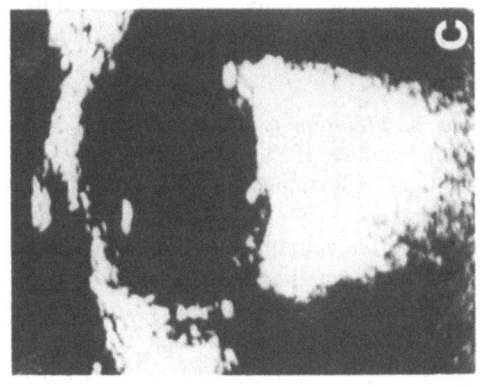

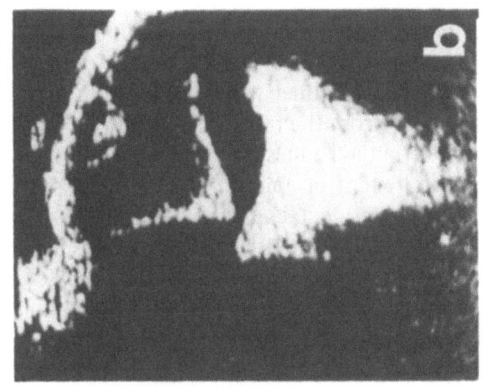

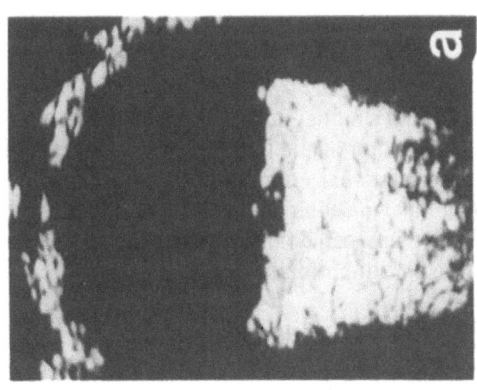

Fig. 2. Horizontal B-scan Sections
(a) Thick epiretinal membranes posteriorly
(b) Ochre membrane tethering to disc
(c) Avulsed edge of epiretinal membrane

23

vitreous gel owing to lack of a scaffolding microstructure in the gel or presence of inhibitory substances. Most diabetic vitreous membranes, whether consisting of fibrous tissue or blood products enmeshed in gel (Fig. 1a), are arranged along the detached posterior hyaloid interface. The flow of blood in preretinal new vessels is generally slow, and pulsation in these vessels is not detectable by ultrasound.

3. Epiretinal fibrovascular proliferation is dependent upon contact of the vitreous gel with the retinal surface. If the gel is completely detached from the retina before vasoproliferation is stimulated, extensive membranes are not formed (though neovascularisation may affect the iris). Similarly, if posterior vitreous detachment occurs after epiretinal proliferation has commenced, there is no further proliferation on the retinal surface — only along the detached posterior hyaloid interface. This necessity for gel/retina contact only applies to *vascular* proliferation: non-vascular epiretinal membranes apparently have a fundamentally different biological behaviour in that they proliferate whether or not the vitreous is detached.

4. Epiretinal fibrovascular proliferation is complicated by incarceration of gel fibrils into the membrane and thence into the retina. The exaggerated vitreo-retinal adhesions at sites of epiretinal vasoproliferation usually prevent complete separation of the gel from the retina following vitreous detachment (Fig. 2b). The degree of vitreoretinal adhesion posterior to the vitreous base is thus dictated largely by the extent of epiretinal vasoproliferation present at the time of posterior vitreous detachment. The residual vitreoretinal adhesions may be focal (Fig. 2b) or extensive (Fig. 2c, 3a), single or multiple (Fig. 3b). The edge of a fibrovascular membrane may be avulsed so that flat vessels become 'forward' vessels (Fig. 2c). In rare instances, complete avulsion of fibrovascular tissue from the retina may occur at the time of posterior vitreous detachment; this may explain some cases of apparently *complete* posterior vitreous detachment in cases of diabetic vitreous haemorrhage.

5. The major complications of proliferative diabetic retionopathy — vitreous haemorrhage and retinal detachment — are associated with, and are (at least in part) dependent upon, vitreous detachment. The cause of vitreous detachment is not entirely clear, i.e. whether due to changes in the cortical gel from leaking new vessels or contraction of the fibrovascular membranes themselves. There is no evidence to suggest that contraction of the gel *as a whole* causes posterior vitreous detachment or complications of proliferative retinopathy. Thus, vitreous detachment has paradoxical effects in protecting the retina from further epiretinal vasoproliferation but causing complications.

6. The degree and persistence of vitreous haemorrhage shows no relationship to the extent of epiretinal vasoproliferation. Disc new vessels have a greater propensity to cause haemorrhage than retinal new vessels; indeed, eyes with extensive retinal new vessels may never go on to vitreous haemorrhage. Conversely, there is no evidence to suggest that fibrovascular proliferation occurs *as a response* to vitreous haemorrhage.

Haemorrhage may occupy the retrohyaloid space, the vitreous gel or both compartments (Fig. 3a, b, c), and the presence of haemorrhage may allow ultrasonic delineation of the vitreoretinal interrelationships, for example, the presence of an incomplete posterior vitreous detachment (Fig. 2b, 3a, b). The posterior hyaloid interface may be mobile (suggesting some degree of gel collapse) or immobile (indicating fibrovascular or fibrous proliferation along the posterior hyaloid interface between the vitreous base anteriorly and neovascular membranes posteriorly). Blood products in a mobile detached cortex may be arranged to form a thick 'ochre membrane' (Fig. 1a, 2b); occasionally, arranged membranes may occur within the gel itself (Fig. 4a), possibly related to "tracts" or other gel microanatomy. Where the fibrovascular membrane is extensive, the vitreoretinal adhesion has a U-shaped configuration in B-scan section (Fig. 3a); in more focal vitreoretinal adhesions, a V-shaped (Fig. 2b) or stalk-like (Fig. 4a, b) attachment to the retina may be seen.

The retrohyaloid space may not necessarily show a homogeneous echo-distribution. Fine (possibly fibrinous) membranes may traverse the retrohyaloid space, and blood may sediment out to form a fluid-level on the retinal surface, especially seen with the patient supine (Fig. 4c).

7. *The occurrence and distribution of traction retinal detachment reflects the extent of epiretinal vasoproliferation.* This relates both to the fact that fibrovascular epiretinal membranes contract (producing tangential traction on the retina) and also to the importance of the vasoproliferation in determining the extent of vitreoretinal adhesion. Since most vasoproliferation occurs in the posterior retina, and since the traction process is 'static', the ensuing retina detachments are generally posterior (usually sparing the equatorial retina) and are immobile on dynamic testing (Fig. 5a, b). The retina beneath an epiretinal membrane is folded and thickened, while the surrounding detached retina is stretched and has an anterior concavity (Fig. 5b). Diabetic detachments also tend to be shallow when contrasted with rhegmatogenous detachments which generally affect the equatorial retina, are mobile on dynamic testing and have an anterior convexity.

8. *Other elements of traction are mediated by contraction along the detached posterior hyaloid interface between areas of vitreoretinal adhesion.* Anteroposterior traction occurs between the vitreous base anteriorly and fibrovascular complexes posteriorly, while bridging traction describes those forces operating between individual fibrovascular complexes. As a result, the detachments tend to be angular in configuration with the posterior hyaloid membrane attached to fibrovascular tissue at the summit of the detachment (Fig. 5b, c). Traction detachments are also seen anteriorly affecting the intrabasal retina (Fig. 6a, b), and also at the base of stalks (Fig. 6c).

The overall configuration of the retinal detachment thus represents the resultant of all elements of traction (anteroposterior, bridging and tangential) and each of these elements is, in the final analysis, dependent on the distribution of epiretinal vasoproliferation. Where the vasoproliferation is modest in extent with individual foci of neovascularisation, the result is an

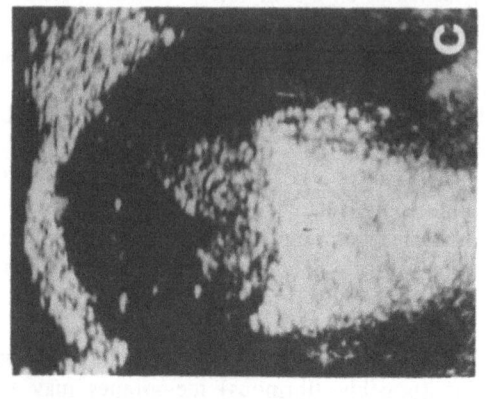
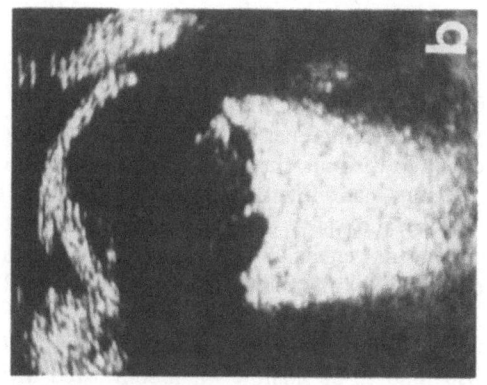
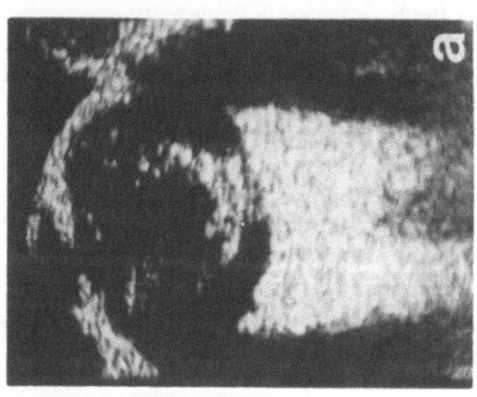

Fig. 3. Horizontal B-scan Sections
(a) Intragel haemorrhage & wide vitreoretinal adhesion
(b) Two vitreoretinal adhesions
(c) Dense retrohyaloid haemorrhage

26

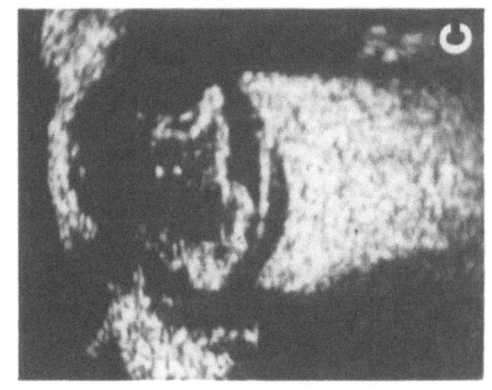
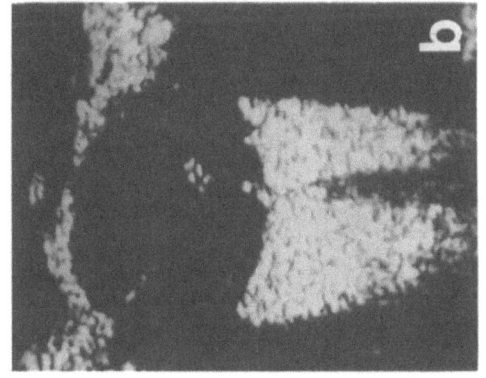
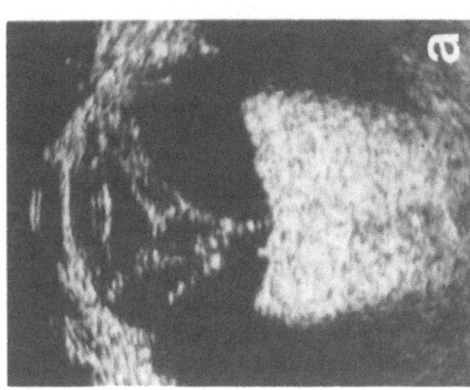

Fig. 4. Horizontal B-scan Sections
(a) Intragel haemorrhage & focal vitreoretinal adhesion
(b) Vitreopapillary adhesion by a stalk
(c) Mobile intragel haemorrhage & fluid level

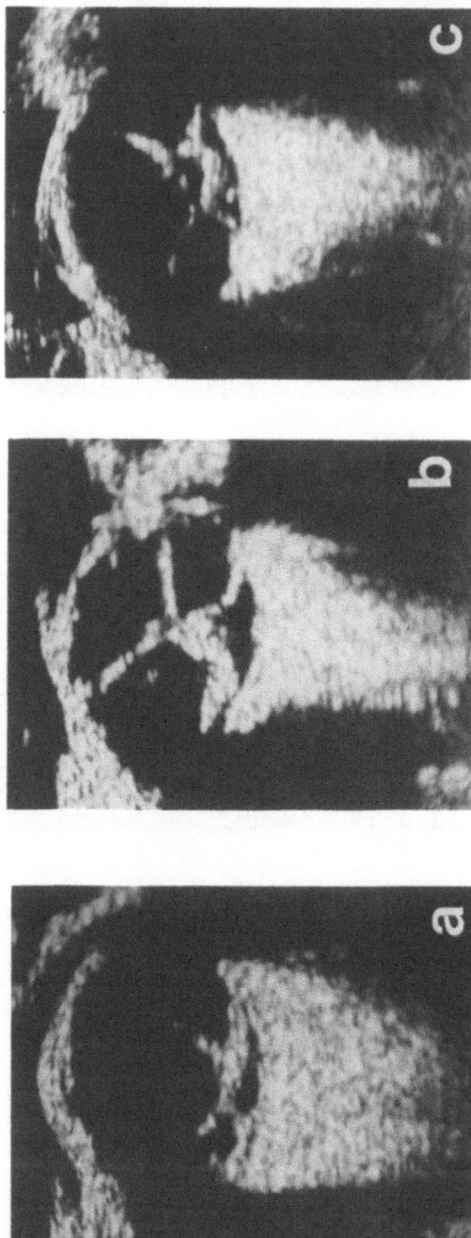

Fig. 5. Horizontal B-scan Sections
(a) (b) (c) Traction retinal detachment

28

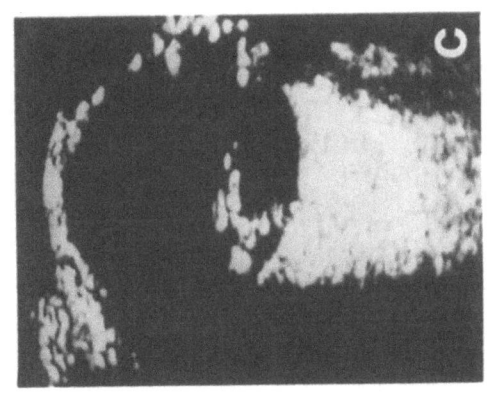

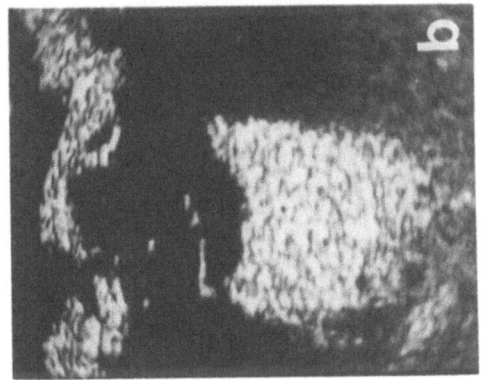

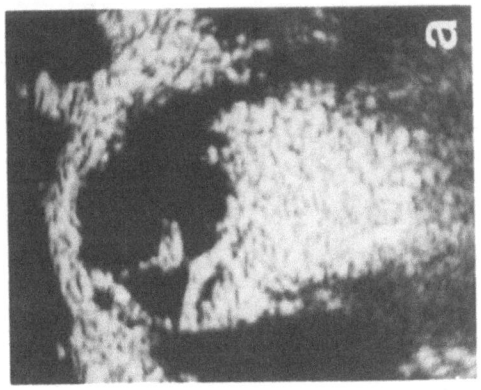

Fig. 6. Horizontal B-scan Sections
(a) Basal & posterior traction retinal detachment
(b) Basal traction detachment
(c) Detachment at base of stalk (eye deviated right)

29

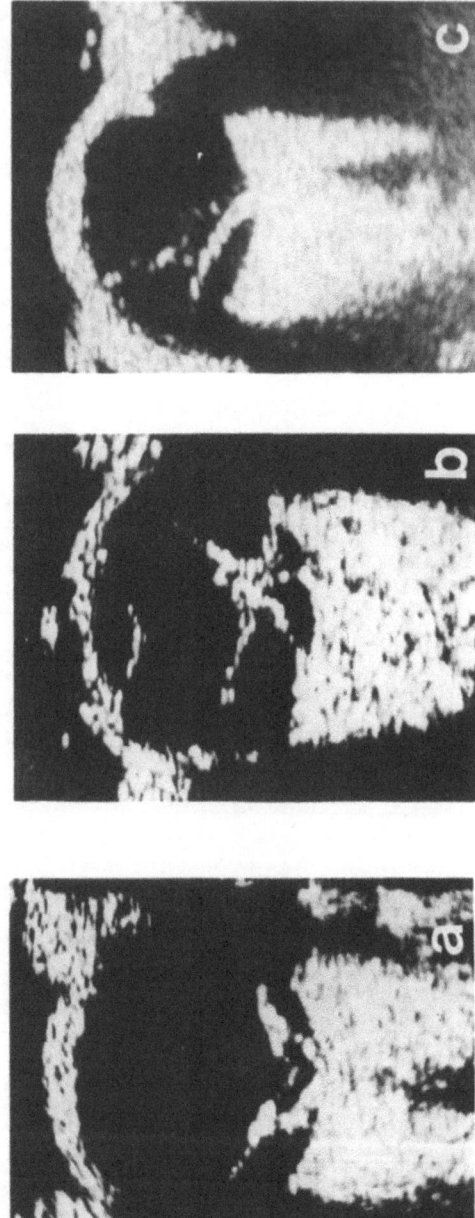

Fig. 7. B-scan Sections
(a) Open configuration of detachment (vertical scan)
(b) Table-top traction detachment
(c) Temporal combined rhegmatogenous & traction detachment

30

'open' or 'hammock' configuration of retinal detachment, often with clearly definable bridging traction (Fig. 5c, 7a). Conversely, where the epiretinal vasoproliferation is very extensive with multiple foci coalescing over the posterior retina, a 'tabletop' configuration of detachment eventually results (Fig. 6a, 7b). In such cases there is massive tangential traction; since this is the most difficult of the elements of traction to manage surgically, many of these detachments are inoperable, especially if the posterior retina is highly elevated.

The configuration of the detachment may also reflect the presence of retinal holes — 'combined rhegmatogenous and traction retinal detachment' — which may sometimes produce a more bullous configuration of detachment with anterior convexity of the retinal surface (Fig. 7c). Such a bullous pattern is generally limited to eyes with relatively focal epiretinal membranes, and in some cases, the detachment may be indistinguishable from a purely rhegmatogenous detachment.

With the above considerations in mind, the clinician managing severe diabetic dye disease generally has three essential questions to be answered by the ultrasonic assessment:
(1) Is a retinal detachment present?
(2) If so, is the macula involved or threatened?
(3) Is the retinal detachment operable?
The answers are vital in that eyes with traction detachment involving the macula should be operated on as soon as possible. Conversely, there is often no urgency to intervene in eyes with vitreous haemorrhage and no retinal detachment, or retinal detachment which is definitely extramacular. However, if there is massive tangential traction producing a severe tabletop detachment, ultrasound may be important in indicating potential inoperability of the retinal detachment as patients subjected to unsuccesful vitreous surgery for diabetic detachment are sentenced to a painful, shrunken and blind eye.

Authors' Address:
Dept of Ultrasound
Moorfields Eye Hospital
London, United Kingdom

PREOPERATIVE EVALUATION OF VITREOUS SURGERY BY ULTRASONOGRAPHY

K. SHIMIZU & K. MINODA

(Tokyo, Japan)

INTRODUCTION

Vitreous surgery has made remarkable progress in recent years, but the procedure for estimating the prognosis of visual function after the vitreous surgery has not been established.

In the present study, ultrasonography was performed on a total of 50 cases before the vitreous surgery and attempt was made to estimate postoperative visual acuity of each case on the basis of ultrasonographic findings.

MATERIAL AND METHODS

A total of 50 cases were selected for the present study and were classified into 25 cases of diabetic retinopathy (DM) and 25 cases of vascular disease (classified as 'others'), the latter group consisting of 22 cases of retinal vein occlusion and three cases of Eales disease.

The average age of the patients was 65 years, and preoperative visual acuity of most of the patients was between finger counting and hand movements (Table 1).

Table 1. Age and preoperative visual acuity of the patients.

Age (years)	•DM	Others	Total
31–40	1	2	3
41–50	4	2	6
51–60	6	7	13
61–70	10	10	20
71–80	4	4	8

Pre-ope V.A.	DM	Others	Total
LS	3	1	4
HM	13	16	29
FC	9	6	15
0.1	0	2	2
(Aphakia)	$\frac{18}{25}$	$\frac{14}{25}$	$\frac{32}{50}$

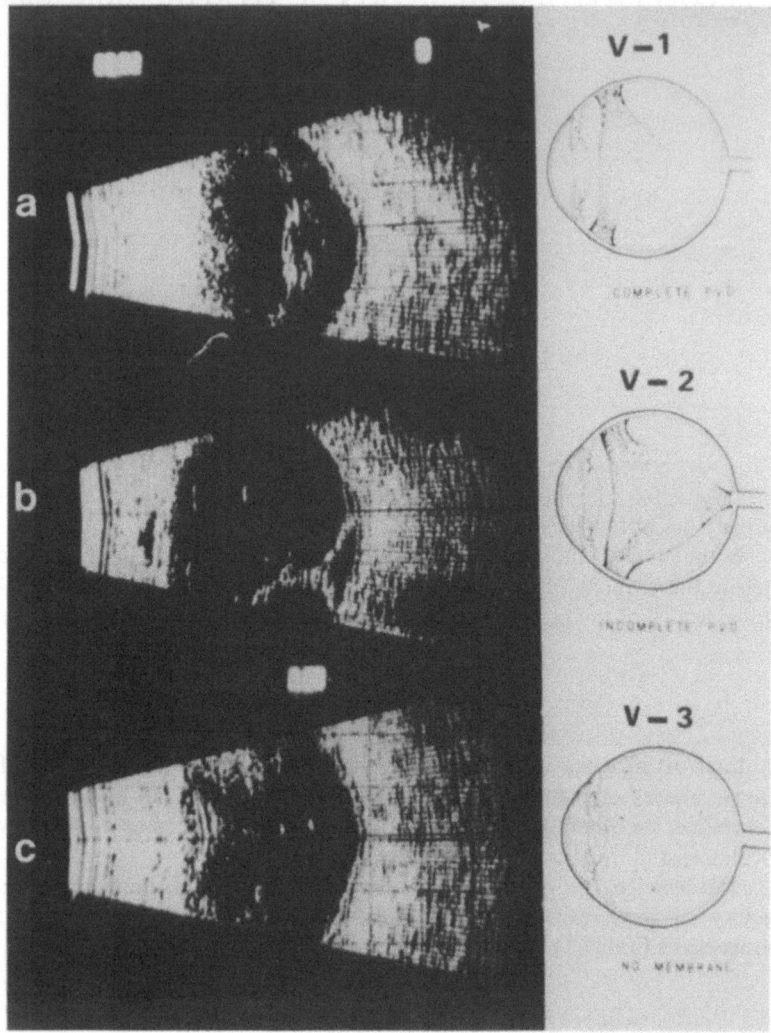

Fig. 1. Horizontal B-scan sections by Ocuscan 400. (a) membrane formation and complete posterior vitreous detachment, (b) membrane formation and incomplete posterior vitreous detachment with vitreoretinal adhesion, (c) no membrane formation and vitreous diffuse opacity.

The instruments for ultrasonography used in the study, were Ocuscan 400 and Xenotec-Ultrascan 500; in the former 5 and 10 MHz probes were used to make A- and B-scan and in the latter a 10 MHz probe was used to make vector A- and D-scan.

The findings obtained by ultrasonography were classified into three types as follows: (Fig. 1 & 2)

    Type V-1: B-scan revealed membranous and massive echoes in the vitreous. There was complete posterior vitreous detachment without adhesion to the retina.

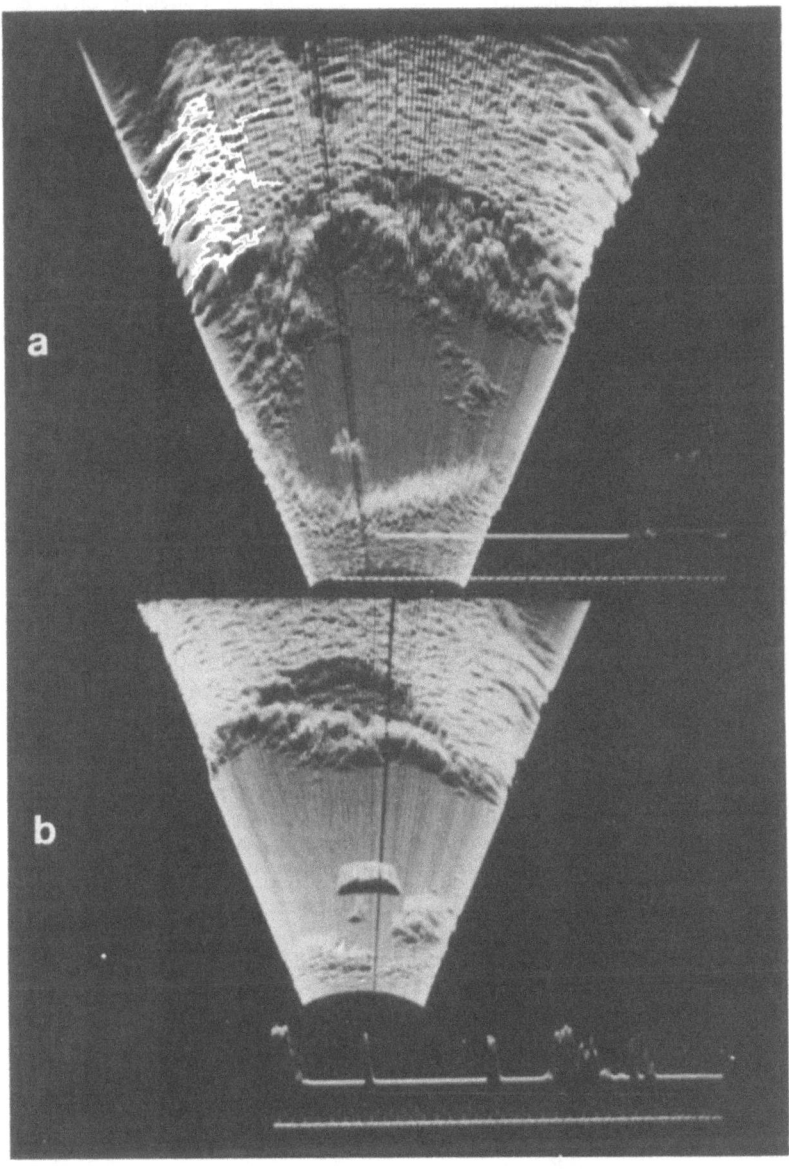

Fig. 2. Horizontal D-scan sections by Xenotec Ultrascan 500. (a) Incomplete posterior vitreous detachment with vitreoretinal adhesion at disc, and retrovitreous hemorrhage (Type V-2) (b) Traction detachment at posterior pole. Vector A-scan shows a high spike (arrow) at retinal detachment (Type V-2).

Type V-2: B-scan revealed membranous and massive echoes in the vitreous. There was incomplete posterior vitreous detachment with retinal adhesion and occasional traction retinal detachment.

Table 2. Correlation of the ultrasonographic classifications and the diseases.

Case	DM	Others	Total
V-1	2	13	15
V-2	20	12	32
V-3	3	0	3

Table 3. Correlation of the postoperative averaging visual acuity and the ultrasonographic classifications.

	DM	Others	Total
V-1	0.4	0.73	0.6
V-2	0.15	0.14	0.14
V-3	0.4		0.4

The patients were examined and classified according to the criteria indicated above within one week before vitreous surgery. Vitreous surgery was performed, using the VISC-X and lactate Ringer solution as the perfusion fluid in all cases.

RESULTS

On the basis of ultrasonographic findings, 20 cases of DM (80%) were classified into type V-2, while 13 (52%) and 12 (48%) cases of the 'others' were classified into types V-1 and V-2, respectively (Table 2).
Type V-1 was more frequently observed in 'others' than in DM.

The postoperative visual acuity of type V-1 ranged from 0.3 to 1.5, averaging 0.6, whereas that of type V-2 ranged from 0 to 0.4, averaging 0.14, and that of type V-3 ranged from 0.3 to 0.5, averaging 0.4 (Table 3, Table 4).

Type V-3: B-scan revealed no membranous or massive echoes in the vitreous but spot-like and diffuse echoes (Fig. 1).

Table 4. Correlation of the postoperative visual acuity (vertical axis) and the ultrasonographic classification (horizontal axis).

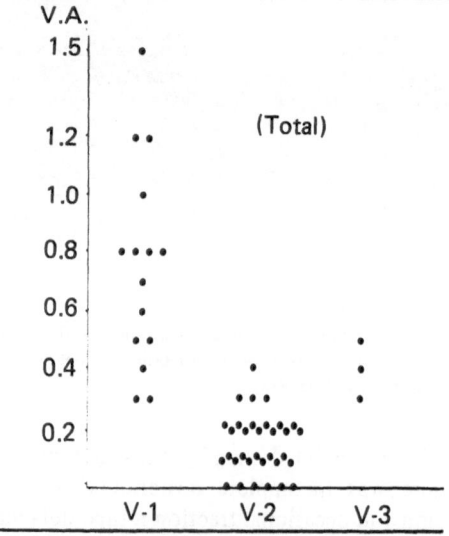

DISCUSSION

The importance of ultrasonography prior to vitreous surgery has been pointed out in many reports (Bigar 1977, Jack 1974, McLeod 1979, McPherson 1977, Takeuchi 1979), which described the procedure for differentiation of vitreous detachment from retinal detachment as well as planning of vitreous surgery by the study of the nature and morphology of the vitreous and indication for vitreous surgery.

However, the procedure for estimating the prognosis of visual acuity after vitreous surgery has not been described yet. In the present study the following considerations were taken into account when classifying 50 cases into three types by ultrasonography.

(1) The adhesion of the vitreous membrane to the retina suggests existence of proliferative change between the vitreous and the retina, which may cause traction to the retina.

(2) In the presence of vitreoretinal adhesion, vitreous surgery may cause considerable mechanical damage to the retina.

(3) Extensive disturbance of retinal circulation may exist more frequently in the eyes with vitreoretinal adhesion than those without adhesion, as often demonstrated by vitreous surgery.

For these reasons the abnormalities revealed by ultrasonography were classified into three types (V-1, V-2, V-3).

Examination during vitreous surgery disclosed there was occasionally mild adhesion of the vitreous to the retina also in types V-1 and V-3, but it was not so remarked as in type V-2. In the types V-1 and V-3 the surgery was easy and the postoperative visual acuity was satisfactory. Type V-2 was observed more frequently in DM cases. This fact seemed to account for the poor postoperative visual acuity in most of DM cases.

As shown in Table 3 cases of DM had better postoperative visual acuity as long they were of V-1 and V-3 types.

Judging from these findings, it appeared that the prognostic determination based on our classification was more accurate than that made according to the type of disease. However, more detailed informations concerning post-operative visual function may be obtained preoperatively by combined study of ultrasonography and ERG.

SUMMARY

Twenty-five patients with diabetic retinopathy, 22 patients with retinal vein occlusion and three patients with Eales disease were examined by ultrasonography prior to vitreous surgery and classified into type V-1 (complete vitreous detachment), type V-2 (incomplete vitreous detachment), and type V-3 (diffuse vitreous opacity), and the postoperative visual acuity was compared among these groups.

(1) The greater part of cases of DM were classified by ultrasonography as type V-2, while cases of 'others' were equally divided between V-1 and V-2. In either case the post-operative visual acuity was better for type V-1 than for type V-2.

(2) In each group classified by ultrasonography the post-operative visual acuity did not differ significantly from one disease to the other, and there was significant correlation between the classification and post-operative visual acuity in the order indicated below:

$$V\text{-}1, \ V\text{-}3 > V\text{-}2$$

The findings obtained in the present study suggest that the postoperative visual acuity can be well estimated by preoperative ultrasonography.

REFERENCES

Bigar, F. *et al.* Combined A- & B-scan echography. Preoperative evaluation of vitrectomy patient. Mod. Probl. Ophthalmol. 18: 2 (1977).

Jack, R.L., Hutton, W.L. & Machemer, R. Ultrasonography and vitrectomy. Am. J. Ophthalmol. 78: 265 (1974).

McLeod D. & Restori, M. Ultrasonic examination in severe diabetic eye disease. Brit. J. Ophthalmol. 63: 533 (1979).

McPherson, A. New and Controversial Aspects of Vitreoretinal Surgery. Part III Pre-operative evaluation. Saint Louis: Mosby (1977) p. 67.

Takeuchi, S. *et al.* The significance of ultrasonic diagnosis prior to vitreous surgery. Jpn. J. Clin. Ophthalmol. 33: 967 (1979).

Authors' Address:
Dept. of Ophthalmology
Tokyo University
Branch Hospital, Faculty of Medicine
Univ. of Tokyo, 3-28-6, Mejirodai,
Bunkyo-ku, Tokyo 112, Japan

DIAGNOSTIC ULTRASOUND IN CASES OF EXPERIMENTAL VITREOUS HEMORRHAGE

L. KOLOZSVÁRI

(*Debrecen, Hungary*)

Acoustic findings in the case of vitreous hemorrhage in humans are as follows: The optically opaque vitreous body is acoustically heterogeneous. Only the surface of larger cell groups can reflect registrable echoes. The bigger the liquifaction of the gel is, the more amplitude of the echoes fluctuates. The peaks become higher parallelly with the increase in cell count and the irregularity of their distribution. The membrane surface reflects high and single spikes. However, in the most cases membraneous cloudiness appears together with corpuscular elements. (Freyler 1974, Ossoinig 1971) Many authors (Forrester 1978) have carried out macroscopic, biomicroscopic and ultrastructural examinations considering the experimental vitreous hemorrhage in rabbit. However, the origin of the vitreous bands following an injection of Formalin and Mohr's salt was examined echographically only by Freyler *et al.* (1974).

This paper presents some ultrasonic appearances of the experimental vitreous hemorrhages.

Intravitreal injection of 0.2 ml autogenous whole blood was given to a total of 18 rabbits bilaterally. The ultrasound examinations were carried out 24 h, three days, 1, 2, 3, 4, 5, 6 weeks following injection according to Freyler's method (Freyler *et al.* 1976) with the apparatus of the Firm Kretztechnik 7100 MA and a slightly focused transducer 6 MHz/5 mm. Two animals i.e. four eyes were examined by each observation interval. The echography of the eyeballs always began with maximum amplification /80 dB/, in the case of quantitative echography the sclera was used as testobject. (Ossoinig 1971) The changes of the vitreous body were followed up ophthalmoscopically. The eyeballs were enucleated and worked up histologically. Ophthalmoscopically, the blood clot was a discrete, opaque mass in the early days which later spreaded and was absorbed in the course of the experiment. The vitreous cleared up, so the fundus could practically be examined in the 6th week in most of the cases.

One day after the intravitreal injection, the blood clot reflected high, manifold echoes which disappeared on lowering the amplification to 6–8 dB and showed an average ΔdB value of 35 and a strong aftermovement. In some animals this echogram was retained. However, in the course of observation the ΔdB value and the aftermovement of the oscillation diminished, the reflection rate became higher. A week later single spikes appeared in the echogram close to the posterior wall. The number of animals with this sign of posterior detachment of the solid vitreous increased as time was going by. Parallel to this, the distance between the retina and the characteristic membrane echo from the posterior surface of the vitreous increased significantly. The ΔR value of these membranes reached an average of 28 ΔdB one week after the intravitreal autogenous whole blood injection, but decreased to 24 ΔdB up to the 6th week of observation.

Our ophthalmoscopic results confirm the findings of Forrester et al.'s 1978 special, macroscopic examinations'. The characteristic membrane echoes appeared at the end of the first week. The decrease of the dB value may indicate the thickening of the posterior vitreal membrane with the elapse of time. The progressing detachment of the posterior hyaloid membrane refers to the retraction of the vitreous body. Despite the presence of the optically opaque media, the state of the retina could be examined echographically. The experimental hemorrhage did not result in retinal detachment during the observation period.

Finally, we have come to the conclusion, that with ultrasonic examination both the various stages and the process of an experimentally induced hemorrhage of the vitreous body can be monitored. Such information can be extremely useful in preparing and carrying out an operation on the vitreous body in humans.

REFERENCES

Freyler, H. & Nichorlis, St. Die Bedeutung der Echographie für die Glaskörperchirurgie Klin. Mbl. Augenheilk. 165: 594 (1974).

Freyler, H., Weiss, H. & Kosmath, B. Echographie bei experimentellen Glaskörpermembranen. Versuch einer Standardisierung. A.v. Graefes. Arch. klin. exp. Ophthalmol. 191: 315 (1974).

Freyler, H., Weiss, H. & Leibl, W. Experimentelle Siderosis bulbi. Eine echographisch-histologische Studie. A.v. Graefes Arch. klin. exp. Ophthalmol. 199: 75 (1976).

Freyler, H., Arnfelser, A. & Weiss, H. Experimentelle Echographie am Kaninchenauge. A.v. Graefes Arch. klin. exp. Ophthalmol. 199: 267 (1976).

Forrester, J.V., Lee, W.R. & Williamson, J. The Pathology of Vitreous Hemorrhage. Arch. Ophthalmol. 96: 703 (1978).

Ossoinig, K. Grundlagen der klinischen Echo-Ophthalmographie. Wien, Verlag der Wiener Medizinischen Akademie (1971).

Kolozsvari, L. Diagnostic Ultrasound in cases of experimental vitreous hemorrhage. UBIOMED IV. 1979. Visegrad. In Press.

Author's Address:
University Eye Clinic
Debrecen, Hungary

A LONG-TERM ULTRASONOGRAPHIC FOLLOW-UP OF INJECTED BLOOD INTO THE VITREOUS

Y. BABA, Y. MASUYAMA, M. FUKUZAKI & A. SAWADA

(Miyazaki, Japan)

Ultrasonic examination in vitreous hemorrhage has been highly evaluated, because this diagnostic method can provide exact information on anatomical changes in the vitreous. The information is very useful in differential diagnosis from retinal detachment as well as in decisions on vitreous surgery. Echographic findings in vitreous hemorrhage in human eyes have been studied by many researchers. Findings have also been studied in experimental eyes. However, changes in findings over a long period of time have barely been studied. It is worthwhile to study with ultrasound changes in the same eye over a long period of time.

Adult pigmented and non-pigmented rabbit eyes were used for experiments. The pupil was contracted with 2% pilocarpine. After retrobulbar injection with 2% Xylocaine of 0.5 ml, the anterior chamber was punctured with a razor knife at the limbus at 12 o'clock meridian and the aqueous was allowed to leak out completely. After the anterior chamber puncture a 0.4 ml sample of whole blood withdrawn from the ear vein was immediately injected with a 27 gauge needle into the vitreous by puncturing the sclera 6 mm posterior to the limbus at 12 o'clock meridian. The blood injection was done in one shot. Heparin was not used.

A-scan echography with Kretztechnik 7200 MA and B-scan echography with Bronson-Turner Ophthalmic B-scan were then done at set periods of time. Echography was done after the eye had been luxated. Quantitative echography was done in eight directions at 12.00, 1.30, 3.00, 4.30, 6.00, 7.30, 9.00 and 10.30. The degree of reflectivity of membrane-like structures in the vitreous after blood injection, was represented as the difference of sensitivity setting (ΔdB) between the target structure and the sclera at 6 o'clock meridian in the same eye. B-scan echograms were taken in four directions, superior, inferior, medial and lateral.

Immediately after blood injection into the vitreous, membraneous to massive echo sources were seen in the upper part of the vitreous in almost all cases. The value of ΔdB measured in quantitative echography was almost the same in each of the eight meridians. The value ranged from 19 to 22. It was ascertained ophthalmoscopically that no retinal detachment developed. Fig. 1 shows B- and A-scan echograms in one eye. A massive echo source was relative highly reflective at tissue sensitivity. The value of ΔdB in quantitative echography was 19. The value of ΔdB after the blood injection into the

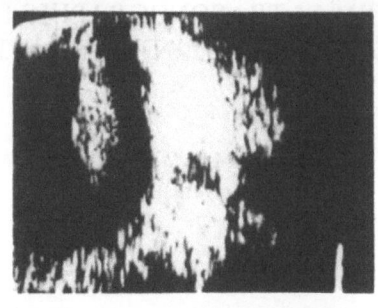

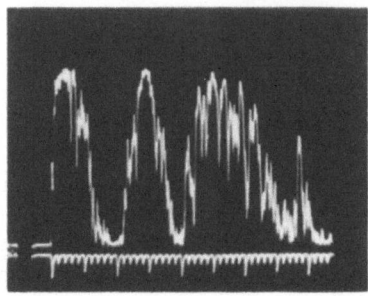

Fig. 1. B- and A-scan echograms immediately after the blood injection.

vitreous in this study was quite similar to that in human vitreous hemorrhage. The sensitivity setting, at which the peak from the sclera reached to the marker line set at the halfway point of the display height, was 31 to 33. Those values were also within the same range as in human eyes.

Changes in the value of ΔdB in eyes which were observed for two or three weeks after blood injection, are shown in Fig. 2.

In six out of seven eyes, the value of ΔdB increased within one week. In

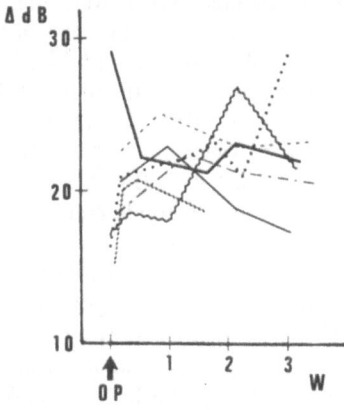

Fig. 2. Changes of the value of ΔdB in eyes observed for two or three weeks after the blood injection.

42

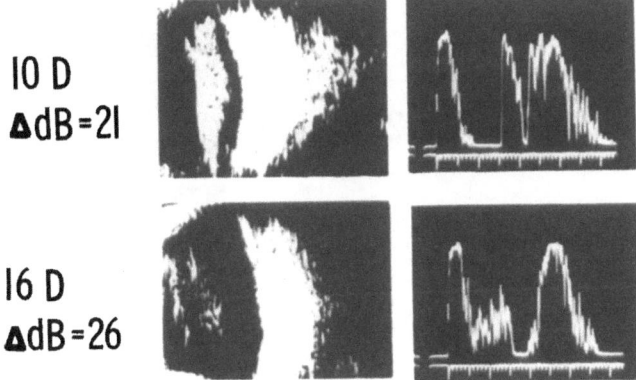

10 D
ΔdB = 21

16 D
ΔdB = 26

Fig. 3. B- and A-scan echograms and the values of ΔdB each time in a short period after the blood injection.

one eye, of which the value of ΔdB decreased in the observation period, the value immediately after blood injection was high (ΔdB = 29). The value in this case decreased once to 21 to 22 and increased again just as in the other eyes.

After two and three weeks the value of ΔdB continued to decrease in some eyes and the value in the other eyes increased. No definite tendency was found.

Fig. 3 shows B- and A-scan echograms with the value of ΔdB in one of the eyes in which values increased. The injected blood into the vitreous inclined to spread downward in parallel with the fundus.

Four eyes were observed for eight weeks after the blood injection. Fig. 4 shows changes of the value of ΔdB. In three to seven weeks, the value of ΔdB in these four eyes was concentrated in a limited range. At seven weeks the values in these eyes showed almost the same value of 18 to 19. Fig. 5

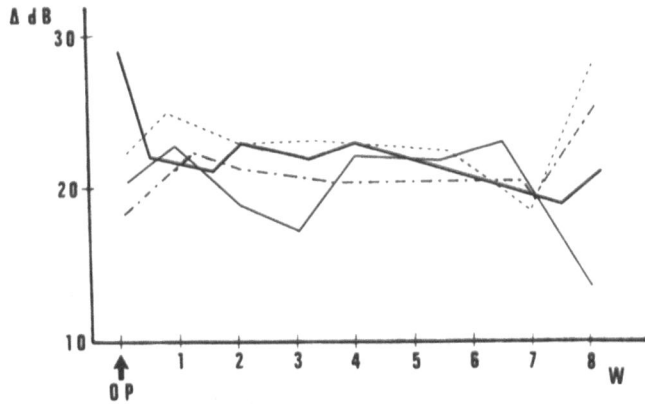

Fig. 4. Changes of the value of ΔdB in four eyes observed for eight weeks after the blood injection.

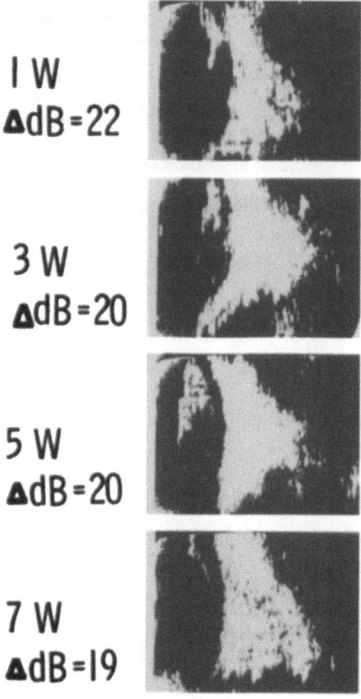

I W
ΔdB=22

3 W
ΔdB=20

5 W
ΔdB=20

7 W
ΔdB=19

Fig. 5. B-scan echograms and the value of dB each time in a longer time period.

shows the variation in B-scan echograms and that of the value of ΔdB. Changes in the B-scan echograms were not the same as those in the reflectivity in A-scan echography. A-scan echography is suggested to be superior to B-scan echography for following the fate of injected blood into the vitreous. After seven weeks the value of ΔdB was no longer confined to the same narrow range. In one of these four eyes, the value of ΔdB decreased to 13 (Fig. 4), while in the other eyes it increased sharply. In the eye with a sharp decrease ΔdB, membraneous structures in B-scan echography were not dense in appearance. They were connected partly to the retina. Based on experience in human eyes and experimental results (Sawada *et al.* 1979), the tendency of the value to decrease means the possibility of organization and traction to cause retinal detachment. This fact might be applicable to the case in the present study. Although histological changes in course of time have not yet been elucidated after long term observation, a study of such changes will provide important information on the cause of dissociation in the value of ΔdB over a period of time.

In a different group of three eyes, A- and B-scan echography was done one year after blood injection into the vitreous. The value of ΔdB in these three eyes ranged from 24 to 28 (Fig. 6). Fig. 7 shows B- and A-scan echograms of these eyes. In all these cases, structures in the vitreous were very faintly presented.

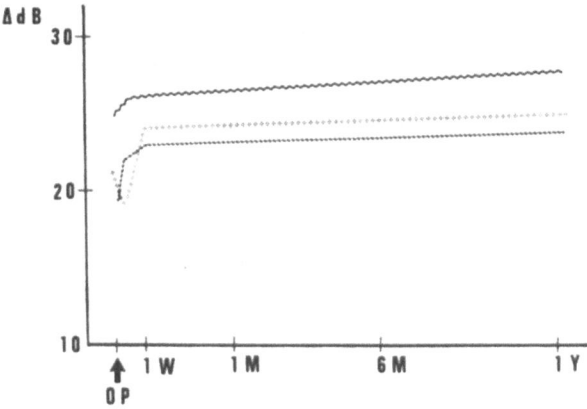

Fig. 6. Changes of the value of dB in eyes observed at one year after the blood injection.

In Summary. Figures of membraneous, or sometimes massive structures, which developed in the vitreous after whole blood injection changed over a period of time. Immediately after blood injection an echo source of a massive structure was displayed in the upper part of the vitreous. Afterward the echo source became membraneous and spread downward in parallel with the retina. No connection to the optic nerve or to the retina was shown in most of the cases. This is in contrast to the results of Tsuboi *et al.* (1979). However, in one case, of which the value of ΔdB decreased to 13, membraneous structures were displayed attaching to the fundus. A relatively rapid change in

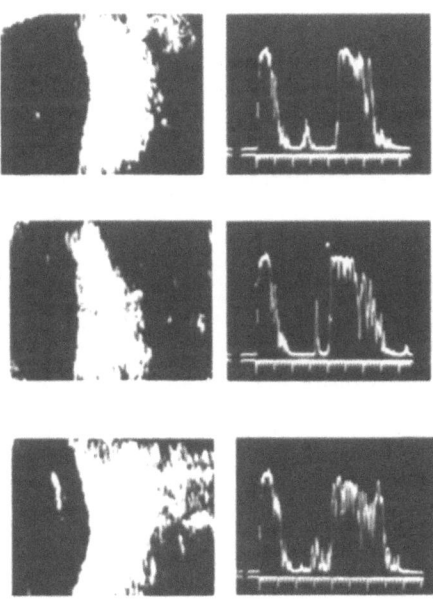

Fig. 7. B- and A-scan echograms in three eyes at one year after the blood injection.

the reflectivity measured by A-scan echography using standardized equipment arouses suspicion of retinal detachment. It is of note that the value of ΔdB in quantitative echography concentrated in a limited range after a long time of four to seven weeks, regardless of high or low reflectivity had been before. After the much longer period of one year, the whole blood injected into the vitreous was mostly absorbed.

Based on the results of the present paper, it is suggested that it is very valuable to trace changes in reflectivity of the target echo sources in case of vitreous hemorrhage rather than to watch the simple changes in echograms figures.

REFERENCES

Sawada, A., Inahara, M., Masuyama, Y. & Baba, Y. Significance of quantitative echography in membrane-like structures in the vitreous. Acta Soc. Ophthalmol. Jpn. 83: 1434 (1979).

Tsuboi, S., Emi, K., Hamada, Y., Hatsukawa, K., Hamada, M., Akena, K., Hohki, T. & Otori, T. Experimental studies of vitreous membrane formation in vitreous hemorrhage. Acta Soc. Ophthalmol. Jpn. 83: 1472 (1979).

Authors' Address:
Dept. of Ophthalmology
Miyazaki Medical College
Kiyotake, Miyazaki 889-16
Japan

ULTRASONIC EXAMINATION OF THE VITREOUS

M. RESTORI & D. MCLEOD

(London, United Kingdom)

Diagnostic ultrasound is now a routine investigation in patients with opacification in the ocular media (Coleman 1972, Ossoinig 1977). The system used at Moorfields Eye Hospital (McLeod, *et al*. 1977) employs a 10 MHz focussed transducer which is coupled to the eye by a saline bath. A Barraquer speculum is used to give good exposure of the eye. The transducer scans mechanically in a linear fashion. Each 4 cm sweep of the transducer takes 150 ms to complete and comprises a B-scan section of the eye and the orbit. Thus the system is capable of producing 8 B-scans/s. The rapid movement of the transducer permits dynamic studies of abnormalities to be performed. The level of the B-scan section is changed by a motor which is activated by pressing buttons close to the display tube. B-scan sections are generally taken at millimetre intervals (serial scanning) in all directions of gaze. Dynamic studies are performed by asking the patient to deviate his eyes laterally and medially during serial scanning. Lateral deviation of the eye takes approximately 0.1 s to complete whereas movements of abnormalities following a deviation of gaze (for example motion of a detached vitreous gel) are considerably slower (of the order of 1 s). Thus B-scanners with frame rates of 8 B-scans/s, or more, have sufficient time resolution to resolve such after-movements in detail. Adequate sensitivity and accurate echo registration allow weak echoes to be detected and displayed.

Rapid B-scanning of the vitreous cavity is most commonly performed in patients being considered for vitrectomy. The main aims of ultrasonic examinations are:

(a) to detect and identify material which has invaded the vitreous cavity.

(b) to determine the presence of posterior vitreous detachment, the extent of vitreo-retinal adhesion, the degree of contraction of gel volume and the mobility of the gel.

(c) to detect the presence of a retinal detachment and determine the nature of the detachment.

SCATTERED ECHOES IN THE VITREOUS CAVITY

Inflammatory cells and vitreous haemorrhage often give rise to low amplitude echoes within the vitreous cavity (Fig. 1a). In general inflammatory debris

Docum. Ophthal. Proc. Series, Vol. 29, ed. by J.M. Thijssen and A.M. Verbeek
© *1981. Dr W. Junk Publishers, The Hague*

47

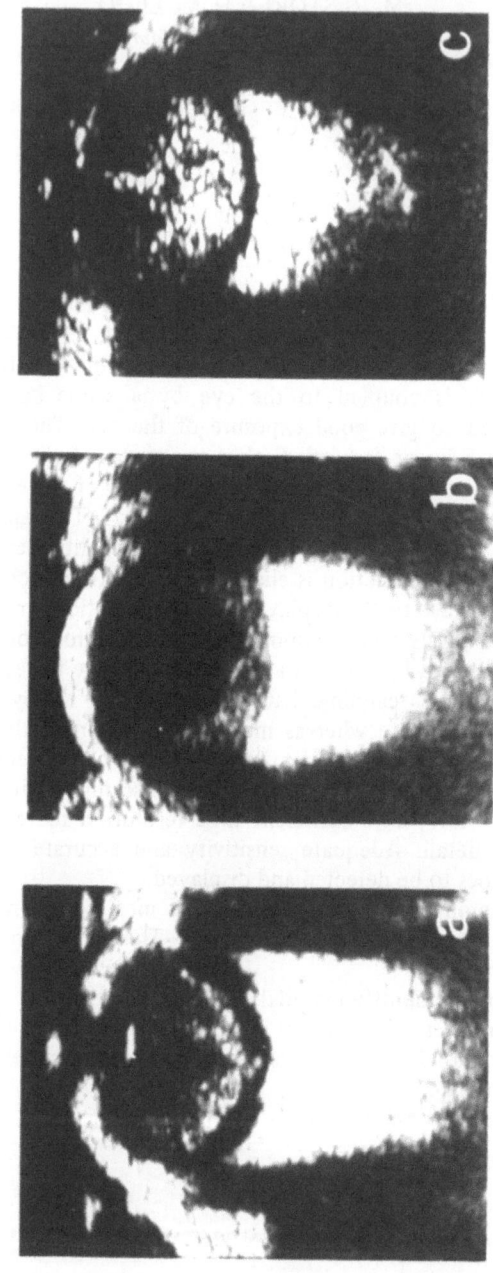

Fig. 1. Horizontal B-scans – Vitreous Opacity.
a. Haemorrhage in detached vitreous gel; b. Retrohyaloid haemorrhage; c. Asteroid bodies.

48

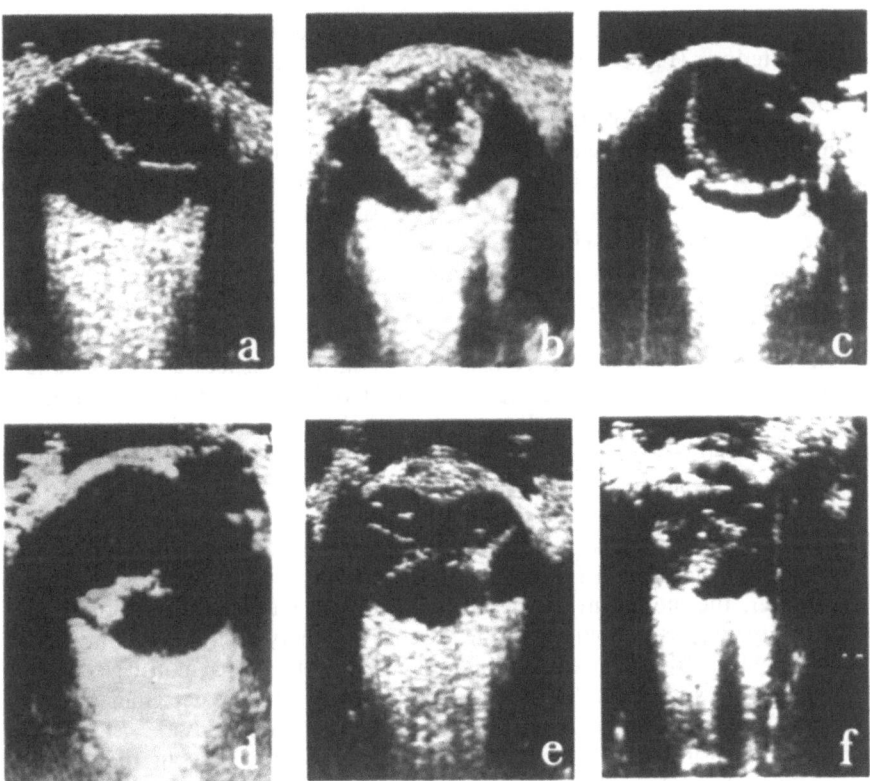

Fig. 2. Horizontal B-scans – Posterior Vitreous Detachment.
a. Echoes along posterior hyaloid interface; b. Detached vitreous gel tethering posteriorly; intra-gel haemorrhage; c. Detached vitreous gel tethering posteriorly ('ochre membrane); d. Detached vitreous gel with fibrous stalk attachment to retina; e. Cataract; detached retracted vitreous gel; two fine stalk vitreoretinal adhesions; f. Detached vitreous gel incarcerated into the retina temporal to optic nerve head; intra-gel haemorrhage.

cannot be distinguished ultrasonically from blood products. Invasion of the vitreous cavity by blood cells sometimes gives rise to low amplitude echoes of relatively uniform echo density (Fig. 1b). Very high amplitude echoes are typical of asteroid hyalitis (Fig. 1c), and individual very high amplitude echoes may arise from foreign bodies.

POSTERIOR VITREOUS DETACHMENT

There are two basic patterns indicative of posterior vitreous detachment:

(1) a sheet of echoes along the posterior-hyaloid interface usually inserting into the retina just anterior to the equator (Fig. 2a). The detached hyaloid sometimes tethers to the posterior retina by a single adhesion (Fig. 2b), which may be stalk like, (Fig. 2c, 2d) or by multiple vitreo-retinal

adhesions (Fig. 2e). After trauma, incarceration of the vitreous gel anteriorly or posteriorly (Fig. 2f) may be suggested by an assymetrical suspension of the vitreous gel.

(2) localisation of dispersed echoes to one or other vitreous compartments, the other compartment being clear or containing a different echo density (Fig. 3a). Intra-gel echoes are often bounded by clear retrohyaloid space (Fig. 1a) or an acoustically clear gel is outlined by diffuse echoes from the retro-hyaloid space (Fig. 1b).

Echoes from one or other vitreous compartment do not necessarily fill that compartment. Commonly, the retro-hyaloid space is completely filled with echoes but only the central part of the gel contains echoes (Fig. 3b). On occasions, an apparent 'compaction' of intra-gel echoes along a mobile posterior hyaloid surface occurs (Fig. 2c); at vitrectomy a dense nonfibrotic 'ochre' membrane is found. Frequently, retro-hyaloid haemorrhage gravitates onto the posterior retinal surface during ultrasonic examination with the patient in a supine position. The resulting fluid-level (Fig. 3c) mimics a shallow posterior retinal detachment.

In some cases the vitreous gel was immobile or moved without significant change in contour indicating gel contraction without collapse. In other cases, however, the movement of the posterior hyaloid interface characterised gel mobility. Extreme mobility of the vitreous gel (as typically seen in myopes with a bleeding retinal tear and in most cases of vitreous haemorrhage due to retinal vein branch occlusion) signifies posterior vitreous detachment with gel collapse. In a minimumly contracted mobile vitreous body the gel tended to settle against the retina under the influence of gravity in the supine position. In such cases dynamic testing is necessary to separate the vitreous from the retina and to identify points of true vitreo-retinal adhesion.

DETACHMENT OF THE RETINA

Detached retina produces a regular continuous sheet of high amplitude echoes. When the retinal detachment is extensive and bullous (fresh rhegmatogenous detachments), the membrane typically shows undulating aftermovements on dynamic testing and is usually characterised by attachments at the ora serrata and optic nerve head. Retinal tears (except when giant) are not detected. In most eyes with rhegmatogenous detachment there are also acoustic signs of invasion of the vitreous cavity by red blood cells or pigment cells or evidence of posterior vitreous detachment. A dense discrete posterior hyaloid membrane tethering by a wide adhesion to the optic nerve head sometimes simulates a total retinal detachment. In such cases, particular attention is paid to the dynamic and tonal features of the membrane.

MASSIVE PRE-RETINAL RETRACTION

(Gregor, *et al*. 1979). When the movements of total retinal detachment appear damped or absent on dynamic testing massive pre-retinal retraction is

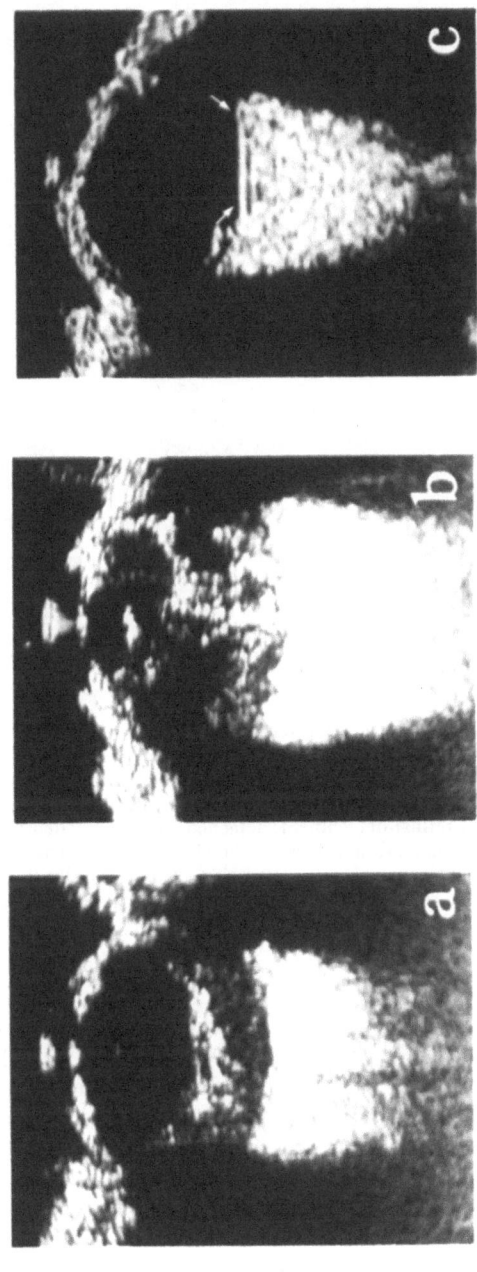

Fig. 3. Horizontal B-scans – Posterior Vitreous Detachment. a. Intra-gel haemorrhage; haemorrhage fills retrohyaloid space. b. Central gel haemorrhage; haemorrhage fills retrohyaloid space. c. Sedimentation of retrohyaloid haemorrphage onto retina (arrows).

51

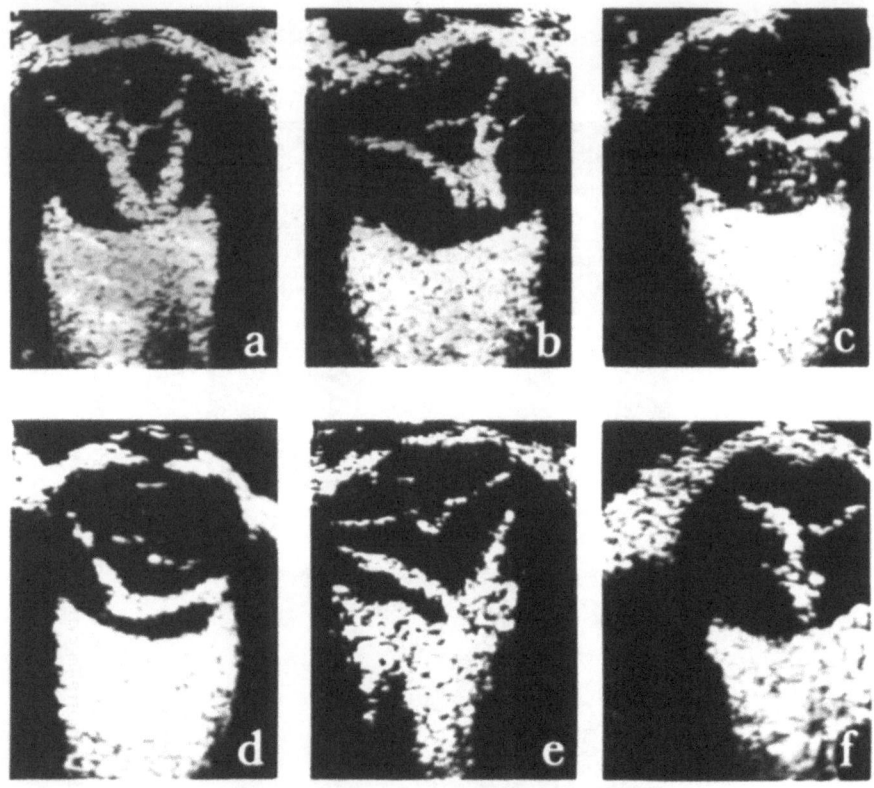

Fig. 4. Horizontal B-scans-Retinal Detachment.
a. Total thickened retinal detachment; detached retracted vitreous gel with taut posterior hyaloid membrane ('triangle sign'); b. Total folded retinal detachment bearing cyst (arrow); detached retracted vitreous gel with taut posterior hyaloid membrane; c. Deviated gaze; total retinal detachment; detached vitreous gel; dense sub-retinal opacity; d. Total retinal detachment; detached mobile vitreous gel; e. Total retinal detachment; detached retracted vitreous gel with herniation of gel centrally through taut posterior hyaloid membrane; f. Total retinal detachment with retinal leaves in apposition.

diagnosed. The retina often appear thickened (Fig. 4a) and folded (Fig. 4b) and retinal cysts (Fig. 4b) or sub-retinal deposits (Fig. 4c), blood products or cholesterol crystals may be detected. Sometimes the vitreous gel remains mobile (Fig. 4d), but usually a taut fibrotic posterior hyaloid membrane bridges between the retinal leaves in the coronal place (Fig. 4b). Thus, the gel occupies only the most anterior part of the vitreous cavity, though some gel may herniate through the gaps in the posterior hyaloid membrane (Fig. 4e).

The angular separation of the retinal leaves at the optic disc varies (Fig. 4e, 4f); juxtaposition of the retinal leaves in front of the optic disc is considered a contra-indication to vitreous surgery, as are the presence of retinal cysts and dense sub-retinal opacities.

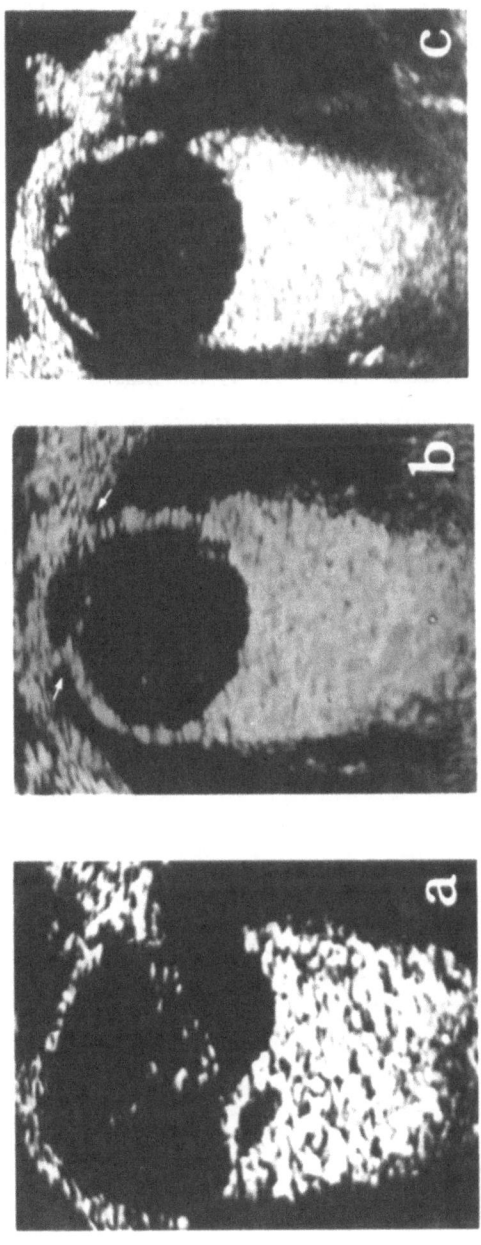

Fig. 5. Horizontal B-scans – Retinal Detachment. a. Detached vitreous gel inserting into posterior retinal detachment; b. Detachment of pars plana/ ora serrata (arrows) 'purse-string' retinal detachment; detached vitreous gel; c. Anterior annular chroidal detachment.

TRACTION RETINAL DETACHMENTS

(McLeod & Restori 1979). In traction detachments, a taut posterior hyaloid membrane typically inserts into the summit of an immobile elevation of the retina (Fig. 5a). Although elevation of the neuro-epithelium sometimes extends anterior to the ora serrata in trans-gel traction retinal detachments (Fig. 5b) there is seldom any real source of confusion with a choroidal detachment (Fig. 5c). However, some difficulty is experienced in differentiating shallow traction detachments of the posterior retina from thick epiretinal membranes or from a taut fibrous minimumly detached posterior hyaloid membrane.

REFERENCES

Coleman, D.J. Ultrasound in Vitreous Surgery. Am. Acad. Ophthalmol. Otolaryngol 76: 467 (1972).

Gregor, Z., Restori, M. & McLeod, D. B-Scan Ultrasound in Massive Pre-retinal retraction, Trans. Ophthalmol. Soc. U.K. 99(1) (1979).

McLeod, D. & Restori, M. Ultrasonic Examination in Severe Diabetic Eye Disease. Brit. J. Ophthalmol. 63: 533 (1979).

McLeod, D., Restori, M. & Wright, J.E. Brit. J. Ophthalmol. 61: 437 (1977).

Ossoinig, K. Echography of the eye, orbit and periorbital region. In: Orbit Roentgenology (P.H. Arger, ed.) New York: Wiley & Sons (1977) p. 223.

Authors' Address:
Dept. of Ultrasound
Moorfields Eye Hospital
London, United Kingdom

PROPHYLAXIS OF RETINAL DETACHMENT IN ENDOVITREOUS HEMORRHAGES EXPERIMENTALLY DRIVEN

A. REIBALDI, V.V. LORUSSO & G. GIANCIPOLI

(Bari, Italy)

INTRODUCTION

It is our everday clinical experience to find endovitreal hemorrhages which, often, can lead to a detachment of the retina. Continuing our research into the prophylaxis of retinal detachment, we have been conducting experiments in the hope of reducing the percentage of cases which actually develop into detachment (Reibaldi *et al.* 1976, Reibaldi *et al.* 1980). These experiments involved the use of encirclement, of vitrectomy and, then of both used in conjunction, on a group of rabbits which had 1 cc. of autogenous blood injected into the eyeball.

Developments were carefully followed, but due to the progressively increasing opacity of the dioptric media mainly by means of echography.

MATERIALS, METHODS AND RESULTS

The research was carried out on 74 rabbits (with an average weight of 3.2 kg) which were divided into four groups and anaesthetized by an infusion of 35 mg/kg sodium nembutal, injected into the marginal vein of the ear.

Then, we disconnected the conjunctiva at the limbus, performed sclerotomy 3 mm away from the limbus and introduced 1 cc of autogenous blood into the vitreous chamber, having first carried out paracenthesis of the anterior chamber to avoid hypertonia.

We checked the progress echographically with A-scan (Kretztechnik 7200) and B-scan (Bronson-Turner) daily for the first two months and every week for the following three months.

When, given the opacity of the media, we were able to detect echographically vitreoretinal adhesions and the formation of dense white vitreal membranes (which immediately precede ˙detachment) we proceeded with the different prophylactic treatments.

In the first group of 23 rabbits we decided to let detachment of retina develop without any prophylactic intervention. Vitreoretinal adhesions and vitreal membranes appeared between the 5th and 11th day, which, with time, got worse.

Between day 19 and day 40 detachment of retina occurred in 21 of the 23 rabbits, a percentage of 91.3%.

With the second group of 14 rabbits we performed an encirclement using a 1 mm-aside band of silicone band, fixed to the sclera with four Dracon stitches and held tight with a ring of silicone. This was carried out between day 6 and day 10 when the echographic trace showed the presence of thick fibrous membranes and vitreoretinal adhesions.

Between day 22 and day 60, detachment of retina appeared in 9 rabbits (64.28%), while in the remaining five rabbits (35.77%) the retina remained adherent in subsequent checks.

In the third group, consisting of 13 rabbits, between day 7 and day 15, echography revealed signs of vitreoretinal adhesions and the formation of dense vitreous bands or membranes. At this point we carried out a vitrectomy through the pars plana: having first disconnected the conjunctiva at the limbus and having performed a sclerotomy about 3 mm away from the limbus, we then inserted through this hole a guide tube, fixed to the sclera with Dracon stitches, and introduced Kloti's vitrotome into the vitreous chamber.

This was followed by dissection and suction of the vitreous which was then substituted by infusion fluid. Between day 27 and day 55, detachment of retina occurred in six rabbits – 46.15%. In three of these cases detachment was only discernable with the aid of echography, due to increasing opacity of the dioptric means. In the other seven cases (53.64%) a gradual clearing-up of the vitreous was observed.

In the fourth group composed of 24 rabbits when, between day 15 and day 32, showed the development of fibrous vitreal bands accompanied by vitreoretinal adhesions, we performed, at the same time, an encirclement and a vitrectomy through the pars plana as described for the preceding groups.

Between days 41 and 73, detachment of the retina appeared in five eyes – a percentage of 20.83. Diagnosis in four eyes was only possible with echography because of advanced opacity of the dioptric means.

CONCLUSIONS

The aim of our study was to find an effective prophylaxis for detachment of retina due to an experimentally induced endovitreal hemorrhage.

While detachment of retina occurred in 91.3% of the rabbits not prophylactically treated in any way, this percentage drops to 64.28% after encirclement, and further to 46.15% after vitrectomy. By far the most attractive result, however, was obtained combining the two operations, encirclement and vitrectomy performed together, after which detachment occurred in only 20.83%. This comes about because the containing-action of the encirclement is reinforced by the resection and removal of the vitreoretinal cusps in the vitrectomy.

In obtaining these results, which in the fourth group of rabbits are very satisfactory, echographic examination proved absolutely invaluable.

Generally, the dioptric means of opaque eyes make ophthalmoscopic examination difficult, if not actually impossible. With echography, however, we were able to follow, day by day, the formation of dense fibrous vitreal bands or membranes, judge their consistency and locate them accurately, thus allowing us to prepare meticolously for operation.

As well as the precise position, we were also able to choose the best moment to operate – that is, when the vitreo-retinal adhesions and vitreal membranes showed signs of imminent detachment of retina.

In conclusion we can affirm that the results obtained in our experiment are owed essentially to echography, thanks to which surgical intervention was made more exact.

All this urges us to use and to rely on echography more and more in clinical practice which every day presents us with pathological cases very similar to those artificially created by us in experiment.

Precisely because vitreal surgery is so very complex and demanding, we believe it unthinkable to proceed to the operating theatre without the help of of a thorough and detailed echographic examination.

REFERENCES

Reibaldi, A., Capotorto, B., Giancipoli, G. & Giummarra, C. Profilassi del distacco di retina nella emorragia massiva del vitreo. Nota III. Bol. Soc. It. Biol. Sper. (1980), p. 56.

Reibaldi, A., Capotorto, B., Giancipoli, G. & Ruggeri, G. Profilassi del distacco di retina nella emorragia massiva del vitreo. Nota I. Bol. Soc. It. Biol. Sper. (1980), p. 56.

Reibaldi, A., Giancipoli, G., Capotorto, B. & Lamorgese, C. Profilassi del distacco di retina nella emorragia massiva del vitreo. Nota II. Bol. Soc. It. Biol. Sper. (1980), p. 56.

Reibaldi, A., Montrone, F. & Balestrazzi, E. Distacco di retina sperimentale. Studio Ecografico. Atti Soc. It. Studi Ultras. Med. Roma (1976).

Authors' Address:
Institute of Ophthalmology
Bari University
Bari, Italy

ECHOGRAPHIC DIAGNOSIS AFTER INTRAOCULAR SILICONE OIL INJECTION

A.M. VERBEEK, A.L. BAYER & J.M. THIJSSEN

(Nijmegen, The Netherlands)

INTRODUCTION

The treatment of severe retinal detachment and of massive vitreous retraction by injection of silicone oil into the vitreous cavity has become a routine surgical procedure in many ophthalmological centers. The early work of Cibis, *et al.* (1962) has been convincingly brought into new light by Scott (1975, 1977), who combined the injection method with vitrectomy procedures. A more recent study by Leaves, *et al.* (1979) showed the complications following the silicone oil treatment. They concluded that these complications did in general not degrade the improvement in visual function. Among the complications two groups, i.e. the cataract cases and the keratopathy, are preventing adequate inspection of the vitreous cavity and it has become evident that echography may be very useful in the assessment of the condition of the retina (cf. Poujol & Massin, 1979). The specific problems arising from the strongly deviating acoustic properties of silicone oil have been partly investigated by these authors. In the present study we will establish the acoustic parameters more accurately and we will qualitatively and quantitatively try to explain the peculiar echographic findings in a silicone oil 'vitreous'.

CLINICAL CASES

Successful oil injection

The A-mode picture (Kretztechnik 7200 MA equipment) in Fig. 1 shows two specific features: the axial length seems to be 38 mm, and the posterior pole echo as well as the orbital tissue are apparently reflecting only weakly. The strongly deviating sound velocity of the oil illustrates the lengthening of the eye. The decreased reflectivity by the attenuation of the ultrasound and the transition of the acoustic impedance from oil to retina.

Air bubbles

A close approximation reveals that air almost totally reflects the ultrasound. As can be seen in Fig. 2, the air bubbles yield a strong first echocomplex

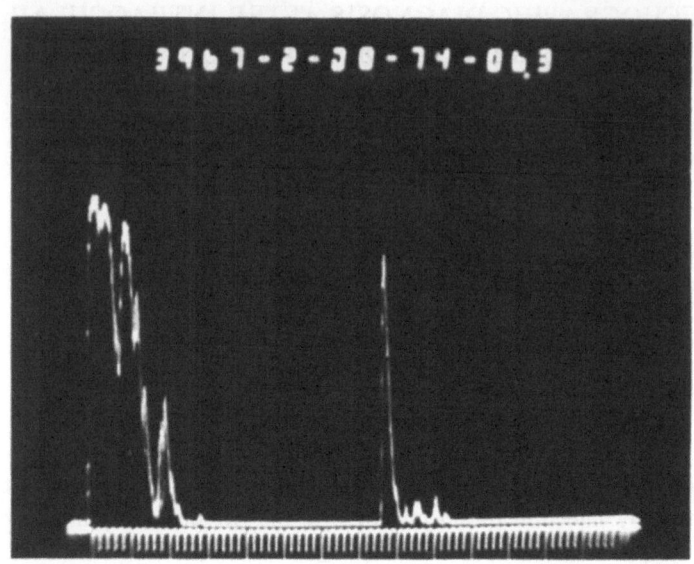

Fig. 1. A-mode picture of silicone 'vitreous'. Note apparent length of 38 mm and weak posterior pole reflectivity.

(Bronson Turner equipment), which is followed by reduplication artifacts. The posterior pole of the eye and the orbital tissue are either not depicted (shadow from air bubble), or only very weakly. This can be explained by the attenuation coefficient of silicone oil.

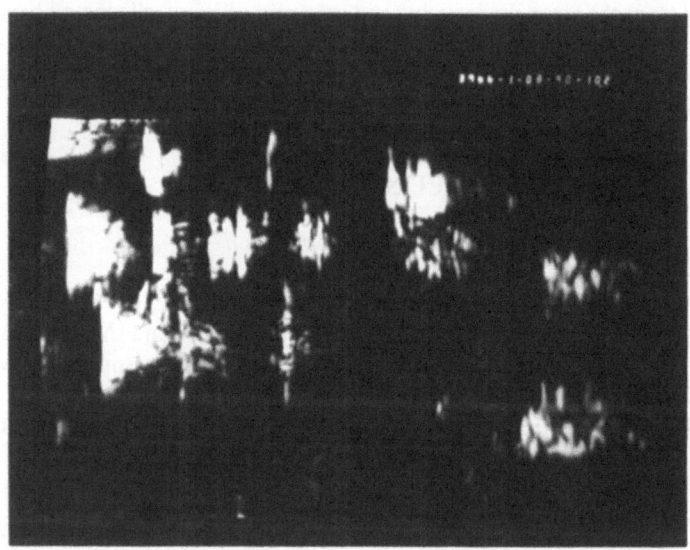

Fig. 2. B-mode picture of silicone filled vitreous cavity with air bubbles.

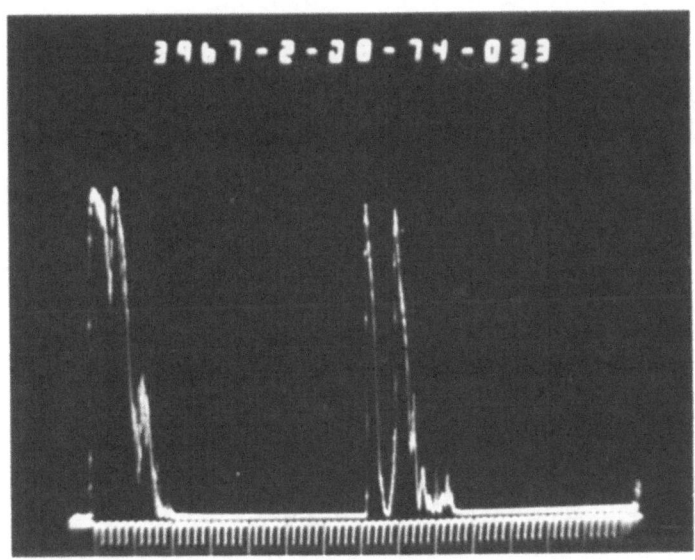

Fig. 3. A-mode picture showing liquid bubble (L) in front of posterior pole.

Fluid in silicone oil

In Fig. 3 the posterior pole echoes are from a transition oil to fluid which is followed by a 'water' bubble and a retina-choroid-sclera complex. The reflectivity of the oil-liquid transition approached that of the normal retinal detachment. Fig. 4 displays the same condition on the B-mode equipment, also in this case no retinal detachment was found.

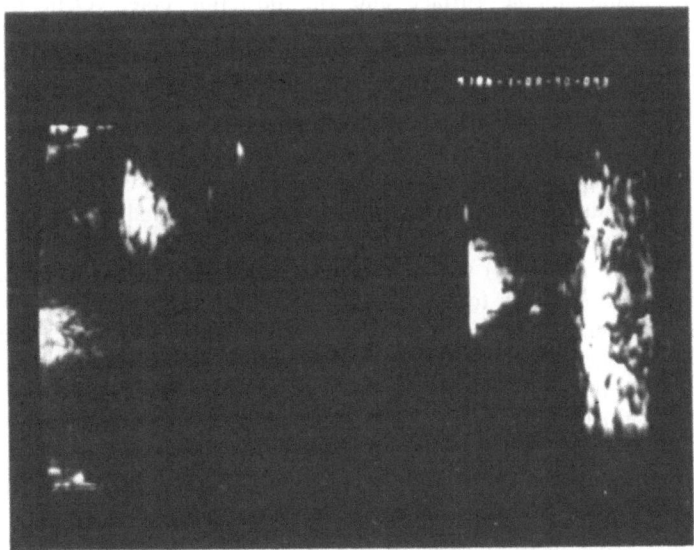

Fig. 4. B-mode picture of liquid bubble in the posterior space of the eye.

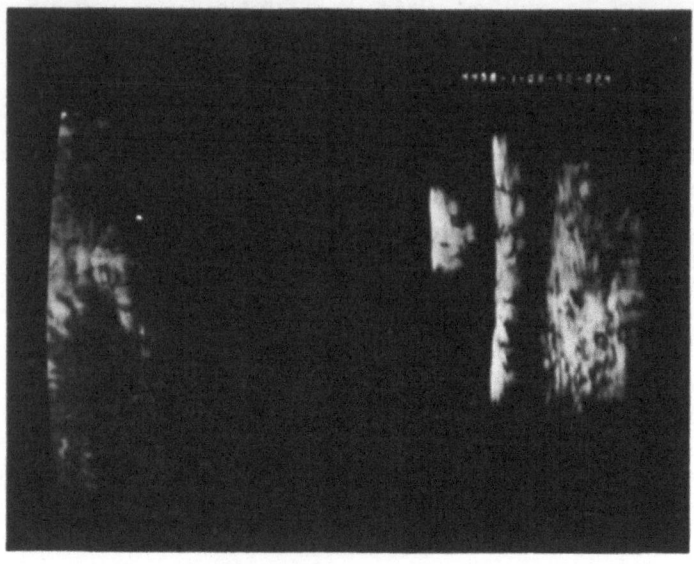

Fig. 5. B-mode picture of posterior liquid bubble anterior to a flat retinal detachment (R).

Fluid in silicone oil and retinal detachment

This condition is shown in Fig. 5. Detachment is clearly visible between the anterior liquid bubble surface and the posterior pole. Again the low reflectivity of the choroid and sclera should be noticed.

PHYSICAL EXPLANATIONS

Before explaining the clinical images obtained from eyes containing silicone oil, a few results from measurements performed with the oil will be shown.

Experimental conditions were as follows: The 8 MHz transducer (Kretztechnik, NM8 5K) was clamped in a vertical micro-manipulator. The readings were accurate to ± 0.02 mm. The transducer was aligned perpendicular to the bottom of a small glass container filled with oil (1000 cSt) which was placed in a thermostatic bath at 37°C. The transducer was then moved − in 0.5 mm steps over a 10 mm distance -- and the time of flight (back and forth) through the oil was measured. This measurement was performed by using a Kretztechnik 7200 MA A-mode apparatus and a transient recorder (Biomation 8100). As can be seen in Fig. 6 the data points can almost exactly be fitted by a straight line with a slope yielding a velocity of 982.8 m/s. This value is close to the result obtained by Poujol & Massin (1979), who found 986 m/s at a non-specified temperature.

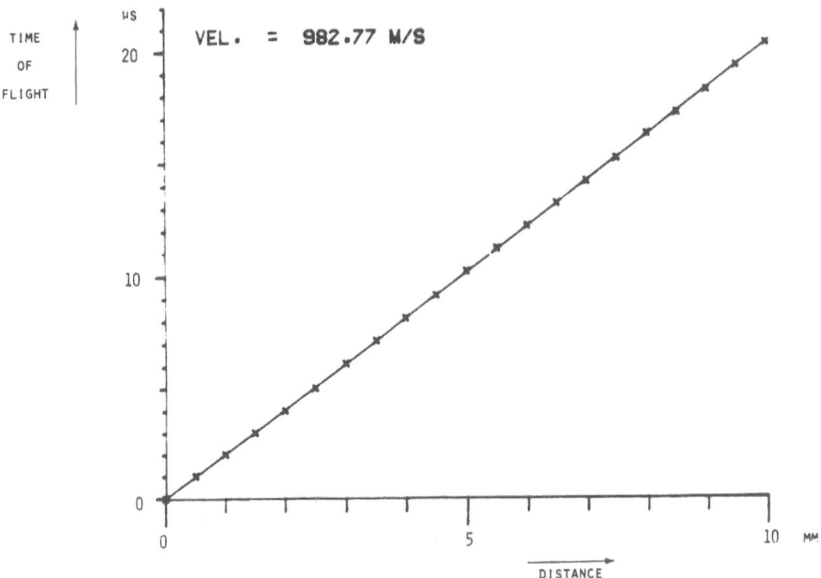

Fig. 6. Graph of measurements to estimate the sound velocity in silicone oil. Abscissa: distance, ordinate: time of flight. Velocity: 982.77 m/s.

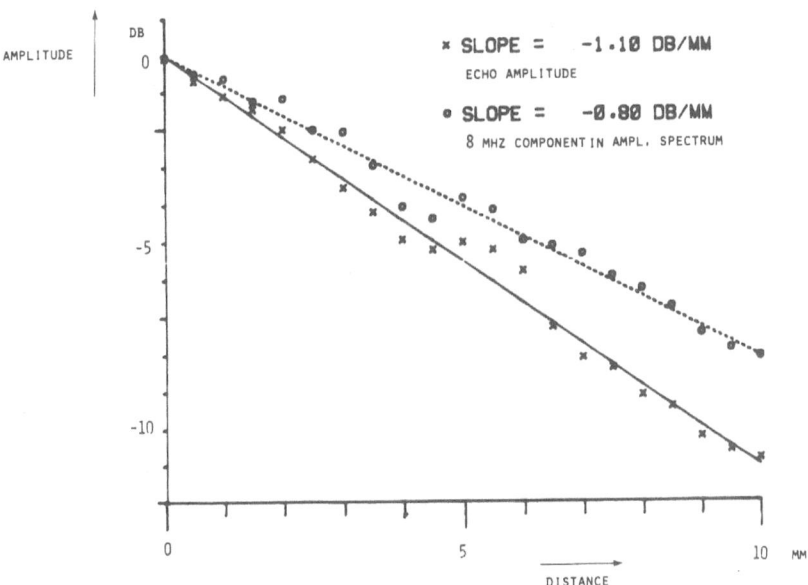

Fig. 7. Graph of measurements to estimate the attenuation in silicone oil. Abscissa: distance, ordinate: amplitude of echo from flat plate. Attenuation coefficient for a 8 MHz transducer (X) 1.10 dB/mm. Attenuation at 8 MHz sharp (0): 0.8 dB/mm.

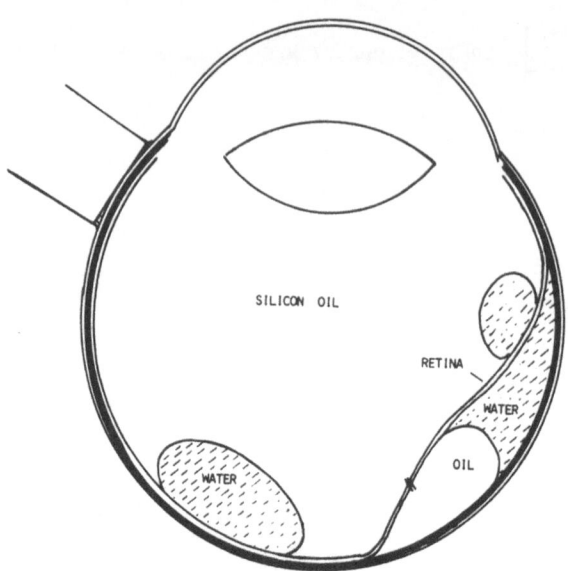

Fig. 8. Various conditions which may be found after silicone oil treatment.

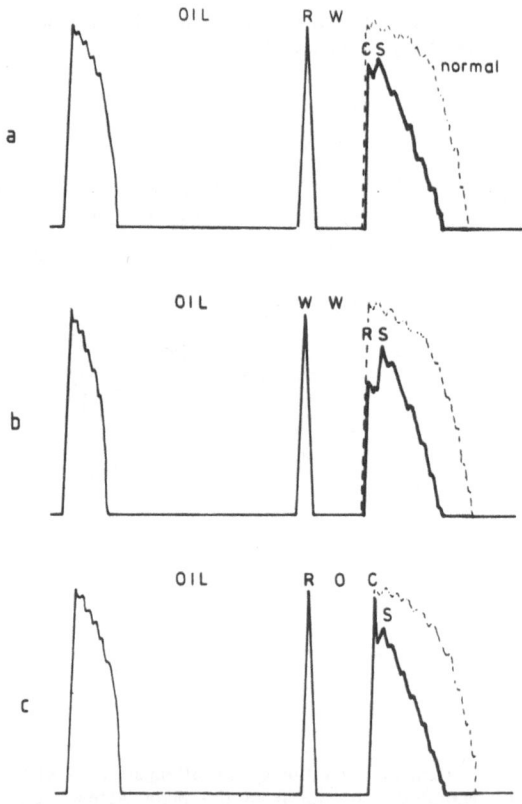

Fig. 9. Semi-quantitative prediction of echopatterns in a few conditions.

Table 1.

	Sound velocity	Impedance
	$(m\,s^{-1})$	$(10^6\ kg\,m^{-2}\,s^{-1})$
Water (35° C)	1539	1.550
Retina	1565	1.610
Silicone oil (35°C)	982 ± 1	0.940

The next measurement concerned sound attenuation. It was also performed with the equipment described above. For this purpose, however, the radiofrequency signal was stored in the transient recorder at 0.5 mm intervals. The spectrum was subsequently calculated by using a digital computer linked with the recorder. We estimated the amplitude of the 8 MHz component in this spectrum as well as the amplitude of the video echogram. The resulting data are summarized in Fig. 7 and a slope of -1.1 dB/mm oil, forth and back, is obtained for the video echoes. This value has to be taken into account in the clinical echograms. Poujol & Massin (1979) measured a value of -1 dB/mm.

With the velocity of silicon oil we are able to calculate the so-called acoustic impedance:

$$Z = \rho \cdot c$$

The mass density ρ is of the order of $956\ kg\,m^{-3}$, so we get an impedance of $0.940\ 10^6\ kg\,m^{-2}\,s^{-1}$.

If we take for retina the values of ρ and c known for brain tissue (Goss et al. 1980) and for water $1007\ kg\,m^{-3}$ and $1539\ m\,s^{-1}$ we obtain the impedance given in Table 1. The reflection coefficients relevant to our clinical data follow from the definition:

$$R_{1,2} = \frac{Z_1 - Z_2}{Z_1 + Z_2}$$

The various coefficients are given in Table 2. The reflection coefficients are independent of the direction of the ultrasound.

Table 2.

	Reflection coefficients
Oil-retina	$R_{o,r} = 0.260$
Water-retina	$R_{w,r} = 0.016$
Oil-water	$R_{o,w} = 0.263$

CLINICAL CASES

The special conditions which may occur are summarized in Fig. 8.

(1) Abnormal axial eye length on A-mode echograms and distortion of the

65

B-mode images can easily be explained by the sound veloctiy. This is almost 2/3 of the velocity in normal vitreous humour. So the real dimensions are obtained if 2/3 of the measured length is taken.

(2) Low posterior pole echoes can be understood from the high attenuation of ultrasound in silicon oil. If we take the average eye length to be of the order of 23 mm we may expect an overall attenuation of *25 dB*, or a factor of 20 ×.

(3) The reflectivity level of the oil-retina transition is much higher than in the normal vitreous (24 dB), and this compensates partly for the enlarged intraocular attenuation. The retinal peak is therefore almost of normal magnitude (Fig. 9a).

(4) Differentiation of retinal detachment from preretinal fluid is practically impossible, because the reflectivity level at the transition oil-retina as compared to oil-water differs only 6%, or 0.5 dB. The posterior wall echocomplex also differs only slightly in these cases, but is considerably reduced relative to normal (Fig. 9b).

(5) If oil is present in the subretinal space not only the retinal echo, but also the choroidal echo will be relatively high. As compared to the situation of subretinal water a 20 dB higher choroidal reflectivity may be observed. The scleral and peri-ocular echoes are still much lower than normal (Fig. 9c).

REFERENCES

Cibis, P.A., Becker, B., Okun, E. & Canaan, S. The use of liquid silicone oil in retinal detachment. Arch. Ophthalmol. (Chicago) 68: 46 (1962).

Goss, S.A., Johnston, R.L. & Dunn, F. Compilation of empirical ultrasonic properties of mammalian tissues II. J. Acoust. Soc. Am. 68: 93 (1980).

Leaver, P.K., Grey, R.H.B. & Garner, A. Complications following silicone-oil injection. Mod. Probl. Ophthalmol. 20: 290 (1979).

Poujol, J. & Massin, M. L'examen échographique des yeux opérés de decollement de rétine avec injection de silicone. In: Diagnostica Ultrasonica in Ophthalmologia (H. Gernet, ed.) Münster: Remy Verlag (1979) p. 111.

Scott, J.D. The treatment of massive vitreous retraction by the separation of pre-retinal membranes using liquid silicone. Mod. Probl. Ophthalmol. 15: 285 (1975).

Scott, J.D. A rationale for the use of liquid silicone. Trans. Ophthalmol. Soc. U.K. 97: 235 (1977).

Authors' Address:
Institute of Ophthalmology
University of Nijmegen
6500 HB Nijmegen, The Netherlands

ROUND TABLE DISCUSSION ON VITREOUS PATHOLOGY

CHAIRMAN: D. MCLEOD
PANELISTS: D.J. COLEMAN, K.C. OSSOINIG, J. POUJOL,
M. RESTORI, A. SAWADA, P. TILL & A.M. VERBEEK

Dr Poujol began the proceedings by considering the diagnosis of vitreous pathology from point-like echoes arising from haemorrhage, inflammation or degeneration of the gel. He emphasized that differentiation between these pathologies is frequently difficult using ultrasonic criteria alone, but inflammatory vitritis tends to produce diffuse low amplitude echoes while echoes from asteroid degeneration usually have a very high amplitude. In discussion, Dr Coleman had calculated that a coagulum of 60 microns (using a 10 MHz probe) is necessary for ultrasonic detection of haemorrhage, while Dr Ossoinig felt that a chain of low amplitude spikes detected with highly sensitive equipment implies considerable opacification and visual obscuration.

Dr McLeod deprecated the use of the term 'organisation' by ultrasonographers to describe the heterogeneous echo-pattern with membrane formation in long standing haemorrhage. Organisation implies invasion of a haemotoma by macrophages, fibroblasts and capillaries (i.e. granulation tissue) with ultimate replacement by a fibrous scar. This is not a feature of haemorrhage in the vitreous where, subsequent to lysis of red cells and and fibrin clots, blood stained vitreous collagen merely becomes arranged in veils or layers, with no new collagen formation or capillary ingrowth.

Miss Restori then discussed the diagnosis of posterior vitreous detachment either from membrane-like echoes along the gel boundary or from the distribution and density of echoes in one or other vitreous compartment i.e. the gel itself or the retrohyaloid space. She stressed that the posterior boundary of a detached gel has a different type of motion on dynamic testing from the retina in a rhegmatogenous detachment where, unless the vitreous remains attached to the detached retina, the membrane undulates as a sheet with tethering points at the ora serrata and optic disc.

Dr Ossoinig discussed the 'posterior ocular hyphema' where red cells in the retrohyaloid space sediment on to the retina and form a fluid level. The high amplitude echoes simulate an immobile detached retina, but the fluid level can be made to 'creep' over the optic disc with changes in eye position. Dr McLeod pointed out that a similar appearance can occasionally be seen in the sub-retinal space after blood-stained retrohyaloid fluid has passed through a retinal break to detach the retina.

Dr Sawada discussed the difficulties in using topographic and quantitative echography to diagnose a retinal detachment and differentiate this from a dense haemorrhagic vitreous membrane tethering at the optic disc; the latter might also have high reflectivity. He felt that quantitative echography is more valuable than the B-scan pattern for such differentiation. This was challenged by Dr Coleman who pointed out that there are no absolute quantitative criteria to distinguish detached retina from a vitreous membrane. Dr Ossoinig conceeded that an atrophic or folded retina might have a relatively low reflectivity, and state that quantitative differentiation is unreliable for localised traction detachment of up to 3 disc-diameters (since part of the sound beam bypasses the small interface). In such cases, the B-scan pattern is more important. With large membranes and borderline results on quantitative echography, the reflectivity of the pre-scleral layer beneath the membrane in question gives useful information.

Dr Verbeek discussed the ultrasonic criteria of operability of a retinal detachment. He pointed out that serous detachment and underlying tumours must first be excluded, while prephthisical changes in the choroid imply urgent surgery. The degree of elevation, folding and mobility of the retina provide useful information for the surgeon, as does the extent of vitreoretinal adhesions. A triangular or T-shaped pattern or the presence of sub-retinal echoes militate against surgery. In discussion, Dr Coleman felt that almost any type of detachment can be managed surgically provided there is evidence of some visual function, and that clinical findings are more important than ultrasonic data in evaluating operability. Dr McLeod stressed the importance of detecting an anterior detachment of the oral retina and pars plana in trauma cases in order to avoid entering the sub-retinal space when introducing instruments through the pars plana.

Dr Coleman then discussed the vitreous pathology in trauma, together with associated damage to the lens, retina and choroid. He felt that isometric scanning was particularly useful for differentiating vitreous and retinal membranes in trauma, and advocated early definitive surgery (i.e. within 48 h). He also advised early surgery for prephthisical eyes with choroidal thickening and cyclitic membranes. However, Dr Coleman suggested that surgery should be delayed for two weeks or more in eyes with haemophthalmos, disorganised topography and gross hyperaemia and thickening of the choroid on initial assessment. Dr McLeod pointed out the difficulty of excluding an oral retinal disinsertion or tear at the posterior border of the vitreous base in cases of blunt trauma with apparently only a vitreous haemorrhage on ultrasound; a small proportion of such patients will detach the retina in the ensuing months.

Dr Till described topographic, kinetic and quantitative echography of the sub-retinal space. A serous detachment gives no sub-retinal echoes, while fluid sub-retinal haemorrhage gives low amplitude echoes showing spontaneous movements. In Coats' Disease, echoes were said to arise from fast moving cholesterol crystals in the sub-retinal space.

In the final discussion period, Dr Ossoinig considered the indications for vitrectomy for example, in vitreous haemorrhage with dense axial membranes or retinal detachment progressing towards the macula. He stressed that ultrasound is only an aid to the surgeon in conjunction with clinical and other data, and emphasized the value of three dimensional documentation of the vitreo-retinal pathology. Dr Ossoinig illustrated the value of ultrasound in indicating to the surgeon the site at which a dense posterior hyaloid membrane should be penetrated in order to avoid damage to underlying detached retina. Dr McLeod emphasized the value of dynamic B-scanning in differentiating complete from incomplete posterior vitreous detachment in cases of spontaneous vitreous haemorrhage. In general, incomplete vitreous detachment is unlikely to be complicated by a retinal detachment, while complete vitreous detachment is frequently associated with a post-basal retinal tear which may subsequently cause the retina to detach. If a tear is suspected from the presence of a complete vitreous detachment, early vitreous surgery may be indicated, while in incomplete vitreous detachment (for example, associated with disc neovascularisation or disciform macula degeneration), spontaneous clearing should be awaited.

Dr Coleman and Miss Restori then discussed real-time scanning and the time resolution necessary to display induced movements of vitreous membranes and detached retina. They pointed out that scanning rates of 8 per second are perfectly satisfactory for this purpose.

THE RELATION BETWEEN HISTOPATHOLOGY AND ULTRASONOGRAPHY IN INTRAOCULAR TUMOURS

Introductory Lecture

W.A. MANSCHOT

(*Rotterdam, The Netherlands*)

When one stands as an ultrasonographic layman before a floor filled by experts, the best way to hide a certain panic seems to tell a story which might be representative for the message a pathologist can carry to his ultrasonographic colleagues.

A friend of mine who is as bald as billiard-ball happened to mention that his brother is even more bald-headed than he himself. When I couldn't help showing some slight incredulity, my friend added: 'But of course, don't forget that his head is larger than mine!'

The message, of course is that everything in life, be it complete baldness or the interpretation of echograms, is to be judged with some sense of relativity.

Naumann & Portwich (1976) encountered in a consecutive series of 1000 eyes 281 globes that had been enucleated because of the suspicion of a neoplastic process. 238 of these eyes harboured a uveal melanoma, 18 contained a retinoblastoma, while choroidal metastases of a carcinoma elsewhere were found in ten eyes. It is to be realized that uveal metastases occur far more frequently than appears from this statistic, because eyes containing a metastatic tumour are rarely enucleated. The real frequency of uveal metastases appears from a study by Bloch & Gartner (1971) who found uveal metastases in 12% of 230 patients who had died of remote carcinoma.

I learned from your literature that macroscopic interfaces as the surface of a tumour, connective tissue septa, large vessels, extensive necrotic areas and the interfaces between large portions of different cell types present significant acoustic interfaces and create high spikes when these interfaces are hit by a perpendicular sound beam. A medium to high reflectivity is provided when these interfaces occur in a dense contribution as, for example, is found in a cavernous hemangioma, or when almost equal amounts of cells and intercellular substances are distributed in such a way that a great number of larger interfaces are formed, as in the intravascular stage of carcinoma metastases to the choroid.

Minimal reflectivity occurs when either cells or intercellular structures are predominant. The first possibility is to be found in melanomas with a compact cellular structure with minimal intercellular substance and vasculature. Predominant intercellular substance is present in, for example, sclerosed disciform macular degeneration.

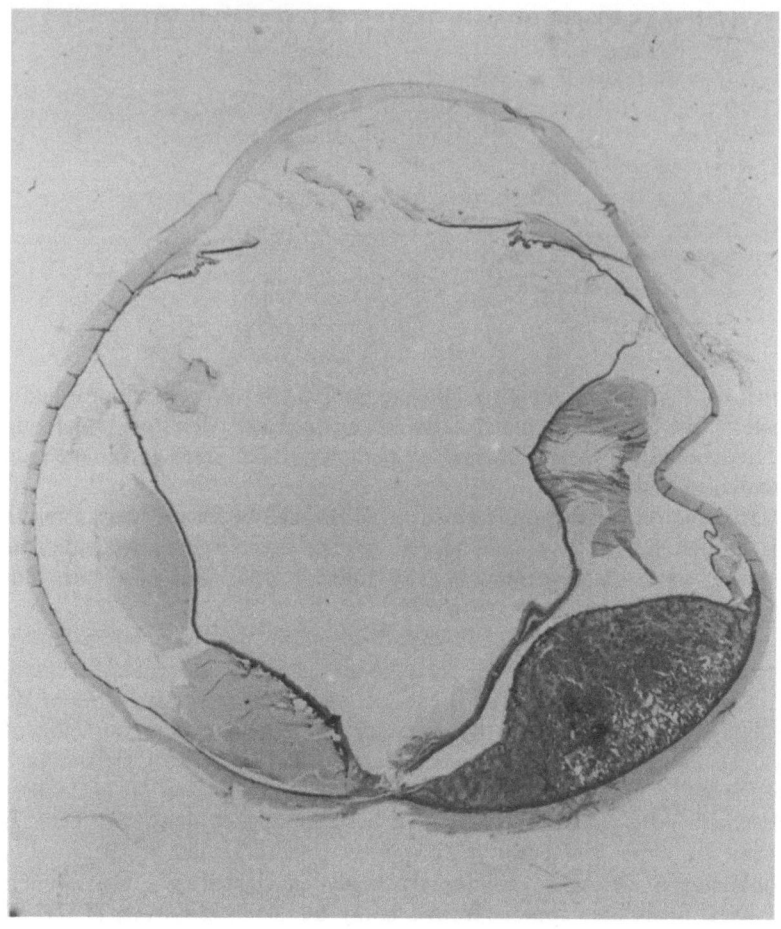

Fig. 1. Choroidal metastasis of adenoid carcinoma (Op. 288, original magnification × 4, neg. 27993-1).

As a pathologist who registers daily through his microscope the individuality of human disease, I noticed a certain liability to generalization in the interpretation of echographic findings in the literature. Therefore, I would like to begin by showing some histopathological examples of the great variability of the microscopic structure of the same type of tumour in various patients and also of one tumour in one patient.

A statement in the literature like: 'in general, metastic tumours have a lower silhouette (i.e. a lower height-to-base ratio) than do malignant melanomas' (Coleman *et al.* 1974) is certainly correct, but is of little value for the interpretation of an echogram in a given patient. Fig. 1 represents a rather prominent choroidal tumour surrounded by an extensive serous retinal detachment. This picture is almost pathognomonic for a choroidal melanoma. Nonetheless, it represents a metastasis of an adenoid carcinoma.

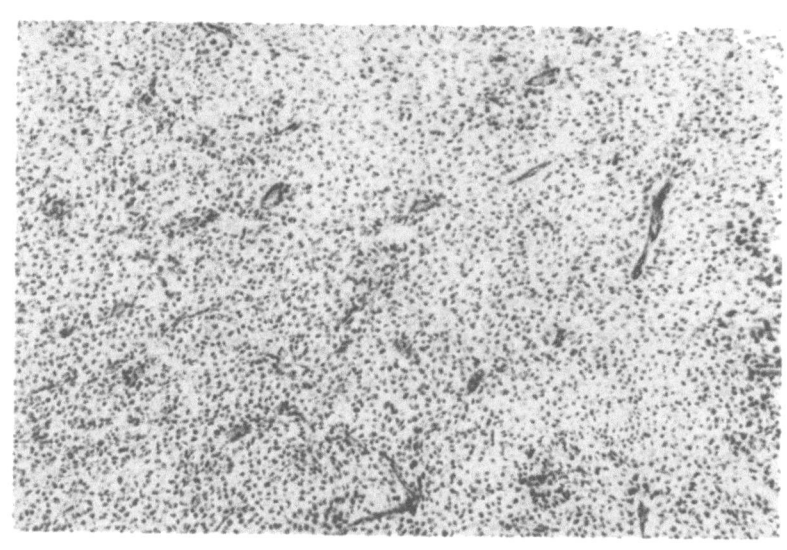

Fig. 2. Details of Fig. 1. Compact cellular structure (Op. 288, original magnification × 95, neg. 27991-2).

Fig. 2 and 3 show two areas of one section of this metastasis; Fig. 2 shows a compact cellular structure with little intercellular substance, small blood-vessels and no intercellular spaces, while Fig. 3, at the same magnification, reveals a similar cell type, but large blood vessels and large intercellular spaces. The reflectivity of these two parts of the same tumour will probably be different.

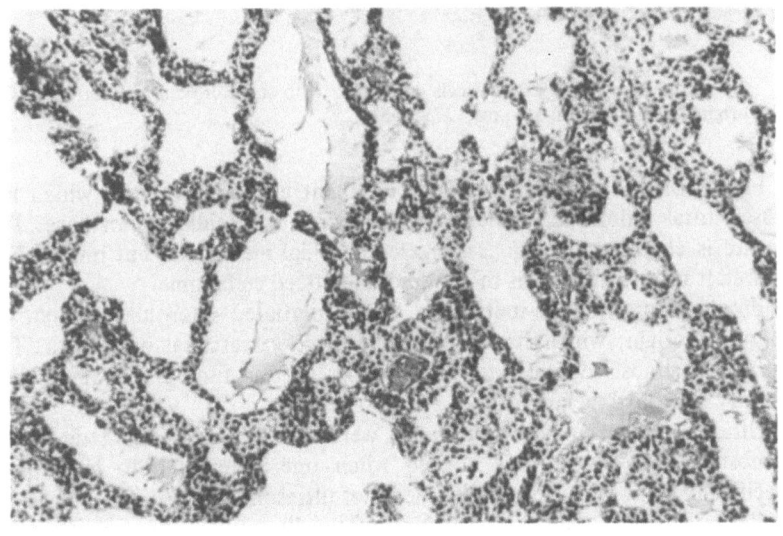

Fig. 3. Detail of Fig. 1. Cystoid structure in same tumour (Op. 288, original magnification × 95, neg. 27991-4).

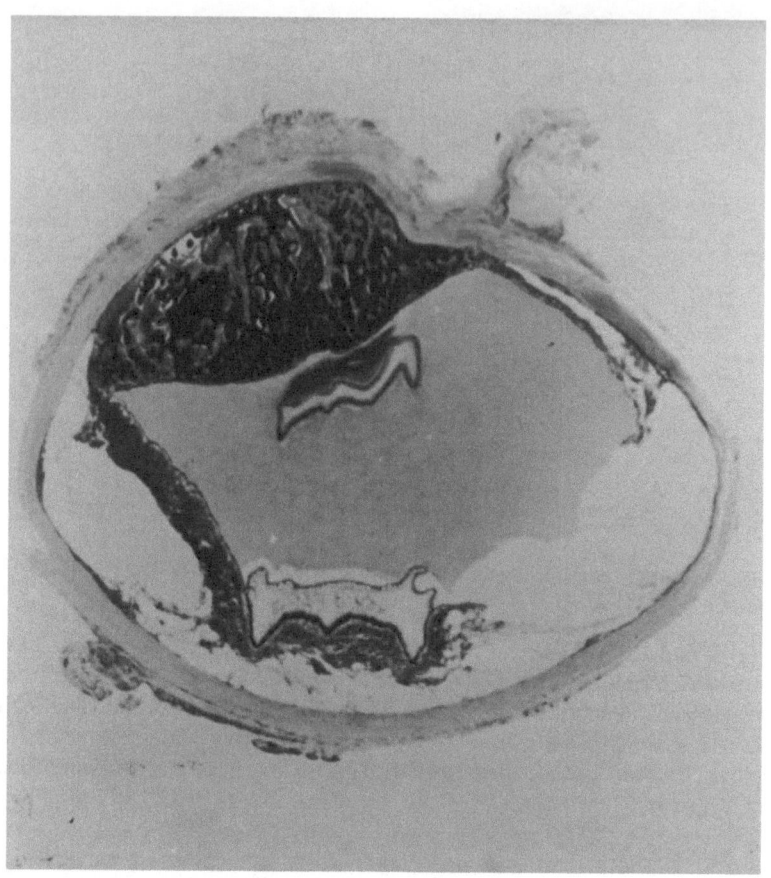

Fig. 4. Choroidal metastasis of oat-cell carcinoma with subchoroidal haemorrhage (Op. 991, original magnification × 4, neg. 27993-5).

Fig. 4 shows a highly necrotic prominent choroidal tumour which has caused total retinal detachment and a large subchoroidal hemorrhage. The picture is characteristic for a necrotic choroidal melanoma, but microscopy showed it to be a metastasis of a pulmonar oat-cell carcinoma.

Fig. 5 represents a metastatic undifferentiated choroidal tumour of unknown origin, which had produced a large extrascleral outgrowth. The picture is almost identical to that of Fig. 6; this tumour, however, is a primary choroidal melanoma.

Other choroidal metastatic tumours were shown, which all illustrated that a most extreme caution is needed when one is tempted to label more specifically a choroidal tumour by means of ultrasonography.

Retinoblastoma seems — according to the literature — not to give much differential diagnostic difficulties in ultrasonography. We have to realize that the presence of the retinoblastoma gen is continuously increasing in our

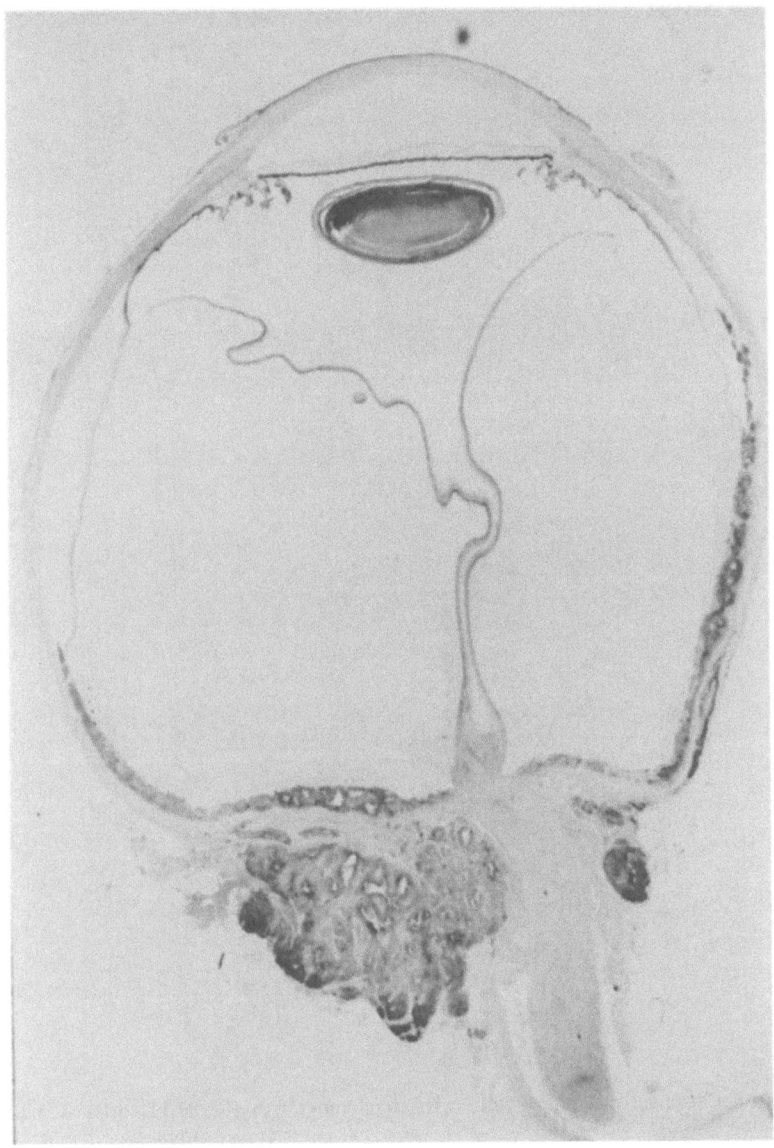

Fig. 5. Choroidal metastasis of undifferentiated carcinoma with extrascleral outgrowth (Op. 1935, original magnification × 4, neg. 27993-2.

populations, because the survival rate of these patients has improved considerably. A morbity of 1 in 14 500 new-borns has recently been reported by Naumann (1980); this morbidity will certainly increase further.

Retinoblastomas may present clinically as one or more small pink or greyish-white retinal tumours, but also as a huge retrolental mass that fills the

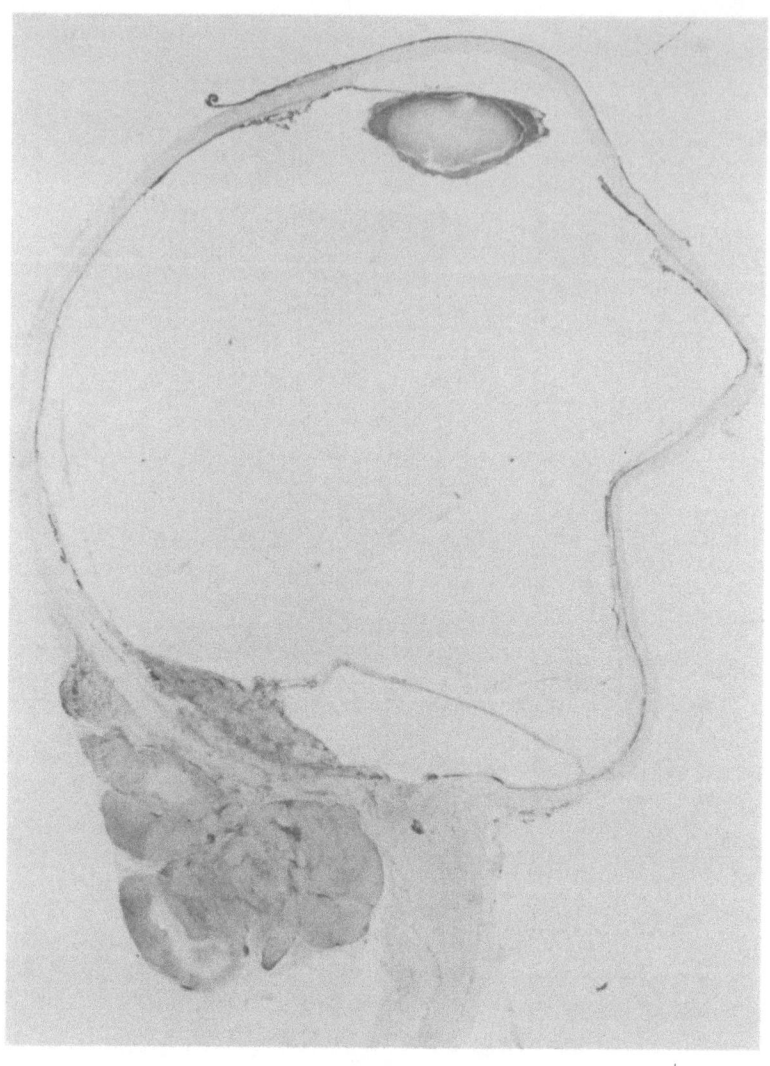

Fig. 6. Choroidal melanoma with extrascleral outgrowth (O. 87-11, original magnification × 4, neg. 27993-3).

entire globe. Fig. 7 shows one of the basic characteristics of retinoblastomas, viz. their multifocal origin. Both halves of the retina reveal a number of isolated tumour foci. The finding of multiple, small retinal tumourous lesions in the echogram of young children is highly suggestive of retinoblastoma. Sometimes, a diffuse infiltrating type of retinoblastoma without circumscribed tumour formations is found. A diffusely thickened retina in childhood has to rouse suspicion for this type of retinoblastoma.

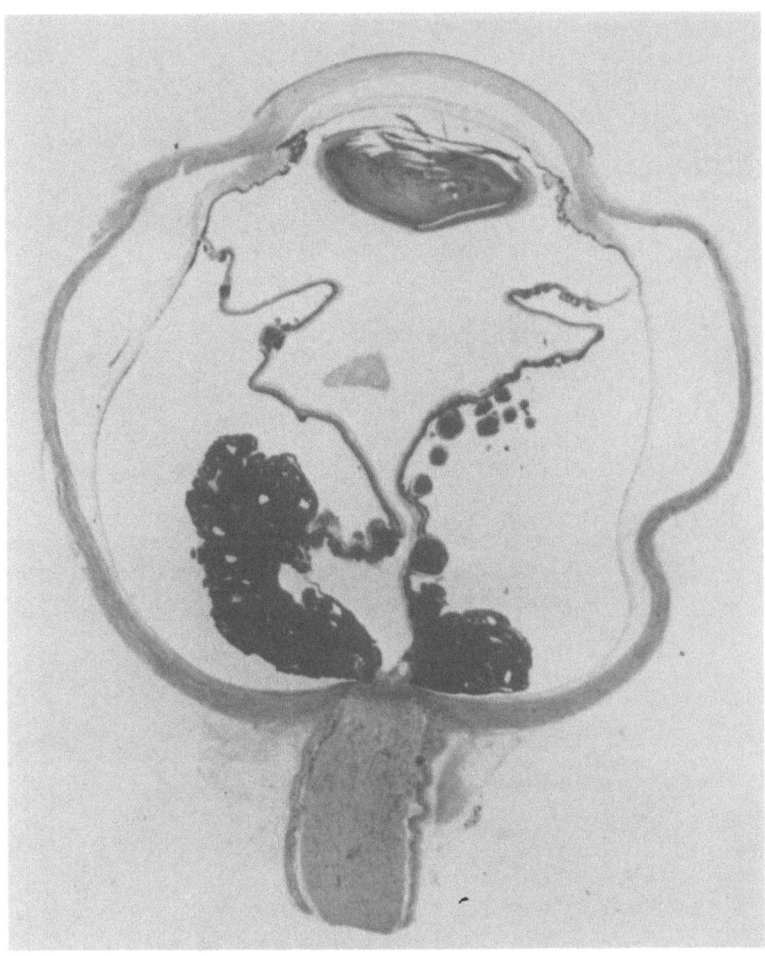

Fig. 7. Retinoblastoma: multiple origins (O. 927-9, original magnification × 4, neg. 27993-4).

Ossoinig & Blodi (1974) have stressed that the acoustic hallmark of retinoblastomas is their extremely highly reflectivity, showing 80% to 100% spike height at tissue sensitivity. The morphological origins of this high reflectivity are (1) rosette formation of the tumour cells, (2) necrosis which produces large interfaces between areas having great acoustic differences and (3) calcifications which behave like foreign bodies which reflect and scatter the sound waves more strongly than any biologic tissues (Fig. 8). These authors also stated that the frequent presence of large vessels forms another reason for the high reflectivity of retinoblastoma tissue. It seems likely that the high reflectivity attributed to the vessels is not caused by the vessels

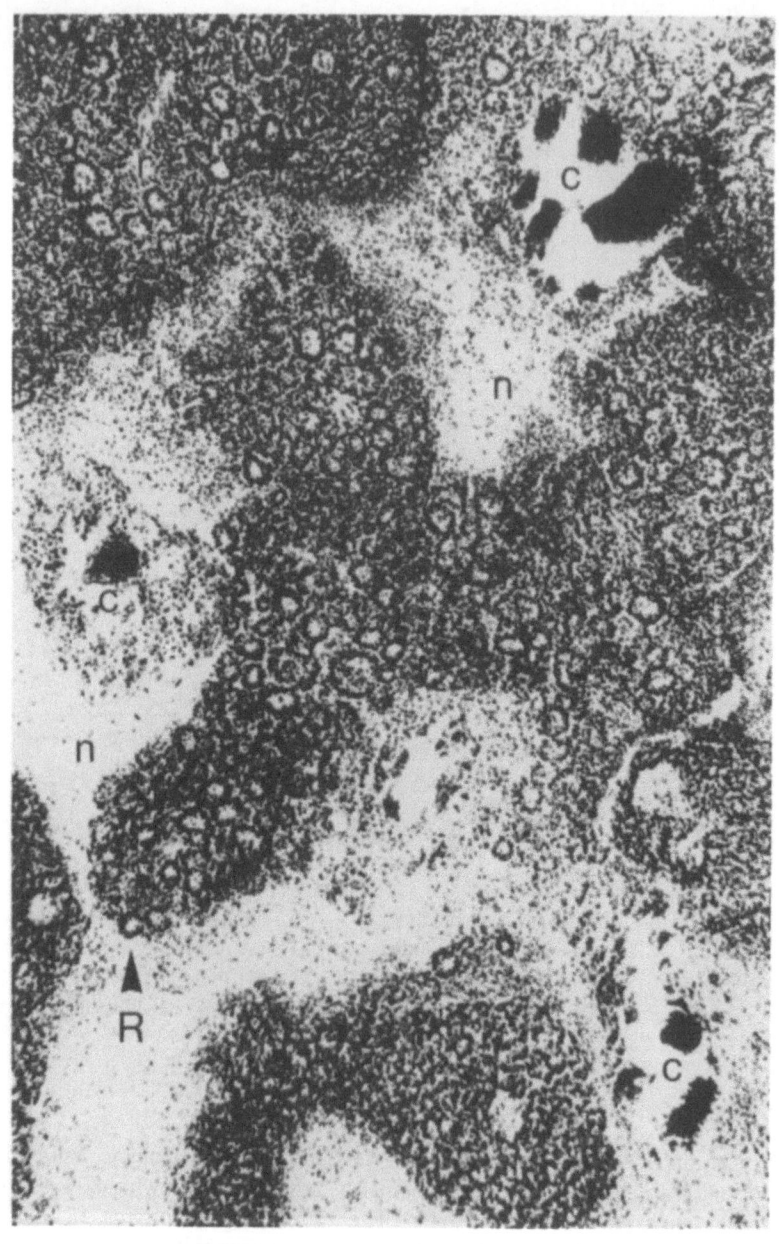

Fig. 8. Retinoblastoma: R = rosette formations; N = necrosis; C = calcifications (O. 904-9, original magnification × 75, neg. 27991-7).

themselves, but by the interfaces between necrotic tumour tissue and the surface of cylindric coats of viable tumour cells around the newly formed — and, therefore, small — tumour vessels (Fig. 9).

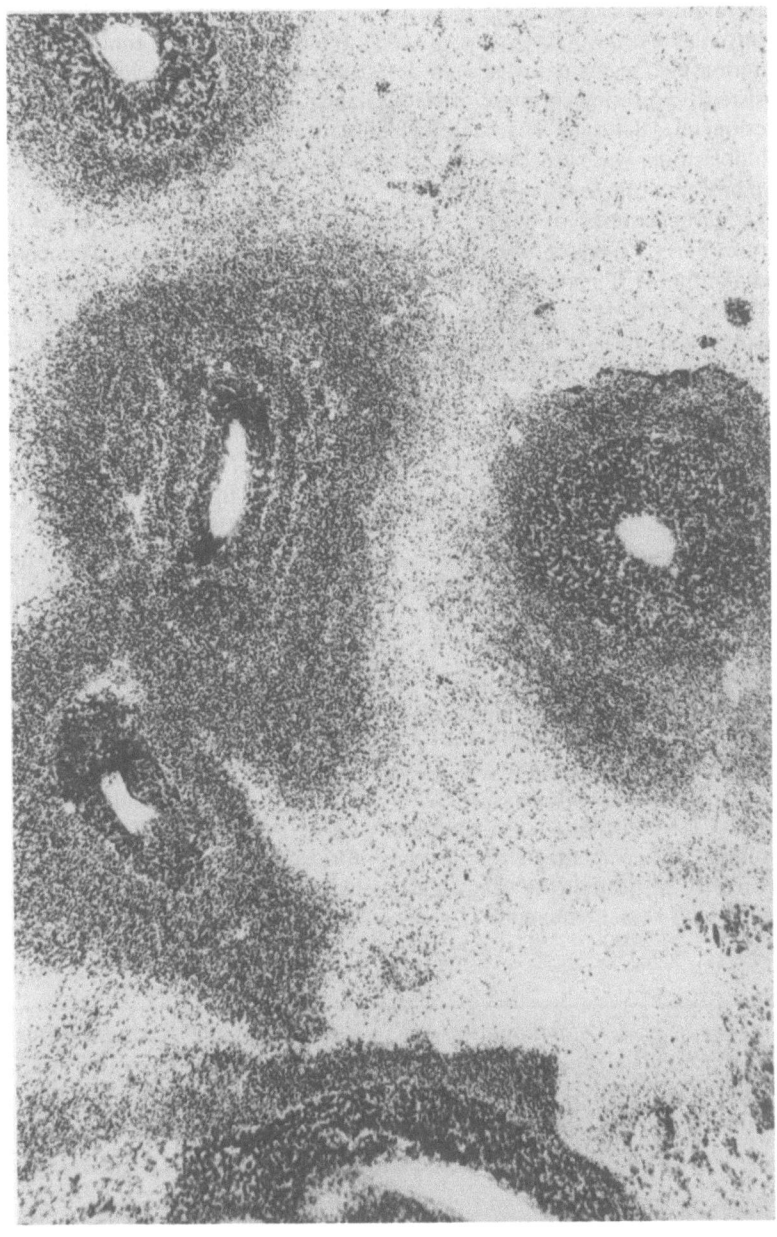

Fig. 9. Retinoblastoma: coats of viable tumour cells around newly-formed vessels (O. 1685-10, original magnification × 16, neg. 27991-10).

It is probable that the high reflectivity of retinoblastomas does not occur in small tumours, which often do not show necrosis and calcifications. Also, rosette formation is not present in all retinoblastomas. For these reasons, ultrasonographic differential diagnosis of a small tumour-like lesion in an infant's eye might cause more difficulties than is suggested in literature. In our files we have specimens of small tumours or pseudo-tumours in the posterior eye segment in children as astrocytic hamartoma, hyperplasia of persistent posterior primary vitreous and granulomatous inflammatory reaction on a larva of Toxa cara, which all have been enucleated because a retinoblastoma was suspected. I am not sure whether ultrasonography would have prevented these enucleations.

Uveal melanomas, of course, constitute the most important subject of this lecture. Ferry (1964) reported that 10% of the enucleated eyes with opaque media in the AFIP material contained a clinically unsuspected melanoma.

Ossoinig (1974) found that 3% of their uveal melanomas had been first detected and diagnosed by echography. This seems a small percentage, but echography might have been life-saving in these patients. Ultrasonography is also important for localizing a tumour for isotope studies. Fuller *et al.* (1979) recently stated that isotope studies for choroidal melanomas have few indications and that they had all but abandoned it. In my opinion, we are obliged to use any possible diagnostic tool in the life-threatening field of uveal melanomas. Shields (1977), although admitting that most uveal melanomas can be easily diagnosed, subjects all patients suspected to have a uveal melanoma to a twelve-step diagnostic procedure – including the P32 uptake test – prior to enucleation. His results are that less than 2% of the eyes which had been removed because of the clinical diagnosis of uveal melanoma did not contain this tumour. On the contrary, the most recent AFIP statistics indicate a false positive melanoma diagnosis of about 20%. The latter material is largely contributed by small ophthalmological centres and individual ophthalmologists who are often not in a position to use all modern diagnostic equipments. In our laboratory, where about half of the material is contributed by ophthalmologists working in smaller general hospitals, the percentage of clinically unsuspected (underdiagnosed) and incorrectly suspected (overdiagnosed) melanomas before and after September 1 1975 have been compared:

	Total number melanomas	Underdiagnosed	Overdiagnosed
Before 1.9.75	213	19 (8.9%)	14 (6.7%)
After 1.9.75	98	10 (10.2%)	3 (3.4%)

A percentage of 10% unsuspected melanomas proves that ultrasonography is still insufficiently used in this country; especially in those cases where a painful blind eye has to be removed. This is unfortunate, because these eyes are often enucleated by inexperienced residents, while surgery on eyes harbouring a melanoma should be performed by an experienced surgeon. On the other hand, the decrease of almost 50% of incorrectly suspected melamonas indicates that modern diagnostic equipments are sufficiently used in patients where the possibility of a melanoma is considered.

It is to be stressed that choroidal melanomas may have any shape, extension and surface. Never generalize on melanomas, except for the fact that they are the most treacherous and life-threatening eye lesion. Not only in adult patients; a choroidal melanoma in a child aged two years has been reported by Scheffer *et al.* (1974). An apparently small, flat melanoma of no more than 1 mm prominence was demonstrated that had been correctly diagnosed by echography. An extensive, clinically undetectable intrachoroidal extension was found microscopically. Another, still more treacherous feature of this melanoma was formed by an intra- and extrascleral extension. This melanoma met all clinical requirements for photocoagulation; this objectionable therapy, however, would never have eliminated the extrascleral extension and would have caused the patient's death.

Also, a prominent melanoma with a clinically undetectable intrachoroidal extension of more than 10 mm was demonstrated. The visible prominent part of a choroidal melanoma often is the tip of the iceberg only; its diameter at the base, as well as its possible intra- and extrascleral extensions can not be diagnosed clinically.

A case of an equatorial melanoma in the right half of the eye was demonstrated, in which the left half of the eye harboured intraretinal and subretinal metastases. Such intraocular metastases are rare, but they do occur, however, and constitute one more reason not to treat a choroidal melanoma otherwise than by enucleation of the eye.

Whether the melanoma is of the spindle cell type, the epitheloid cell type or the mixed cell type will, most probably, have no influence on the tissue echogram. More important is the presence of vessels within the tumour. Generally, vessels near the surface and in the periphery of the tumour are larger than those more centrally in the tumour. Most melanomas show little vascularization and their vessels are small. Sometimes, numerous small vessels are seen within the tumour. It is difficult to understand how these minute vessels can be responsible for the ultrasonographic phenomenon of spontaneous movements, also because these spontaneous movements are said not to be synchronic with the pulse. The low vascularity of most choroidal melanomas may constitute one of the reasons for their low to medium reflectivity. Another reason is the general finding that melanoma cells are densely packed without substantial intercellular connective tissue septa. A case was presented of a rather prominent choroidal melanoma with a possible acoustic interface at a sharp delineation of a heavily pigmented area within an otherwise almost unpigmented tumour. The unpigmented cells were smaller than the pigmented cells. The melanoma also showed so-called blood lakes within the pigmented part of the tumour. These blood lakes are frequently found in melanomas. Their lumen is not covered by endothelium and detaching melanoma cells can enter freely into the blood. These blood lakes will cause acoustic interfaces; it is not known whether there is a regular blood flow within them.

Necrosis is another etiology of acoustic interfaces. Necrosis is often found in large melanomas, but seldom in small ones. Melanomas grow slowly. The

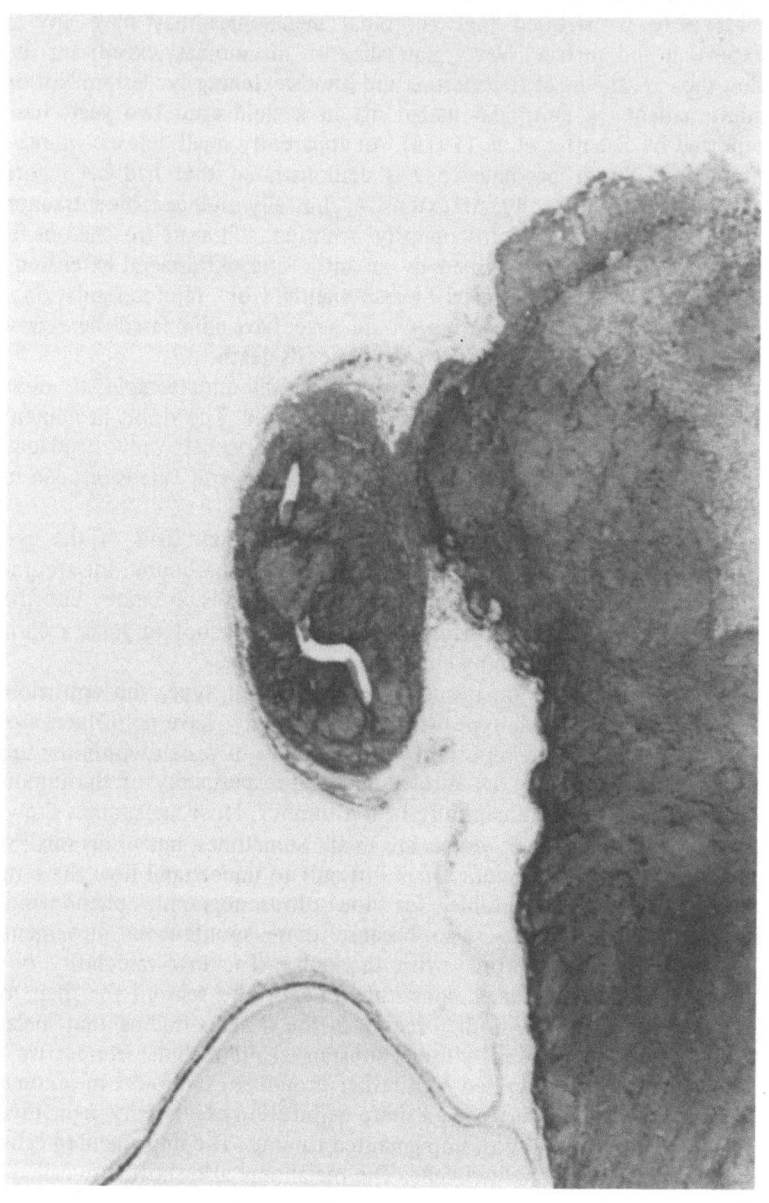

Fig. 10. Choroidal melanoma with irregular surface (O. 107-10, original magnification ×
8, neg. 27993-7).

occurrence of necrosis in melanomas cannot – as in retinoblastoma – be due
to the circumstance that the speed of tumour growth surpasses the growth
of its vessels. A distinct enlargement of a fundus lesion suspect for

melanoma within a short time forms a strong argument against this diagnosis. Only a haemorrhage within a necrotic melanoma can cause a rather sudden enlargement. However, small melanomas, the only ones liable of causing diagnostic difficulties, will seldom or never be necrotic. The occurence of acoustic interfaces in necrotic melanomas probably depends on the formation of tissue defects within the necrotic tissue and on the interfaces between necrotic and viable tissue within the tumour.

Pictures of two melanoma containing eyes with many abnormal large acoustic interfaces were demonstrated. The clinical history of the first eye revealed that the melanoma probably had been present for 36 years. This phthisic eye showed an extensive intraocular ossification. It is likely that a spontaneous regression of the tumour had occurred. Such a spontaneous regression had certainly occurred in the melanoma of the second eye; fibrous scar tissue and calcerous deposits had developed within the remnants of the tumour.

Even the surface of melanomas may refute the generalization that they are always smooth. When the retina has been infiltrated or perforated by the tumour, the latter may show an irregular surface and may protrude into the vitreous. (Fig. 10).

One more echographic feature needs to be discussed, viz. *choroidal excavation.* Coleman (1974) wrote: 'The acoustic quiet zone in the interior of a choroidal tumour on B-scan gives the appearance of an excavation in the posterior walls of the globe. The area of the tumour that has replaced the surrounding choroid is thereby demonstrated.' When I understand this quotation correct, it means that a choroidal excavation is due to both sound absorption and to a difference in reflectivity between melanoma tissue and normal choroidal tissue. The question arises why all choroidal excavations reproduced in the literature are localized centrally behind the prominent part of the melanoma, and never sideward from this prominence. It has already been said that the visible prominent part of a choroidal melanoma often is the tip of the iceberg only and that the base of the tumour not seldom infiltrates the choroid over a large distance. When the answer should be that the central location of the choroidal excavation is largely due to sound absorption which cannot occur in the peripheral intrachoroidal part of the melanoma, then the question arises why flat choroidal nevi can cause choroidal excavations, as has recently been reported by Fuller *et al.* (1979).

Finally, the differential diagnostic potential of ultrasonography between choroidal melanoma and disciform macular degeneration was discussed. Coleman *et al.* (1974) wrote on the subject of macular degeneration that these hemorrhagic lesions in the first stage show low amplitude internal echoes on A-scan. The fibrosed stage of disciform macular degeneration will also show a low reflectivity, which makes a differential diagnosis with melanomas difficult.

SUMMARY

The significance of some of the histopathological characteristics of intra-ocular tumours for ultrasonographic interpretation was demonstrated. There is a danger of generalization of echographic findings: in a given intraocular tumour, differential diagnosis by means of echography may often be a risky procedure.

REFERENCES

Bloch, R.S. & Gartner, S. The incidence of ocular metastatic carcinoma. A.M.A. Arch. Ophthalmol. 85: 673 (1971).

Coleman, D.J., Abramson, D.H., Jack, L.J. & Franzen, A. Ultrasonic diagnosis of tumours of the choroid. A.M.A. Arch. Ophthalmol 91: 344 (1974).

Ferry, A.P. Lesions mistaken for malignant melanoma of the posterior uvea: a clinico-pathologic analysis of 100 cases with ophthalmoscopically visible lesions. A.M.A. Arch. Ophthalmol. 72: 463 (1964).

Fuller, D.G., Snyder, W.B., Hutton, W.L. & Vaiser, A. Ultrasonographic features of choroidal malignant melanomas. A.M.A. Arch. Ophthalmol. 97: 1465 (1979).

Naumann, G.O.H. Pathologie des Auges. Berlin: Springer Verlag (1980) p. 626.

Naumann, G.O.H. & Portwich, E. Ätiologie und letzter Anlass zu 1000 Enukleationen. Klin. Mbl. Augenheilk. 168: 622 (1976).

Ossoinig, K.C. Physical principles and morphologic background of tissue echograms. In: Current concepts in ophalmology (F.C. Blodi, ed). St. Louis, Missouri: Mosby (1974) p. 264.

Ossoinig, K.C. & Blodi, F.C. Diagnosis of intraocular tumours. In: Current concepts in ophthalmology (F.C. Blodi, ed.) St. Louis, Missouri: Mosby (1974) p. 296.

Scheffer, C.H., Binkhorst, P.G. & Hamburg, A. Malignant melanoma of the choroid in a 2-year-old infant, Ophthalmologica 169: 401 (1974).

Shields, J.A. Current approaches to the diagnosis and management of choroidal melanomas. Surv. Ophthalmol. 21: 443 (1977).

Author's Address:
W.A. Manschot, Ph.D.
Institute of Pathology
Erasmus University
P.O. Box 1738
3000 DR Rotterdam
The Netherlands

THE ROLE OF ULTRASOUND IN THE INVESTIGATION AND MANAGEMENT OF SUSPECTED OCULAR MELANOMA

M. LEMAY, S.T.D. ROXBURGH & W.R. LEE

(Glasgow, United Kingdom)

The ultrasonic appearances of malignant melanoma of the uveal tract have been described (Baum 1967, Chang *et al.* 1978, Coleman 1972, 1973, Coleman & Jack 1972, Coleman *et al.* 1974, Hodes & Chromokos 1977).

In Glasgow Western Infirmary ultrasonography has been used for the past six years as part of a detailed assessment of all patients presenting with suspected ocular melanoma. The examination of a patient with an intraocular mass includes binocular indirect ophthalmoscopy, fluorescein angiography and radioactive phosphorus (^{32}P) test (Moseley & Foulds 1980).

The accuracy of ultrasound in the diagnosis of ocular melanoma has been the subject of a previous report (Roxburgh & LeMay 1980). The review of all patients presenting to the ultrasonography clinic has led to a further study of all cases of ocular melanoma submitted to pathology in a similar period. The value of ultrasound in the pre-operative assessment of those tumours suitable for local excision is under review.

MATERIALS AND METHODS

Ultrasonic examination includes A and B-scanning with the 'Coleman' Sonometrics 100 Ophthalmoscan using the water bath technique (Coleman *et al.* 1969).

Retrospective study has been performed on both the photographic records of the examination and on the written reports on the ultrasonic files. The assessment of the accuracy of a report was not by the author who had performed the scans.

The pathology files were also reviewed and the reports were compared with the ultrasonic results. The original sections of all cases presenting with extraocular extension were re-examined and the size of the extraocular extension was measured. If tumour was outwith the sclera it was classified as *macroscopic* (visible to the naked eye) or *microscopic* (not visible to the naked eye) and in practice there were no macroscopic tumours smaller than 1 mm.

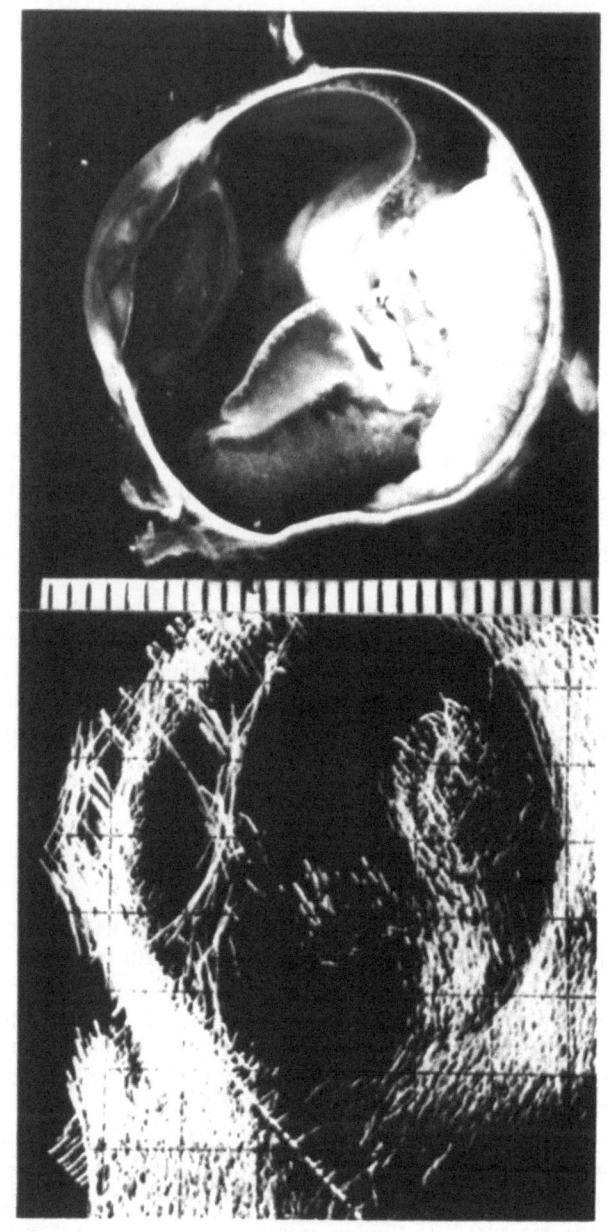

Fig. 1. Ultrasound (left) and excision (right) of a case of metastatic cervical carcinoma. The ultrasound was erroneously thought to be a melanoma.

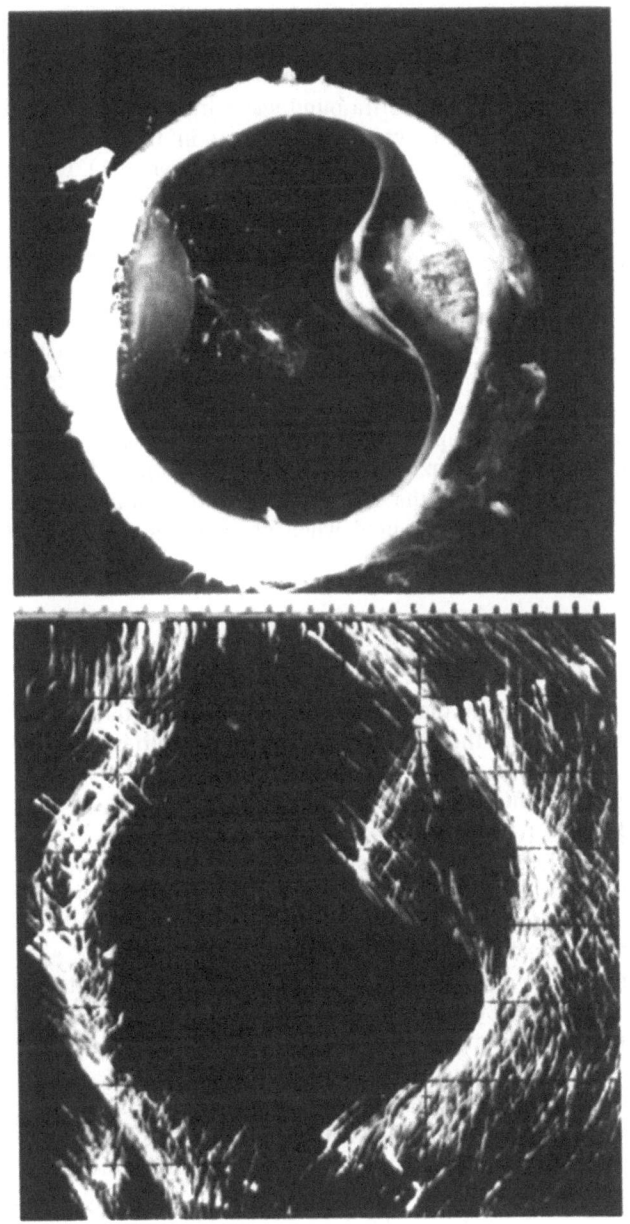

Fig. 2. Ultrasound (left) and excision (right). An ocular melanoma with an overlying disciform response. The separation in the right hand illustration is artefactual.

RESULTS

In a five year period there were 175 patients with suspected ocular melanoma. After all investigations 88 (50.3%) were considered to have an ocular melanoma and 78 patients in this group had a surgical excision performed, the remaining ten had alternative treatment. Seventy-five excised eyes (96.2%) contained melanoma and of the three remaining the ultrasound was only incorrect in one (Fig. 1). Ultrasound was correct in 70 of the 75 eyes containing melanoma (93%), was unsatisfactory in four and erroneously diagnosed only one tumour as a disciform lesion (Diagram 1). One eye contained tumour covered by a disciform lesion (Fig. 2) and this was diagnosed as a melanoma on ultrasound.

There was a high success rate for the pre-operative diagnosis of extraocular extension of tumour when extensions were greater than 1 mm. in diameter and a reasonable degree of success was achieved even in the diagnosis of microscopic extensions. When small anterior extensions were excluded from the survey, 11 out of a total of 13 cases (85%) of extraocular extension were diagnosed by echography.

Ophthalmic ultrasonography has also been used to assess a total of 26 patients who had a local excision of tumour performed (Foulds 1973). Ultrasound was of value in the measurement and accurate siting of such tumours. This information was used when deciding on the suitability of a patient for this type of surgery.

CONCLUSION

The experience gained in the examination of almost 200 cases of ocular melanoma has enabled the reasons for referral for ultrasonography to be classified as follows:

(1) Diagnosis of melanoma.
(2) Assessment of extraocular extension.
(3) Assessment of size and site before local excision.

Early diagnosis depends on the use of ultrasound as part of detailed programme of assessment. This must include binocular indirect ophthalmoscope, fluorescein angiography and ^{32}P uptake.

The management of melanoma is the subject of a current controversy (Zimmerman et al. 1978, 1980, Manschot & Van Peperzeel 1980) with regard to enucleation or observation, but whatever the management, early diagnosis is desirable.

The role of extraocular extension is less controversial. Survival rates are poorer (Shammas & Blodi 1977); exenteration as a primary procedure may affect the prognosis and ultrasound is currently the only practicable method of assessing extension before surgery although detection is theoretically possible with computed tomography.

Local excision of tumour is now technically possible and does not apparently affect the prognosis for life adversely (Foulds 1980). Although the excision of the tumour is excised under direct vision at the time of surgery,

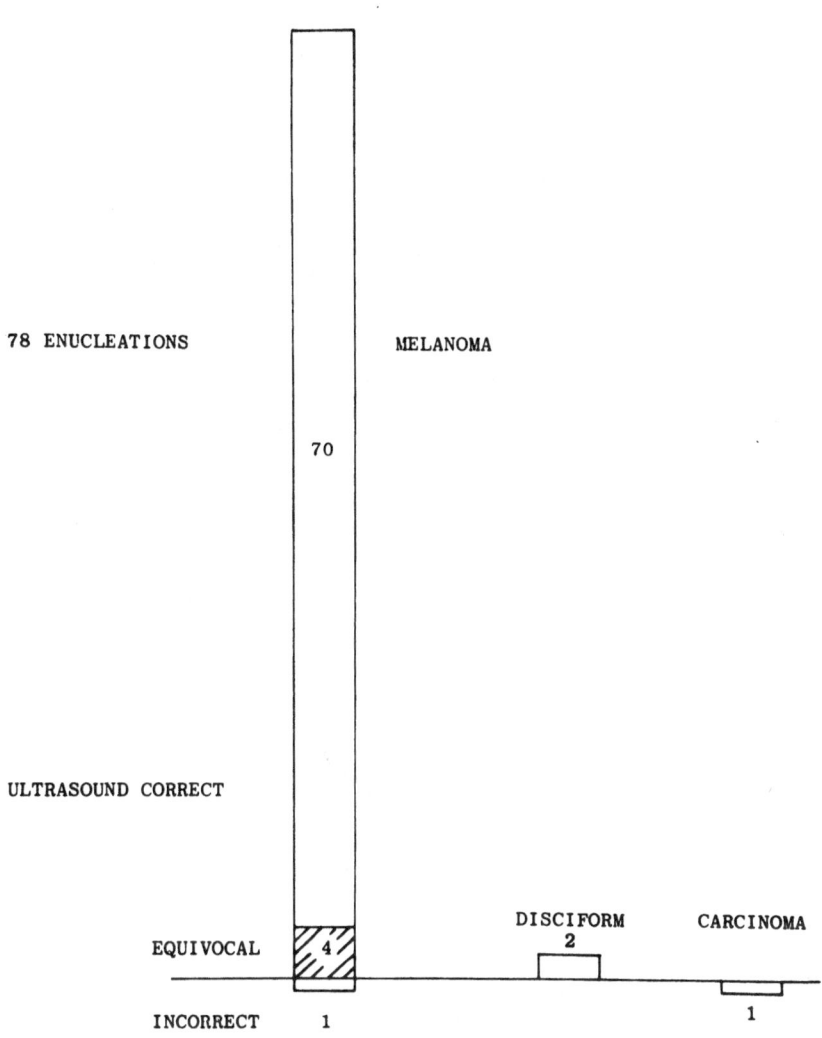

Diagram 1. Bar diagram summarising the ultrasonic and pathological diagnosis in 78 excised eyes.

the decision to undertake this type of surgery and the technique in the initial stages of the operation are dependent on pre-operative ultrasonic assessment. Char *et al.* (1980) suggest that there is a good correlation between the ultrasonic and pathological size of tumours if shrinkage artefact due to fixation is considered.

ACKNOWLEDGEMENTS

The authors express their thanks to Mrs. Anne Currie for the illustrations and to Miss Olive M. Rankin who typed the manuscript.

REFERENCES

Baum, G. Ultrasonographic characteristics of malignant melanoma. Arch. Ophthalmo. 78: 12 (1967).

Chang, S., Dallon, R., Coleman, D.J. Ultrasonic evaluation of intraocular tumours. In: (Jakobiec F.A., ed.) Ocular and Adnexal Tumours P. 281 Birmingham Ala., U.S.A.: Aesculapius Publishing Co.

Char, D.H., Stone, R.D., Ruine, A.R., Crawford, J.B., Milton, G.F., Lonn, L.I. & Schwartz, A. Diagnostic modalities in choroidal melanoma. Am. J. Ophthalmol. 89: 223 (1980).

Coleman, D.J. Reliability of ocular and orbital diagnosis with B-scan ultrasound 1) ocular diagnosis. Am. J. Ophthalmol. 74: 501 (1972).

Coleman, D.J. Reliability of ocular tumour diagnosis with ultrasound. Trans. Am. Acad. Ophthalmol. Otolaryngol. 77: 677 (1973).

Coleman, D.J., Abramson, D.H., Jack, R.L. & Franzen, L.A. Ultrasonic diagnosis of tumours of the choroid. Arch. Ophthalmol. 91: 344 (1974).

Coleman, D.J., Konig, W.F. & Katz, L. A hand operated ultrasound scan system for ophthalmic evaluation. Am. J. Ophthalmol. 68: 256 (1969).

Foulds, W.S. The local excision of choroidal melanomata. Trans. of Ophthalmological Soc. U.K. 93: 343 (1973).

Foulds, W.S. Personal Communication (1980).

Fuller, D.G., Snyder, W.B., Multon, W.L. & Vaiser, A. Ultrasonographic features of choroidal and malignant melanomas. Arch. Ophthalmol. 97: 1465 (1979).

Hodes, B.L. & Choromokos, E. Standardised A-scan echographic diagnosis of choroidal malignant melanomas. Arch. Ophthalmol. 95: 593 (1977).

Jack, R.L. & Coleman, D.J. Detection of retinal detachments secondary to choroidal melanomas with B-scan ultrasound. Am. J. Ophthalmol. 74: 1057 (1972).

Manschot, W.A. & Van Peperzeel, H.A. Choroidal melanoma: Enucleation or observation? A new approach. Arch. Ophthalmol. 98: 71 (1980).

Moseley, H. & Foulds, W.S. Observations on the ^{32}P uptake test. Brit. J. Ophthalmol. 64: 186 (1980).

Roxburgh, S.T.D. & Lemay, M. Ultrasonic investigation of malignant melanoma. Proc. of the VI Cong. Europ. Soc. of Ophthalmol. (in press) (1980).

Shammas, H.F. & Blodi, F. Orbital extension of choroidal and ciliary body melanomas. Arch. Ophthalmol. 95: 2002 (1977).

Zimmerman, L.E., McLean, I.W. & Foster, W.D. Does enucleation of the eye containing melanoma prevent or accelerate the dissemination of tumour cells? Brit. J. Ophthalmol. 62: 420 (1978).

Zimmerman, L.E., McLean, I.W. & Foster, W.D. Statistical analysis of follow-up data concerning uveal melanomas and the influence of enucleation. Ophthalmology 87: 557 (1980).

Authors' Address:
Dept. of Ophthalmology
Glasgow Western Infirmary
Glasgow, United Kingdom

DIFFERENTIAL DIAGNOSTIC RESULTS OF CLINICAL ECHOGRAPHY IN INTRAOCULAR TUMORS

P. TILL & W. HAUFF

(*Vienna, Austria*)

Since 1963 the echographic department of 2nd University-Eye Clinic in Vienna performed more than 9000 echographic examinations of the globe. Five hundred ninety-three intraocular tumors were diagnosed and differentiated with standardized echography. The results of the years 1963–1973 are published (Till & Ossoinig 1975). In this study we are reporting the results of the years 1973–1980.

METHOD

Acoustic differential diagnosis is based on the specific design of the A-scan equipment. The first and, so far only standardized A-scan instrument, the 7200 MA unit (Kretztechnik) was used by four different examiners of our laboratory. Structure, reflectivity, consistency, vascularity, exact measurements of prominence and growth of intraocular lesions were determined with this standardized A-scan unit and with the help of the standardized examination techniques (Ossoinig). A contact B-scan unit (Bronson-Turner) demonstrated the location, shape and lateral extension of a lesion.

RESULTS

Since 1973 we performed 4924 echographic examinations of the globe, nearly 30% because of the suspicion of an intraocular tumor. 301 intraocular tumors were differentiated with standardized A-scan Echography. Two hundred eight-three tumors are verified histologically or by means of follow up examinations. Two hundred-seventy-seven echographic diagnoses were correct and six incorrect. Table 1 demonstrates the results of echographic differential diagnoses. In our series 125 malignant melanomas were correct and three incorrect false positive; these identical three false positive cases were not detected as malignant melanomas and indicate on the table as false negative cases the true nature of these tumors (two metastatic carcinomas of the choroid and one vortex vein): Two false positive echographic diagnoses of malignant melanomas were verified histologically after enucleation as metastatic carcinomas of the choroid. One false positive case was verified

Table 1. Results of echographic differential diagnoses of intraocular tumors (1973–1980).

Echographic diagnoses Total	unverified	verified correct	verified incorrect false +	incorrect false −
142 malignant melanoma	14	125	2▲ + 1△	1●
3 choroidal hemangioma	2	0	1▲	1●
14 retinoblastoma	2	12	0	0
2 astrocytoma	0	2	0	0
112 disciforme degen.	0	110	2●	0
23 metastat.carcinoma	0	23	0	3▲
5 Coats' disease	0	5	0	0
301	18	277	6	1△(Vo)

Vo: Vortex vein of circumscribed choroidal detachment.

clinically during follow up examinations as vortex vein in a circumscribed area of choroidal detachment. This failure was caused by the fact, that only single differential diagnostic criteria were considered by the examiner; the fast spontaneous movements of low echos in this circumscribed area of choroidal detachment were interpreted as vascularization of a tumor. The one false negative case of malignant melanomas stems from one of the two false positive cases of disciforme macula degeneration; histologically this tumor was verified as cystic malignant melanoma (Till 1979). Table 2 demonstrates the histologic diagnoses of the false positive echographic tumor diagnoses.

Malignant melanomas of the choroid and ciliary body can be detected reliably, provided their prominence is at least 0.75 mm in the choroid and 1.5 mm in the ciliary body. Melanomas can be differentiated from all other

Table 2. Histologic diagnoses of the six false positive echographic tumor diagnoses.

Echographic diagnoses	false +	histologic diagnoses
malignant melanoma	3	metastatic carcinoma
		metastatic carcinoma
		vortex vein (clinical diagnosis)
choroidal hemangioma	1	metastatic carcinoma
disciforme degeneration	2	malignant melanoma
		choroidal hemangioma

Fig. 1. A-scan echograms from various choroidal tumors obtained with 7200 MA (Kretztechnik) at tissue sensitivity:
(A) normal retino-choroidal layer.
(B) malignant melanoma of the choroid.
(C) choroidal hemangioma.
(D) metastatic carcinoma of the choroid with detachment of the retina.
(E) disciforme degeneration of the macula
(F) Coats' disease (typical spontaneous movements of cholesterol crystals in the sub-retinal fluid).
(G) subchoroidal hemorrhage and vitreous hemorrhage.

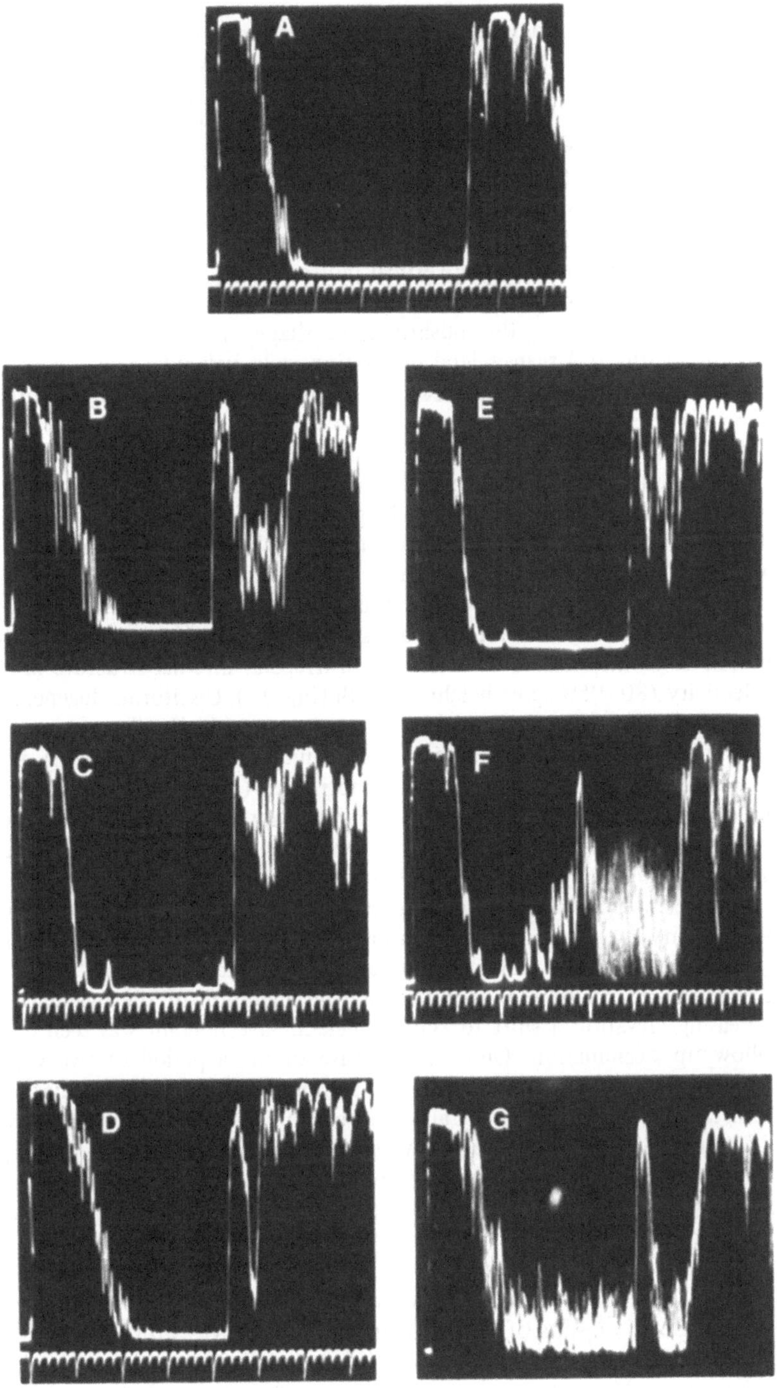

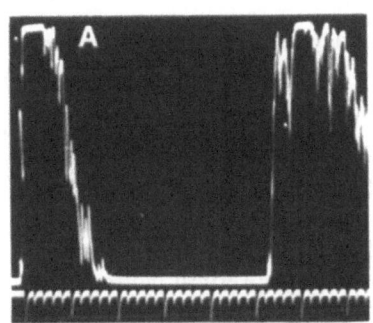

lesions with an accuracy of 97% if their elevation from the inner sclera surface is at least 1.5 mm (choroid) or 3 mm (ciliary body). The acoustic hallmarks of a malignant melanoma are: (1) a regular internal structure (the inner tumor spikes show a similar height or regular decrease in height from left to right); (2) low to medium reflectivity (the height of the inner tumor spikes is 5–60% of display height); (3) a solid consistency with no after-movement of tumor spikes; (4) vascularization (more than 90% of malignant melanomas show the echographic sign of vascularization – a fast, spon-taneous, continuous, flickering vertical motion of single tumor spikes). These four cardinal signs are A-scan criteria, but B-scan is occasionally very helpful in documenting the mushroomlike shape of some of these tumors. With standardized A-scan, scleral infiltration and small extraocular extension can be detected; with both A-scan and B-scan methods, massive orbital involvement can be demonstrated.

Fig. 1b shows the A-scan echogram of a malignant melanoma; in contrast to malignant melanomas, hemangiomas of the choroid display very high reflectivity (95–100% of display height) as can be seen in Fig. 1c. A histologic section explains the high reflectivity because of the blood filled endothelium lined spaces; malignant melanomas consist histologically of single cells and cell groups without large acoustic interfaces, accordingly reflectivity is low to medium. In contrast to malignant melanomas, carcinomas metastatic to the choroid demonstrate an irregular internal structure or high reflectivity (80–95% spike height) or both (Fig. 1d). Disciforme degeneration of the macula produces two or three narrowly spaced high spikes representing the surfaces of the retina, pigment epithelium and choroid (Fig. 1e). While Coats' disease or fresh choroidal hemorrhages (Fig. 1f, g) may have an internal structure and reflectivity similar to that of malignant melanomas, these conditions are showing aftermovements following small eye movements and that should not be confused with a solid tumor.

In cases with borderline acoustic criteria careful follow up examinations often clarify the situation by indicating the growth. In our series four times a malignant melanoma developed under the echographic signs of 'membrane like' lesion as can be seen in disciforme degeneration of the macula. With increasing elevation a shift to typical melanoma echogram was seen during follow up examination. Only in one case during a period of five years a membrane like lesion was found to be stationary; this tumor was diagnosed as disciforme degeneration (paramacular choroidal edema). After the 84 year old patient died from uremia following an attack of acute pyelonephritis, his eyes were examined histologically and the choroidal lesion was proven to be a cystic malignant melanoma (see Table 1 – false negative case of malignant melanomas).

In cases of disciforme degeneration of the macula a regression of the lesion is often seen during follow up examinations. Table 3 demonstrates the echographic results of malignant melanomas in eyes with opaque media; all 15 cases are histologically verified as malignant melanomas. These malignant melanomas of the choroid were detected and diagnosed with echography although not even suspected with clinical examinations. Dense cataracts, maximal miosis, vitreous hemorrhages or dense vitreous opacities

Table 3. Echographic differential diagnoses of malignant melanomas of the choroid in eyes with opaque media (10%).

Echography	total	histologically verified correct	incorrect
mal.melanoma	15	15	0

were the main reasons that these tumors remained undetected with ophthamoscopy and slit lamp examination. The clinical diagnoses in such cases were 'posttraumatic uveitis', 'angle closure glaucoma', 'intumescent cataract with secundary glaucoma'. In these cases echography applied as a routine examination was absolutely necessary for correct diagnosis.

REFERENCES

Ossoinig, K.C. Standardized Echography: Basic Principles, Clinical Applications, and Results. In: Ophthalmic Ultrasonography: Comparative Techniques (R.L. Dallow, ed.) Int. Ophthalmol. Clinics 19 (4), Boston Little, Brown & Co. (1979) p. 127.

Ossoinig, K.C. Preoperative Differential Diagnosis of Tumors with Echography: III. Diagnosis of Intraocular Tumors. In: Current Concepts in Ophthalmology 4, (F.C. Blodi, ed.), St. Louis: Mosby (1974) p. 296.

Till, P. & Ossoinig, K.C. Ten-year study on clinical echography in intraocular disease. Bibl. Ophthalmol. 83: 49 (1975).

Till, P. Echography in intraocular tumors. In: Diagnostica Ultrasonica in Ophthalmologia (H. Gernet, ed.) Münster: R.A. Remy-Verlag, (1979).

Authors' Address:
II. Univ.-Augenklinik
Alserstrasse 4
A-1090 Wien

ABSOLUTE ABSORPTION AND REFLECTANCE CONSTANTS OF OCULAR TISSUE

D.J. COLEMAN & F.L. LIZZI
(New York, U.S.A.)

ABSTRACT

The constants for acoustic absorption for a series of patients with malignant melanoma, metastatic carcinoma, choroidal hemangioma, and organized subretinal hemorrhage have been determined through the use of power spectrum analysis. These values, combined with conventional A- and B-scan display dynamics have provided a distinction among these tumor types.

Improved display detail allows us to deduce the sources of internal tumor reflections far more reliably than previously possible. For example, the vascular channel dimensions of a tumor can be determined and quantified. The absorption components can be determined for specific and sequential areas of the tumor, as well as the averaged absorption constants for total tumor volume.

The quantifiable values obtained by this computer analysis technique provides an improved dimension of confidence to tumor diagnosis.

Authors' Addresses:

Dr. D.J. Coleman
The New York Hospital-Cornell Medical Center
New York

Dr. F.L. Lizzi
Riverside Research Institute
New York

A-MODE ULTRASONOGRAPHY IN CASES OF LEUKOKORIA

A. BERTÉNYI & M. FODOR

(*Budapest, Hungary*)

The white pupillary reflex called leukokoria can be caused by different diseases. Our foremost task is if leukokoria is present — to rule out, or demonstrate the presence of retinoblastoma. Since leukokoric eyes cannot be optically examined, echo-ophthalmography is the only method we can use for diagnosing it. (Isotope examination is generally contraindicated in the diagnostics of children).

Neither Kogan & Boniuk (1962) nor Howard & Ellsworth (1965) mentioned ultrasonography in their publications on leukokoria. According to Kogan & Boniuk (1962) 30% of the eyes enucleated because of suspected retinoblastoma proved to be only pseudogliomatic. Howard & Ellsworth (1965) did not find a tumour in 50% of the suspected eyes. Since echo-ophthalmography was introduced (Mundt & Hughes 1956) the rate of unnecessary enucleations has significantly decreased and there have been many papers dealing with the problem of leukokoria (Buschmann 1966, Gitter, *et al.* 1968, Oksala 1971, Ossoinig 1972, Hamard, *et al.* 1973, Kaneko 1975, Till & Ossoinig 1975, Fridman, *et al.* 1977, Kaneko, *et al.* 1978, Bertényi, *et al.* 1980).

METHOD AND MATERIAL

Our examinations were carried out with the A-mode equipment Kretztechnik type 7000, calibrated by the test reflector from HEMA soft corneal lens material (Buschmann, *et al.* 1977). The working frequency was mostly 8 MHz. Sometimes, however, we also had to work with 6 and 10 MHz.

Local anaesthesia was used, but small children were usually examined through the eyelids. We applied narcosis only in exceptional cases — when it was necessary for other examination, or operation.

We measured the axial length of the globe in every case of leukokoria because it is known that eyes with retinoblastoma are usually not smaller than normal eyes (Till & Ossoinig 1975). In cases of retrolental fibroplasia (RLF) we repeated the measurements several times because we found that the growth of the globe is of prognostical importance in this disease (Bertényi, *et al.* 1980).

Echo-ophthalmography was performed in 126 eyes of 91 children younger than 14 years. Table 1 shows the diseases causing leukokoria and the number of cases in our material.

Table 1.

Diagnosis	Leukokoria Children	Eyes
RLF	31	62
Uveitis	19	20
Cataract	10	10
Pseudoglioma	10	10
Retinoblastoma	6	8
Coats' disease	5	5
A. hyal. persist.	3	4
PHPV	4	4
Retinitis prolif.	3	3
All	91	126

RESULTS

RLF was found in 62 eyes of 31 premature babies. From among the remaining 64 leukokoric eyes (60 children) massive tissue was found in 11 cases. (Table 2) Histology proved retinoblastoma in eight and Coats' disease in two eyes. One case could not be verified.

Table 2.

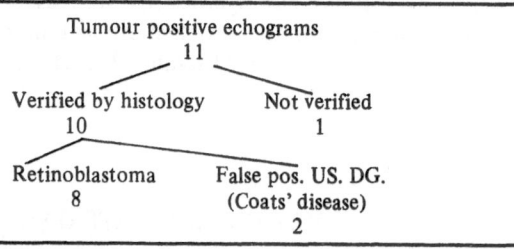

Tumour could be excluded echographically in 53 eyes (Table 3). Forty-one cases were proved tumour negative (four histologically, 37 clinically) and 12 could not be verified. We had no false negative ultrasound diagnosis in our leukokoria material.

Table 3.

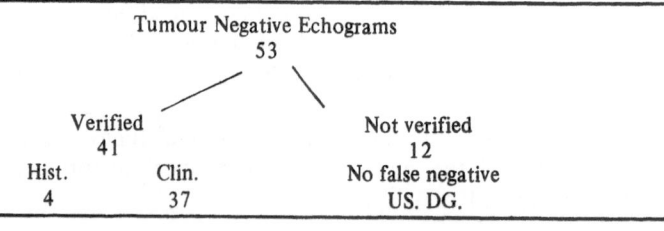

DISCUSSION

Differential diagnosis in cases of leukokoria is based upon the following echographical characteristics:

RLF (Fig. 1) usually occurs in both eyes of premature babies treated with oxygen. A dense white fibrous tissue is formed directly behind the lens reflecting relatively high echo peaks. The posterior part of the vitreous is acoustically clear except when the retina is detached. Microphthalmus was found in 54% of the RLF cases.

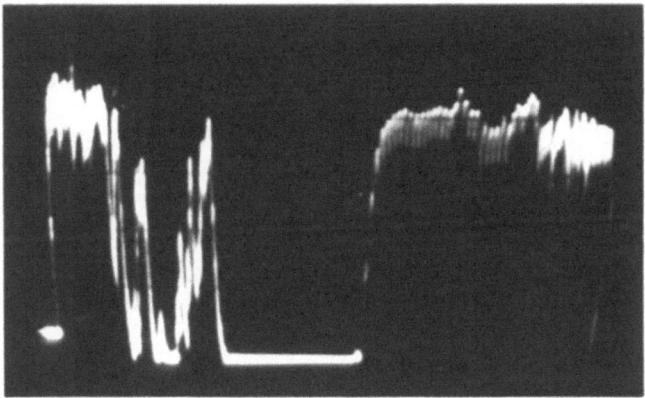

Fig. 1. Echogram of retrolental fibroplasia (RLF).

Uveitis: pathological echoes may arise from any part of the vitreous; however, their amplitude does not reach that of a tumour.

Cataract: the echogram is normal if no other disease is present.

Pseudoglioma is a collective term for white masses in the vitreous which are of different — mostly unknown — etiology (Fig. 2). Localisation and

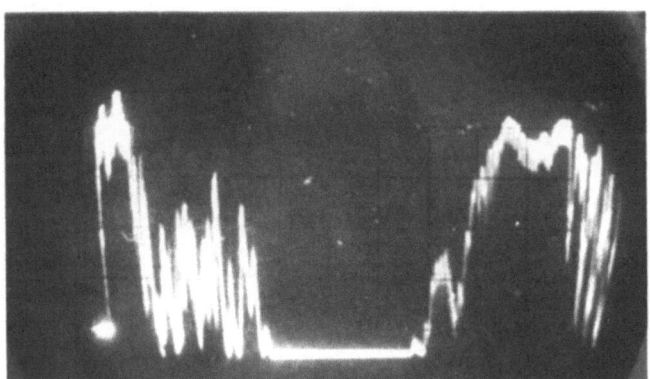

Fig. 2. Echogram of pseudoglioma.

amplitude of the pathological echoes can greatly vary but the sound attenuation is smaller than in retinoblastoma.

Retinoblastoma (Fig. 3) is discovered usually between the age of one and three. The echogram shows multiple echoes of high amplitudes which are connected with the scleral echo. The tumour has great attenuating effect. The axial length of the globe is normal or longer, microphthalmus is extremely rare.

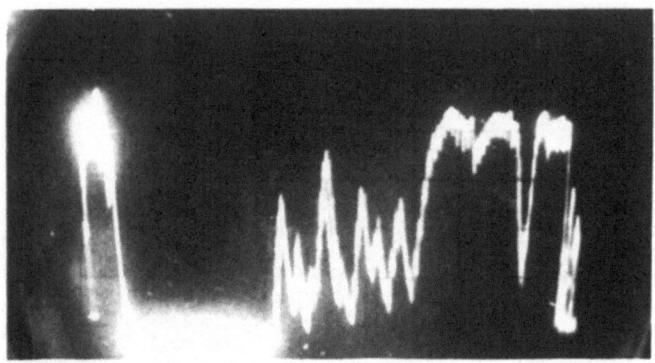

Fig. 3. Echogram of retinoblastoma.

Coats' disease (retinitis exudativa externa) (Fig. 4). Multiple echo peaks are reflected from the vitreous space and if reflectivity is high enough, it can be confused with a tumour. Both of our false positive diagnoses were proved histologically as Coats' disease.

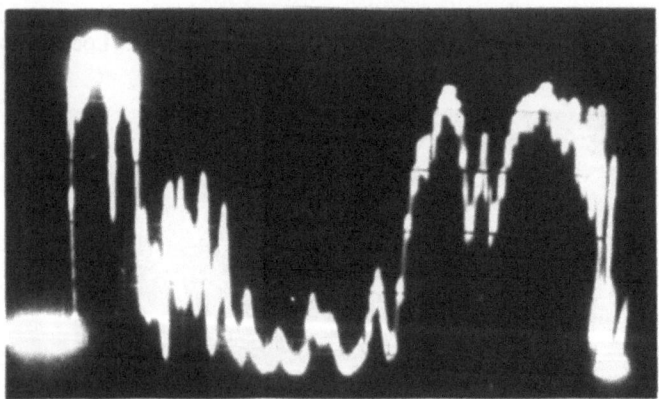

Fig. 4. Echogram of Coats' disease.

Arteria hyaloidea persistens (Fig. 5) in itself does not cause leukokoria but was incidently found in leukokoric eyes as well. There are no problems

100

involved in differentiating it from a tumour by means of the echogram since there is a sagittal fascicle in the vitreous.

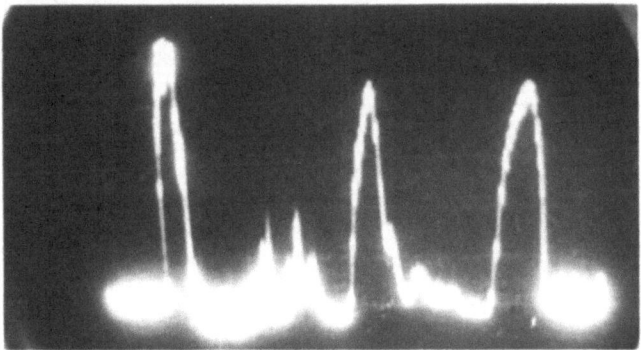

Fig. 5. Echogram of arteria hyaloidea persistens.

Persistent hyperplastic primary vitreous (Fig. 6) is a usually monocular congenital disorder. The echogram looks similar to that of RLF.

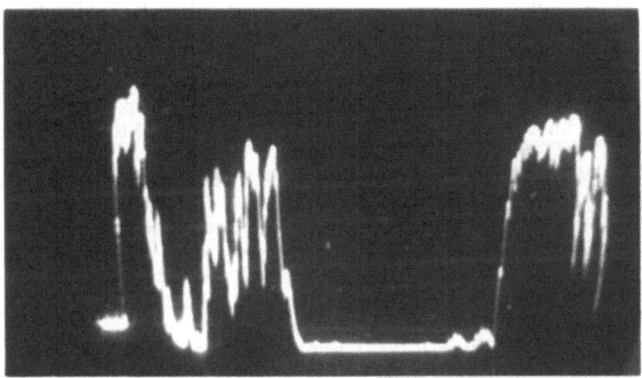

Fig. 6. Echogram of persistent hyperplastic primary vitreous (PHPV).

Retinitis proliferans (Fig. 7) may cause pathological echoes of medium or high amplitude. Differentiating it from a tumour by means of the echogram is not always easy.

Retinal detachment was proved in 23 leukokoria cases, eight of which in RLF.

SUMMARY

On the basis of literary data and our own experiences we can conclude that in order to demonstrate or exclude retinoblastoma echo-ophthalmography has

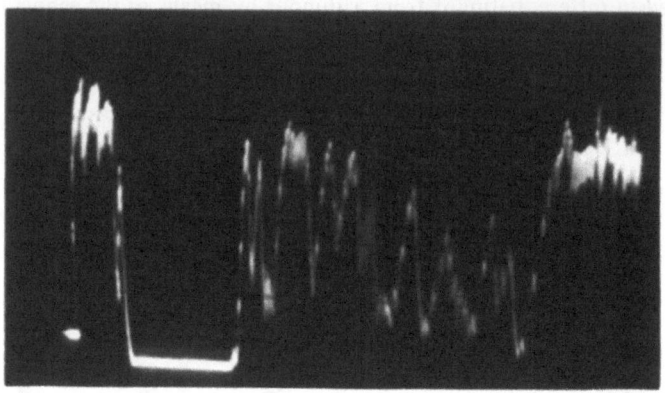

Fig. 7. Echogram of retinitis proliferans.

to be performed on every leukokoric eye. Ultrasonographically retino-blastoma can be differentiated with great certainty from other diseases causing leukokoria. In this way many unnecessary enucleations can be prevented.

REFERENCES

Bertényi, A., Véli, M. & Fodor, M. Ultrasound in Med. & Biol. 6: 19 (1980).

Buschmann, W. Einführung in die ophthalmologische Ultraschalldiagnostik, Leipzig: G. Thieme (1966).

Buschmann, W., Linnert, D. & Eysholdt, E. Ultrasound in Med. & Biol. Vol. 2 (3B) (D.N. White & R.E. Brown, eds.) New York: Plenum (1977) p. 1925.

Fridman, F.E., Khvatova, A.V., Timakova, V.J. & Sorokina, M.N. Vestn. Oftal. (Mosk.) 1: 65 (1977).

Gitter, A.K., Meyer, D., White, R.H., Ortolan, G. & Sarin, L.K. Am. J. Ophthalmol. 65: 190 (1968).

Hamard, H., Massin, M. & Poujol, J. Echographie de l'oeil et de l'orbite. Rapport annuel. Bull. Soc. Ophtal. Fr. suppl. (1973).

Howard, G.H. & Ellsworth, R.M. Am. J. Ophthalmol. 60: 610 (1965).

Kaneko, A. Ultrasonography in Ophthalmology (J. Francois & F. Goes, eds.) Bibl. Ophthalmol. No. 83. Basel, Karger (1975) p. 119.

Kaneko, A., Inone, H. & Hiroe, J. Jap. J. Clin. Ophthalmol. 32: 917 (1978).

Kogan, K. & Boniuk, M. Int. Clinics of Ophthalmol. 507 (1962).

Mundt, G.H. & Hughes, W.F. Am. J. Ophthalmol. 41: 488 (1956).

Oksala, A. Ultrasonographia Medica (J. Böck & K. Ossoinig eds.) Vol. II. Wien: Verl. d. Wiener Med. Akad. (1971) p. 209.

Ossoinig, K.C. Current Concepts in Ophthalmology (F.C.Blodi ed.) Vol. III. St. Louis: Mosby (1972) p. 101.

Scheie, H.G. & Albert, D.M. Textbook of Ophthalmology Philad., London, Toronto: W.B. Saunders (1977) p. 329.

Till, P. & Ossoinig, K.C. Ultrasonography in ophthalmology (J. Francois & F. Goes, eds) Bibl. Ophthalmol. No. 83. Basel: Karger (1975) p. 49.

Author's Address:

M. Fodor

2nd Eye Dept. of Semmelweis Medical School

Maria u. 39

Budapest, Hungary H-1085

ECHOGRAPHIC RESULTS IN THE DIAGNOSIS OF RETINOBLASTOMA

K.C. OSSOINIG, G. CENNAMO, R.L. GREEN & N.L. WEYER

(Iowa City, Iowa, U.S.A.)

With standardized echography, a combination of standardized A-scan and contact B-scan, more than 80 types of intraocular lesions, mostly of the posterior segment, can be detected and differentiated. Standardized A-scan is used in the basic examination to detect or rule out a lesion. If a lesion is found, special techniques, i.e., topographic echography, quantitative echography and kinetic echography, are applied to localize, measure and differentiate the lesion.

Some lesions of the posterior ocular segment frequently produce pathognomonic patterns. Retinoblastoma is one of them. In this presentation, two acoustic key criteria, which enable the diagnosis of retinoblastoma to be made, will be discussed, using one case of retinoblastoma as an example. And the results obtained with standardized echography in the evaluation of 35 consecutive cases of (unilateral or bilateral) retinoblastoma will be presented.

Both key criteria are quantitative in nature. One is *extremely high reflectivity* of at least a part of the tumor. This is caused by calcium deposits that are typical of retinoblastoma, and are assumed to originate from the many necrotic foci within the tumor. The calcium deposits are very small, but are multiple and closely spaced. At the standardized tissue sensitivity, they produce a chain of very high (overloaded) spikes in A-scans (Fig. 1). As illustrated in Fig. 2, the calcium-induced echoes in this case were so strong that one had to reduce system sensitivity to better show the individual calcium foci as single echo spikes. Correspondingly, one had to decrease system sensitivity in B-scan (Fig. 3) to show the calcium deposits as single echo spots, which persisted at lower system sensitivity due to their high echo intensities. The calcium deposits in retinoblastomas are also responsible for the second key criterion, *shadowing*. When the calcification is heavy, B-scan is the more impressive method in showing the dense shadows (Fig. 4). In the case used as an example, however, the shadowing was relatively weak, and one had to decrease system sensitivity to show it in the B-scan echograms (Fig. 3). In such cases, the A-scan method is more sensitive and clearly shows lower spikes from the orbital tissues behind the tumor (Figs. 1, 2). When evaluating relatively weak shadowing in B-scan echograms, one must be aware of lower-reflective structures, such as the optic nerve and the extraocular muscles, as well as artefacts caused by total reflection at the lateral wall, that may simulate shadowing. The A-scan method is more sensitive in clearly

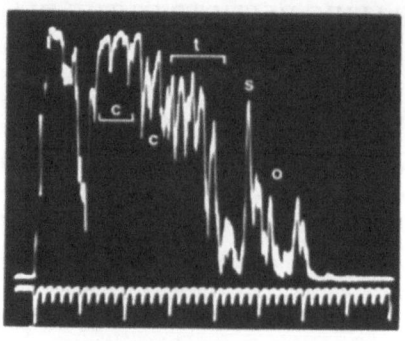

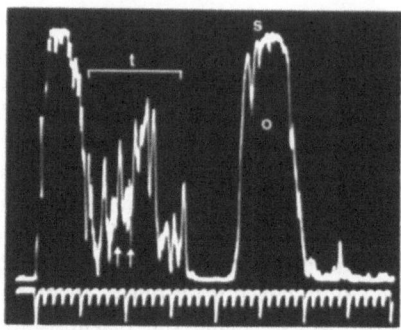

Fig. 1. A-scan echograms from a case of unilateral retinoblastoma, obtained at tissue sensitivity. Sound beam was directed through calcified central portion of tumor (above) and through calcium-free peripheral portion (below). Note the extremely high 'calcium-spikes' (c) and the marked shadowing as indicated by lower tumor spikes (t), scleral signal (s) and orbital spikes (o) behind the tumor (top echogram). Compare with normally high scleral and orbital spikes in bottom echogram. → fast flickering spontaneous movement caused by blood flow in tumor vessels.

identifying true shadows in these cases. Other A-scan findings in retino-blastoma are a regularly-seen shortening of the axial eye length (in contrast to traditional textbook wisdom) and occasionally-noted fast-flickering movement of lower tumor spikes indicating blood flow in the tumor. The shortening of axial eye length is relative to the normal globe (unilateral cases) or the eye with the lesser tumor masses (bilateral cases), and on an average amounts to about to 1 mm.

The combination of high reflectivity, typical spacing of the strong echo signals, and shadowing is pathognomonic for retinoblastoma. Only the calcification within the tumor produces these patterns. Neither the rosette formation, nor the pseudo-rosettes or the many vessels in a retino-blastoma, can cause such strong echoes and sound attenuation. Calcification may occur only in small portions of the tumor, and one must scan the tumor carefully from different sides. When doing so, calcification and the corresponding typical echograms are found in the great majority of cases of retinoblastoma. In 35 consecutive cases seen in the Eye Department of The

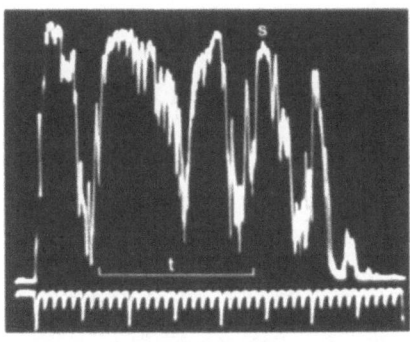

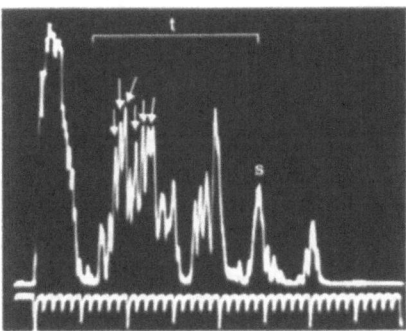

Fig. 2. A-scan echograms from eye with retinoblastoma (beam direction similar to top echogram in Fig. 1), obtained at tissue sensitivity (top) and at reduced sensitivity to better demonstrate the individual spikes (arrows) from the calcium deposits (bottom echogram). t tumor pattern; s sclera.

University of Iowa, 97% were calcified and consequently diagnosed correctly with echography (Table 1.) 32 (91%) of the cases were so heavily calcified that pathognomonic echographic patterns were obtained. In two of the cases, calcification was borderline and shadowing was not clearly shown; nevertheless, the echograms in these cases were still consistent with retinoblastoma. Calcification was absent in only one of the cases, and low to medium reflectivity of the tumor resulted; in this case, the erroneous echographic diagnosis of Coats' disease was made. But 97% of all retinoblastoma cases seen by us showed echographic signs of calcification. Thus, standardized echography is more sensitive in detecting calcification than plain X-rays. Also, the incidence of calcification in these tumors is obviously much higher than was previously suspected from X-ray data, which showed such calcification in only about 60% of the cases. It must, however, be emphasized that a careful and complete scanning of all portions of an intraocular tumor is necessary to find pockets of calcification, which may be relatively small and may lie eccentrically, and to achieve such a high success rate.

In addition to the important aid standardized echography provides as an independent and objective method in the primary diagnosis of retinoblastoma,

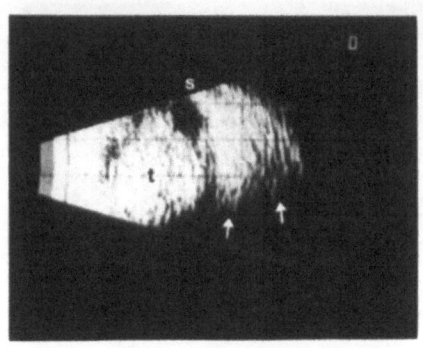

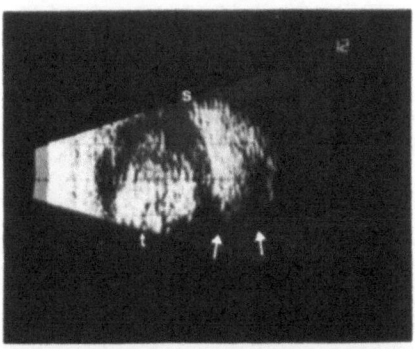

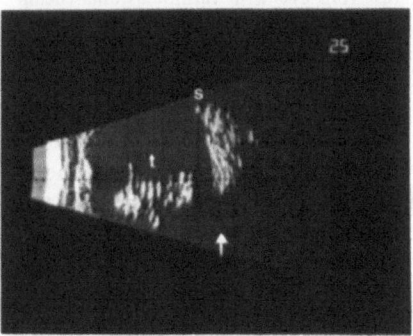

Fig. 3. B-scan echograms from retinoblastoma (same case as in *Figs. 1, 2*), displayed with maximum sensitivity (0 db setting) and with 12 and 25 db lower settings. Note the persistence of several individual echo spots at reduced sensitivity (calcium foci). → moderate shadow (enhanced by artefact due to total reflection of sound beam at lateral ocular wall and tumor surface) t tumor; s sclera.

Table 1. Results of standardized echography.

Histologically proven cases of retinoblastoma 35	Echographic diagnosis	
	'Retinoblastoma' (correct) 34 (97%)	'Coats' Disease' (incorrect) 1 (3%)

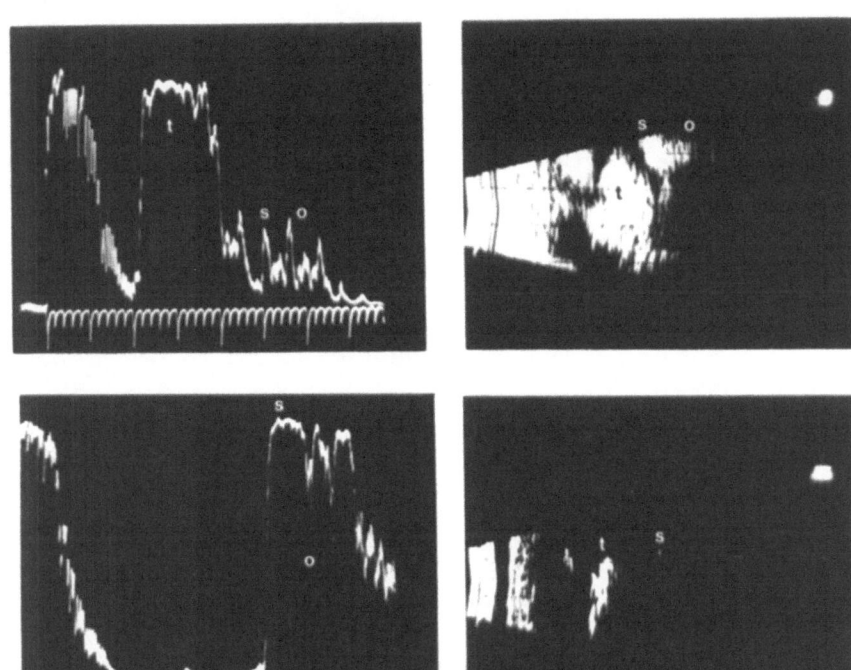

Fig. 4. A-scan and B-scan echograms from heavily calcified retinoblastoma demonstrating massive shadowing. t tumor pattern; s sclera; o orbital pattern. Bottom A-scan echogram was obtained with sound beam bypassing tumor (normally high signals from sclera and orbit).

echography is also helpful in detecting or confirming growth or regression of the tumor following radiotherapy or chemotherapy. Echography is also important in ruling out retinoblastoma in cases of leukokoria. In early stages of this condition, echography often helps to specify the underlying condition, be it retrolental fibroplasia, persistent hyperplastic primary vitreous, endophthalmitis, Coats' disease or retinal displasis. Although echography may fail to differentiate the underlying disease process in advanced cases, the echograms still clearly differ from those produced by retinoblastoma. Even when calcification or bone formation occurs in phthisical eyes, the patterns are different from the focal calcification observed in retinoblastomas.

In summary, standardized echography is very helpful in confirming the primary diagnosis of retinoblastoma (usually by producing pathognomonic patterns), in following the course of retinoblastoma during and following treatment and, more frequently, in ruling out retinoblastoma in cases of leukokoria.

Authors' Address:
Dept. of Ophthalmology
University of Iowa
Iowa City, IA 55242 U.S.A.

CONSIDERATIONS OF TWO CASES OF
MEDULLO-EPITHELIOMAS

V. MAZZEO, R. SCORRANO, L. RAVALLI & F. PISTOCCHI

(Ferrara, Italy)

The medullo-epithelioma whether 'congenital' or 'acquired' is an extremely rare tumor. The history of the 'Primary tumors of the non pigmented ciliary epithelium' dates from the beginning of this century and many reports in the past have given their contribution to the understanding of the nature and the exact histogenesis of this kind of neoplasms. Many names were attributed to them: 'Teratoneuroma' (Verhoeff 1904); 'Diktyoma' (Fuchs 1908) and 'Medullo-epithelioma' (Grinker 1931), because of the difficulties in classifying them (Vogel 1974, Reese 1976). In the last years Zimmerman (1971), in the fourth Verhoeff Lecture, after having discussed extensively history, terminology and genesis of these tumors suggested a classification, based on their embryonic nature now widely accepted (Broughton & Zimmerman 1978). According to this classification our two cases dealing with a baby and one adult, should be properly classified as medullo-epithelioma the child's one, and as a carcinoma (malignant ephithelioma) the second one.

CASE REPORT

A 15 months old male baby was referred to the Clinic because of a right eye exotropia of four months duration. The family history was negative concering ocular malignancies.

Examination: both pupils were round, but the right one was irregular on the temporal side. A white-greyish mass was seen through the pupil. The slit-lamp examination under general anesthesia revealed peripheral anterior synechiae at 8 o'clock and posterior synechiae at 9–10 o'clock where the lens showed sector opacities. The lens itself was slightly displaced nasally. Behind the lens there was a whitish mass with neovascularisation which occupied almost completely the anterior vitreous. The fundus was unexplorable, except nasally where a reddish reflex was seen. The ocular tension was normal.

Ultrasound examination (A-scan made by Kretztechnik 7200 MA equipped with an 8 MHz non-focused probe): in paralimbar projections, from the temporal side of the bulbus, it was possible to see a series of

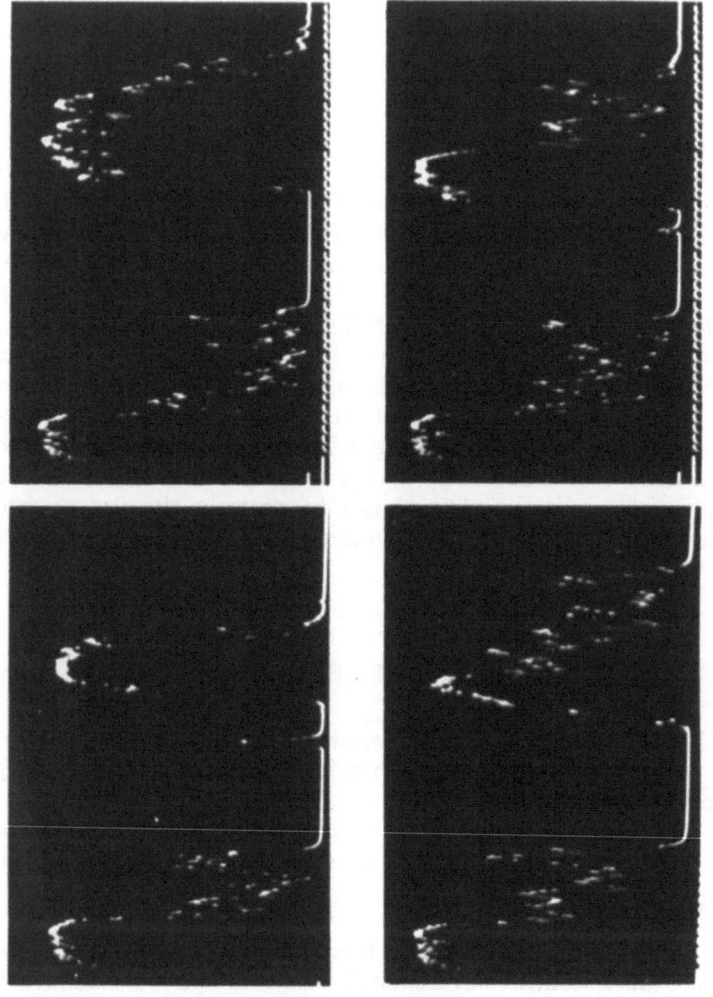

Fig. 1. Medullo-ephithelioma. Paralimbar echograms. Solid zone at the level of the ciliary body.

echoes of low to medium reflectivity (Fig. 1). The lesion was unexplorable from the opposite side, owing to its anteriority. Exploring more temporally it was possible to find a retinal detachment with a slight solid zone behind the retina. Since neither the echographic pattern nor the physical examination were characteristic it was decided to wait before any surgical procedure.

After three months the eye had become painful and the examination revealed an almost complete seclusio. Therefore enucleation was performed. Unfortunately u.s. examination was not repeated before the enucleation because the equipment was out of order. At gross examination a white mass, occupying the anterior vitreous, with an appearance like nervous tissue was seen. A retinoblastoma was considered.

Histopathological findings

The tumor arising from ciliary body was composed of cylindrical epithelial cells arranged in tube-like and net-like formations. Several solid mass of these cells could be seen. Several cells contained dark granular pigment. The arrangement of these elements resembled the primitive medullary epithelium (Fig. 2). No atypical cells were observed, but the initial involvment of the contiguous retina was suggestive of malignancy. The lens, cornea, slera and optic nerve were free of involvment. *Diagnosis*: medullo-epithelioma of the ciliary body.

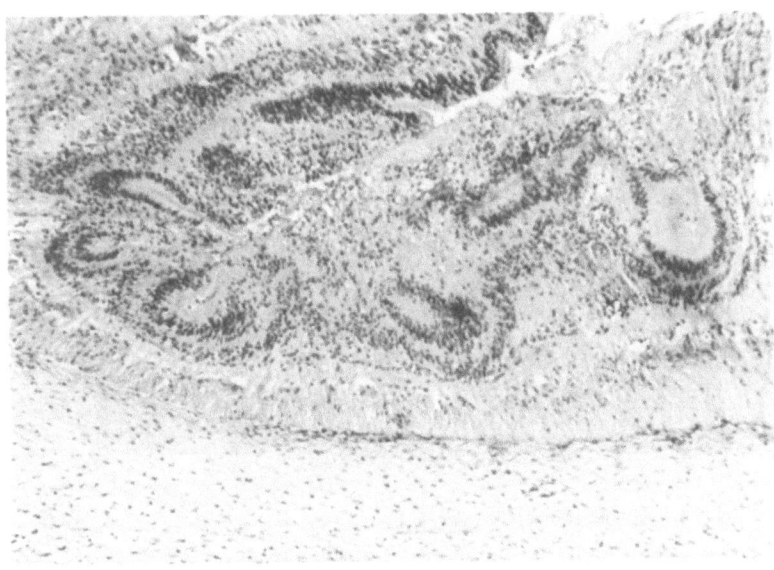

Fig. 2. Medullo-epithelioma. The neoplastic proliferation shows typical aspect resembling embryonic medullary epithelium; this zone is divided from the others tumoral areas by a basal membrane (H & E × 30).

111

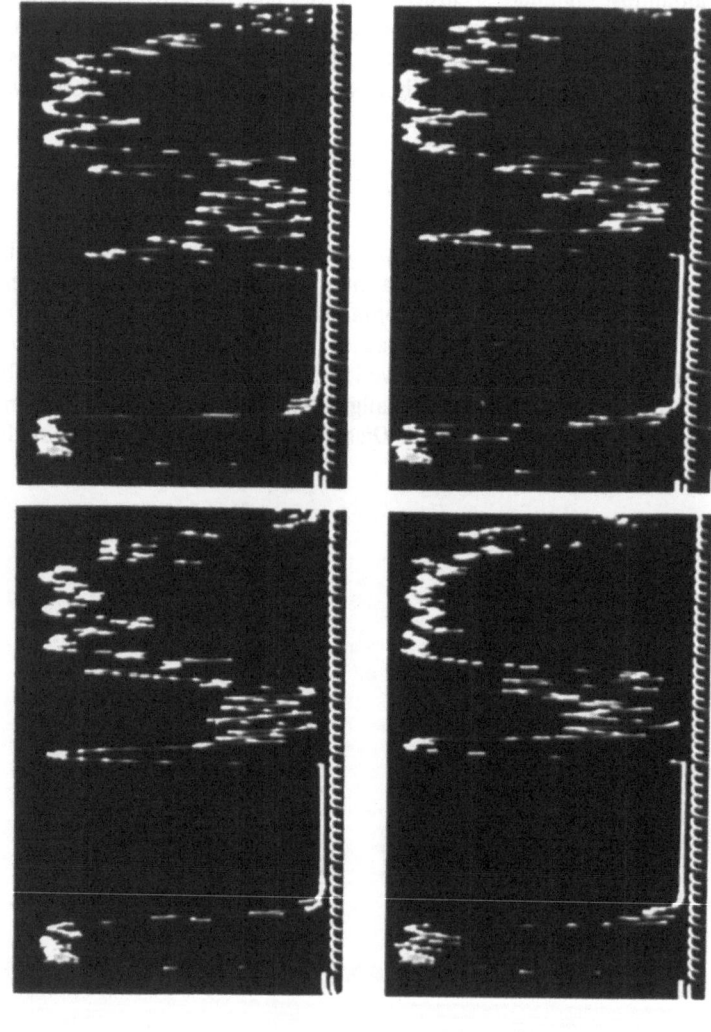

Fig. 3. Solid retinal detachment. High surface signal, low internal reflectivity with some high spike (upper) regular disposition of internal spikes.

CASE REPORT II

The second case dealt with an out patient sent by a private practitioner to undergo an u.s. examination because of peripheral solid retinal detachment at about 6 o'clock.

The A-scan disclosed that the lesion was approximately 10 μsec. thick. The internal reflectivity was from low to medium. Mobile spikes indicating vascularisation could not be demonstrated; attenuation (Poujol 1973) was 0,8 db/μsec (Fig. 3). The echographic diagnosis was of a choroidal malignant melanoma. The patient was enucleated by the ophthalmologist who had sent him. The pathologist's diagnostic answer was sent with a slide.

Histopathologic findings

Corresponding to the anterior choroid, starting from the ciliary body, a well-outlined tumor was found. It was composed of a fibrous stroma associated with anastomized ropes and nests of cuboidal-cylindrical epithelia.

The epithelial cells showed a poor badly-outlined, sometimes pigmented cytoplasm and large dysmorphic and hypercromatic nuclei. Many mitotic figures were present. In some places the neoplastic elements were arranged to form structures resembling the Flexner-Wintersteiner rosettes. Phologistic-necrotic areas were present (Fig. 4). The neoplasm did not infiltrate the sclera and retina. *Diagnosis*: carcinoma of the nonpigmented epithelium of the ciliary body.

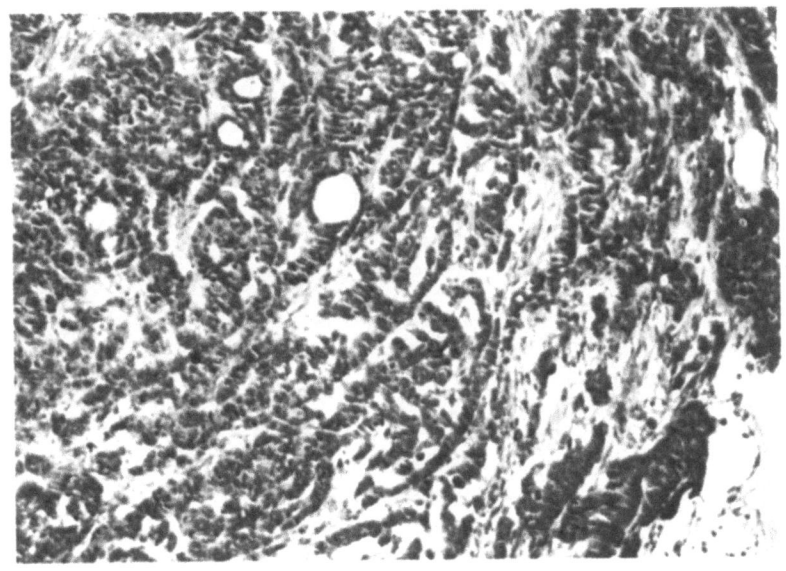

Fig. 4. Carcinoma. Many mitosis meaning malignancy are present. Among cells ropes, sometime resembling rosettes, some pigmented cell is found (H & E × 120).

113

CONCLUSIONS

These two cases have been discussed together because of their common origin from the ciliary neuroepithelium and their rarity. But considering their clinical-pathologic findings they are completely different. From an echographic point of view, as regards the first case we can say that we performed the examination in an unfavorable position having the tumor proximal to the transducer. This situation does not allow any precise evaluation of the echo amplitudes.

The comparison between the frequency dependence of the echogram and the histologic structure, which has been constantly done in the last few years to explain the echo features of tissues, is extremely difficult.

In the first case there are two main types of tissues irregularly mixed in the mass. In the zone shown in the Fig. 5 (right) one can see structures generally smaller than the wave-length and threfore the low-medium reflectivity can be explained.

In the second case it is possible to see (Fig. 5, left) rare large interfaces, larger than the wave-length, mixed with homogeneous zones. Thus the pattern shows a rather low internal reflectivity. Of course we cannot think that only one case is enough to reveal characteristic echo pattern. Some other echographist's experience may confirm or refute these findings.

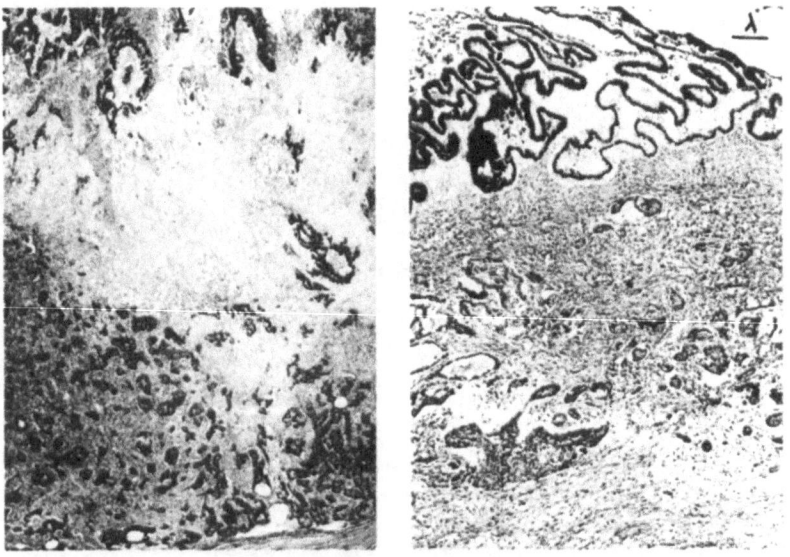

Fig. 5. Hystological section from medullo-epithelioma (right) ($\times$ 63; λ = wavelength). Hystological section from carcinoma of the nonpigmented ciliary epithelium ($\times$ 25; λ = wavelength) (left).

REFERENCES

Broughton W.L. & Zimmerman L.E. A Clinicopathologic study of 56 cases of intraocular medulloepitheliomas. Am. J. Ophthalmol. 85: 407 (1978).

Fuchs E. Wucherungen und Geschwülste des ziliarepithels. Von Grafe's Arch. Ophthalmol. 68: 534 (1908).

Grinker R.R. Gliomas of the retina, including the results of studies with silver impregnation. Arch. Ophthalmol. 5: 920 (1931).

Poujol J., Iris L. & Armand M.J. Corrélations entre la réflectivité et l'atténuation ultrasonore des tumeurs intraoculaires et leur structure histologique. Bibl. Ophtalmol. 83: 172 (1975).

Reese A.B. Epithelial tumors of the uvea. In: Tumors of the eye (A.B. Reese ed.). New York, Harper & Row (1976) p. 63.

Verhoeff F.C. A rare tumor arising from the pars ciliaris retinae (terato-neuroma), of a nature hitherto unrecognized, and its relation to the so-called glioma retinae. Trans. Am. Ophthalmol. Soc. 10: 351 (1904).

Vogel M.H. Tumoren des Ziliarkörperepitheis. Klin Mbl. Augenheil. 165: 458 (1974).

Zimmerman L.E. Verhoeff's 'Terato-neuroma'. A critical reapparaisal in light of new observation and current concepts of embryonic tumors. The fourth Frederick H. Verhoeff lecture. Am. J. Ophthalmol. 72: 1039 (1971).

Authors' Address:
Clinica Oculistica
Università di Ferrara
Corso Giovecca, 203
I-44100 Ferrara, Italy

REFERENCES

THE ROLE OF ECHOGRAPHY IN THE CONSERVATIVE TREATMENT OF ENDOBULBAR TUMOURS

P.E. GALLENGA, T. DALIA, G. BELLONE*, G. CENNAMO**,
V.MAZZEO*** & A. ROSSI***

(Chieti, Torino*, Napoli**, Ferrara***, Italy)

The diagnosis of endobulbar tumour and the identification of their nature being made (Bellone & Gallenga 1970–1971, Gallenga & Mazzeo 1974–1975, Ossoinig, et al. 1975, Mazzeo, et al. 1979) echography plays a fundamental role even in the subsequent strategy (Table 1).

Table 1.

The role of echography in antitumourous strategy	
Diagnosis	presence/absence nature location dimensions – volume scleral infiltration
Indication,	enucleation conservative treatment
Control of conservative treatment	

The measurement of the neoplastic mass dimensions and the identification of their location, limits and connections i.e. topography, emphasized by B-scan requests either the enucleation or may support the optic evaluation of the tumour and its contention inside the scleral wall.

According to Ossoinig (1977), an irregular behaviour of the scleral peak behind the malignant choroidal tumour points out a scleral infiltration exactly justifying the fall of the internal reflectivity of this membrane. In our data this happens only in the tumours of the third group according to Meyer-Schwickerat (1968). When the conservative treatment is decided, echography, because of its uninvasiveness becomes the method of choice in the following controls especially when media opacity induced by the treatment itself handicaps any other observation.

Having considered tumours treated by Stallard's cobalt plaque, photocoagulation and or chemo- or- hormonotherapy, we cannot summarize in an unique behaviour the acoustic response of tumours treated in different conservative ways.

The first echographic observation of changes in tumoural echo pattern after therapy we know is the one by Riccardo Gallenga and coworkers (Fig. 1).

In 1971 he showed an image of a melanoblastoma treated by application of cobalt plaque obtained by a Kretztechnik 7900 S equipment. Later on, Soriano and coworkers (1975) presented another melanoblastoma where echoes of increased reflectivity appear in the tumoral trace and are pointed out as typical.

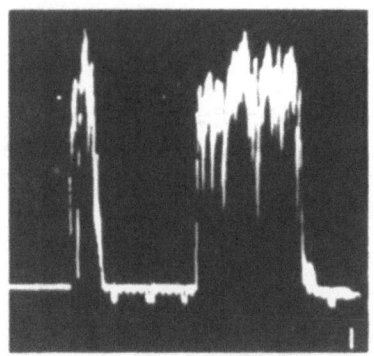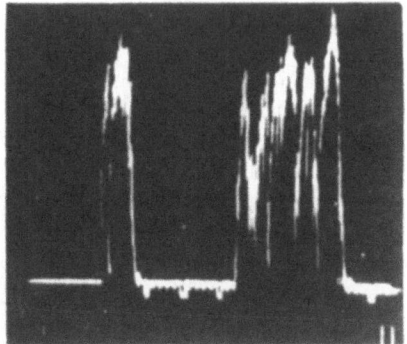

Fig. 1. Melanoblastoma treated by Co⁶⁰ plaque. Iₜ after 30 days (Gallenga *et al.* 1971).

A *succesful* conservative treatment modifies the echographic pattern of retinoblastoma and melanoblastoma, hemangioma and metastatic carcinoma of the choroid as concern thickness, height, attenuation and morphology of the tumoral trace (Table 2). Hemangiomas have a fast and tremendous evolution while retinoblastomas need some weeks. Metastatic carcinomas need a few months evolution. Melanoblastomas (Fig. 2) are the slowest; the reduction of the maximal thickness is about 30% and 50% from seven months until one year after the treatment; the smaller tumour being more reduced in a shorter time. In 1978 Coleman and co-workers presented a tumour regression of 39% after 17 months.

Table 2.

Echographic control of conservative treatment
Efficacious
reduction of tumor thickness change of internal reflectivity appearance of progressively extending cicatricial areas reduction of attenuation exerted on the sclera (may be erroneous because of reduction of scleral reflectivity)
Unefficacious
increasing of tumor thickness persistence of tumourous echo-pattern

118

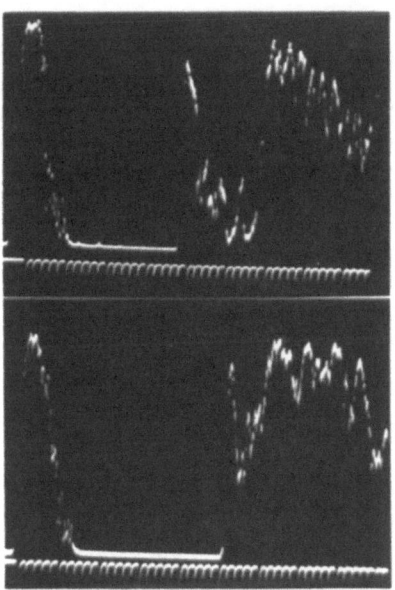

Fig. 2. Melanoblastoma of the choroid (top) Conservative treatment with Argon laser photocoagulations. After 1 year thickness reduction (bottom).

Hemangiomas and retinoblastomas exhibit a reduction in the height of the tumour peaks (Fig. 3), while melanoblastomas show an increase of it. After treatment with polichemiotherapy metastasis variate only their dimensions as it is easily demonstrated by subsequent fluorangiographies and echography indicate the thickness decrease until disappearance.

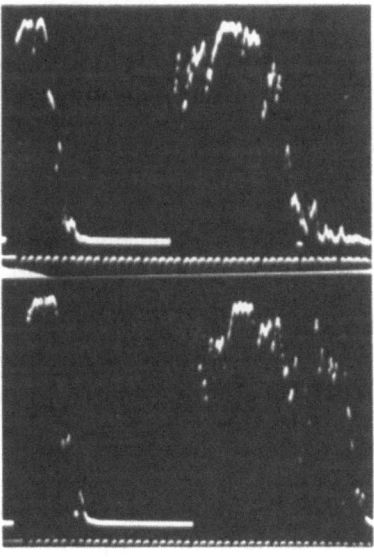

Fig. 3. Retinoblastoma (top). Conservative treatment by Xenon photocoagulation. After 30 days it is evident a slight reduction (bottom).

Cicatricial expanding areas progressively substitute the neoplastic tissue in melanoblastomas (Fig. 4) and modify the pattern; furthermore the attenuation induced by the tumoural mass on the echo of the sclera changes. This phenomenon may be altered by a lowering of scleral reflectivity in the site of treatment due perhaps to an excessive permanence of the plaque. We noticed, moreover, that this reduction is clearly inferior to the one provoked by diatermy.

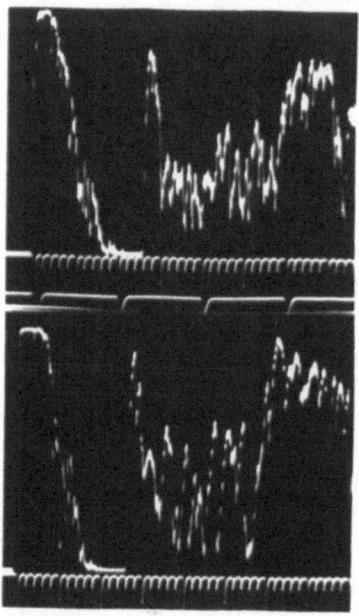

Fig. 4. Melanoblastoma of the choroid. Conservative treatment (one-eyed patient). Echopattern before insertion of a Co⁶⁰ plaque (top): low internal reflectivity. After 40 days (bottom) increase of internal reflectivity 'teeth comb' pattern.

The treatment is to be considered *unsuccessful* when the above mentioned conditions are not realized, that is, when the tumoural thickness increases or, when remaining unreduced, the echo pattern will keep the tumoural aspect without any substitution with cicatricial areas. (Fig. 5) In these cases treatment was *unsuccessful*: on the right in a retinoblastoma we obtained the complete disappearance of the mass, but the echographic control after five months allowed to individuate a $2 \mu sec$ relapse in the already treated zone. On the left in a melanoblastoma three months after the treatment we observed a $2 \mu sec$ increased thickness with persistence of tumoural pattern.

This induced us to the enucleation and the histological specimen confirmed the presence of tumoural nests in a partially hyaline tissue without scleral infiltration. The presence of melanophora indicated the loss of melanine by the neoplastic suffering cells.

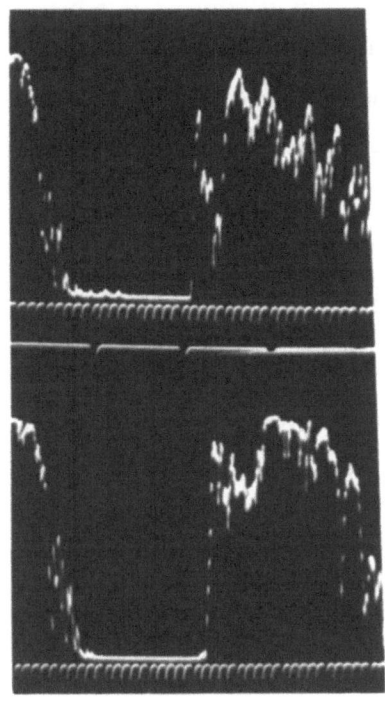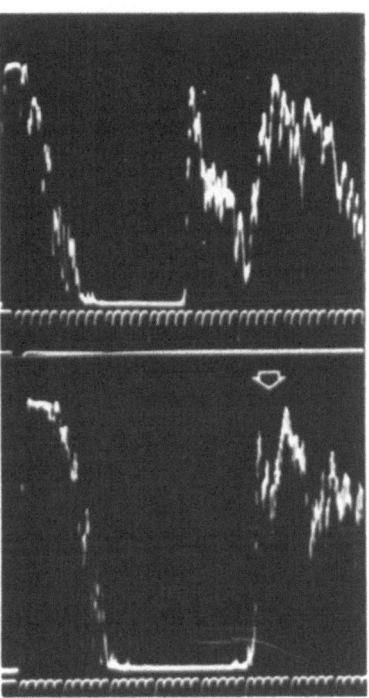

Fig. 5. Unsuccessful conservative treatment. (Co⁶⁰ applicator and Xenon photocoagulation). Top left: 4 μsec Thick melanoblastoma of the choroid. Bottom left: after three months increase of 2 μsec. Top right: retinoblastoma. After treatment the mass had totally disappeared. Bottom: the echographic control after five months allowed to find a 2 μsec thick relapse in the already treated area.

We must point out as *complications* of the treatment the relative frequence of endovitreal haemorrhages, the appearance of whitish scar tissue which can mask the tumour below and a moderate reduction of the thickness of the retrobulbar trace even without enophtalmos (Gallenga, *et al.* 1976). It is therefore possible today to effect such conservative treatment basing the diagnostic precision and the therapeutical strategy on echography.

REFERENCES

Bellone G. & Gallenga P.E. Diagnostica ecografica del retinoblastoma. Arch. Rass. Ital. Ottal 1: 241 (1970–71).

Chang S., Dallow R.L. & Coleman D.J. Ultrasonic evaluation of intraocular tumors. In Ocular and Adnexal tumors. (Jakobiec F. ed.) Aesculapius Publ. Co. (1978) p. 281.

Dalia T., Aiello F., Di Censo B. & Baquis G. Echographic and fluorangiographic study of metastatic choroidal tumours.

In: P.E. Gallenga *et al.*, Current concepts in Ultrasound Vol. II italo jugoslavian days, Chieti, Novappia Publ. Co. (1980) p. 71.

121

Gallenga R., Bellone G., Gallenga P.E. & Pasquarelli A. Ultrasonografia clinica dell'occhio e dell'orbita. In Recenti acquisizione di semeiotica oculare (SOI ed.) Firenze (1971).

Gallenga P.E. & Mazzeo V. Semeiotica dei tumori melanici della coroide. Arch. Rass. Ital. Ottal. IV: 72 (1974–75).

Gallenga P.E., Mazzeo V. & Cennamo G. Semeiotica ultrasonica dei tumori endobulbari. Atti X Congresso S.O.M. 222 (1976).

Mazzeo V., Scorrano R., Gallenga P.E. & Rossi A. Echography in choroidal metastatic tumors. Second WFMB Myiazaki 22–27 July 1979. Abstract book (1979) p. 159.

Meyer-Schwickerath C. Malignes melanoblastom der chorioidea. Mod. Probl. Ophthalmol. 7: 7 (1968).

Ossoinig K. Echography of the Eye, Orbit and Periorbital Region. In Orbit Roentgenology (P.H. Arger, ed.) New York, Wiley (1977) p. 224.

Ossoinig K., Bigar F. & Kaefring S.L. Malignant melanoma of the choroid and Ciliary Body. A differential diagnosis in Clinical Echography. Bibl. Ophthal. 83: 141 (1975).

Soriano H., Psilas K. & Houber J.P. Valeur et limites de l'examen echographique métode A, dans le diagnostic des affections intraoculaires. Bibl. Opthalmol. 83: 68 (1975).

Till P. & Ossoinig K. Ten year study on Clinical Echography in Intraocular Disease. Bibl. Ophthalmol. 83: 49 (1975).

Author's Address:
P.E. Gallenga
Dept. of Ophthalmology
University of Chieti
Chieti, Italy

COMPUTER ANALYSIS OF A-MODE ECHOGRAMS FROM CHOROIDAL MELANOMA

J.M. THIJSSEN & A.M. VERBEEK

(Nijmegen, The Netherlands)

INTRODUCTION

The potentials of A-mode echography have been recognized in ophthalmology from the very start of diagnostic applications. In particular the work of Poujol, Oksala, Ossoinig and others yielded valuable criteria for the differentiation of intra-ocular pathology and of ocular and orbital tumours. A serious drawback of A-mode echography is its dependance on the technical specifications of the equipment and on the skill of the examiner. In our attempts to remove these limitations we have developed an on-line system of computer analysis of A-mode echograms (Thijssen, *et al.* 1979, 1981). The involvement of the equipment characteristics is reduced by correction of the echogram for compression by the amplifier. The dependance on skill is reduced by collecting a series of echograms in a single record and by introducing statistical evaluation of the data.

For that purpose quantitive parameters like amplitude distribution, attenuation, variability of the echogram and peak density are calculated. In this paper our work on the diagnosis of choroidal melanoma will be presented and the results compared with other kinds of intraocular tumours. Preliminary data from orbital pathology will also be discussed.

TECHNIQUES

The equipment consists of an ophthalmological A-mode apparatus (Kretztechnik 7200 MA), a home-made trigger unit connected to a Polaroid camera, a transient recorder (Biomation 8100) and a digital computer system (Digital Equipment PDP 11/34), that is on-line connected to the transient recorder. When a polaroid photo is taken the trigger unit 'enables' the transient recorder and the next coming transmission pulse of the A-mode apparatus triggers the acquisition by the recorder and the subsequent storage into the computer memory. This cycle is repeated then automatically 24 times in 3 seconds. The echogram is stored digitally in the transient recorder by taking samples (Fig. 1) at 0.1 μs intervals (i.e. 10 MHz sampling rate). The examination technique is the following: after localization of the pathology by

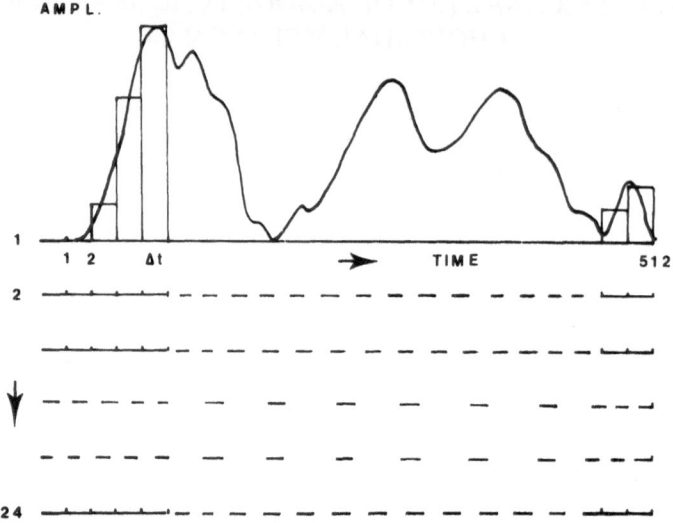

Fig. 1. Scheme of data acquisition. Digital sampling of video A-mode echogram in a 10 MHz rate up to 512 samples. Sequence of 24 echograms collected by computer in three seconds (Thijssen, *et al.* 1980).

A-scan and B-scan procedures the A-scan probe is transocularly directed towards the lesion. When the optimum position is obtained (e.g. maximum diameter of lesion) a photograph is taken and during data acquisition the probe is slightly moved in a tremor-like fashion. The result of this procedure may be a kind of 'tissue sampling', i.e the sound beam is transmitted through different parts of the pathology and by this means more or less statistically independent tissue echograms are collected.

The computer program then produces a copy of the first echogram stored and the examiner may insert the region of interest by positioning the cursor lines at the display of the computer terminal. The complete record of 24 echograms is then checked visually (cf Thijssen, *et al.* 1979, 1980) and if satisfactory the proper analysis may either start, or another record collected.

RESULTS

The output of the statistical analysis program is shown in Fig. 2. This is a typical example of a melanoma of the choroid. The tumour region under the retina is indicated by the dotted vertical lines in the upper left part. The lower left part is a display of the average of 24 successive echograms (see Techniques) and it may be used to visually evaluate the amplitude level and the attenuation. The latter is also indicated by the oblique line on top. The upper right picture represents an extended display of the lesion (single echogram) and of the attenuation. As indicated in the data to the right of the latter picture the amplitude level is rather high in this case (52%). The attenuation is 0.9 dB/mm tissue (forth and back through the lesion).

124

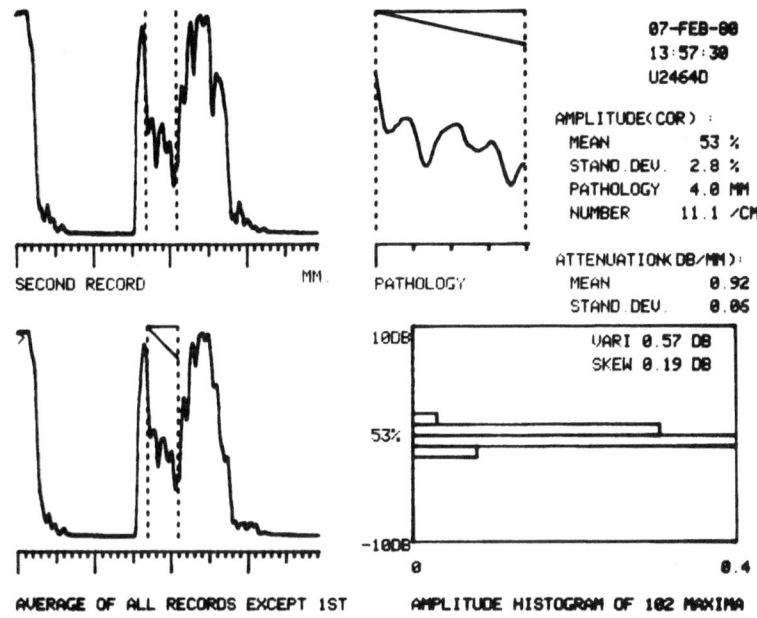

Fig. 2. Output of computer main program for statistical analysis of echograms. For description see text (Thijssen, *et al.* 1980).

Another typical feature of the melanoma is the great regularity of the echopattern, which is given by the amplitude histogram and by the variability measure (i.e. the standard deviation of the peak values relative to the regression line). Other characteristics like the number of peaks per millimeter tissue and the skewness of the histogram are not typical.

The melanomas we have investigated (20 eyes, 30 records) had a prominence of at least 3.5 mm, because this is needed for a reliable estimation of the attenuation. The echographic diagnosis was histologically verified in all cases. Most of the lesions enable an estimation of the attenuation. In a few cases however, the echopattern did not decrease over the whole region (Fig. 3), possible causes: either the sound beam was not exclusively hitting the tumour, or the tumour was atypical because of necrosis. We have concluded that in only one case the latter cause was valid, so we have to conclude that sometimes the echograms were not adequately recorded. This of course is a principal problem of A-mode echography.

The results are further elucidated in Figs. 4–6. It can be concluded that the spread in the amplitude levels (Fig. 4) is not extremely high, so these may be expected to yield a differentiation parameter. The mean value is given in Table 1, together with the standard deviation of the mean. The attenuation shows a relatively high spread (Fig. 5) but if we consider the extreme high values to be influenced by the examination technique the picture becomes much more positive. The average of 0.8 dB/mm (Table 1) is significantly different from water (0.15 dB/mm) as one extreme and of orbital fat (1.5 dB/mm) as the other. The variability of those records yielding an estimate of the attenuation (Fig. 6) is expressed by the standard deviation of

125

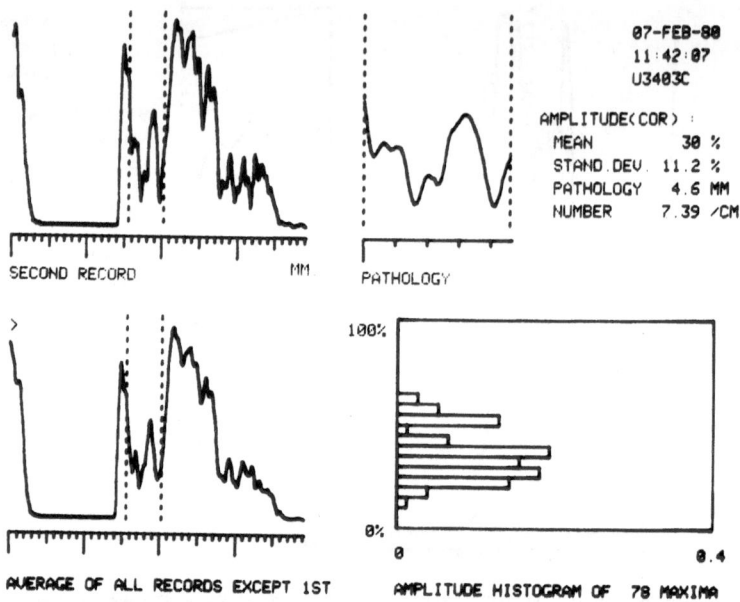

Fig. 3. Atypical example of a melanoma of the choroid. Note the irregular texture and the lack of decrease of the echoes within the pathological region.

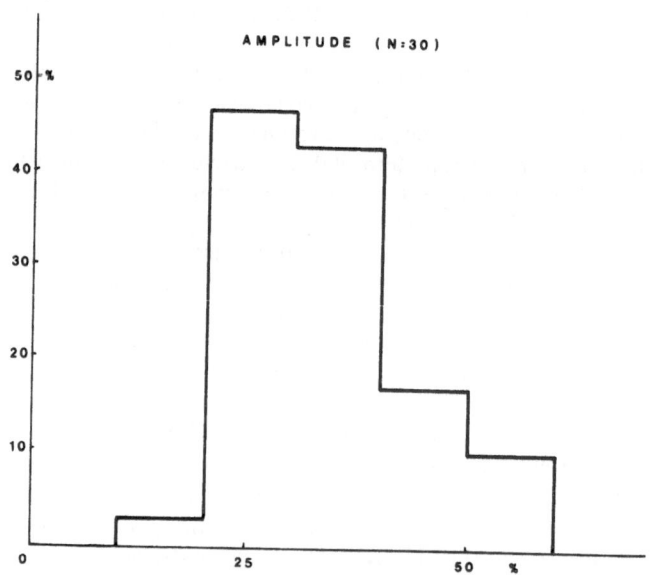

Fig. 4. Amplitude levels of melanomas (20 eyes, 30 records), mean and standard deviation: (33 + 3)%.

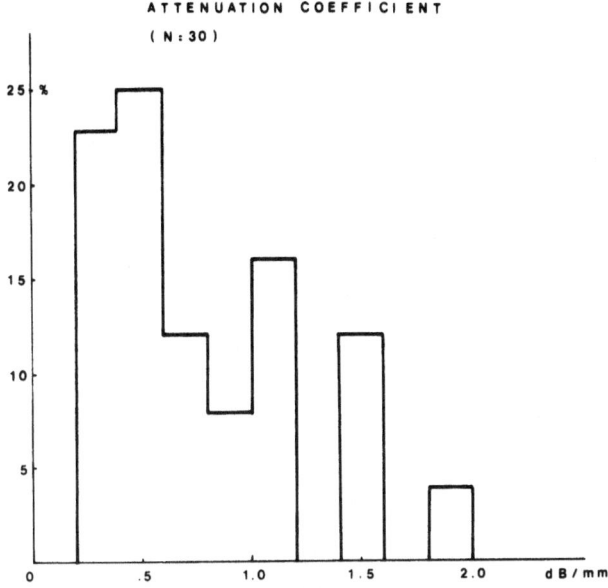

Fig. 5. Attenuation values of melanomas. Mean and standard deviation (0.8 + 0.1) dB/mm tissue.

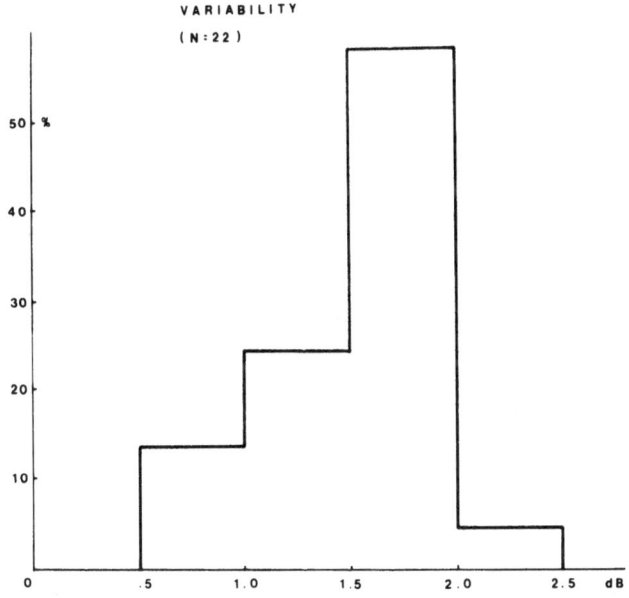

Fig. 6. Variability (standard deviation) of amplitudes after correction for the attenuation. Mean value 1.7 dB, i.e. regular texture.

Table 1.

	Amplitude %	Attenuation dB/mm	Number of peaks	Variability dB
Melanoma chor.	33 ± 3	0.8 ± 0.1	7.5 ± 0.5	1.7 ± 0.2
Metastasis	80	?	8	?
Oatcell carcinoma	38	?	8	?
Normal orbit	90	1.5	10.5	2.5
Pseudo tumour	27	0.6	8	1.0
Mixed tumour	60	0.6	10	3.0
Meningo-encephalocele	90	1.6	11.5	1.6

the amplitudes after correction for the attenuation. A rather low value of 1.7 dB is obtained on average (cf. Table 1).

The data of two other kinds of lesion are given in Table 1. Both displayed a rather irregular texture, so the attenuation, or the variability, could not be measured. The best differential parameter of a metastasis appears to be the amplitude level, although it is known that e.g. a heamangioma yields a comparable, or still higher level (Ossoinig 1974). A rather rare lesion, the Oatcell carcinoma could not be differentiated from a melanoma because except for the texture there was no differing parameter. The number of echoes per cm tissue is also given in Table 1 though it appears not to be a differentiation parameter in these kinds of intraocular lesions. We have, however, some indications that it may be useful in the differentiation of orbital tumours, but the amount of data gathered at present is too low to allow for conclusions.

DISCUSSION

The statistical parameters selected to investigate the computer support of echographic tissue differentiation are giving quantitative and reliable tissue characteristics. Additionally, the procedure of what is called tissue sampling gives a objective means of averaging out inhomogeneities within a lesion. The results of the melanomas presented in this paper have to be complemented by data on subretinal haemorrhages, because in our experience this is often the most difficult differentiation. It should be kept in mind that additional data like the shape of the lesion and the vascularity may be very typical as well. So a more complete decision scheme has to be used anyway. Our experience with orbital lesions, although limited, is very promising and we will proceed with our work in the detection and subsequent differentiation of focal and diffuse orbital lesions.

ACKNOWLEDGEMENT

This work has been supported by the Health Organization TNO. The authors are very much indepted to A.L. Bayer, M. Eng. Sc. and M. Cloostermans, M. Sc., who recently improved the computer softwae.

128

REFERENCES

Ossoinig, K.C. Quantitative echography, the basis of tissue differentiation. J. Clin. Ultrasound 2: 33 (1974).

Thijssen, J.M., Kruizinga, R., Dooren, H.A.F. van, & Verbeek, A.M. Computer assisted echographic analysis. Quantitative and statistical analysis of the video signal. In: Diagnostica Ultrasonica in Ophthalmologia. (H. Gernet, ed.) Münster: Remy Verlag (1979) p. 12.

Thijssen, J.M., Bayer, A.L., & Verbeek, A.M. Computer support for Ultrasonic diagnosis. Doc. Ophthalmol. 48: 315 (1979).

Thijssen, J.M., Bayer, A.L. & Cloostermans, M. Computer assisted echography: statistical analysis of A-mode video echograms obtained by tissue sampling. In press: Med. Biol. Eng. & Comp.

Authors' Address:
J.M. Thijssen Ph. D. & A.M. Verbeek M.D.
Biophysics Laboratory and Ultrasonography Unit
Institute of Ophthalmology, Nijmegen University,
6500 HB Nijmegen, The Netherlands

129

REFERENCES

A CHOROIDAL OAT-CELL CARCINOMA METASTASIS MIMICKING A CHOROIDAL MELANOMA

Case history

A.M. VERBEEK

(Nijmegen, The Netherlands)

One and a half years ago, a thirty-eight-year old male patient was referred to us because of a prominent process in the upper temporal fundus quadrant of his right eye. The patient had complained of blurred vision and metamorphopsia for two weeks. The patient was in good general condition. Ocular examination revealed a visual acuity of 25/200 in the right eye and 20/20 in the left eye. The left eye showed no abnormalities. Slitlamp examination of the right eye showed pigment-cells in the vitreous. Applanation pressure was normal. Ophthalmoscopy of the right eye revealed a very prominent yellow-gray lesion with a small haemorrhage on its surface. Below the lesion the retina was partly detached. Visual field examination showed an aboslute scotoma in the area of the lesion and fluorescein angiography showed a picture most consistent with a choroidal melanoma. Echographic A mode examination with the Kretztechnik 7200 MA (Ossoinig 1974) revealed a mass lesion with a smooth surface and maximal prominence of 7 mm of solid consistancy, low to medium reflectivity with spontaneous movements (vascularity), B-scanning with the Bronson-Turner unit showed a spherical shaped lesion with choroidal excavation and retinal detachment at its base. (Fig. 1a, b)

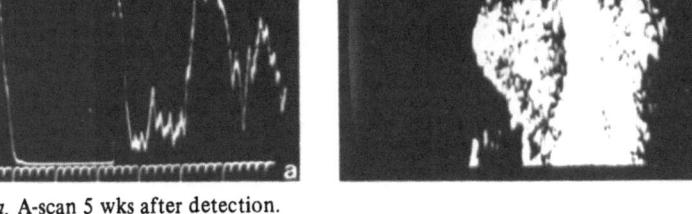

Fig. 1a. A-scan 5 wks after detection.
Fig. 1b. B-scan 5 wks after detection.

After these investigations were completed, we were almost convinced that this process should be a melanoma of the choroid, but during physical examination signs suggesting a process in the left lung were found. X-rays, cytological examination on sputum, bronchoscopy, biopsy and pathological anatomical examination revealed a strong vascularised oat-cell carcinoma in the upper quadrant of the left lung without, at that moment, signs of metastasis elsewhere than (may be) the choroid. No enucleation was performed and the patient got cythostatic therapy. (Vincristin, Cyclofosfamide, Procarbazine). The follow-up is schematically shown in Table 1.

Table 1. Case History.

Ultrasonografic examination	Prominence of the tumor	Therapy
0 wk	7 mm	–
5 wk	8.5– 9 mm	–
8 wk	8.5– 9 mm	chemotherapy
11 wk	11 mm	chemother./radioth.
20 wk	6 – 7 mm	chemotherapy
26 wk	5 mm	chemotherapy
32 wk	6 –6.5 mm	chemotherapy
36 wk	8 –8.5 mm	–
40 wk	explosive growth general metastasis	–
52	death	

On chemotherapy alone no benificial effect, even growing of the tumor was seen. In combination with radiotherapy on the primary and choroidal process (3000 rad telecobalt) the process reduced, then escaped from the therapy followed by an explosive growth. (Fig. 2a, b) 52 weeks after the first ocular examination the patient died from cardiorespiratory insufficiency due to extensive metastasis. Post mortem investigation showed a very large oat-cell carcinoma of the left lung with multiple metastasis in the choroid as well. In the literature there are more reports of lesions accoustically mimicking choroidal melanoma such as tuberculoma, adenoma, or adeno-

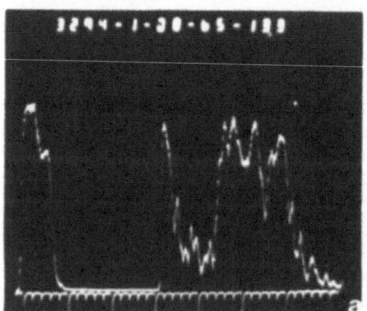 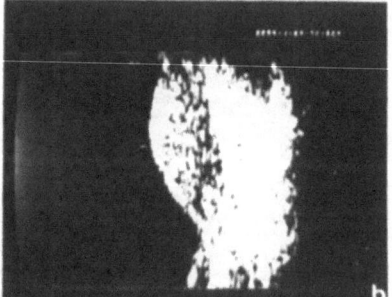

Fig. 2a. A-scan 20 wks after detection.
Fig. 2b. B-scan 20 wks after detection.
A-scan shows no changes in the reflectivity of the tumor.

carcinoma of the pigment epithelium, melanocythoma, atypical retino-blastoma, subretinal haemorrhage and choroidal metastasis of a seminoma, all having in common a dense cellular packing like melanoma. (Blodi 1977, Freyler 1977, Hodes 1977, Meimei Chung 1979). We may now add to this series an oat-cell carcinoma metastasis.

REFERENCES

Blodi, F.C. Ein Tuberkulom der Aderhaut, ein Melanom vortauschend. Klin. Mbl. Augenheilk. 170: 845 (1977).
Freyler, H. & Egerer, I. Echography and histological studies in various eye conditions. Arch. Ophthalmol. 95: 1387 (1977).
Hodes, B.L. & Chromokos, E. Standardized A-scan echographic diagnosis of choroidal malignant melanomas. Arch. Ophthalmol. 95: 593 (1977).
Meimei Chung & Shields, J.A. Adenoma of the pigmentepithelium of the ciliary body dimulating a malignant melanoma. Am. J. of Ophthalmol. 88: 40 (1977).
Ossoinig, K.C. & Blodi, F.C. Preoperative differential diagnosis of tumors with echography. Part. III. Diagnosis of intra ocular tumors. Current Concepts in Ophthalmology, Vol. 4 (F.C. Blodi, ed.) St Louis: Mosby (1974) p. 296.

Author's Address:
Institute of Ophthalmology
University of Nijmegen
Philips van Leydenlaan 15
6500 HB Nijmegen
The Netherlands

OCULAR BIOMETRY

Introductory Lecture

J. FRANÇOIS
with the collaboration of F. GOES
(*Ghent, Belgium*)

1. HISTORY

The first oculometry was made by Pourfour de Petit, who, in 1728, demonstrated his ophthalmometer at the Academy of Sciences in Paris. In the 19th century many anatomical measurements were performed, but they were not accurate because of the post mortem changes. The first optical measurement in vivo of the anterior chamber depth and of the lens thickness was made in 1856 by von Helmholtz, who, using his ophthalmometer, found a lens thickness between 3.41 and 3.80 mm in adult eyes. In 1938, Rushton used a radiological method for the measurement of the eye-length. In 1940 Schoute used the chromatic aberration of the lens for the same purpose, while in 1941 Goldmann & Heim published their photographic method for the determination of the anterior chamber depth and the lens thickness.

In 1956, ultrasonography, which is based on an entirely different principle, was introduced in ophthalmology by Mundt and Hughes. The two main clinical applications of ultrasonic biometry are the axial measurements for anatomic or physiologic correlative studies, and the morphologic comparative studies of size and growth for intra- or retroocular tumours (Fig. 1), as well as of extraocular muscle thickness.

In 1974, Vanysek found use for ultrasonography to measure experimentally the intraocular pressure by exerting an external pressure on the globe, which shortens its axial length.

2. TECHNIQUE

The ultrasonic measurement of intraocular distances depends on the ultrasound velocity in the various parts of the eye, the elapsed time and the direction of the sound beam in the eye.

In order to obtain a maximal accuracy, the transducer must be perfectly aligned along the desired *axis of measurement* (optical axis, visual axis, tumour height). In oculometry the axis is usually the visual one. An error of five degrees in the transducer orientation results in an error of 0, 1 mm in the axial length measurement (Coleman 1977).

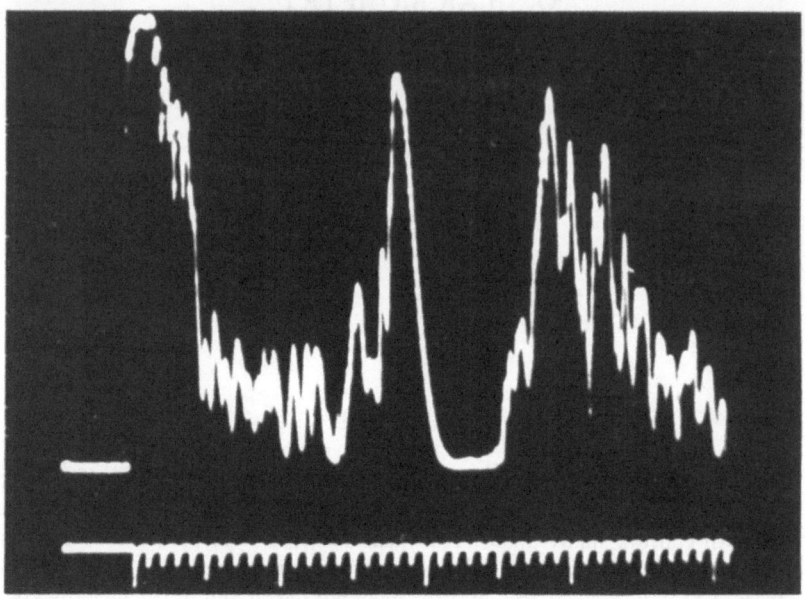

Fig. 1. Proximal echo of a malignant melanoma of the ciliary body. The biometric comparative study allows the observation of the tumor growth (pers. obs.).

Different fixation devices have been used by various observers in order to obtain an alignement with the visual axis (Yamamoto, *et al.* 1961, Buschmann 1963, Rivara 1963, Gernet 1964, Leary 1965, Giglio & Ludlam 1967; Coleman, *et al.* 1975). We have used the Rivara's technique. A cup having the shape of the sclera and an open bottom is fitted between the lids. It is filled with saline or methylcellulose, which serves as a delay column, and the transducer is dipped into the front of the cup.

Clinically, the technique, whereby the ultrasound beam is aimed at the macular region, under control of the echoes on the screen, while the patient's eye is aligned with a light source, is the most useful.

The measurement is performed along the optical axis (Fig. 2), when:

(1) The lens echoes are maximally separated.

(2) When the posterior lens echo amplitude is maximal for the adjusted amplification, and nearly as high as the anterior lens echo and as the corneal echoes.

(3) When the echo rise is perpendicular to the base line.

(4) When the vitreous dimension from the posterior lens echo to the internal retinal membrane is maximal, while the posterior lens echo remains maximal.

In practice the accuracy can be enhanced by averaging the measurements. In order to avoid errors in the measurement of the paramacular curved surface, a narrow beam focused transducer should be used. Otherwise, the rays arriving at the extreme of the beam are reflected before those arriving at the macula.

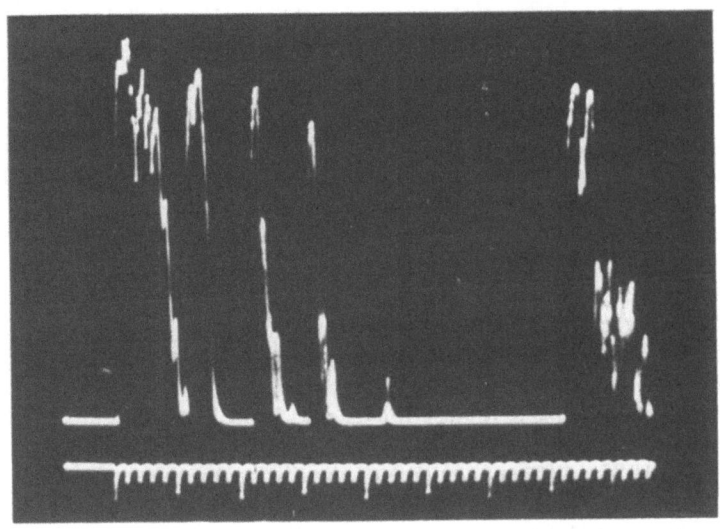

Fig. 2. Biometric axial measurement with focalised narrow beam and 15 MHz transducer (pers. obs.).

In order to avoid a deformation of the eyeball by compression of the globe, the transducer should not be applied directly to the cornea. As already said, we use Rivara's technique. Other investigators use a combined optical-echographic method, the anterior eye segment being measured optically and the posterior segment echographically (Gernet 1964).

The higher the frequency, the shorter the wave length and the more accurate the resolving power of the system. A frequency of 20 MHZ provides high resolution and sensitivity and has still sufficient penetration to detect echoes from the posterior wall surface.

The *time distance* between the echoes must be accurately determined. On photographs, the reading of this distance introduces always an error, as the echoes are represented as lines with a certain thickness. More accurate readings can be made electronically with an interval counter, which gives the number of pulses occurring during the interval between the echoes. With frequencies of 20 MHZ. the accuracy of the method can be approximately 0.02 mm, when the conditions are optimal. Because of the iris thickness the pupil must be dilated.

The *velocity of the ultrasounds* is different in the various parts of the eye. Usually, 1641 m/sec for the lens and 1532 m/sec for the vitreous are accepted (Jansson & Köck 1962), although the range is rather large (1615–1657 m/sec for the lens, 1523–1539 m/sec for the vitreous). For the biometric study of intraocular tumours, Coleman (1975) used a constant velocity of 1600 m/sec.

Concerning the Scan system we prefer the A-Scan for biometric measurements. Weinstein, *et al.* (1966) & Baum (1967) prefer, nevertheless, the B-scan because this system allows measurements of structures, which are not along the visual axis and because volumes as well as curvatures can be visualised.

137

What is the accuracy of ultrasonographic oculometry? In comparative studies we obtained an accuracy of 0.2 mm (1%) for the axial length, of 0.1 mm for the anterior chamber depth and the lens thickness and of 0.25 mm for the vitreous, using the Kretz 7200 MA equipment and a 15 MHZ focused transducer (François & Goes 1976). Most of the investigators obtained more or less the same accuracy values (Jansson 1963, Rivara 1963, Gernet 1963, Leary, *et al.*, 1963, Leary 1965, Nakajima & Kimura 1967, Itin & Braward 1968, Lowe 1968, Bechetoille & Saraux 1970, Fledelius 1976). Threfore, it may be said that in clinical conditions the accuracy of ultrasonic biometry is 0.2 mm.

The accuracy with ultrasonography is higher than with optical phakometric and radiologic measurements (Araki 1961, Kanki, *et al.* 1961, Otsuka, *et al.* 1961, Jansson 1963, 1965, Sorsby, *et al.* 1963, Leary 1965, Young and Leary 1966, Nakajima & Kimura 1967, Lowe 1968, Kimura, *et al.* 1969).

Finally, it must be stressed that one has to use a standardised equipment (Fledelius 1975): different equipments give different results.

Some disparity can be found, because not all authors use cycloplegia under a certain age and because they add a different corrective factor (0.3 mm Gernet 1964, 0.6 mm, Luyckx 1966, Bechetoille & Saraux 1970, 0.35 mm, François & Goes 1970) or without corrective factor (Larson 1971, Perez Llorca 1971) owing to the uncertainty of the site of reflection in the posterior pole and the distance between the internal limiting membrane and the receptor layer of rods and cones.

3. GROWTH OF THE EYE

The average eye length *at birth* (Fig. 3 and Table 1) was found to be between 16.40 and 17.85 mm, the mean value being 17.0 mm (Gernet 1964, Luyckx 1966, Grignolo & Rivara 1968, Larsen 1971), Gernet (1964) & Luyckx (1966) did not mention sex differences. Larsen (1971) found, nevertheless, a longer eye length in boys, the difference being 0.38 mm.

The mean value for the anterior chamber depth at birth is between 2.38 and 2.90 mm (Luyckx 1966, Gernet 1970, Larsen 1971). The average lens thickness at birth is between 3.60 and 3.65 mm (Luycks 1966, Gernet 1970), while the vitreous length is between 10.22 and 10.80 mm (Luyckx 1966, Gernet & Hollwich 1971, Larsen 1971).

In *premature children* (Table 2) the eye is myopic (Gleiss & Pau 1952, Graham & Gray 1963, Grignolo & Rivara 1968). This myopia is caused by a still incomplete development of a spherical highly refractive thick lens. It is directly proportional to the degree of prematurity: − 6.24D at six months and − 1.015D at eight months (Rivara & Gemme 1965, Grignolo & Rivara 1968). In premature children, the eye length is very short: 12.08 mm at six months (Grignolo & Rivara 1968).

Tane, *et al.* (1979), examining 22 eyes of premature children, found a mean refraction of − 5.75D. The axial length was shorter than in myopia of the same degree (22.16 mm), the lens thicker than normal (4.38 mm) and the corneal curvature increased (7.28 mm).

138

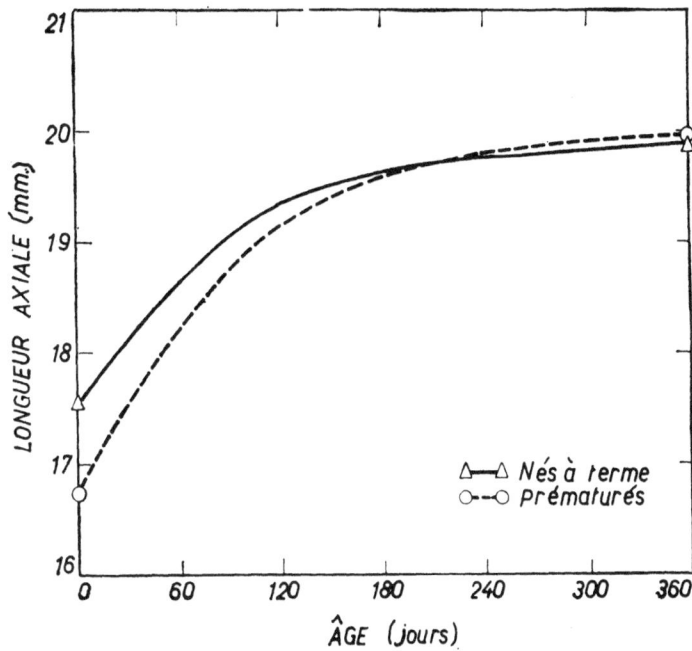

Fig. 3. Axial eye length (mm) in premature newborns and fullborn children (after Grignolo & Rivara 1968).

Table 1.

At birth	
Eye length	16.40–17.85 mm
Anterior chamber depth	2.38– 2.90 mm
Lens thickness	3.60– 3.65 mm
Vitreous length	10.22–10.80 mm

Table 2.

Prematurity (6 months)	
Myopia	– 6.24 D
Eye length	12.08 mm
4 Months after birth	= Full term children

Fledelius (1976) studied the influence of prematurity (or low birth weight) on the subsequent development and function of the eyes: 302 children whose birthweight was less than 2000 g, were examined at the age of ten years. He found 13.3% myopias, while in a control group it was only 9.3%. In the premature group the axial eye length was 0.3 mm shorter, the corneal curvature 0.18 mm smaller and the lens significantly thicker, while the anterior chamber depth was the same in both groups. On a whole, the eyes of premature children were harmoniously smaller than the eyes of mature children (Table 3).

Table 3.

Prematurity
Harmonious small eye
Axial length shorter
Lens thicker (highly refractive)
Corneal curvature increased

After birth the eye becomes progressively emmetropic and later on even hypermetropic because of a fast reduction of the lens refractive power, although the axial length increases. At 4 months after birth there is no more difference between eyes of premature and full-term children (Rivara & Gemme 1965, Grignolo & Rivara 1968).

In full-term newborns (Table 4) the *eye length* increases especially during the first 18 months of life (± 3.7 mm) (Gernet & Hollwich 1968). Larsen (1971) found an increase of 1.4 mm/year from birth to the 3rd year of age. From the 3rd year to the 6th year Delmarcelle & Luyckx (1971) found an increase of 0.4 mm/year and from the 6th till the 15th year 0.1 mm/year.

Table 4.

Growth	
Eye length increases	0– 3Y, 1.4 mm/year 3– 6Y, 0.4 mm/year 6–15Y, 0.1 mm/year
Lens thickness unchanged from 0 to 20Y, Then increases 0.2 mm every decade	
Anterior chamber depth	2.0 mm at birth 3.25 mm at adulthood then decreases 0.1mm per decade

The anterior segment increases also progressively, especially during the first year of life (0.9 mm) (Gernet & Hollwich 1971, Larsen 1971). The normal growth of the eye is finished between 13 and 15 years of age (Delmarcelle & Luyckx 1971, Larsen 1971). In conclusion, the normal lengthening especially of the posterior eye segment, is more or less 2% a year and ends shortly after ten years of age (Saraux & Bechetoille 1972).

The *lens thickness* remains unchanged from birth till the age of 20 (François & Goes 1970, Gernet 1970). Afterwards there is an increase of 0.2 mm every decade.

The *anterior chamber depth* increases progressively from birth (2.0 mm) till adulthood (3.25 mm). Afterwards it decreases 0.1 mm every decade (Delmarcelle & Luyckx, 1971).

The *eye length* becomes shorter with age, the values being between 0.4 and 0.9 mm (Gernet 1964, François & Goes 1971, Leighton & Tamlinson 1972).

140

4. EMMETROPIA (Table 5)

It is a fact that (1) the total refraction of the eye changes only a little after birth, although its dimensions are very strongly modified, and (2) that there is an impressive range of eyelengths in emmetropic adult eyes, between 20.12 and 25.94 mm, the mean value being 23.50 mm (Delmarcella, *et al*. 1976), although emmetropic eyes of the same subject have the same eye length (Karantinos, *et al*. 1974). On the other hand, the eye-length is shorter in women than in men, the difference being between 0.21 and 0.77 mm (Gernet 1964, 1969, Nover & Grote 1965, François & Goes 1968, 1970, Fridman 1968, Fledelius 1976). This sex difference exists also in ametropia (Larsen 1971, Levchenko & Drukman 1976).

Table 5.

Emmetropisation

Excess of emmetropia in population
Eye length varies in emmetropia
Corrective factor depending on lens
Refractive power
Decrease of this refractive power
Exists also in ametropia

We know that there is an excess of emmertropic eyes in the normal population (Straub 1909, Wibaut 1926, Betsch 1929) and that the eye length varies enormously in emmetropic eyes. Therefore, there must be a corrective factor depending on the lens refractive power (Tron 1929, Strömberg 1936, Stenström 1946). This *emmetropisation* was first demonstrated by Gernet (1964) and afterwards by Franceschetti & Gernet (1965), Friedman & Savitskaya (1966), Franceschetti & Luyckx (1967), François & Goes (1968, 1973) & Friedman (1969), who found a different lens refractive power according to the eyelength. It could be demonstrated that an eye length between 20.12 and 25.94 mm may still result in emmetropia because of different lens refractive powers. This phenomenon is also observed in ametropia, so that a partial compensation of the different eye lengths either in hypermetropia or myopia is found following a decrease or an increase of the lens refractive power (Franceschetti & Gernet 1965, Franceschetti & Luyckx 1967, François & Goes 1968, 1970, 1973, Fridman 1968) and that finally the total degree of the ametropia is diminished. The emmetropisation exists also in premature children: as we have already said, there is a fast decrease of the lens refractive power from 96D at six months prematurity till 33D three months later (Grignolo & Rivara 1968), so that a premature myopic eye becomes emmetropic, although the eye length increases with age.

5. AMETROPIA (Table 6)

Ultrasonography confirmed the known fact that the anterior chamber is shallower in hypermetropia than in myopia. Extreme differences up to

Table 6.

Ametropia

	Hyperopia	Myopia
Anterior chamber	Shallower	Deeper
Lens thickness	Same	Same
Eye length	Shorter	Longer

Changes of posterior segment
1D myopia = elongation 0.4 mm
1D hyperopia = shortening 0.4 mm

0.8 mm may be observed between both refractive states. The change in depth does not progress with the ametropia value (Delmarcelle, *et al.* 1976).

There is no significant change in *lens thickness* according to the ametropia and most authors found the same lens thickness increase with age in ametropia and emmetropia (Luyckx & Weekers 1966, Delmarcelle & Luyckx 1971), although Levchenko & Druckman (1976) found sometimes a thinner lens in myopia. The different lens refractive powers must be explained by a change in curvature or index.

The changes responsible for the degree of ametropia involve especially the *posterior segment of the eye* (Fig. 4 and 5). There is a highly significant negative correlation between the axial length and the refraction (Jansson

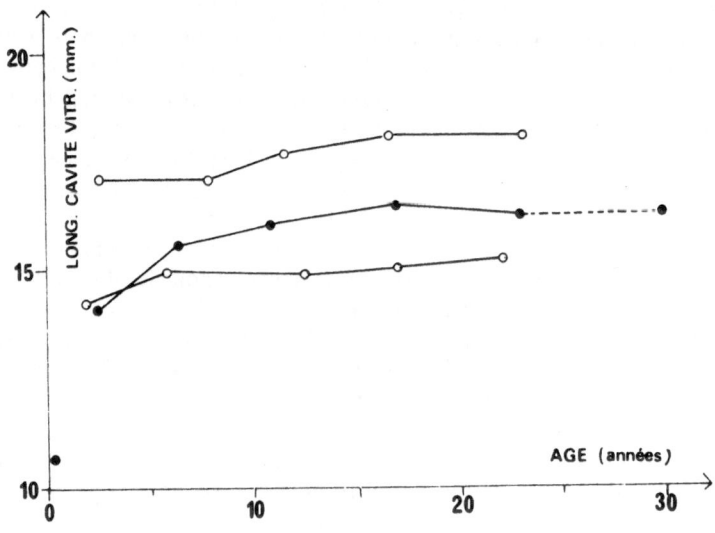

Influence de l'âge et de la réfraction sur la longueur de la cavité vitréenne :

● yeux emmétropes;

○ yeux myopes;

◐ yeux hypermétropes.

Fig. 4. Influence of age and refraction on the vitreous length (after Luyckx & Delmarcelle 1973).

142

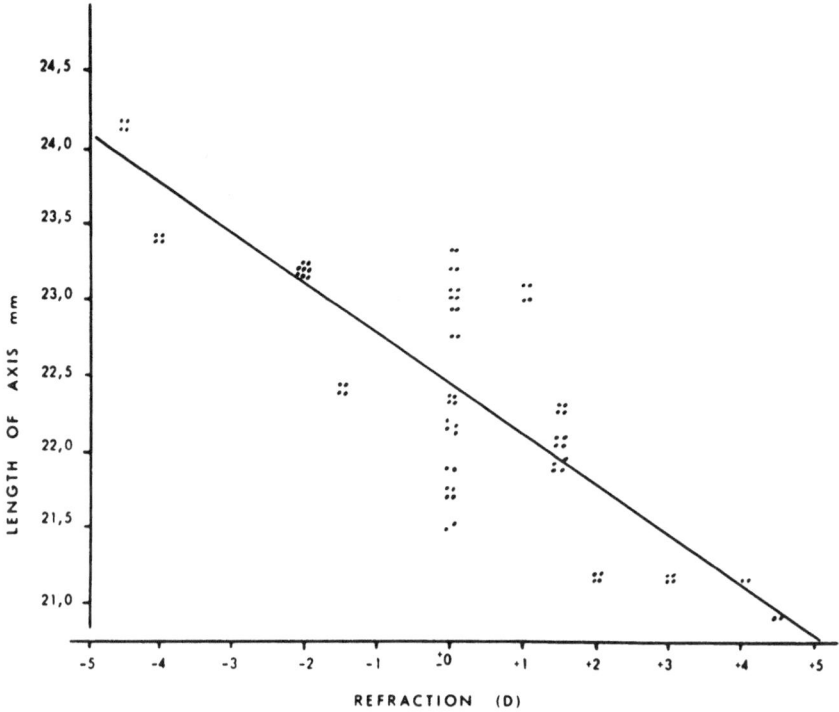

Fig. 5. Correlation between the axial length and the refraction in 12 years old girls. R: — 0.824, Y: 22.44–0.32 mm (after Larsen 1971).

1963, Rivara & Cambiaggi 1964, Luyckx & Weekers 1966, Franceschetti *et al.* 1968, Gernet 1969, Larsen 1971, Machekin 1972) and this correlation is already present in the immediate postnatal period (Larsen 1971). At the age of 1–3 years the eye length is in myopic eyes 0.35 mm longer and in hypermetropic eyes 0.25 mm shorter than in emmetropic eyes. Moreover, it seems that a myopic eye is still becoming longer, when the normal eye growth stops in emmetropic eyes (11–13 years), while the growth of a hypermetropic eye stops earlier before the age of ten years. Finally, Fledelius (1979) examined 50 high myopic eyes at the age of 24 years. He found no significant difference between the anterior segment of low or high myopic eyes.

Ultrasonography can differentiate the various refraction entities according to the *causative factor* (axial, index and curvature ametropia). The correlation between the axial length and the degree of myopia can be calculated and it has been shown that one diopter of myopia corresponds to an elongation of ± 0.40 mm in juvenile as well as in adult eyes (Franceschetti & Luyckx 1967, Fridman 1968, Franceschetti, *et al.* 1968, François & Goes 1968, 1973). In hypermetropia, the eye is shorter, but the correlation between the degree of ametropia and the axial length is the same as in myopia (Franceschetti & Gernet 1965, Luyckx 1967, Fridman 1968, François & Goes 1970, Gavrilenko 1974).

The correlations between the refraction and the vitreous are the same as between the refraction and the eye length, because the changes responsible for the ametropia are especially pronounced in the posterior segment.

Ultrasound oculometry demonstrated in vivo the elongated form of the eye in high myopia (Gernet & Boateng 1967, Mozherenkov 1974, François & Goes 1976, Karetskaya, et al. 1976). This fact is particularly demonstrative in cases of posterior staphyloma (François, et al. 1969, Fledelius 1970, Makabe 1975).

In low ametropia there exists a harmonious increase or decrease of the eye volume, while in high ametropia there is a dysharmonious change of the eye form with an elongated posterior segment in myopia and a spherical eyeball in hypermetropia.

In emmetropia, the axial length and the transversal diameter of the eye have nearly the same value, the quotient being 1.015. In high myopia the quotient is 1.186 and in high hypermetropia only 0.969 (Gernet & Boateng 1967).

In our series of 126 myopic eyes (Table 7) we found an axial myopia in 92% of cases, a compound myopia (curved cornea and elongated vitreous) in 4% of the cases, a corneal myopia in 2.4% of cases and a mixed myopia (flat cornea and elongated vitreous) in 1% of cases (François & Goes 1975).

Table 7.

126 myopic eyes	
Axial myopia	92%
Compound myopia	4%
Corneal myopia	2.4%
Mixed myopia	1%

6. CATARACT (Table 8)

In cataract a mean decrease of 0.60 mm in the lens thickness is mostly observed (Delmarcelle & Luyckx 1970, 1971) (Fig. 6). But when the cataract is intumescent, there is of course an increase of the lens thickness and a decrease of the anterior chamber depth (Fig. 7). This biometric study could be helpful for the prevention of qlaucoma.

Cataractous lenses have also a different ultrasound velocity varying from 1665 m/sec to 1691 m/sec (Jansson & Sundmark 1962, Jansson & Köck 1962, Nover & Glandschneider 1965), what implies a maximal measurement

Table 8.

Cataract
Decrease in lens thickness
Change in ultrasound velocity

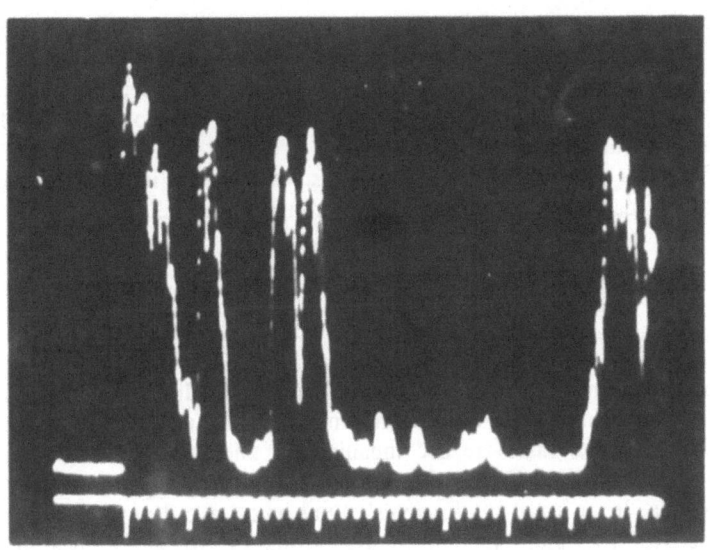

Fig. 6. Cataract with secondary phacolytic glaucoma (Po 40 mm Hg) in a 67 years old man. Anterior chamber depth: 4.13 mm. Lens thickness: 2.12 mm. Vitreous length: 17.2 mm. Axial eye length: 24.0 mm (pers. obs.).

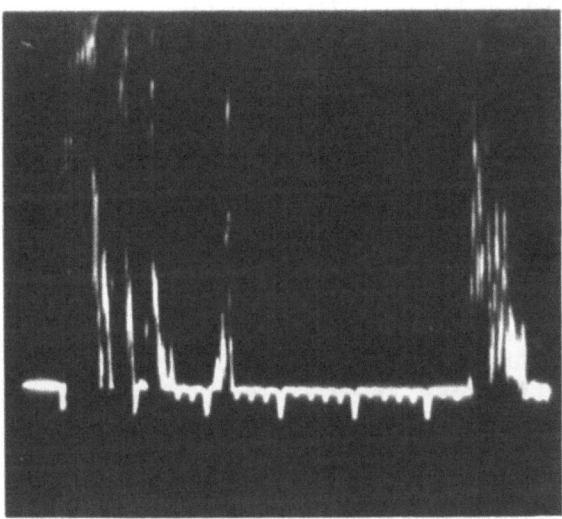

Fig. 7. Intumescent cataract with glaucoma, (Po 35 mm Hg) in a 54 years old woman. Anterior chamber depth: 2.4 mm. Lens thickness: 6.04 mm. Axial eye length: 26.3 mm (pers. obs.).

error of 0.3 mm for a lens of 4.0 mm. Coleman, *et al.* (1975) admit an ultrasound velocity of 1629 m/sec in cataract lenses, which have a lower density than normal lenses, although in the case of very thin sclerotic lenses,

145

they admit a velocity of 1660 m/sec. Forgie, *et al.* (1979) found that the more dense the cataract is, the lower the velocity. In any case more studies on the ultrasound velocity in cataractous eyes have to be scientifically carried out in order to be able to calculate more precisely the power needed for an intraocular implant lens.

Fledelius & Larsen (1979) found also a decrease in lens thickness of unilateral cataractous eyes (24 eyes, range from 0.2 to 1.6 mm, mean 0.6 mm).

7. MICROCORNEA AND MICROPHTHALMOS

Before ultrasonography the diagnosis of microphthalmia was only based on the corneal diameter. At the present time we know, nevertheless, that not all the microcornea cases are accompanied by microphthalmos (Fig. 8) and vice-versa. In 1964, Gernet demonstrated for the first time a real micro-phthalmia in a case of François' syndrome: eye length of both eyes respectively 14.9 and 14.5 mm, hypermetropia of 26D and corneal diameter of 9.0 mm.

The first cases of microcornea without microphthalmia but with coloboma were diagnosed ultrasonographically by Gernet (1965) & Itin (1965). In 1965, Franceschetti & Gernet reported five cases of microphthalmia without microcornea in eyes affected by a tapeto-retinal degeneration. On the contrary, François & Goes (1974) observed the association of an important shortening of the axial length (20.6 and 20.72 mm) with an hypermetropia of + 9.5D and 8.50D and a megalocornea (corneal diameter of 13 mm). Boynton and Purnell (1975) diagnosed also a bilateral microphthalmia with microcornea in high hypermetropia (+ 16.75D and + 16.50D).

During the last seven years we have examined 79 eyes with *microcornea* and classified them according to the oculometric measurements and the associated disease (Table 9). In 33 eyes the microcornea was associated with a congenital cataract. In half of these cases the anterior segment was reduced,

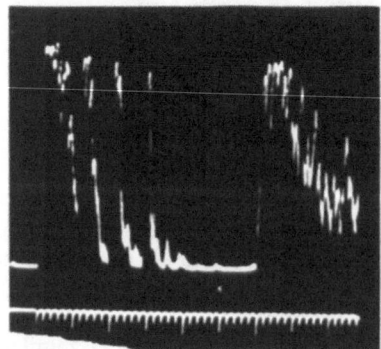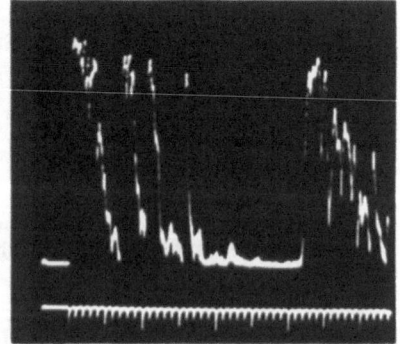

Fig. 8. Microcornea (9.5 mm) with uveal coloboma in a 5 months old child. Axial eye length: 19.73 mm, which is longer than the normal value at this age (pers. obs.).

146

Table 9.

Microcornea (79 cases)	
With congenital cataract	33 eyes
With coloboma	26 eyes
With persistant hyperplastic primary vitreous	5 eyes
With retrolental fibroplasia	7 eyes
With Francois syndrome	4 eyes
With congenital toxoplasmosis	4 eyes

but the lens thickness was mostly normal, although sometimes very small (extreme value 1.17 mm). In 12 eyes the vitreous length was diminished, in 14 normal and in seven increased. In 12 of these 33 eyes we found a real microphthalmos, but in seven of them there was an increase in the axial length, which was sometimes important: in a rubeola case an axial length of 24.88 and 27.68 mm could be measured.

In 26 eyes there was an association of microcornea and coloboma. In half of these cases a zonular or nuclear cataract was also present. The anterior segment was normal or reduced, the lens thickness slightly increased and the axial length normal in more than 50% of the cases. The eye length varied between 16.66 and 28.64 mm, demonstrating a pseudo-microphthalmia or an anterior microphthalmos in 20 out of the 26 eyes. In five cases a persistent hyperplastic primary vitreous was responsible for the microcornea. The axial length was normal in four of them. In seven cases there was a retrolental fibroplasia. In nearly half of these cases the axial length was shortened.

In two cases of François' syndrome the axial length was normal or even increased. In one of these cases the increased eye length (27.94 and 25.66 mm) was associated with an important thickening of the lens (5.77 and 5.54 mm), a very short anterior segment (2 and 2.1 mm), a high myopia ($-16.5D$) and a closed angle glaucoma. In 2 cases there was a congenital toxoplasmosis. In one of them a high myopia was found ($-11.5D$).

This personal statistics shows that a classification of microcornea and microphthalmia and a better understanding of the underlying factors is only possible thanks to ultrasonographic oculometry.

8. MEGALOCORNEA

In eyes with *megalocornea* without ocular hypertension, the biometric measurements show an important change of the anterior segment, the lens thickness and the vitreous length remaining normal. We could distinguish two entities (Table 10):

Table 10.

Megalocornea with:
(1) Increased anterior corneal curvature radius, normal anterior chamber depth, normal lens thickness, normal vitreous length
(2) Anterior megalophthalmos, elongation of anterior segment, normal lens thickness, normal vitreous length

(1) Simple megalocornea with an increased anterior corneal curvature radius, the anterior chamber depth, the lens thickness and the vitreous length remaining normal (Delmarcelle, *et al*. 1976).

(2) Anterior megalophthalmos with an important elongation of the anterior segment, the lens thickness and the vitreous length remaining normal. We could examine nine eyes with such an anterior megalophthalmos. We found an extreme anterior chamber depth of 5.7 mm, but the vitreous length was normal (extreme values 12.42 to 15.82 mm).

9. PRIMARY GLAUCOMA

In *congenital glaucoma* (buphthalmos) the increase of the eye volume results from a genetic factor (megalocornea with a flat corneal curvature radius) and from an acquired factor, which is the distention of the scleral wall under the influence of the ocular hypertension (Luyckx & Delmarcelle 1968, Gernet & Hollwich 1969 Ustimenko 1972). The posterior eye segment is involved as well as the anterior segment and there is a parallelism between the elongation of the eye and the duration or the severity of the ocular hypertension. Consequently, there is a myopia, which is partly compensated by an increase of the corneal curvature, the lens thickness remaining normal (Table 11). In an ultrasonographic study, where the vitreous growth was compared with age in 108

Table 11.

Buphthalmos

(1) Anterior and posterior segments involved
(2) Parallelism between elongation and duration or severity of hypertension
(3) Myopia

normal eyes and 81 buphthalmic eyes, the close correlation between the duration of the ocular hypertension and the vitreous length was graphically illustrated by Gernet & Hollwich (1969, 1971). The lens thickness was usually normal and similar in both groups. In the buphthalmic eyes there was an important elongation of the anterior and of the posterior eye segment, as compared with the normal eye growth. The consequence was a myopia, which was partly compensated by an increase of the corneal curvature.

Buschman & Bluth (1974), Machekin & Krivolpolova (1979) used the axial eye length measurement for the postoperative control of buphthalmic eyes. They observed a stretching of the posterior segment when the intraocular pressure was insufficiently reduced.

Zingirian & Rossi (1975) studied 14 buphthalmic eyes and found a frequently unsuspected aniseiconia, which causes amblyopia. Therefore, a biometric evaluation of these myopic eyes should regularly be carried out.

In *open angle glaucoma* (Table 12), the axial length, the anterior chamber depth, the lens thickness, the corneal curvature and the refraction remain normal (Tane, *et al*. 1973, Delmarcelle, *et al*. 1976), although Tomlinson & Philips (1970) found a positive correlation between the intraocular pressure and the eye length ($r = + 0.367$) in 75 adult subjects. Machekin (1972) made the same observation.

Table 12.

Open angle glaucoma	
Axial length	
Anterior chamber depth	
Lens thickness	Normal
Corneal curvature	
Refraction	

In *closed angle glaucoma*, (Fig. 9; Table 13) ultrasonography is very important. The most obvious fact is a *shallow anterior chamber* (2.5 mm or less). Moreover, the *lens thickness is increased*, the mean increase being 0.55 mm (Gernet & Jürgens 1965, Luyckx-Bacchus & Weekers 1966, Hollwich & Boateng, 1969, Lowe 1969, 1972, Weekers, *et al.* 1969, Storey & Philips 1971, Tomlinson & Leighton 1973, Tane *et al.* 1973, Machekin 1975, Massin, Lesroux-Lesjardins, *et al.* 1977). The situation becomes critical, when the ratio lens thickness versus axial eyelength is more than 1/4.

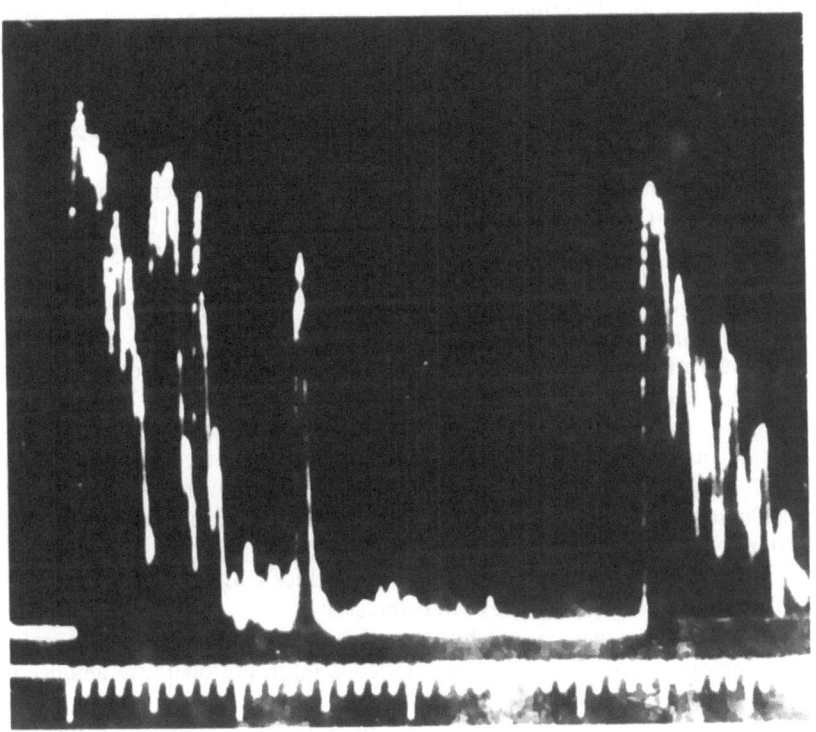

Fig. 9. Acute closed angle glaucoma in a 21 years old woman with a congenitally thick lens, resulting in a high myopia of − 14d, and a shallow anterior chamber. Anterior chamber depth: 1.96 mm. Lens thickness: 4.84 mm. Vitreous length: 15.82 mm. Axial eye length: 22.97 mm (Pers. obs.).

Table 13.

Closed angle glaucoma
Occurs in a small eye with
shallow anterior chamber and thick lens
1. Closed angle by abnormal thick lens
2. Closed angle by anterior lens displacement

The *lens* is also *in forward position* (Lowe 1969, Delmarcelle, *et al.* 1969, 1971, Tomlinson & Leighton 1973). The distance between the lens center and the limbus is reduced, because the total eye-length is diminished (Delmarcelle, *et al.* 1976). The mean reduction of the axial eye-length is 1.09 mm according to Lowe (1969), 1.14 mm according to Delmarcelle, *et al.* (1971), 0.52 mm according to Tomlinson & Leighton (1973) and 2.6% according to Alsbink (1973). This shorter eye-length explains the frequency of hypermetropia. The vitreous cavity is also reduced and the difference is at least 1.0 mm (Gernet & Jürgens 1965, Luyckx-Bacchus & Weekers 1967, Hollwich & Boateng 1969, Pelletier 1971).

In conclusion, closed angle glaucoma occurs in a small eye with a shallow anterior chamber and a thick lens. The relative importance of the lens thickness for the determination of the anterior chamber depth has been stressed by Delmarcelle, *et al.* (1969, 1970), who found a 0.37 mm shallowing of the anterior chamber (y) for every mm increase of lens thickness (x) ($Y = 4.44 - 0.37 X$) in 151 emmetropic eyes at the age of 40 years. François & Goes (1976) found the same relationship in 203 emmetropic eyes at the same age ($Y = 4.35 - 0.36 X$).

The lens thickening which may amount to 0.97 mm versus a group of normal eyes (Delmarcelle, *et al.* 1971) is partly caused by an absolute difference of 0.55 mm with a corresponding age group and partly by an age difference. This fact explains the importance of older age in the closed glaucoma group, because with age the lens thickness still increases and surpasses the critical point. Moreover, the lens has a relative forward displacement of 0.35 mm due either to an acquired displacement or to a change in the lens shape with age.

Angle closure glaucoma may be due either to a direct closure of the angle by the lens (lens block) or by a pupillary block, the contact between the lens and the iris being enhanced by the forward position of the lens.

The biometric findings allow to classify closed angle glaucoma in two main groups.

    (1) Closed angle caused by an abnormal thick lens (congenital, excessive growth with age, intumescent cataract).

    (2) Closed angle caused by an anterior lens displacement (congenital ectopia, acquired traumatism, vitreous push, postoperative absence of the anterior chamber).

These causes may be combined with predisposing factors (short eye) and some trigger mechanisms (mydriasis, accommodation), although the essential biometric finding remains the shallow anterior chamber.

An interesting study on *malignant glaucoma* was made by Lesioux-Lesjardins *et al.* (1977), who found in 12 cases (mean age 49½ years) more pronounced characteristics as in closed angle glaucoma, except for the lens thickness, which was normal or reduced (mean 4.2 mm).

In conclusion, at least three factors contribute to the narrowness of the anterior chamber angle, which predisposes to angle closure glaucoma.

(1) The increase of the lens thickness causes on one hand a reduction of the depth of the anterior chamber and on the other hand a shortening of the vitreous length, the change being the same on both sides.

(2) The reduction of the corneal height, which is usually correlated with a reduction of the total volume of the globe (short hypermetropic eye with a mean eye-length of 22.0 mm), with a small vitreous, a small cornea diameter (mean 10.85 mm) and a small anterior (mean 7.64 mm) and posterior corneal radius. While the corneal height is 2.61 mm in normal eyes, it is only 2.27 mm in closed angle glaucoma (Delmarcelle et al. 1976).

(3) The forward position of the lens, due to ageing, has little significance, but in closed angle glaucoma it is usually due to a genetic factor and much more important (difference 0.35 mm).

These three factors may be combined to cause a reduction of the anterior chamber depth, which amounts to 1.19 mm when compared with a normal eye.

10. OPERATIONS

In *retinal detachment surgery* or *cataract surgery*, ultrasonography can of course measure the occasional changes in eye length. More interesting is the calculation of the *refractive indices of the eye components* (Zingarian & Rivara 1971, Gernet 1971), the *total refractive power of the eye* and the *lens refractive power*, according to the formulas of Sorsby *et al.* (1963), Sopanen (1963), Rivara & Zingirian (1963), Gernet (1964, 1965), Gernet & Franceschetti (1964), Belkin, *et al.* (1973), Gernet & Ostholt (1973), Grignolo, *et al.* (1974), Oguchi & Van Balen (1974), Merlin & Rossi (1975). The accuracy can reach ± 0.5 diopter (Gernet & Ostholt 1973).

Consequently, the *optic correction of the aphakic eye* (Elenius & Sopanen, 1963; Gernet & Granceschetti 1964, Gernet & Ostholt 1973, Grignolo, *et al.* 1974, Oguchi & Van Balen 1974) and the *power of the implant lens* can be precisely calculated (Fedorov & Kolinko 1967, Colenbrander 1969, 1973; Gernet 1970; Ostholt, *et al.* 1970, Oguchi & Van Balen 1974, Van der Heyde 1975, Thÿssen 1975). A precision of ± 0.5 diopter can be obtained (Gernet, *et al.* 1970, Oguchi & Van Balen 1974). Since Ostholt & Gernet (1973) developed a formula to calculate the posterior facal length, the measurement of aniseikonia became also possible. The mean posterior focal distance in emmetropia is 21.6 mm (Gernet & Ostholt 1973, 446 eyes).

The calculation of the retinal image size in ametropia or aphakia permitted to Gernet (1974, 1975, 1979) to introduce his combined correction (iseikonic glasses and contact lens). The aniseikonia can so be reduced from 11% to 6% in cases of unilateral aphakia.

The intraocular lens power can also be calculated taking into account the position of the lens, the change in axial length and the posterior focal length (Gernet & Ostholt 1975, Van der Heyde 1975, Binkhorst 1977).

The more anterior position of the lens results in a higher effective power, while the more posterior position results in a lower effective power, the change being 0.5 D for every 0.3 mm difference in position.

The nomogram developed by Van der Heyde (1975) gives an error of 0.25 D for the power of the implanted lens, when there is an error of 0.1 mm in the calculation of the axial length or 0.2 mm in that of the anterior chamber depth or 0.25 D in that of the power of the cornea.

11. BIOMETRIC EFFECTS OF PHARMACODYNAMIC DRUGS

1. Pilocarpine. (Table 14). There exists a definite correlation between the biometric effects of voluntary accommodation and pilocarpine induced accommodation. Abramson *et al.* (1972, 1973, 1974) demonstrated also that in young subjects of 18–30 years of age the shallowing of the anterior chamber (mean − 0.29 mm) was caused by a lens thickening (mean + 0.32 mm) and in some cases by a forward displacement of the lens. In older subjects of 60–80 years of age there is still a shallowing of the anterior chamber (− 0.19 mm). Moreover, there is a positive correlation between the concentrations of pilocarpine (1,4 and 8%) and the changes in the anterior segment.

Table 14.

Pilocarpine
Shallowing of anterior chamber
Lens thickening and lens displacement
Accomodative myopia

2. Aceclidine. François & Goes (1975) compared the biometric effects between aceclidine (glaucostat (R) and pilocarpine. In similar age group subjects (40–45 years) aceclidine, which has the same tension lowering effect, produced much less shallowing of the anterior chamber (0.09 mm versus 0.27 mm), lens thickening (0.07 mm versus 0.24 mm), and myopisation (0.2 D versus 3.0 D) than pilocarpine 2%. Aceclidine is thus a much safer product for the treatment of closed-angle glaucoma with a shallow anterior segment and a thick lens, because it gives much less lens displacement. This fact is illustrated by the observation of Leydhecker (1953), François, *et al.* (1971), and others, who could observe an acute closed angle glaucoma with pupillary block caused by the instillation of pilocarpine in an eye with a shallow anterior chamber (2 mm) and a thick lens (5.5 mm).

3. Ocusert P20. François, *et al.* (1978) compared the side effects of Ocusert P20 and Pilocarpine 2%, which have the same antiglaucoma effect. Accommodative myopia and changes in the anterior chamber depth and the lens thickness were much less pronounced in the group treated by Ocusert

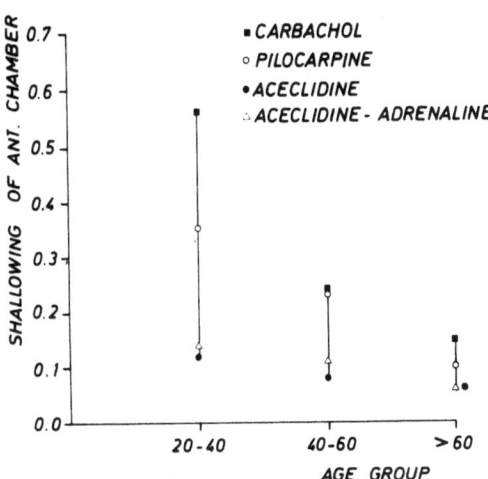

Fig. 10. Influence of different miotics on the depth of the anterior chamber (after François & Goes 1977).

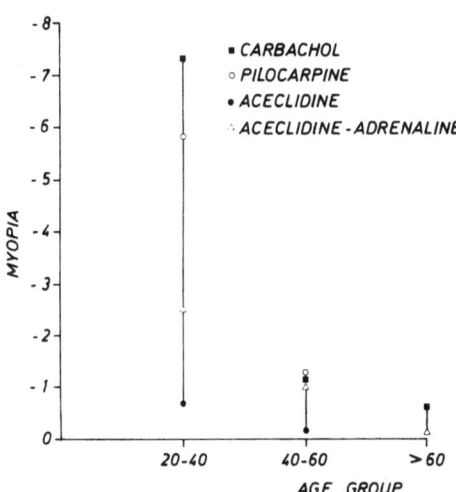

Fig. 11. Influence of different miotics on accomodative myopia (after François Goes 1977).

delivery system P20 than in the group treated by 2% pilocarpine. The mean difference for the shallowing of the anterior chamber was 0.18 mm, for the lens thickening 0.21 mm, and for the accomodative myopia 2.65 diopters. François & Goes (1977) compared also carbachol 3%, aceclidine 2% with adrenaline 1%, pilocarpine 2% and Ocusert P20. Aceclidine had a negligible effect on the ocular parameters, and Carbachol had the strongest side-effects. It caused, together with pilocarpine, an important lens forward displacement, the maximal myopisation being – 11.50 D.

4. Beta blocking agents. François & Goes (1979) studied the biometric effects of timolol. They could not demonstrate any significant change. The maximal changes for the anterior chamber depth and for the eye length never exceeded 0.1 mm.

5. Succinylcholine. The injection of this drug produces a relaxation of the ciliary muscle and the opposite effect of pilocarpine (Abramson 1971): a deepening of the anterior chamber of 0.71 mm, a lens thinning of 0.63 mm, and sometimes a backward displacement of the lens.

6. Accommodation. Coleman (1970) & Manabe (1974) studied the voluntary accommodation mechanism and demonstrated an important forward movement of the lens center in 92% of cases.

7. Parasympathicolytic agents. Atropine causes a relaxation of the ciliary muscle with deepening of the anterior chamber (till 0.38 mm), thinning and sometimes backward displacement of the lens (Bechac 1957; Delmarcelle & Luyckx 1969, 1971, Forsius 1971, Storey & Philips 1971).

8. Diuretic agents. Pallin & Ericson (1965) measured an important lens thickening (0.3 mm) and a myopisation of − 2.5 D after general administration of chlorthalidolone (Hygroton[R]). Acetazolamide (Diamox[R]) may produce a shallowing of the anterior chamber (Kronning 1957).

Vucicevic, *et al.* (1971) demonstrated an important vitreous shortening after administration of osmotic agents. The maximal effect was observed after mannitol administration, the shortening being as important as 30%. François & Goes (1974) studied also the changes after administration of mannitol in normotensive subjects. They could not demonstrate any significative change of the anterior chamber depth, the lens thickness or the vitreous, the maximal differences being 0.1 mm. After 5 min digital massage they could only registrate minor biometric changes, the maximal vitreous shortening being 0.20 mm.

12. PHTYSIS BULBI

Ultrasound biometry may be important in the initial phase of phtysis bulbi, as for example after retinal detachment or vitreous surgery or after ocular injury or severe uveitis, since it is an excellent method for the early determination of eye length shortening. This shortening concerns essentially the vitreous.

13. PSEUDO-EXOPHTHALMOS (Fig. 10)

Ultrasound biometry may become extremely important for the differential diagnosis of exophthalmos, especially in case of cloudy ocular media. Combined with exophthalmometry, the echographic biometry allows the

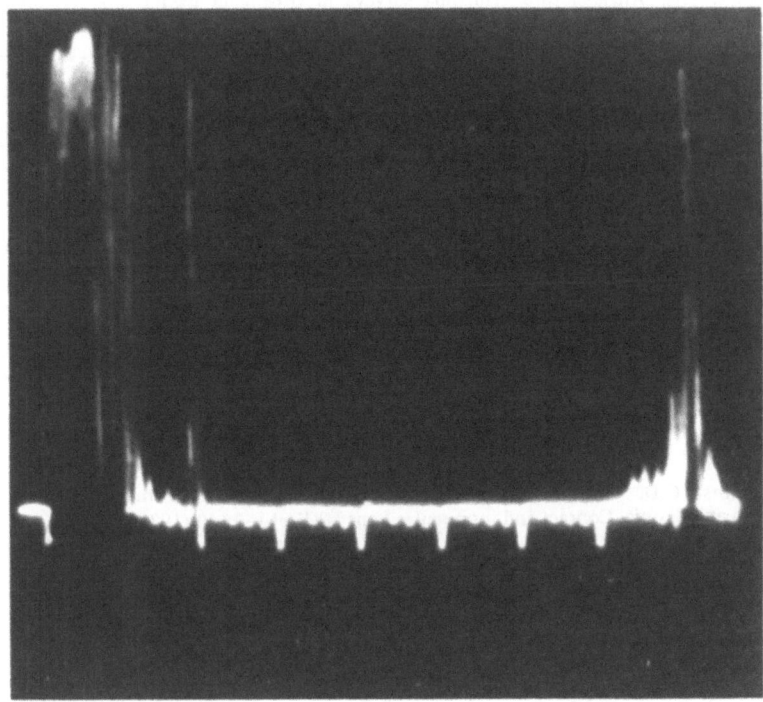

Fig. 10. **Pseudo-exophthalmos.** Nuclear cataract. Exophthalmometry: 27 mm. Axial eye
length: 39.13 mm (Pers. obs.).

determination of the position of the centre of the globe in regard to the outer
orbital rim (Herrmann & Buschmann 1968).

SUMMARY

Ultrasound biometry is of utmost importance in the study of the eye growth,
emmetropia and ametropia, cataract, microcornea and microphthalmos,
megalocornea and buphthalmos, open-angle or closed angle glaucoma, refractive power of the lens and the eye, as well as of the biometric effects of anti-
glaucomatous or other drugs.

REFERENCES

Abramson, D.H. Anterior chamber and lens thickness changes induced by succinylcholine. Arch. Ophthalmol. 86: 643 (1971)
Abramson, D.H., Chang, S., Coleman, J. & Smith, M.E. Pilocarpine-induced lens
changes. An ultrasonic biometric evaluation of dose response. Arch. Ophthalmol. 92:
464 (1974).
Abramson, D.H., Coleman, J., Forbes, M. & Franzen, L. Pilocarpine. Effect on the
anterior chamber and lens thickness. Arch. Ophthalmol. 87: 615 (1972).
Abramson, D.H., Franzen, L.A. & Coleman, J. Pilocarpine in the presbyope. Arch.
Ophthalmol. 89: 100 (1973).

155

Alsbirk, P.H. Angle-closure glaucoma surveys in Greenland Eskimos. A preliminary report. Can. J. Ophthalmol. 8: 260 (1973).

Araki, M. Studies on refractive components of human eye by means of ultrasonic echogram. Report I. Accuracy of the measurement of ocular axial length by ultrasonic echography. Jap. J. Clin. Ophthalmol. 15: 111 (1961).

Babel, J., Panarello, A. & Psilas, K. La biométrie oculaire dans les cataractes congénitales. In: Siduo round table (Massin M. & Poujol, J., eds.) Paris: Centre National d'ophtal. des Quinze-Vingts (1974) p. 11.

Baum, G. The effect of ultrasonic radiation upon the eye and ocular adnexa. Am. J. Opthalmol. 42: 696 (1956).

Baum, G. An evaluation of ultrasonic techniques used in measurements of eye size. Am. J. Ophthalmol. 64: 926 (1967).

Bechac, G. Contribution à l'étude de la profondeur de la chambre antérieure. Variations physiologiques et au cours des amétropies. Thèse, Toulouse, 1–73 (1957).

Bechetoille, A. & Saraux, H. Biométrie oculaire ultrasonique. Etude de 100 yeux appartenant à une population homogène jeune. Ann. Oculistique, 203: 131 (1970).

Belkin, M., Ticho, U., Susal, A. & Levinson, A. Ultrasonography in the refraction of aphakic infants. Brit. J. Ophthalmol. 57: 845 (1973).

Betsch, A. Über die menschliche Refraktionskurve. Klin. Mbl. Augenheilk. 82: 365 (1929).

Binkhorst, C.D. Where contactology and pseudopathology meet, with special reference to aniseikonia. Contact and intraocular Lens Medical J. 3: 40 (1977).

Binkhorst, C.D. & Loones, L.H. Intraocular Lens Power. Trans. Am. Acad. Ophthalmol. Otolaryng. 81: 70 (1976).

Boynton, J. and Purnell, E. Microphthalmos without microcornea associated with unusual papillomacular retinal folds and high hypertropia. Am. J. Ophthalmol. 79: 820 (1965).

Buschmann, W. Technische Fortschritte in der ophthalmologischen Ultraschalldiagnostik. Wiss. Zbl. Ernst Moritz Arndt Univ., Greifswald 1: 59 (1963).

Buschmann, W. Die Ultraschall Exophthalmometrie. In: Diagnostica Ultrasonica in Ophthalmologia (Massin M. & Poujol J. eds.), Paris: Centre National Ophtal. Quinze Vingts (1973) p. 303.

Buschmann, W. and Bluth, K. – Regelmässique echographische Messung der Achsenlänge des Auges zur Kontrolle der Druckregulierung bei Hydrophthalmie. Klin. Mbl. Augenheilk., 165, 878–886, (1974).

Coleman, D.J. – Unified model for accommodative mechanism. Amer. J. Ophthal., 69, 1063 (1970).

Coleman, D.J., Lizzi, F.L., Franzen L. & Abramson D. – In Ultrasonography in ophthalmology. François J. et Goes F. (eds.) Bibl. Ophthal., Basel, 83, 246, (1975).

Colenbrander, M.C. On the measurement of the power of the lens and the accommodation. Ophthalmologica, 99: 402 (1940).

Colenbrander, M.C. In: (H. Gernet & J.G.F. Worst, eds.) Klinische Oculometrie und Linseneinplanzung nach Binkhorst (1973).

Collins, Roy. Lond. Ophthal. Hosp. Rep. 13: 81 (1890).

Delmarcelle, Y., Collignon, J. & Luyckx, J. La profondeur de la chambre antérieure de l'oeil normal et ses facteurs constituants. Bull Soc. Belge Ophtal. 152: 447 (1969).

Delmarcelle, Y., Collignon, J. & Luyckx, J. Rôle de la cornée et du cristallin sur la biométrie de la chambre antérieure du sujet normal. Arch. Ophtal. Paris, 30: 291 (1970).

Delmarcelle, Y., Collignon, J., Luyckx, J. & Weekers, R. Etude Biométrique du globe oculaire dans le glaucome à angle fermé. Bull. et Mém. Soc. Franç. Ophtal. 84: 449 (1971).

Delmarcelle, Y. & Luyckx-Bacus, J. Influence de la cataracte sénile sur l'épaisseur du cristallin et la profondeur de la chambre antérieure. Bull. Soc. Belge Ophtal. 155: 465 (1970).

Delmarcelle, Y. & Luyckx-Bacus, J. Evolution biométrique de la chambre antérieure chez l'enfant. Etude de 1960 globes. Bull. Soc. belge Ophtal. 158: 451 (1971).

Delmarcelle, Y., François, J., Goes, F., et al. Biométrie oculaire clinique. Bull. Soc. Belge Ophtal. 172: 1–608 (1976).

156

Elenius, V. & Sopanen, V. Power of the correcting lens of the aphakic eye as calculated from the keratometric measurement of the corneal radius and ultrasonically measured axial length of the eye. Acta Ophthalmol., Kbh. 41: 71 (1963).

Enoch, J., Rabinowicz, I. & Campos, E. Visual correction of infants with sensory deprivation amblyopia, post surgical management in unilateral aphakia. In: Diagnostica ultrasonica in Ophthalmologia; Gernet H., Münster: R.A. Remy Verlag (1979) p. 209.

Federov, N., Kolinko, A.I. & Kolinko, A.I. Estimation of optical power of the intraocular lens. Vestn. Oftal., 80: 27 (1967).

Flament, J. Aspects échographiques des poches sclérales. Etude expérimentale (note préliminaire). Bull. Soc. Ophtal., France, 70: 165 (1970).

Flament, J. Etude opticoéchographique des modifications biométriques de l'axe antéropostérieur de l'oeil provoquées par quelques techniques de la chirurgie choriorétinienne. Arch. Ophtal., Paris, 33: 397 (1973).

Flament, J. & Gerhard, J.D. Influence biométrique respective et comparative de quelques techniques de chirurgie chorio-rétinienne. In: Ultrasonography in ophthalmology (J. François & F. Goes eds.) Bibl. Ophthal., Basel, 83: 328 (1975).

Fledelius, H. Ultrasound (A-mode) in a case of nasal posterior scleral ectasy. Acta Ophthal., Kbh. 48: 502 (1970).

Fledelius. H. Prematurity and the eye. Copenhagen: J.J. Trykteknik ALS (1976).

Fledelius, H. Oculometry in high myopia in a representative sample of young adults aged 24. In: Diagnostica Ultrasonica in Ophthalmologia (H. Gernet, ed.) Münster: R.A. Remy Verlag (1979) p. 195.

Fledelius, H. & Alsbirk, P.H. Comparative ultrasound oculometry. In: Ultrasonography in ophthalmology (J. François & F. Goes, eds.) Bibl. Ophthal., Basel, 83: 263 (1975).

Fledelius H. & Laursen A. Cataract and lens thinning. In: Diagnostica Ultrasonica in ophthalmologia (H. Gernet ed.) Münster: R.A. Remy Verlag (1979) p. 184.

Franceschetti, A. & Gernet, H. Diagnostic ultrasonique d'une microphtalmie sans microcornée, avec macrophakie, haute hypermétropie associée à une dégénérescence tapéto-rétinienne, une disposition glaucomateuse et des anomalies dentaires. Nouveau syndrome familial. Arch. Ophtal., Paris, 25: 105 (1965).

Franceschetti, A. & Gernet, H. Importance of ultrasonic echography for measurements of the optical components of the eye. Trans. Am. Acad. Ophthalmol. Otolaryng. 69: 465 (1965).

Franceschetti, A. & Gernet, H. Über optische Grössen bei leichter und höher Myopie auf Grund echografischer Befunde. Graefe's Arch. Ophthalmol. 168: 1 (1965).

Franceschetti, A. & Luyckx, J. Etude de l'effet emmétropisant du cristallin par la méthode d'échographie ultrasonique. Ann. Oculistique 200: 177 (1967).

Franceschetti, A. Th., Linder, A. & Franceschetti, A. New results concerning the problem of axial lengths of the eye in anisometropia. In: Diagnostica Ultrasonica in Ophthalmologia, (J. Vanysek, ed.) Brno: Universita J.E. Purkinje (1968) p. 235.

François, J. & Goes, F. L'ultrasonographie dans le diagnostic des affections oculaires. Possibilité et limitations de la technique. Bull. Soc. belge Ophtal. 150: 600 (1968).

François, J. & Goes, F. Comparative study of ultrasonic biometry of emmetropes and myopes with special regard to the heredity of myopia. In: Ophthalmic Ultrasound (Gitter K., Keeney A., Sarin L. & Meyer D., eds.) New York: Mosby Co., (1969) p. 165.

François, J. & Goes, F. Etude échographique de la myopie. Bull. Soc. belge Ophtal. 154: 415 (1970).

François, J. & Goes, F. Oculometry in emmetropia and ametropia. In: Ultrasonographia Medica (Böck J. & Ossoinig K., eds.,) Wien: Verlag der Wiener Med. Akademie, (1971) p. 473

François, J. & Goes, F. Ultrasonography in pediatric ophthalmology. J. Ped. Ophthalmol. 8: 221 (1972).

François, J. & Goes, F. Biométrie de la myopie. Ophthalmologica, Basel, 147: 49 (1973).

François, J. & Goes, F. Biométrie de la myopie juvénile. In: Diagnostica Ultrasonica in Ophthalmologia (Massin M. & Poujol J., eds.) Paris: Centre National d'Ophtal. des Quinze-Vingts (1973) p. 277.

157

François, J. & Goes, F. Ultrasonic Biometry in ophthalmology. In: Ultrasonics in Medicine, M. De Vlieger, D.N. White & V.R. McReady, Amsterdam: Excerpta Medica (1974) p. 128.
François, J. & Goes, F. Oculometry of progressive myopia. In: Ultrasonography in Ophthalmology. François J. and Goes F., Bibl. Ophthal., Basel, Karger, 83: 277 (1975)
François, J. & Goes, F. Ultrasonographic comparative study of the effect of pilocarpine and aceclidine on the eye components. Ophthalmologica, Basel, 168: 299 (1974).
François, J. & Goes, F. Diagnostic ultrasound in ophthalmology. In: Present and future of diagnostic ultrasound (I. Donald & Stevi, eds.) Amsterdam: Kooyker Scientific Publications (1976) p. 109.
François, J. & Goes, F. Ultrasonographic study of the effect of Timolol on the eye components. In: Diagnostica Ultrasonographica in Ophthalmologia (Gernet H., ed.) Münster: R.A. Remy Verlag (1979) p. 204.
François, J., Goes, F. & Stockmans, L. Glaucome aigu secondaire à une instillation de pilocarpine. Ann. d'Oculistique, 204: 481 (1971).
Fridman, F.E. Bedeutung der Ultraschallbiometrie beim Studium der Anatomooptischen Elemente der Augen verschiedener Refraktionen. In: Diagnostica Ultrasonica in Ophthalmologia, (Vanysek J., ed.) Brno: Universita J. Purkinje, (1968) p. 259.
Fridman, F.E. & Savitskaya, N.F. Ultrasound Biometry in the study of anatomooptic elements of the eye in myopia. Vestn. Oftal. 79: 30 (1966).
Gavrilenko, I.N. Ultrasonic Biometry of eyes with differing refraction. Oftal. Zh. 29: 61 (1974).
Gerke, E. Ultraschallechographische Untersuchungen bei Scleraeinfaltungen. In: Diagnostica Ultrasonica in Ophthalmologia (H. Gernet, ed.) Münster: R.A. Remy Verlag (1979) p. 107.
Gernet, H. Über Achsenlänge und Brechkraft emmetroper lebender Augen. Graefe's Arch. Ophthalmol. 166: 424 (1964).
Gernet, H. Achsenlänge und Refraktion lebender Augen von Neugeborenen. Graefe's Arch. Ophthalmol. 166: 530 (1964).
Gernet, H. Ueber Mikrophthalmus, Macuaveränderung und Refraktion bei einem Fall von Dysostosis mandibulo-facialis. Klin. Mbl. Auganheilk. 144: 887 (1964).
Gernet, H. Microcornée sans microphtalmie. Bull. et Mém. Soc. Franç. Ophtal. (178) 368 (1965).
Gernet, H. Klinische Ultraschalluntersuchungen an Emmetropen – Emmetropisation und Akkommodationsbreite. Wiss. Z. Humboldt-Univ., Berlin (14) 201 (1965).
Gernet, H. Datensammlung in der klinischen Oculometrie. Doc. Ophthal., (27) 42 (1969).
Gernet, H. Résultats oculométriques à propos du glaucome infantile. Bull. et Mém. Soc. franç. Ophtal. (92) 41 (1969).
Gernet, H. Oculometriedaten bei Augengesunden. Ber. dtsch. Ophthal. Ges. (70) 597 (1969).
Gernet, H. Valeur de base en oculométrie clinique. Bull. et Mém. Soc. franç. Ophtal. (83) 379 (1970).
Gernet, H. Oculométrie zur Erkennung von Anomalien der Bulbusdimension. In: Ultrasonographia Medica, (Böck J. & Ossoinig K. eds.) Wien, Verlag der Wiener Akademie (1971) p. 455.
Gernet, H. Neue Entwicklungen am Echometrie und Oculometrie. Die Augenseitige Optik. In: Siduo. Table ronde, (Massin M. & Poujol J. eds.) Paris, Centre nat. Ophtal. des Quinze-Vingts, (1974) p. 3.
Gernet, H. Objective Aniseikoniemessung. In: Ultrasonography in Ophthalmology, (François J. & Goes F., eds.) Bibl. Ophthal., Basel (83) 294 (1975).
Gernet, H. Kontaktlinsen, Brillen, Kombinationen bei einseitiger Aphakie jüngener Patienten. In:Diagnostica Ultrasonica in Ophthalmologia, (Gernet H., ed.) Münster, R.A. Remy Verlag (1979) p. 245.
Gernet, H. Kontaktlinsen, Brillen, Kombinationen bei einseitiger Aphakie Presbyopen. In: Diagnostica Ultrasonica in Ophthalmologia, (Gernet H., ed.) Münster, R.A. Remy Verlag (1979) p. 239.

158

Gernet, H. & Boateng, A. Zur Dimension des Glaskörperraumes. Dtsch. Ophthal. Ges., Heidelberg (68) 31 (1967).

Gernet, H. & Franceschetti, A. Zur Voraussage der Rekraktions- und des Vergrösserungseffektes nach Fukala-Operation auf Grund von Ultraschalluntersuchungen. Ophthalmologica, Basel (148) 393 (1964).

Gernet, H. & Hollwich, F. Oculometrie des kindlichen Glaukoms. Ber. dtsch. Ophthal. Ges. (69) 341 (1969).

Gernet, H. & Hollwich, F. Résultats oculométriques à propos du glaucoma infantile. Bull. et Mém. Soc. franç. Ophtal. (82) 41 (1969).

Gernet, H. & Hollwich, F. Oculometrie beim kindlichen Glaukom. In: Ultrasonographia Medica. (Böck J. & Ossoinig K., eds.,) Wien, Verlag der Wiener Medizinischen Akademie (1971) p. 579.

Gernet, H. & Jürgens, V. Echographischer Befunden beim primärchronischen Glaukom. Graefe's Arch. Ophthal. (168) 419 (1965).

Gernet, H. & Ostholt, H. Augenseitige Optik. Ophthalmologica, Basel (166) 120 (1973).

Gernet, H. & Ostholt, H. Objective Aniseikoniemessung: Grundlagen und Möglichkeiten. In: Ultrasonography in Ophthalmology, (François J. and Goes F., eds.,) Bibl. Ophthal., Basel (83) 287 (1975).

Gernet, H., Ostholt, H. & Werner, H. Zur Bildangleichung bei einseitiger Apkakie. In: Diagnostica Ultrasonica in Ophthalmologia (Gernet H., ed.) Münster, R.A. Remy Verlag, 221 (1979).

Gernet, H. & Worst, J.G.F. Klinische Oculometrie und Linseneinplanzung nach Binkhorst. In: Diagnostica Ultrasonica in Ophthalmologia (Massin M. & Poujol J., eds.) Paris, Centre National Ophtal. des Quinze-Vingts, (1973) p. 247.

Giglio, E.J. & Ludlam, W.M. High resolution ultrasonic equipment to measure intraocular distances. J. Am. Optom. Assoc. (38) 367 (1967).

Gleiss, J. & Pau, H. Die Entwicklung der Refraktion vor der Geburt. Klin. Mbl. Augenheilk., (121) 440 (1952).

Goldmann, H. Spaltlampphotographie und -photometrie. Ophthalmologica, Basel (98) 257 (1939).

Goldmann, H. Eine Methode zur Volumbestimmung der Vorderkammer des lebenden Menschen. Ophthalmologica, Basel (102) 7 (1941).

Graham M.V. & Gray O.P. Refraction of premature babies' eyes. Brit. Med. J. (1) 452 (1963).

Grignolo, A. & Rivara, A. Biometry of the human eye from the sixth month of pregnancy to the tenth year of life, measurements of the axial length, retinoscopy, refraction, total refraction, corneal and lens refraction. In: Diagnostica Ultrasonica in Ophthalmologia (Vanysek J., ed.) Brno, Universita J.E. Purkinje (1968) p. 251.

Grignolo, A., Rivara, A. & Zingirian, M. Evaluation of errors in optical and ultrasound methods employed in ocular biometry. In: Ultrasonics in Medicine, (De Vliegler M., White D.N. & McReady V.R. eds.) Amsterdam, Excerpta Medica (1974) p. 154.

Grignolo, A., Rivara, A. & Zingirian, M. Recherches sur certains problèmes oculométriques à l'aide de méthodes ultrasonographiques et optiques. In: Functional examinations in ophthalmology (François J., ed.) Basel, S. Karger (1974) p. 250.

Heim, M. Photografische Bestimmung der Tiefe und des Volumens der menschlichen Vorderkammer. Ophthalmologica, Basel (102) 193 (1941).

Heine, L. Beiträge zur Anatomie des myopischen Auges. Arch. Augenheilk, (38) 177 (1899).

Heine, L. Weitere Beiträge zur Anatomie der myopischen Auges. Arch. Augenheilk. (40) 160 (1900).

Helmholtz, H. von. Handbuch der Physiologischen Optik. Leipzig, Leopold Voss, 1st ed. (1866) p. 873. Traduction française: Optique physiologique, par Javal E. et Klein, Paris, 1–1058 (1867).

Hippel, E. von. Über das normale Auge des Neugeborenen. Graefe's Arch. Ophthal. (45) 286 (1898).

Hollwich, F. & Boateng, A. Ultrasonographic measurements in primary glaucomas. In: Ophthalmic ultrasound (Gitter et al., eds.) St. Louis, Mosby Co. (1969) p. 187.

Itin, W. Longueur axiale de l'oeil dans deux cas de microcornée mesurée à l'aide de l'échographie ultrasonique. Ann. Oculistique (198) 465 (1965).

Itin, W. & Brawand, L. Etude échographique de la longueur axiale de l'oeil avant at après l'extraction du cristallin. Ophthalmologica, Basel (156) 256 (1968).

Jaeger, E. von. Über die Einstellungen des dioptrischen Apparates im menschlichen Auge. Wien, L.W. Seidel u. Sohn und Paris, V. Masson (1861) p. 10.

Jansson, F. Measurement of intraocular distances by ultrasound and comparison between optical and ultrasonic determinations of the depth of the anterior chamber. Acta Ophthal., Kbh. (41) 25 (1963).

Jansson, F. Determination of the axis length of eye roentgenologically and by ultrasound. Acta Ophthal., Kbh. (41) 236 (1963).

Jansson, F. Measurements of intraocular distances by ultrasound. Acta Ophthal., Kbh., Suppl. (74) 1 (1963).

Jansson, F. Intraokulare Messungen mit Ultraschall. Wiss. Z. Humboldt-Univ., Berlin (14) 205 (1965).

Jansson, F. and Kock, E.- Determination of the velocity of ultrasound in the human lens and vitreous. Acta Ophthal., Kbh., 40, 420, (1962).

Jansson, F. and Sundmark, E.-Determination of the velocity of ultrasound in ocular tissues at different temperatures. Acta Ophthal. Kbh., 39, 899, (1961).

Kanki, K., Yoshimoto, M., Uesugi, T. and Kimura T.- Measurement of the axial length of the eye by the application of ultrasonic waves. Acta Soc. Ophthal. Jap., 65, 1877, (1961).

Karantinos, D., Papacharalampous, E., Theodossiadis, G. and Velissaropouos, P.- Biométrie oculaire par échographie A. Arch. Ophtal., Paris, 34, 581, (1974).

Katz, D. and Ledoux, A.C.- Measurement of antero-posterior diameter of the eyeball in situ correlated with micrometer measurement following enucleation. Amer. J. Ophthal., 18, 914, (1935).

Kimura, T., Yamazaki, M., Nakajima, A., Hayashi, C. and Nagata, Y.- Analysis of errors in ultrasound biometry and phacometry. In: Ophthalmic Ultrasound (Gitter K., Sarin L. and Meyer D., eds.) Saint-Louis, C.V. Mosby, Co. (1969) p. 190.

Koretskaya, Y.M., Mozhrenkov, V.P. and Ukhaneva, G.L.- A table for determining the volume of the vitreous body from ultrasonic biometric data. Vestn. Oftal., 92, 63, (1976).

Larsen, J.S.- The saggital growth of the eye. Acta Ophthal., Kbh., 49, 239, 427, 441, 873, (1971).

Larsen, J.S. and Syrdalen, P.- Ultrasonic studies on changes in axial eye dimensions after encircling procedure in retinal detachment surgery. Acta Ophthal., Kbh., 57, 337, (1979).

Leary, G.A.- Ultrasonographic measurement of the comoponents of ocular refraction in life. Wiss. Z. Humboldt-Univ., Berlin, 14, 217, (1965).

Leary, G.A., Sorsby, A., Richards, M.J. and Chaston, J.- Ultrasonographic measurement of the components of ocular refraction in life. I. Technical Considerations. Vision Res., 3, 487, (1963).

Leighton, D.A. and Tomlinson, A.- Changes in axial length and other dimensions of the eyeball with increasing age. Acta Ophthal., Kbh., 50, 815, (1972).

Leighton, D.A. and Tomlinson, A.- Ocular tension and axial length of the eyeball in open-angle glaucoma and low tension glaucoma. Brit. J. Ophthal., 57, 499, (1973).

Leonard, P.A.M.- Ultrasonography and Lens Implantation, Ophthalmologica, Basel, 171, 276, (1975).

Lesroux, Lesjardins, S., Massin, M. and Poujol, J.- Etude biométrique du glaucome malin. Arch. Ophtal., 37, 523, (1977).

Levchenko, O.G. and Drukman, A.B.- Ultrasonic biometry in the eyes of children with varying refraction. Vestn. Oftal., 92, 47, (1976).

Leydhecker, W.- Gonioskopische Beobachtungen über Tenzionsansteige nach Miotics und nach Lesen. Dtsch. Ophthal. Ges., Heidelberg, 58, 326, (1953).

Lindstedt, F.- Über die Messung der Tiefe der vorderen Augenkammer mittels eines neuen für klinischen Gebrauch bestimmten Instruments. Graefe's Arch. Augenheilk., 80, 104, (1916).

160

Lowe, R.F.- Time-amplitude ultrasonography for ocular biometry. Amer. J. Ophthal., 66, 913, (1968).

Lowe, R.F.- Causes of shallow anterior chamber in primary angle-closure glaucoma. Ultrasonic biometry of normal and angle-closure glaucoma eyes. Amer. J. Ophthal., 67, 87, (1969).

Lowe, R.F.- Corneal radius and ocular correlations in normal eyes with primary angle-closure glaucoma. Amer. J. Ophthal., 67, 864, (1969).

Lowe, R.F.- Primary angle-closure glaucoma. Inheritance and environment. Brit. J. Ophthal., 56, 13, (1972).

Lowe, R.F.- Anterior lens curvature. Comparisons between normal eyes and those with primary angle-closure glaucoma. Brit. J. Ophthal., 56, 409, (1972).

Luyckx, J.- Mesure des composantes optiques de l'ceil du nouveau-né par échographie ultrasonique. Arch. Ophtal., Paris, 26, 159, (1966).

Luyckx, J.- Relation entre le coefficient de rigidité et la longueur de l'oeil mesurée par échographie ultrasonique. Ophthalmologica, Basel, 153, 355, (1967).

Luyckx-Bacus, J. and Weekers, J.F.- Etude biométrique de l'oeil humain par ultrasonographie, 2e partie: les glaucomes. Bull. Soc. belge Ophtal., 144, 913, (1966).

Luyckx-Bacus, J. and Weekers, J.F.- Contribution à l'étude des glaucomes par l'ultrasonographie. Ann. Oculistique, 200, 489, (1967).

Luyckx, J. and Delmarcelle, Y.- Recherches biométriques sur des yeux présentant une microcornés ou une mégalocornée. Bull. Soc. belge Ophtal., 149, 433, (1968).

Luyckx, J. and Delmarcelle, Y.- Contribution of ultrasonography to the study of microcornea and megalocornea. In Ophthalmic Ultrasound, (Gitter K., Keeny A., Sarin L. and Meyer D., eds.) Saint-Louis, Mosby Co., (1969) p. 149.

Machekhin, V.A.- Ultraschallbiometrie bei Augen mit unterschiedlicher Refraktion. Oftal. Zh., 27, 204, (1972).

Machekhin, V.A.- Ultrasound biometry in subjects suspected of having glaucoma. Vestn. Oftal., 92, 5, (1975).

Machekhin, V.A. and Krivopaluva.- The possibilities of ultrasonic biometry in assessing the extent of stabilisation of glaucoma. Vestn. Oftal., 96, 17, (1979).

Makabe, R.- Echographische Untersuchungen bei excentrischen hinteren Skleraektasien. Klin. Mbl. Augenheilk., 167, 97, (1975).

Manabe, T.- Studies of dynamic changes in the lens due to accommodation. 1. The Principle of a new recording. Acta Soc. Ophthal. Jap., 78, 1213, (1974).

Marschke, E.- Beiträge zur pathologischen Anatomie der Myopie und der Hydrophthalmus. Klin. Mbl. Augenheilk., 39, 705, (1901).

Massin, M., Poujol, J. and Hieronimus.- Etude statistique de différents facteurs influant sur la précision des mesures biométriques. In Ultrasonographia Medica, Böck- J. and Ossoinig K., Wien, Verlag Wiener Med. Akad., (1971) p. 467.

Merkel, F. and Orr, A.W.- Das Auge des Neugeborenen an einem schematischen Durchschnitt arlaufert. Anatom. Hafte 3, 315, Ref. Nagels, Jahresber. 4, (1892). Arb. anat. Inst. Wiesbaden, 1, 271, (1892).

Merlin, U. and Rossi, A.- Sur la validité des formules de biométrie fonctionnelle. In: François J. and Goes F., Ultrasonography in Ophthalmology. Bibl. Ophthal., Basel, 83, 301, (1975).

Miettinen, P. and Ursin, K.V.- Ultrasound studies on changes in the length of cerclage operated eyes. In: Diagnostica Ultrasonica in Ophthalmologia, (Vanysek J. ed.) Brno, Universita J.E. Purkinje, (1968) p. 239.

Mozherenkov, V.P.-Ultrasonic data concerning the relationship between the shape of the globe and the degree of refraction. Oftal. Zh., 29, 127, (1974).

Mundt, G.H. and Hughes, W.F.- Ultrasonics in ocular diagnosis. Amer. J. Ophthal., 42, 488, (1956).

Nakajima, A. and Kimura, T.- Ultrasonography and phacometry in study of refractive elements of the eye. In Ultrasonics in Ophthalmology (Oksala A. and Gernet H., eds.) Basel, Karger, (1967) p. 226

Nover, A. and Glanschneider, D.- Untersuchungen über die Fortpflanzungs-geschwindigkeit und Absorption des Ultraschalls im Gewebe. Graefe's Arch. Ophthal., 168, 304, (1965).

Oguchi, Y. and Van Balen, Th.M.- Prepupillary pseudophakos and iseikonisation. Doc. Ophthal., 37, 295, (1974).

Ostholt, H.- Objektive Messung der Brennweiten und Netzhautbildes lebenden Augen. Genauigkeitsanforderungen. In: Diagnostica Ultrasonica in Ophthalmologica, (H. Gernet, ed.) Münster, R.A. Remy Verlag, (1979), p. 234

Ostholt, H. and Gernet, H.- Die hinters Brennweite linsenhaltiger emmetropen Augen. In Diagnostica Ultrasonica in Ophthalmologia. (Massin M. and Poujol J., eds.) Paris, Centre National d'Ophtal. des Quinze-Vingts, Paris, (1973), p. 250.

Ostholt, H., Gernet, H. and Werner, H.- Ein neues Haftschalen Nomogramm für Aphakie. Sitz. 122 Versammlung Ver. Rhein. West. Augenärzte, (1970).

Otsuka, J., Tokoro, R. and Araki, M.- Comparison of phacometry with ultrasonic method in the measurement of human refractive elements. Acta Soc. Ophthal. Jap., 65, 1777, (1961).

Pallin, O. and Ericsson, R.- Ultrasound studies in a case of hygroton induced myopia. Acta Ophthal., Kbh., 43, 692, (1965).

Pelletier,.- Contribution à l'étude ultrasonique du vitré glaucomateux. Thése, Nancy, (1971).

Perez-Llorca-Rodriguez, R.- Biométrie échographie statique du segment antérieur et axe antéro-postérieur de l'ceil humain vivant, du nouveau-né prématuré au vieillard chez les habitants de Cadix. Bull. Mém. Soc. franç. Ophtal., 84, 275, (1971).

Pflugk, K.A. von.- Die Fixierung der Wirbeltierlinsen insbesondere der Linse der neugeborenen Menschen. Klin. Mbl. Augenheilk., 47, 1, (1909).

Pourfour du Petit, F.P.- Mémoires sur les yeux gelés dans lesquels on détermine la grandeur des chambres qui renferment l'humeur aqueuse. Mém. Acad. Roy. Sci., 38, (1723).

Pourfour du Petit, F.P.- Mémoires sur le crystallin de l'oeil de l'homme, des animaux à 4 pieds, des oiseaux et des poissons. Mém. Acad. Roy. Sci., (1730) Lité par Scammon, (1950).

Pourfour du Petit, F.P.- Cité par Jansson, F., Acta Ophthal., Kbh., 41, 25, (1963).

Priestley-Smith,- On the size of the cornea in relation to age. Diseases of the cornea. Trans. Ophthal. Soc. U.K., 10, 68, (1890).

Raeder- Untersuchungen über die Lage und Dicke der Linse im menschlicher Auge bei physiologischen und pathologischen Zustanden nach einer neuen Methode gemessen. Graefe's Arch. Ophthal., 110, 73–108, 1922; 112, 20, (1923).

Rivara, A.- Ricerche sull impiego degli ultrasuoni nelle misurazione dell'asse oculare antero-posteriore. Atti Soc. Oftal. Lombarde, 48, (1963).

Rivara, A.- Misurazione dell'asse oculare antero-posteriore per mezzo degli ultrasuoni. Ann. Ottal., 89, 195, (1963).

Rivara, A. and Gemme, G.- Misurazione dell'asse oculare antero-post riore e del potere diottrico oculare nei prematuri. Ann. Ottal., 91, 1328, (1965).

Rivara, A. and Gemme, G.- Miopia degli immaturi. Atti XLIX Cong. Soc. Ital., 23, 395, (1965).

Rivara, A. and Sanna, G.- Determinazione della velocità degli ultrasoni nei tessuti oculari di uomo e di maiale. Ann. Ottal., 88, 675, (1962).

Rivara, A. and Zingirian, M.- Calculation of total refractive ocular power and refractive lens power. An ultrasonic optical procedure. Ophthalmologica, Basel, 159, 202, (1969).

Rosengren, B.- Studien über die Tiefe der vorderen Augenkammer. Teil II. Acta Ophthal., Kbh., 9, 103, (1931).

Rushton, R.H.- The clinical measurements of the axial length of the living eye. Trans. Ophthal. Soc. U.K., 58, 136, (1938).

Saraux, H. and Bechetoille, A.- Etude en temps réel de la croissance de 30 yeux d'adolescents amétropes. Ann. Oculistique, 205, 1103, (1972).

Schnabel, and Herrnheiser,- Zeitschr. f. Heilk., 16, 1, (1895).

Schoute, G.J.- Le phénomène d'Finthoven et la longueur de l'oeil vivant. Ophthalmologica, Basel, 99, 282, (1940).

Shibata, H. and Amano, K.- Objective measurement of ocular axis by X-ray photograph. Jap. J. Ophthal., 2, 263, (1958).

Sorsby, A., Leary, G.A., Richards, M.J. and Chaston, J.- Ultrasonographic measurement of the components of ocular refraction in life. II. Clinical procedures. Vision Res., 3, 499, (1963).

Stenström, S.- Untersuchungen über die Variation and Kovariation der optischen Elemente des menschlichen Auges. Acta Ophthal., Kbh., Suppl., 26 (1946).

Stenström, S.- An apparatus for measuring the depth of the anterior chamber, based on Lindstedt's principle. Acta Ophthal., Kbh., 31, 265, (1953).

Storey, J.K. and Phillips, C.I.- Ultrasonic investigation on mobility of crystalline lens. In Ultrasonographia Medica. (Massin M. and Poujol J. eds.) Paris, Centre Nat. Ophtal. Quinze-Vingts (1971) p. 261.

Storey, J.K. and Phillips, C.I.- Ocular dimensions in angle-closure glaucoma. Brit. J. Physiol. Optics, 26, 228, (1971).

Straub, M.- Über die Aetiologie der Brechungsanomalien des Auges und dem Ursprung der Emmetropie. Graefe's Arch. Ophthal., 70, 130, (1909).

Stromberg, E.- Über Refraktion und Achsenlänge des menschlichen Auges. Acta Ophthal., Kbh., 14, 281, (1936).

Szczypinski, J.- Ultrasonography in operations for shortening of the globe. II. Late Investigations. Klin. Oczna, 44, 33, (1974).

Tane, S., Kawago E.M. and Takemoto, N.- Studies on Ultrasonographic diagnosis in ophthalmology. 5. Ultrasonographic measurements in normal and glaucomatous eyes. Rinsho Ganka, 27, 471, (1973).

Tane, S., Kushiro, H. and Kohno, J.- Echographic biometry in myopia of prematurity in Japan. In Diagnostica Ultrasonica in Ophthalmologia (Gernet H. ed.) Münster, R.A. Remy Varlag (1979) p. 190.

Tane, S. and Takemoto, N.- Studies on ultrasonic diagnosis in ophthalmology. Echographic findings in glaucomatous eyes. Folia Ophthal. Jap., 24, 49, (1973).

Thijssen, J.M. The emmetropic and iseikonic implant lens: Computer calculation of the refractive power and its accuracy Ophthalmologica 171, 467 (1975).

Tomlinson, A. and Leighton, D.A.- Ocular dimensions in low tension glaucoma compared with open angle glaucoma and the normal. Brit. J. Ophthal., 56, 97 (1972).

Tomlinson, A. and Leighton, D.A.- Ocular dimensions in the heredity of angle-closure glaucoma. Brit. J. Ophthal., 57, 475, (1973).

Tomlinson, A. and Leighton, D.A.- Ocular tension and axial length of the eyeball in open-angle glaucoma and low tension glaucoma. Brit. J. Ophthal., 57, 499, (1973).

Tomlinson, A. and Phillips, C.I.- Applanation tension and axial length of the eyeball. Brit. J. Ophthal., 54, 548, (1970).

Tomlinson, A. and Phillips, C.I.- Unequal axial length of eyeball and ocular tension. Acta Ophthal., Kbh., 50, 872, (1972).

Tschewnenko, A.A.- Über die Ausbreitungsgeschwindigkeit des Ultraschalls in den Augengeweben. Wiss. Z. Humboldt-Univ., Berlin, 14, 67, (1965).

Ustimenko, L.L.- Zehnjßrige Erfahrungen im Studien des diagnostischen Wertes der Ultraschallbiometrie in der Ophthalmologie. Oftal. Zh. Moscou, 27, 487, (1972).

Van der Heijde, G.L.- A nomogram for calculating the power of the prepupillary lens in the apkakic eye. In: François J. and Goes G., Ultrasonography in Ophthalmology. Bibl. Ophthal., Basel, Karger, 83, 273, (1975).

Van der Heijde, G.L. and Stilma, J.S.- Biometrie und Aphakie. Klin. Mbl. Augenheilk., 169, 289, (1976).

Vucicevic, M., Scheie, G. and Ralston, J.- Ultrasonic evaluation of osmotic agents. In: Ultrasonographia Medica. (Böck J. and Ossoinig K., (eds.) Wien, Verlag der Wiener Med. Akad., (1971) p. 587.

Weekers, R., Luyckx, J. and Weekers, J.F.- Engwinkelglaukom infolge einer kongenitalen Anomalie der Linsendicke. Klin. Mbl. Augenheilk 155, 625, (1969).

Weinstein, G.W., Baum, G., Binkhorst, R.D. and Troutman, R.C.- A comparison of ultrasonographic and optical methods for determining the axial length of the apkakic eye. Amer. J. Ophthal., 62, 1194, (1966).

Wibaut, F.- Über die Emmetropisation und den Ursprung der sphßrischen Refraktionsanomalien. Graefe's Arch. Ophthal., 116, 596, (1926).

Yamamoto, Y., Namiki, R., Baba, M. and Kato, M.- A study of the measurement of ocular axial length by ultrasonic echography. Jap. J. Ophthal., 5, 134, (1961).

Young, F.A., Leary, G.A. and Farrer, D.N.- Ultrasound and Phakometry measurements of the primate eye. Amer. J. Optom., 43, 370, (1966).

Zingirian, M. and Rivara, A.- Über die Anwendung der Echographie zur Bestimmung des Brechungsindex des Kammerwassers und des Glaskörpers. In Ultrasonographia Medica. (Böck J., and Ossoinig K., eds.) Wien, Verlag der Wiener Med. Akademie, (1971) p. 517.

Zingirian, M. and Rossi, P.L.- Biometrical investigation of the hydrophthalmic Eye. In: Diagnostica Ultrasonica in Ophthalmologia, (Gernet H., ed.) Münster, R.A. Remy Verlag, (1979) p. 200.

Zürkendürfer, S.- Nachzusatz und Netzhautbildorösse. In, Diagnostica Ultrasonica in Ophthalmologia. (H. Gernet, ed.) Münster, R.A. Remy Verlag, (1979) p. 229.

Author's Address:
Prof. dr. J. François
Dept. of Ophthalmology
University of Ghent, De Pintelaan, 135
B-9000 Ghent, Belgium

DETERMINATION OF SOUND VELOCITY IN DIFFERENT FORMS OF CATARACTS

I. PALLIKARIS & H. GRUBER,

(Zürich, Switzerland)

The increasing use of intraocular lens implants has given a practical value to biometric measurements. The preoperative calculation of the refraction of intraocular lenses allows a good prediction of postoperative refraction (Jaffe 1978). The precision of i.o.L calculation depends mostly on the accuracy of axial length determination with ultrasound (Binkhorst 1976).

To calculate the length of the eye from the biometric data the velocity of ultrasound in the ocular media must be known. The velocity of sound in the aqueous and vitreous (1532 m/sec) (Willard 1947) can be assumed as a constant. The velocity in the opaque lenses, however, can have quite different values (Coleman, *et al.* 1975).

Not only the determination of axial length but perhaps also the accuracy of the postoperative anterior chamber depth prediction might be improved with a more precise knowledge of the sound velocity in cataract. Oguchi & van Balen (1974) have shown that there is a relation between the change in anterior chamber depth after lens implantation and lens thickness. The low correlation between the two sets of data may be in part due to the assumption of a constant velocity of sound in different cataracts.

An improved correlation between the change in the anterior segment depth and lens thickness could however be practically used to predict the postoperative position of an implant. The aim of this work was to measure the velocity of ultrasound in human lenses shortly after intracapsular extraction to obtain a relation between the slitlamp aspects of the cataract and the velocity of ultrasound, in that lens.

METHODS

The experimental procedure tried to avoid premeasurement degeneration of the lens upon its removal from the eye by placing it in isotonic solution heated to the physiological temperature of 37°C and beginning study as soon as possible after the cataract extraction, that is, no later than 20 min. It must be noted, however, that two lenses measured again after 2 h immersion in isotonic sodium solution at 37°C did not increase in thickness.

A total of 37 cataractous lenses were measured. Lenses were obtained from patients undergoing uncomplicated intracapsular cataract extraction. A

© 1981. Dr W. Junk Publishers, The Hague

slit-lamp photography was made of the cataract the day before surgery. The lenses were divided into four classes according to their morphological appearance (Table 1). The principles of measurement were similar to those applied by Coleman, *et al.* (1975). The only difference was that we used a photographic procedure. (Fig. 1). The transducer was fixated in a vertical position in normal saline at 37°C temperature. The transducer was moved only in a horizontal plane, always at the same distance from the base of the water bath.

Table 1. Various kinds of cataracts involved in this study.

○	intumeszent
○	nuclear sclerosis
	nucl. scler.
◐	——————————
	post. caps. opac.
●	posterior capasular opacity
△	minimal cataract

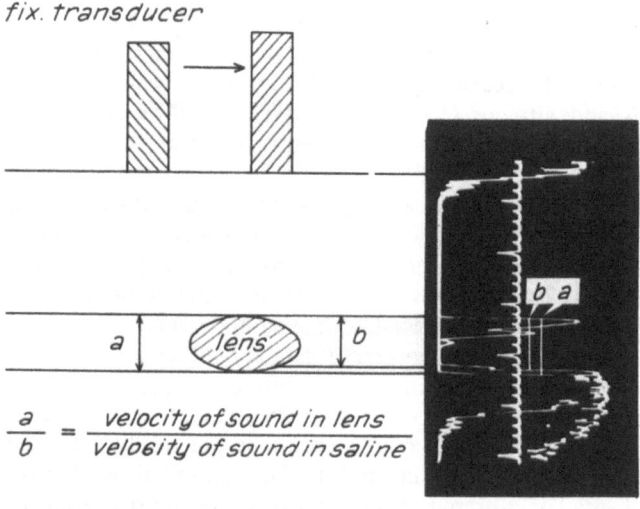

$$\frac{a}{b} = \frac{\text{velocity of sound in lens}}{\text{velocity of sound in saline}}$$

a = saline transit time through the space the lens previously

b = lens transit time

Fig. 1. Measuring procedure: The A-mode echogram is recorded twice at two different locations, which do or do not include the lens. The lens thickness is also measured optically.

First we made a picture without lenses and then another with the ultra-sound beam through the lens. Both pictures were taken on the same polaroid film. Eight such picture were taken for each lens. The transducer was moved in the horizontal plane to obtain a reading of the thickest part in the middle of the lens. The distances a and b were measured with the help of a micro-scope (Wild M7A) with a calibrated eye piece at a magnification of $20 \times$.

When the lens was introduced in the sound beam the base of the water bath seemed to move upward due to the faster sound velocity in the lens. The only changes detected when introducing the lens were below the level of the anterior lens surfac and the first lens echo. Thus, the distance *a* is equal to a length of water equal to the thickness of the lens. The distance *b* is the length of the lens itself. The difference between the two measurements may be used to calculate the sound velocity in the lens if the velocity in the water bath is known (cf. Coleman, *et al.* 1977):

$$V_l = V_w \frac{a}{b}$$

In this procedure we used an A-scan instrument (7200 M.A. Kretz-Technik) with a 8 MHz probe. The scale on the screen was spread as far as possible. The velocity of sound in our 9% saline solution is assumed as 1352 m/sec (Willard 1947).

RESULTS

The 37 cataracteous lenses were classified. Of the 37 studied lenses four where intumescent cataracts, nine had a nuclear sclerosis, in 12 cases the opacity was limited to the capsula, ten lenses had a combination of nuclear sclerosis and posterior capsula opacification. In two lenses there was only a minimal sclerosis. Other factors controlled in this experiment were temperature, duration of the time between lens removal and measurement, the medium in which the lens was supported and the integrity of the lens capsule. The temperature was $37°C \pm 0.5°C$. Transport time was at maximum 20 min. Transport medium was 9% normal saline. Only those lenses with an intact capsule were used. The velocity of sound was computed for each lens. The values obtained range from 1588 to 1692, the average velocity was 1641.35 m/sec, with a standard deviation ± 28 m/sec. The relationship between the thickness of the lens, sound velocity and slit-lamp aspect has been shown.

DISCUSSION

Jansson & Kock (1962) measured a series of 12 cataracts, Yamamoto, *et al.* (1961) made another sound determination and Coleman, *et al.* (1975) have done an extensive study with 50 lenses. The average velocity in cataracts was found to be between 1640.5 (Jansson) and 1629 (Coleman). Coleman, *et al.* (1975) write in their paper: 'The relationship between water content and velocity has not been proven, this explanation seems to be a good working hypothesis'. Oguchi & van Balen (1974) however found that the post-operative anterior chamber depth is dependant upon the thickness of cataracteous lens before extraction. The significance of the lens thickness, therefore, was known but could not be precisely measured. On the other hand the morphological aspect of the cataracteous lens was not recorded.

From our data a relation between lens morphology and sound velocity can be seen. (Fig. 2)

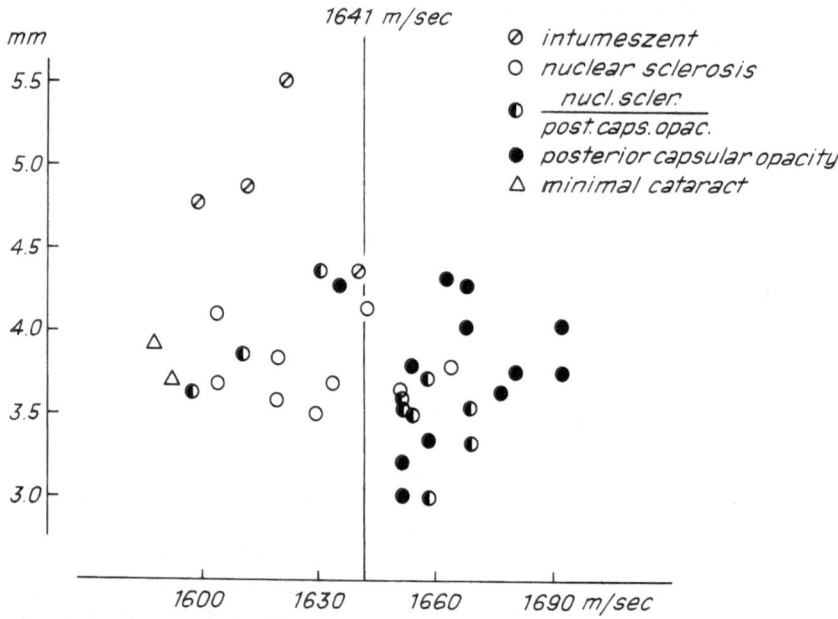

Fig. 2. Resulting sound velocity of 37 lenses. For symbols see Table 1.

If one does exclude the intumescent lenses there is no reasonable correlation between sound velocity and lens thickness. In all thick intumescent lenses however the sound velocity is below average. Sound velocity decreases in lenses with nuclear sclerosis and increases in lenses with opacity of the posterior capsula. The lowest speed is measured in lenses with minimal cataract.

How can those values be used to improve axial length determination? Deviation from the mean sound velocity can be up to 40 m/sec. An error of 40 m/sec in sound velocity – assuming a lens of 5 mm thickness is used – will result in an error of around one tenth of a millimeter in axial length determination. This potential error lies in the same range of error given for the best ultrasound equipment available. The dioptric effect of a 1/10 mm error in i.o. lens calculation is about 1/3 D (cf. Thÿssen 1975). It is therefore not a negligible error and thus seems worth reducing.

CONCLUSIONS

Without knowledge of the lens morphology an average sound velocity of 1641 m/sec should be used. In cases of thick intumescent cataracts as well as in cases of pure nuclear sclerosis an assumed velocity of 1610 is preferable. In the presence of an isolated capsular opacity a higher velocity of 1670 m/sec is a better average. If both nuclear sclerosis and capsular opacities are present one should again use the average velocity of 1641 m/sec.

REFERENCES

Jaffe, N. A-scan calculation of exact desired intraocular lens. In: Current Progress in Cataract surgery: selected proceedings of the 5th biannual Cataract surgical Congress. St. Louis: Mosby (1978).

Binkhorst, K. Pitfalls in the determination of intraocular lens-power without ultrasound. Ophthalmic Surg. 7: 69 (1978).

Willard, G.W. Temperature coefficient of ultrasonic velocity in solutions. J. Accoustic Soc. Am. 19: 235 (1947).

Coleman, J-D., Lizzi, L.F., Franzen, L.A. & Abramson, H.D. Ultrasonography in Ophthalmology. Bibl. Ophthalmol. 83: 246 (1975).

Oguchi, V. & van Balen, Th. Ultrasound in medicine. Biol. 1: 267 (1974).

Coleman, J.D., Lizzi, F.L. & Jack, R.L. Ultrasound velocity of tissue. Philadelphia 124 (1977).

Jansson, F. & Kock, E. Determination of the velocity of ultrasound in the human lens and vitreous. Acta Ophthalmol. Kbh. 40: 420 (1962).

Yamamoto, Y., Namici, R., Baba, M. & Kato, M. A study on the measurement of ocular axial length by ultrasonic echography. Jap. J. Ophthal. 5 (2): 50 (1961).

Thijssen, J.M. The emmetropic and the isokonic implant lens: Computer calculation of the refractive power and its accuracy. Ophthalmologica 171: 467 (1975).

Author's Address:
I. Pallikaris
University Eye Clinic
Kantonsspital
Zürich, Switzerland
Present address:
Philellinon 9, GR-Thessaloniki, Greece.

ULTRASONOGRAPHIC STUDY OF THE OCULAR PARAMETERS AFTER GLAUCOMA SURGERY

F. GOES, J. FRANÇOIS & J. BENOZZI

(Ghent, Belgium)

With the help of A-Scan ultrasonography, we examined the ocular parameters in glaucoma eyes before and after surgery. The aim of the study was to determine, on the one hand, the biometric characteristics of glaucoma eyes, and, on the other hand, the eventual postoperative changes. The ultrasonographic biometry was performed a few days before and one to two weeks after surgery. The technique with a focused narrow beam transducer of 15 MHz yielded an accuracy of 0.1 mm for the anterior eye segment and of 0.2 mm for the posterior segment (François & Goes 1973). The anterior chamber was measured both optically and ultrasonographically. The results were discarded, when the difference between both measurements exceeded 0.1 mm. In open angle glaucoma, trabeculectomy was performed, while closed angle glaucoma cases were surgically treated either by a trabeculectomy or by a transcorneal iridectomy. At the moment of the postoperative measurements all the eyes were under the influence of topic cortisone and atropine.

OPEN ANGLE GLAUCOMA

We could examine 25 open angle glaucoma eyes. In 16 cases we could obtain pre- and postoperative measurements (Table 1). The mean age of the patients was 66 years ($\sigma = 11$). There were ten women and five men. Pre-operatively, the mean refraction was -0.5 D ($\sigma = 2.3$). The mean ocular tension was 28.0 mm ($\sigma = 7.6$). The eyes were under topical pilocarpine, adrenaline or timolol or combined treatment, and in many cases acetazolamide per os was given.

From previous biometric studies we know that the mean value of the anterior chamber depth in emmetropic adult eyes is 3.25 mm. This value is reduced by 0.1 mm every decade (Delmarcelle & Luyckx 1971, Delmarcelle, et al. 1976). The mean value of the lens thickness is 3.65 mm at birth till 20 years. Afterwards, it increases by 0.2 mm every decade (François & Goes 1970, Delmarcelle, et al. 1976). The ocular eye length has a mean value of 23.30 to 23.50 mm in emmetropic eyes (Delmarcelle, et al. 1976). It slightly decreases with age (François & Goes 1971).

The mean interval between surgery and the biometric measurements was 8.8 days (extremes 4–14 days).

Table 1. Open angle glaucoma. Biometric measurements of 16 open angle glaucoma eyes before and after trabeculectomy.

	Pre-operative values	Post-operative values
I.O. Pressure	28.0 mmHg	13.0 mmHg
Corneal Refractive Power	43.96 D	44.30 D
A.C. depth	2.68 mm	2.67 mm
Lens thickness	4.86 mm	4.76 mm
Vitreous length	15.14 mm	15.21 mm
Eye length	23.05 mm	23.00 mm
Refraction	− 0.5 D	− 0.55 D

In the surgically treated group, the corneal diameter (mean value 10.90 mm; $\sigma = 0.30$) and the corneal refractive power (mean value 43.96 D; $\sigma = 1.72$) were normal. The mean anterior chamber depth was 2.68 mm ($\sigma = 0.48$), what is in the range of normal values for an age group between 65 and 70 years, the mean anterior chamber depth being 2.75 mm at the age of 70 years (Delmarcelle & Luyckx 1971). The lens thickness was also normal (mean value 4.86 mm, $\sigma = 0.58$), the mean lens thickness being 4.65 mm in the normal population at the age of 70 years (François & Goes 1970). The mean values of the vitreous length (mean value 15.14 mm; $\sigma = 1.5$) and of the axial eye-length (mean value 23.05 mm; $\sigma = 1.70$) were also normal for a mean ocular refraction of − 0.5 D (extreme values − 6 to + 4 D). In a normal emmetropic population, the mean ocular length is between 23.30 and 23.50 mm (Delmarcelle, François, Goes, *et al.*, 1976).

Postoperatively no significant changes of the mean values of the ocular parameters could be observed, although important individual changes could be seen. The mean intraocular pressure (IOP) was 13.0 mmHg ($\sigma = 3.0$). The mean corneal refractive power did not change significantly (44.30 D versus 43.96^D). The mean change of the anterior chamber depth (− 0.01 mm) was not significant (mean value 2.67 mm; $\sigma = 0.58$), although important individual changes were measured (− 0.62 to + 0.65 mm). The mean lens thickness (4.76 mm; $\sigma = 0.58$) was slightly but not significantly shortened by − 0.10 mm, although here also important individual changes were observed (− 0.43 to + 0.34 mm). The mean vitreous length remained unchanged (mean value 15.21 mm; $\sigma = 1.21$), the individual extreme changes being between − 0.94 and + 0.78 mm. The mean total eye length remained also unchanged (mean value 23.0 mm), the mean change being of − 0.05 mm, but here also important individual changes between − 0.96 and + 1.40 mm could be observed. The mean refractive change was insignificant (− 0.05 D), but in one case we noticed a refraction change of − 3.0 D (Table 1).

When analysing the individual cases, we found in three eyes important changes, concerning mostly the vitreous: in one case, a vitreous lengthening of 0.8 mm accompanied by a myopisation of − 3D, and in two other cases, a vitreous shortening of 0.8 and 0.9 mm with a resulting slight hypermetropia. The shortening of the vitreous length can be explained by a backwards displacement of the lens as a consequence of the zonular fibres relaxation caused by the atropine.

Nine other open angle glaucoma eyes could only be studied preoperatively. The mean age was 68 years. The mean anterior chamber depth was 2.8 mm, the mean lens thickness 4.69 mm, the mean vitreous length 15.10 mm, the mean ocular eye-length 22.94 mm, the mean refraction + 0.75 D (extremes values − 2 D and + 4.5 D), and the mean corneal refractive power 43.0 D. These are normal biometric values for this age group.

The analysis of the mean values of the different ocular parameters in open angle glaucoma showed a slightly shorter eye length and a slightly thicker lens than could statistically be expected. In normal emmetropic eyes, these variations are nevertheless not statistically significant. We may conclude that open angle glaucoma eyes have no specific biometric characteristics, although some authors found a slight eye lengthening (Tomlinson & Phillips 1972, Leighton & Tomlinson 1972, 1973).

The analysis of the postoparative changes showed that trabeculectomy had only a minor and not significant influence on the ocular parameters. The anterior eye segment, the lens thickness, the vitreous length and the refraction were not changed. This is in favour of trabeculectomy in open angle glaucoma.

In three glaucoma cases we could measure an important eye-shortening after surgery, followed by a normalisation of the pressure. One was a buphthalmic eye in a 19 years old boy (tension of 50 mmHg). A shortening of the eye length of 1.94 mm was measured after glaucoma surgery (1.34 mm anterior chamber shallowing, from 4.66 to 3.32 mm, vitreous shortening of 0.76 mm). In two hemorrhagic glaucoma cases, treated by cyclodiathermy, the shortening of the eye length amounted respectively to 0.38 mm and 0.21 mm after surgery. These observations demonstrate the expansive effect of the intraocular hypertension on the eye-ball volume, as was also seen by Buschmann & Bluth (1974) in their follow-up study of congenital glaucoma eyes.

ANGLE CLOSURE GLAUCOMA

We could examine ten eyes with angle-closure glaucoma (eight women, two men) (Table 2). The mean age was 79 years (extremes 75 and 84, $\sigma = 7$). *Preoperatively*, the mean tension was 45 mmHg ($\sigma = 9$). The eyes were under the influence of miotics.

The mean corneal diameter was 10.9 mm (σ: 0.25), the mean corneal refractive power being 45.0 D ($\sigma = 0.9$). The mean anterior chamber depth was 1.80 mm ($\sigma = 0.15$), what is obviously shallower than the normal depth (2.65 mm at the age of 79 years). The mean lens thickness was 5.48 mm ($T = 0.35$), which is much thicker than the normal value/4.85 mm at the age of 79 years). The vitreous length was 15.0 mm ($\sigma = 0.9$) and the mean eye length 22.70 mm ($\sigma = 0.7$) for a mean ocular refraction of + 0.75 D ($\sigma = 0.5$), what is only slightly shorter than the normal eye-length.

We know already that angle-closure glaucoma is characterised by important biometric findings. The most striking characteristic is the shallow anterior chamber (mean value 1.19 mm, Delmarcelle, *et al.* 1976). The second important characteristic is the lens thickening, which amounts to + 0.55 mm

Table 2. Angle closure glaucoma. Biometric results in six eyes before and after glaucoma surgery (three iridectomies, three trabeculectomies).

	Pre-operative values	Post-operative values
I.O. Pressure	45 mmHg	11 mmHg
Corneal refractive power	45.0 D	45.20 D
A.C. depth	1.80 mm	2.85 mm
Lens thickness	5.48 mm	5.0 mm
Vitreous length	15.0 mm	14.4 mm
Eye length	22.70 mm	22.60 mm
Refraction	+ 0.75 D	

compared to corresponding age groups (Delmarcelle, *et al.* 1971). This lens thickening is accompanied by an abnormal forward position of the lens, so that the distance between the lens centre and the limbus is reduced, the mean difference being 0.35 mm (Delmarcelle, *et al.* 1976). The axial eye length is reduced by more or less 1.0 mm (Lowe 1969: 1.09 mm, Delmarcelle *et al.* 1971: 1.14 mm), the disease being more frequent in hypermetropic eyes and in female patients.

Six cases could be examined *postoperatively* after a mean interval of five days. The mean postoperative IOP was 11 mmHg ($\sigma = 4$). In three cases a trabeculectomy was performed and in three an iridectomy. The corneal refractive power change never exceeded 0.5 D (mean value 45.20 D, $\sigma = 0.8$). On the other hand, the anterior chamber always deepened significantly, the mean change being a deepening of 1.05 mm in the trabeculectomy cases and of 0.27 mm in the iridectomy ones. The mean anterior chamber depth was 2.85 mm ($\sigma = 0.7$). The mean lens thickness was 5.0 mm ($\sigma = 0.5$). An important decrease of the lens thickness was seen in the trabeculectomy cases (mean $- 0.75$ mm). The mean vitreous length was 14.4 mm ($\sigma = 0.3$), a mean shortening of 1.90 mm, being observed in the trabeculectomy cases. The mean eye-length was 22.60 mm ($\sigma = 0.05$), the mean change being 0.5 mm in the trabeculectomy cases (Table 2).

When we consider these results, we see that there is an important difference between the effect of the trabeculectomy and of the iridectomy on the postoperative eye parameters in closed angle glaucoma. The iridectomy does not produce fundamental changes, and in many cases there was only a slight refraction change. The postoperative change was a slight deepening of the anterior chamber, with a little backwards displacement of the lens. In most cases this fact can already be seen peroperatively, when the anterior chamber suddenly deepens at the moment of the perforating iridectomy. We must also take into account the effect of the preoperative pilocarpine instillations, although their effect on the anterior chamber shallowing is reduced at an older age.

On the contrary, the trabeculectomy in closed angle glaucoma resulted in important changes of the eye parameters. There was a very pronounced anterior chamber deepening, which could partly be explained by a decrease of the lens thickness, and partly by a backwards displacement of the lens, what produced a shortening of the vitreous cavity.

Very interesting was the ultrasonographic study of the same eye first at the moment of acute intraocular hypertension (50 mmHg, notwithstanding a topical miotic treatment), and afterwards at the moment of the normalisation of the tension by medical therapy (mannitol, miotics, timolol, 17 mmHg). We found changes similar to these observed after surgical normalisation of the IOP, namely a deepening of the anterior chamber of 1.14 mm (versus 1.67 mm post-surgery), a change in lens thickness of − 0.24 mm (versus − 0.47 mm post-surgery), a vitreous shortening of 1.32 mm (versus 1.54 mm post surgery) and a total eye-length shortening of − 0.42 mm (versus − 0.34 mm post surgery). This observation illustrates the importance of the forward position of the lens for the etiology of angle-closure glaucoma.

DISCUSSION AND CONCLUSION

The biometric study of open angle glaucoma eyes did not reveal any specific biometric characteristic. After trabeculectomy no significant changes of the ocular parameters could be observed, although some important individual changes were sometimes seen.

The angle-closure glaucoma eyes are characterized by a too thick lens in a too short eye with a shallow anterior chamber. After trabeculectomy important changes could be observed and more particularly the backwards displacement of the lens. The forward position of a thick lens in a small eye is therefore very important in producing an acute glaucoma attack. Successful glaucoma surgery replaces the eye in the pre-crisis condition. Iridectomy never resulted in important parameter changes, but this operation was only performed in mild or recent forms of angle-closure glaucoma.

Ultrasound biometry brings important informations concerning the different glaucoma forms. It may aid to a better understanding of the causative factors in angle-closure glaucoma. The change of the lens position and of the lens shape may explain an acute glaucoma attack.

REFERENCES

Buschmann, W. & Bluth, K. Regelmässige echographische Messung der Achsenlänge des Auges zur Kontrolle der Druckregulierung bei Hydrophthalmie. Klin. Mbl. Augenheilk. (165) 878 (1974).

Delmarcelle, Y., Collignon, J. & Luyckx, J. and Weekers, R. Etude biométrique du globe oculaire dans le glaucome à angle fermé. Bull. Soc. Franç. Ophtal. (84) 449 (1971).

Delmarcelle, Y., François, J., Goes, F. et al. Biométrie oculaire clinique. Bull. Soc. Belge Ophtal. (172) 1 (1976).

Delmarcelle, Y. and Luyckx, J. Biométrie du segment antérieur dans la cataracte sénile. Acta Ophthalmol., Kbh. (49) 454 (1971).

Delmarcelle, Y. & Luyckx-Bacus, J. Evolution biométrique de la chambre antérieure chez l'enfant. Etude de 1960 globes. Bull. Soc. Belge Ophtal. (158) 451 (1971).

François, J. & Goes, F. Etude échographique de la myopie. Bull. Soc. Belge Ophtal. (154) 415 (1970).

François, J. & Goes, F. Oculometry in emmetropia and ametropia. In: Ultrasonographica Medica (Böck J. & Ossoinig K. ed.) Verlag der Wiener Med. Akademia 473 (1971).

François, J. & Goes, F. Ultrasonic Biometry in ophthalmology. Proc. 2nd World Congress on Ultrasonics in Medicine (De Vlieger, M., ed.) Excerpta Medica. Amsterdam, (1973) p. 128.

Leighton, D.A. & Tomlinson, A. Changes in axial length and other dimensions of the eye-ball with increasing age. Acta Ophthalmol., Kbh. (50) 815 (1972).

Leighton, D.A. & Tomlinson, A. Ocular tension and axial length of the eye-ball in open angle glaucoma and low tension glaucoma. Brit. J. Ophthalmol. (57), 499 (1973).

Lowe, R.F. Causes of shallow anterior chamber in primary angle closure glaucoma. Ultrasonic biometry of normal and angle-closure glaucoma eyes. Am. J. Ophthalmol. (67) 87 (1969).

Tomlinson, A. & Phillips, C.I. Unequal axial length of eyeball and ocular tension. Acta Ophthalmol., Kbh., (50) 872 (1972).

Author's Address:
Dr. F. Goes
Ophthalmological Clinic
University of Ghent
Ghent, Belgium

OCULAR ECHOMETRY IN THE DIAGNOSIS OF CONGENITAL GLAUCOMA

R. SAMPAOLESI

(*Buenos Aires, Argentina*)

ABSTRACT

Thirty-three eyes of 18 normal infants and children and 22 eyes of 15 infants and children in whom congenital glaucoma had been diagnosed were measured by echometry. The anterior chamber depth, vitreous length and axial length were significantly greater in glaucomatous eyes, while the lens thickness was smaller in glaucomatous eyes. The axial length of normal eyes was found to increase with age according to the equation: axial length = 18.7 + 2.245 log (age in months.) The confidence interval of the normal growth curve allows the prediction of the maximum normal axial length for any given age. In congenital glaucoma cases, in which the visual fields and daily pressure curve cannot be evaluated, clinical echometry is proposed as a very valuable diagnostic and follow-up procedure.

INTRODUCTION

It is well known that the diagnosis of congenital glaucoma and the consequent indication of surgical treatment depend upon two factors: (1) the clinical symptoms, and (2) the intraocular pressure measured by applanation tonometry (Sampaolesi 1969, 1979). In 1971 we started performing echometries on eyes with congenital glaucoma, and it became apparent that in those cases with borderline pressure levels which did not show any meaningful deviation from the normal, echometry seemed to furnish us with a new and helpful parameter. This led us to undertake a systematic study of ocular echometry in normal children in order to establish the mean values and their dispersion in relation to age. We further studied a group of congenital glaucomas by means of echometry, applanation tonometry, and the usual diagnostic procedures, and thus we were finally able to establish the comparative value of echometry and tonometry.

MATERIAL

First group: Normal eyes (without ophthalmic symptoms, and showing normal applanation tonometry values). Thirty-three eyes of 18 children of ages ranging between two and 72 months; seven male and eleven female.

Second group: Glaucomatous eyes (with characteristic symptoms and pathological ocular pressure). Twenty-two eyes of 15 children of ages ranging from 2 to 24 months; ten male and five female. This group was subjected to preoperative as well as immediate postoperative echometry.

METHOD

The case history plays an important role in the clinical study of a child in whom congenital glaucoma is suspected, and, as far as this study is concerned, one of the main aspects to be considered is that of the time-span between the earliest symptoms, and surgery. The child is then put under general anesthesia with pentrane (methoxifluorane), and the hroizontal diameter of the cornea is measured. The anterior segment is examined with the slit lamp, paying particular attention to the chamber angle. Applanation tonometry is used to determine intraocular pressure (IOP); an eye-fundus examination is performed (optic disc), and the last step is an ultrasound study (echometry) under cyclplegics.

ECHOMETRY

Our echograph is a Kretz 7200 MA (A scan) model with 10 MHz probe. We use an immersion device consisting of a plastic cylinder (Fig. 1) fitted to the sclera (Ossoinig Scleral Shell N°20, manufactured by Hansen Ophthalmic Development Laboratory, Iowa City) in which we first instil four drops of 2.5% 4000 centipoise viscosity methylcellulose to seal off the scleral contact area. The cylinder is then filled with isotonic saline solution. The mehtoxifluorane anesthesia procedure we have described allows for the accurate centering of the eye with the child in dorsal position, an absolute prerequisite to a correct measurement. The probe is then inserted into the cylinder up to within approximately 5 mm from the cornea and in this manner we proceed to obtain 4 echograms of each eye at varying attenuation levels (Fig. 2).

Fig. 3 shows a characteristic echogram. Here measurements are obtained with dividers points resting on the base line of the echogram, precisely on the point where each echo arises. Thus we measure the anterior chamber, the lens, and the vitreous body. Only in the event of a corneal edema do we take the pertinent value into consideration as measured from the echoes pertaining to the anterior and posterior faces of the cornea. Otherwise we assume a 0.5 mean value for it.

Since our measurements are obtained in microseconds, we convert these to millimeters by taking into account the velocity of ultrasound in the various transparent media (Jansson & Kock 1962). On the basis of the above data we have developed a program to calculate the following echometric parameters (see Fig. 4).

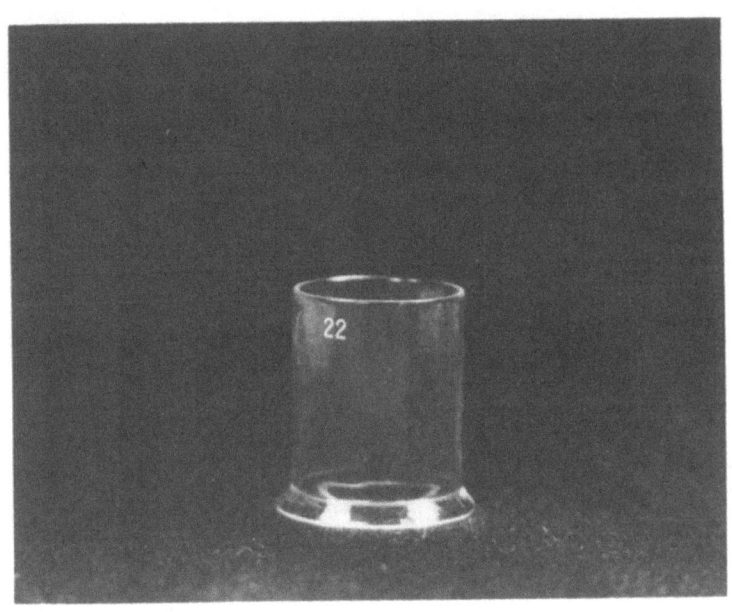

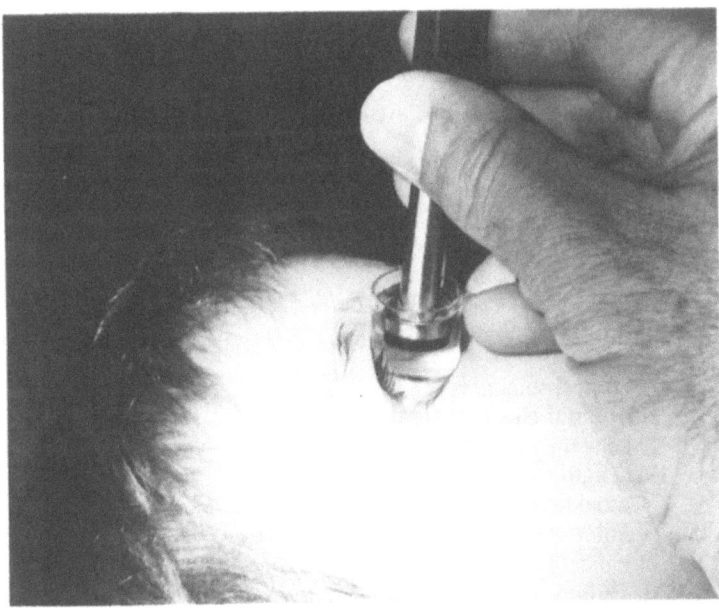

Fig. 2. Echometry procedure: the ultrasonic probe is immersed in the scleral shell filled with saline solution.

179

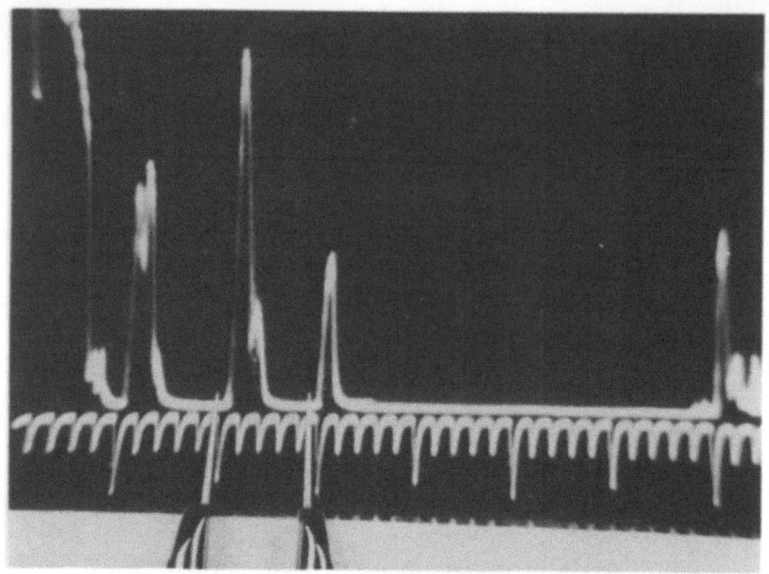

Fig. 3. The echogram is measured with dividers which point at the anterior and posterior lens surfaces in the figure.

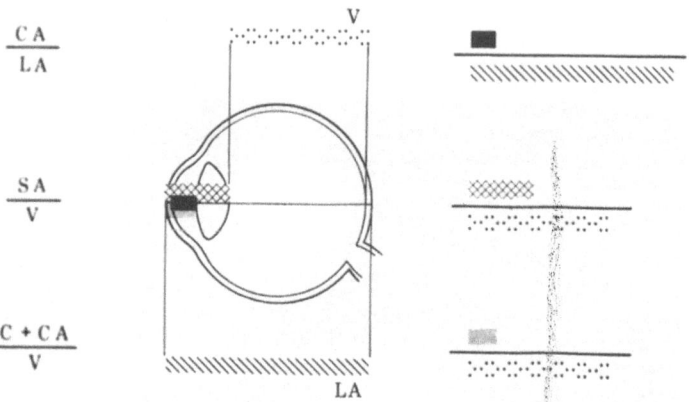

Fig. 4. Outline of the indices inter relating the measured segments. (See description in text).

I Corneal thickness
II Anterior chamber depth
III Lens thickness
IV Length of the vitreous body
V Axial length
VI $\dfrac{\text{Anterior chamber}}{\text{axial length}}$
VII $\dfrac{\text{Anterior segment (cornea + anterior chamber + lens)}}{\text{vitreous}}$
VIII $\dfrac{\text{Cornea + anterior chamber}}{\text{vitreous}}$

VI, VII, and VIII are three different indices. It must further be taken into consideration that the axial length is made up of the summation I + II + III + IV the thickness of the retina considered constant at 0.35 mm (François & Goes 1975).

STATISTICAL METHODS

The growth curve of normal and glaucomatous eyes in relation to age was calculated according to the least squares method. The statistical significance of the echometric differences found in both groups were evaluated with Student's t-test.

RESULTS

(a) *Correlation between axial length and age in normal eyes*

A logarithmic growth curve of the type y = a + b (log x) was plotted for the reviewed population of 33 eyes, in accordance with the following equation:

$$y = 18.7 + 2.245 \ (\log x)$$

where y is equal to axial length in mm and x is equal to the age in months (Fig. 5).

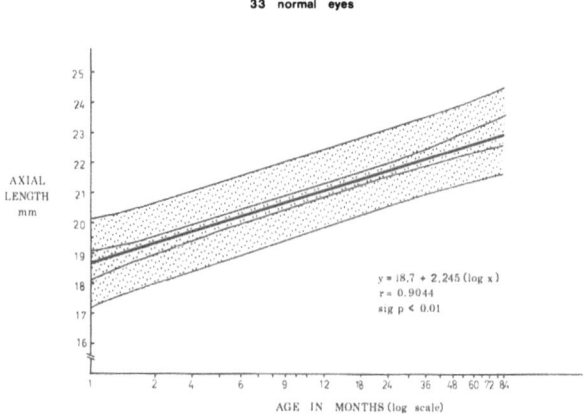

Fig. 5. Growth of normal eyes, abscissa logarithmic.

The correlation coefficient r is 0.9044 (p < 0.001 significance). Also calculated were the line confidence interval (related to each normal eye studied), and the prediction confidence interval (related to the population of normal children) (see Table 1). The diagnostical value of the prediction confidence interval shall be referred to in the discussion.

Table 1. Correlation between axial length and age in normal eyes.

Age in months	Y Axial length	95% Confidence interval Line	Prediction
1	18.7	18.2–19.1	17.3–20.1
2	19.4	19.0–19.7	18.0–20.7
3	19.8	19.4–20.1	18.4–21.1
4	20.0	19.8–20.3	18.7–21.4
5	20.3	20.0–20.5	19.9–21.6
6	20.4	20.2–20.7	19.1–21.8
7	20.5	20.3–20.8	19.3–21.9
8	20.7	20.5–20.9	19.4–22.0
9	20.8	20.6–21.1	19.5–22.2
10	20.9	20.7–21.2	19.6–22.3
11	21.0	20.8–21.3	19.7–22.4
12	21.1	20.9–21.3	19.8–22.4
18	21.5	21.3–21.8	20.2–22.8
24	21.8	21.5–22.1	20.5–23.1
30	22.0	21.7–22.3	20.7–23.3
36	22.2	21.9–22.5	20.8–23.5
42	22.3	22.0–22.7	21.0–23.7
48	22.5	22.1–22.8	21.1–23.8
54	22.6	22.2–22.9	21.2–23.9
60	22.7	22.3–23.1	21.3–24.0
66	22.8	22.4–23.2	21.4–24.1
72	22.9	22.5–23.3	21.5–24.2
78	22.9	22.5–23.3	21.6–24.3
84	23.0	22.6–23.4	21.6–24.4

(b) *Correlation between axial length and age in glaucomatous eyes*

A linear growth curve of the type y = a + b. x was plotted for the population of 22 eyes surveyed according to the following equation:

$$y = 22.10 + 0.13 x$$

where y is equal to axial length in millimeters and x is equal to age in months (see Fig. 6). The correlation coefficient r is 0.666 ($p < 0.01$ significance).

(c) *Value of the prediction confidence interval for normal eyes in the differential diagnosis between normal and glaucomatous eyes*

In Fig. 7 the values for the glaucomatous eyes surveyed are superposed on the data of Fig. 5 (prediction confidence interval for normal eyes). It can be clearly seen that of 36 eyes with congenital glaucoma, only one falls within the upper limit of the prediction interval.

(d) *Comparison between the echometric values of normal and glaucomatous eyes*

In paragraphs (a) (b) and (c) above, we have dealt with the axial length of normal and glaucomatous eyes in children up to age two. We shall now refer

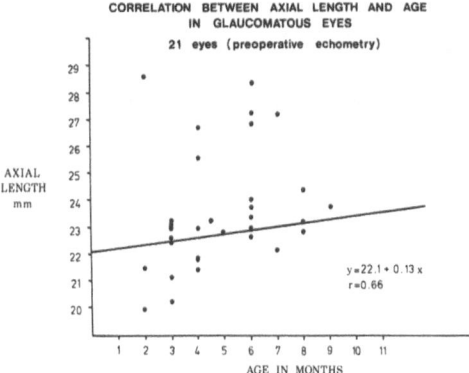

Fig. 6. Growth of glaucomatous eyes, abscissa linear.

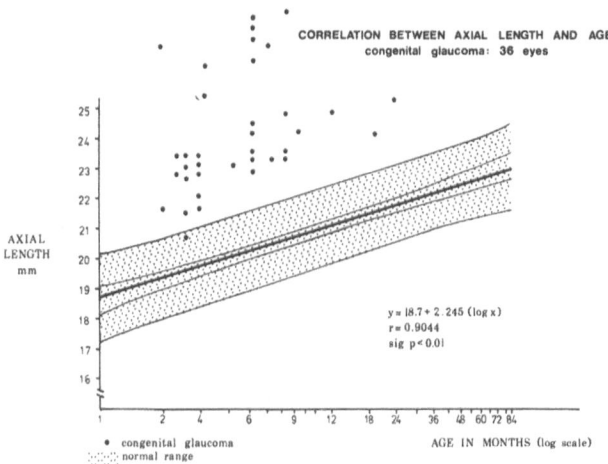

Fig. 7. Growth of normal eyes (from Fig. 5) compared to glaucomatous eyes (data different from those in Fig. 6).

to the comparison of echometric values pertaining to the two groups surveyed. In the first place, the length or thickness of each of the transparent media will be considered, and secondly, three indices interrlating the transparent media will be discussed.

(d) (i) *Anteroposterior length of the different transparent media in normal and glaucomatous eyes.* (Table 2).

As clearly emerges from this table, the values of the measurements of the anterior chamber depth, length of the vitreous body, and axial length, are significatively higher in the group of glaucomatous eyes. This fact has been established by Gernet and Hollwich (1969) and Espildora Couso (1979), and reflects the effect of an increased intraocular pressure on a distensible eye.

Table 2. Echometry in normal and glaucomatous eyes.
Arithmetical mean ± standard deviation

Echometry	Normal	Glaucomatous	Independent Student's t-test
Number of eyes	33	22	
Cornea	0.54	0.64 ± 0.24	
Anterior chamber	3.04 ± 0.51	3.57 ± 0.53	− 3.71[*]
Lens	3.85 ± 0.24	3.50 ± 0.25	5.30[*]
Vitreous	13.25 ± 1.18	14.70 ± 0.93	− 4.82[*]
Axial length	20.97 ± 1.48	22.75 ± 1.05	− 4.84[*]

[*]Significant difference (p < 0.001)

In our opinion, however, the most interesting finding is that the lens thickness of glaucomatous eyes is significantly reduced in the groups. This is an important contributing factor in the emmetropization of the glaucomatous eye, the axial length of which, when considered as an isolated factor, would warrant a higher myopia than that corresponding to the actual refractive state of the patients. (The other emmetropia-inducing factors are the larger corneal radius, and the deeper anterior chamber.)

(d) (ii) *Indices interrelating the segments examined above.* Fig. 4 summarizes the three indices which interrelate the segments referred to in the Echometry section, i.e. VI = CA/LA, VII = SA/V, VIII = C + CA/V.

The statistical study of the above indices shows that no significant difference exists between normal and glaucomatous eyes as far as indices VI and VIII are concerned. However, index VII, reveals a highly significant difference. In Table 3 the numerical values of these indices are given.

Table 3. Echometry in normal and glaucomatous eyes.
Arithmetical mean ± standard deviation

Echometry	Normal	Glaucomatous	Independent student's t-test
Anterior chamber / Axial length	0.15 ± 0.02	0.15 ± 0.02	− 1.28[**]
Anterior segment / Vitreous	0.57 ± 0.04	0.53 ± 0.05	3.51[*]
Cornea + Anterior chamber / Vitreous	0.27 ± 0.04	0.28 ± 0.03	− 1.27[**]

[*]Significant difference (p < 0.001)
[**]Non significant difference

Index VI and index VIII show no significant variation between the two populations surveyed, because when the eye is subjected to increased IOP the anteroposterior length increases accordingly in most cases. i.e., there is an increase in both anterior chamber depth and vitreous length. As to index VIII, this is significatively lower inglaucomatous children because it comprises the lens, the thickness of which decreases in eyes with congenital glaucoma.

(e) *Echometric asymmetry in bilateral congenital glaucoma.*

Of 60 cases surveyed, 20 are unilateral and 40 bilateral. In the latter we have found a manifest asymmetry in both the axial length, and each of the segments corresponding to the transparent media, and this is probably related to the fact that in glaucomatous children there is usually a difference between the intraocular pressures of the two affected eyes. This finding is in marked contrast to the values obtained for both normal children (33 eyes), and bilateral megalocorneas (ten eyes), where symmetry is characteristical. (Examples 1, 2 and 3)

We shall discuss three cases, the first being the one which induced us to consider echometry in the clinical study of congenital glaucoma, and which was therefore the starting point of this paper; the second and third more recent case which demonstrate the value of this new diagnostic parameter.

First example: Case History N°1382, K.R. 4 months, female.

The child is referred to us by an ophthalmologist with the presumptive diagnosis of congenital glaucoma.

First IOP measurement	OD 15 mm Hg	OS 9 mm Hg.
Second IOP measurement one month after the first	OD 15 mm Hg	OS 6 mm Hg
Third IOP measurement 45 days after second	OD 15 mm Hg	OS 6 mm Hg

The symptoms persist, and the eye fundus shows physiological cupping of the optic disc. Fig. 8 shows the echogram obtained at the age of six and a half months. The echograms have been arranged as mirror images in order to allow for the comparison of the difference between both eyes. The vitreous segment of the OD measures 19 microseconds, or 14.55 mm, whereas in OS it is 16 microseconds, or 12.66 mm.

Second example: (See Table 4) *Glaucoma case history N°2645, S.M. male, age three months.*

Observing this table we note that the child is brought in for examination in 10/78. It shows symptoms of unilateral congenital glaucoma, with a 12 mm corneal diameter in the normal eye, and 12.4 in the diseased one. IOP under anesthesia with Pentrane is 10 mm Hg in the healthy eye, and 29 mm Hg in OS. Corneal thickness measurements are above normal due to edema, and vitreous and axial length are higher in the diseased eye with respect to the healthy one. The child returns for a second examination in 12/78, after surgery had been performed on OS (trabeculotomy). At this time the IOP is completely normal. Another examination in 2/79 shows increased pressure in the previously normal eye, i.e., the IOP has risen to 25 mm Hg in OD, whereas it is found to be normal in the operated eye. We perform surgery on the latter, and in 5/79 the child's pressure is normal in both eyes. At that time we had not yet analysed the results of the research described in this paper, so that we were still unaware of these factors bearing on normality and its limits.

185

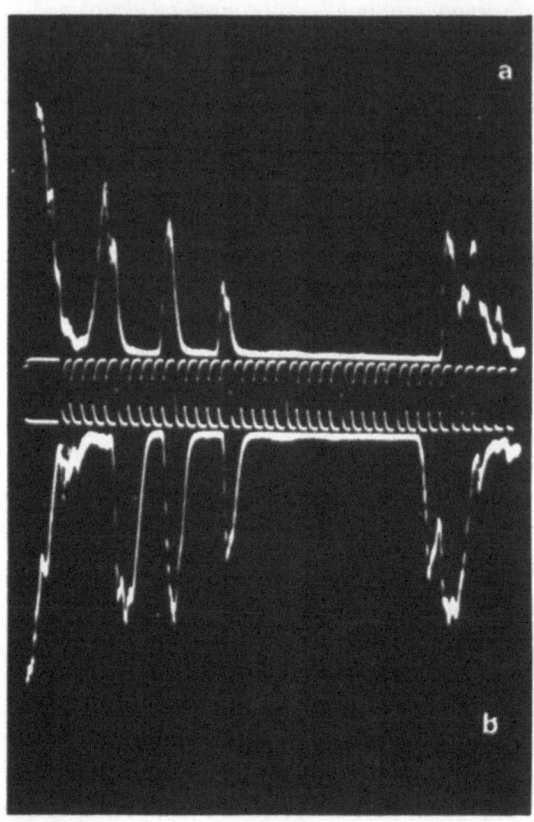

Fig. 8. Echograms of the right eye (a) and the left eye (b) of first example case, arranged as mirror images.

Table 4.

G: 2645 S.M. ♂ 3 m.						Echometry					
Date	D.C.	P.O.	C	C.A.	Cris	V	L.A.	*C.A.* L.A.	*S.A.* V	*C + CA* V
X/78	12	10	.54	3.45	3.69	12.26	20.29	.17	.63	.33
*	12.5	29	.78	3.06	3.94	13.02	21.15	.15	.60	.29
XII/78	12	8	.54	3.45	3.69	*13.41*	*21.44*	.16	.57	.30
	12.5	8	.54	3.06	3.96	12.64	20.53	.15	.60	.29
II/79*	13.5	25	.54	3.83	3.28	*13.79*	*21.71*	.18	.56	.32
	12.5	12	.54	3.06	3.69	12.64	20.29	.15	.58	.29
V/79	13.5	10	.54	3.83	3.69	13.79	22.20	.18	.58	.32
	12.5	10	.54	3.06	3.69	12.64	20.29	.15	.58	.29

*Trabeculotomy

It can be seen clearly that, during the first postoperative checkup in 12/78, despite a normal IOP in both eyes—8 and 8 mm Hg—the length of the vitreous was 13.41 mm in the eye which was hitherto considered normal, and 12.64 mm in the eye which had undergone surgery, the axial length being 21.44 mm in the so-called healthy eye, and 20.63 mm in the trabeculotomized one. Intraocular pressure was obviously normal in both eyes, yet the echometrical values were already pointing toward glaucoma in the eye hitherto believed to be healthy, which upon further examination, two months later, shows a distinctly pathological intraocular pressure.

Third example: Glaucoma case history N° 2204, P.F. male, age three months.

The child is referred with the classical symptoms of congenital glaucoma, ephora and photophobia, at age three months. The following measurements were obtained:

	IOP	Vitreous length	Axial length
OD	20 mm Hg	13.79	22.59
OS	24 mm Hg	14.67	22.97

A bilateral trabeculotomy was subsequently performed.

At the age of four years while the IOP was apparently under control the axial length was significantly increased, as can be seen in the following values:

	IOP	Vitreous length	Axial length
OD	15 mm Hg	16.47	25.27
OS	15 mm Hg	15.70	24.50

Finally, at five years of age the IOP values were markedly increased. It is worth noting that the increase in axial and vitreous length has apparently preceded the rise of the IOP:

	IOP	Vitreous length	Axial length
OD	38 mm Hg	16.85	25.68
OS	32 mm Hg	16.85	25.68

DISCUSSION

The enlarged dimensions of the eyes of children with congenital glaucoma is certainly not a recent discovery, since the word 'buphthalmos' designating this abnormality, was coined by Ambroise Paré as far back as 1661.

The value of echometry for an accurate description of the comparative growth of normal and glaucomatous eyes was pointed out by Gernet of Hollwich (1969), and its importance in the follow-up of congenital glaucoma case histories was recently stressed by W. Buschmann & Karin Bluth (1974 a, b).

On the basis of the results described above, it is the purpose of this paper to propose the echometric measurement of the axial length of childrens' eyes as a highly valuable variable in the diagnosis of congenital glaucoma.

Our results confirmed the clinical value of echographic biometry both for the diagnosis of congenital glaucoma in cases with borderline IOP (see Example 1) and to detect a glaucoma in the fellow eye of patients with presumed unilateral disease (see Example 2). Also the mehtod proved its efficiency in the follow-up of operated cases of congenital glaucoma (see Example 3).

Until this time ocular pressure was considered to be the fundamental variable in the diagnosis of congential glaucoma. The essential difference between tonometry in adults and children resides in the practical impossibility of ascertaining the daily pressure curve of the latter.

The second difference is the need to measure a child's ocular pressure under general anesthesia, since even when using a reliable method such as that described in our previous paper (Sampaolesi 1976), the intraocular pressure is never measured more than once daily. The daily ocular pressure variability in hypertensive eyes is a characteristic of the disease occurring over a relatively short period (24 h), whereas increased axial length in congenital glaucoma reflects variations occurring over prolonged periods (days, months, or years) as result of the increased mean intraocular pressure acting on a distensible eye.

Summarizing, intraocular pressure values hold true only for a given moment in time, whereas axial length furnishes information about what has happened in the course of the disease over a prolonged period of time up to a given moment. Furthermore, while intraocular pressure is a variable influenced by the anesthetic agents which are necessary for its measurement in children, echometric measurements are not altered by these agents.

Our experience leads us to consider axial length as the fundamental factor for the diagnosis of congential glaucoma, when occurring in conjunction with clinical symptoms, and it has the most direct bearing on whether surgery is indicated or not. Thus the fundamental basis for diagnosis are, in the first place, axial length, and secondly, ocular pressure in the presence of clinical symptoms.

REFERENCES

Buschmann, W., & Bluth, K. Regelmassige echographische Messung der Achsenlange des Auges zur Kontrolle der Druckregulierung bei Hydrophthalmie. Klinische Monatsblatter fuer Aguenheilkunde 165: 878 (1974a).

Buschmann, W. & Bluth, K. Eine Echographische Methode zur Verlaufskontrolle angeborener Glaukome. Albrecht v. Graefes Arch. Klin. Exp. Ophthalmol. 192:.313 (1974b).

Espíldora Couso, J., Vicuña, & Gormaz, A. Alteraciones biométricas en el control tardío del ojo con glaucoma congénito operado. Glaucoma Symposium. The Panam. Cong. Ophthalmol. (1979).

François, J., & Goes, F. Oculometry of progressive myopia. In: Ultrasonography in Ophthalmology (François J. & Goes, E., eds.) Bibl. Ophthalmol. Basel: Karger 83: 277 (1975).

Gernet, H., & Hollvich, F. Oculometrie des kindlichen Glaukoms. Ber. dtsch. Ophthalmol. Ges. 69: 341 (1969).

Jansson, F., & Kock, E. Determination of the velocity of ultrasound in the human lens and vitreous. Acta Ophthalmol. Kbh. 39: 899 (1962).

Luyckx & Delmarcelle. Contribution of ultrasonography to the study of microcornea and megalocornea. In: Ophthalmic Ultrasound (Gitter, et al., eds) The Saint Louis: Mosby (1969) p. 149.

Sampaolesi, R. La pression oculaire et le sinus camerulaire chez l'enfant normal et dans le glaucome congénital au-dessous de l'age de cinq ans. Documenta Ophthalmologica 26: 497 (1969).

Sampaolesi, R., Reca, R., Carro, A., & Armando, A.: Normaler intraocularer Druck bei
    Kindern bis zu 5 Jahren mit und ohne Allgemeinnarkose. Seine Wichtigkeit für die
    Frühdiagnose des angeborenen Glaukoms.
Glaukom-Symposion Wüzburg, 1974. Stuttgart: Ferdinand Enke Verlag. (1976) p. 278.

Author's Address:
Dept. of Ophthalmology
School of Medicine
University of Buenos Aires
Parana 1239. 1° A
1018 Buenos Aires, Argentina

OCULAR DIMENSIONS OF EYES WITH FUCHS' SPOT PROVIDED BY ULTRASONIC BIOMETRY

M. FRIED, A. SIEBERT, A. WESSING & G. MEYER-SCHWICKERATH

(Essen, F.R.G.)

INTRODUCTION

The shape of the eye and its size have been shown to be of great importance in the manifestation of eye disease, for instance such as retinal detachment (Gernet 1965, Dominguez 1977, Gerke 1979) and Glaucoma. Fuchs' spot which is a well defined clinical entity is another condition with specific ocular dimensions. Whereas some valuable studies have been carried out on the refractive, clinical, morphological and fluorescein angiographic characteristics of Fuchs' spot (Förster 1862, Fuchs 1901, Lehmus 1875, Aiello & Master 1953, Lloyd 1954, Campos 1957, Gass 1967, D'hoine *et al.* 1974, Levy, Pollock & Curtin 1974, 1977), very little information is available on its oculometric features provided by ultrasound. Ultrasonic axial length measurements of 28 eyes with Fuchs' spot were first produced by Curtin & Karlin (1971). In the framework of a follow-up study (Fried *et al.* 1980) we were able to determine the ocular dimensions by ultrasound in 55 eyes with Fuchs' spot. We herein report the findings in this regard.

SUBJECTS AND METHODS

For this purpose all patients on record at the Essen University Eye Hospital with the confirmed diagnosis Fuchs' spot were reviewed in 1980. 145 patients (206 eyes) were documented to have Fuchs' spot (= Group A). Up to date 36 patients living within a reasonable travel distance answered to our check-up call, comprising those 55 eyes which we were able to examine by ultrasound. In addition a complete ocular examination, including fundus photography and fluorescein angiography was performed.

For ultrasonic oculometry we used the Kretz Technik 7200 MA with a plan 8 MHz transducer (probe NM 8–5 k). A contacts lens was used with a sterile water column between the transducer and the cornea for axial length measurements. The equatorial diameters were measured by placing the transducer upon the conjunctiva at the equator at 12 o'clock, 1:30, 3, 4:30, 6, 7:30, 9 and 10:30. Five Polaroid photos were taken of both eyes of each person at every reading and averaged. Differences between the five readings were usually minimal. Calculations were then based on the different sound velocities in the aqueous (1532 m/sec.), lens (1641 m/sec.) and vitreous (1532 m/sec.) as reported by Jansson (1963). In this way anterior chamber depth (ACD), lens thickness (LT), axial length of the vitreous body (VL) and total axial length (AL) as well as the horizontal and vertical equatorial diameter were obtained. No correction for retinal thickness was made.

B-Scan was performed with the Ocuscan 400 system to detect posterior staphylomata by moving the probe systematically into all explorable positions. The 36 patients were 12 males and 24 females. Age ranged from 15–66 years with a mean of 43.2 ± 13.7 years when Fuchs' spot first appeared.

RESULTS AND DISCUSSION

(1) Table 1 gives the range, mean a standard deviation (SD) for anterior chamber depth (ACD), lens thickness (LT), vitreous length (VL) and axial length (AL). Compared to the normal values for the emmetropic adult eye vitreous length and axial length are grossly enlarged, while anterior chamber depth and lens thickness are well within normal limits. This confirms the well established fact that Fuchs' spot is a condition in pathological myopia, which in its nature is of axial origin. Vitreous length and axial length were highly correlated, the correlation coefficient being 0.9 ($p < 0.001$).

Table 1. Ultrasonic measurement results in 55 eyes with Fuchs' spot (Kretz Technik 7200 MA). The axial length and its components are given.

| | Ultrasonic biometry in 55 eyes with Fuchs' spot | |
	Mean ± SD	Range
ACD	3.76 ± 0.36	3.06– 4.60
LT	4.27 ± 0.35	3.69– 4.92
VL	21.17 ± 2.01	18.38–27.19
AL	29.11 ± 2.19	26.31–35.91

ACD = Anterior chamber depth
LT = Lens thickness
VL = Vitreous length
AL = Axial length

(2) The mean equatorial diameter horizontally was 26.42 ± 1.21 mm and vertically 26.26 ± 1.33 mm in the eyes with Fuchs' spot. These increased diameters reveal that in pathological myopia axial elongation and equatorial expansion are combined.

(3) Posterior staphylomata were detected by ophthalmoscopy in 15 of the 55 eyes (27.3%). It was not in all cases possible to confirm this finding by A- and B-Scan ultrasound. Especially in shallow posterior staphylomata this proved difficult.

(4) Table 2 shows the frequency of Fuchs' spot in our material at each axial length. The large majority of eyes are distributed between an axial length of 26.5 and 31.4 mm. This interval makes up 91.5% of all eyes with

Table 2. Frequency distribution of 55 eyes with Fuchs' spot from 26.5 to 36.4 mm of axial length. Incidence below and above these values was zero.

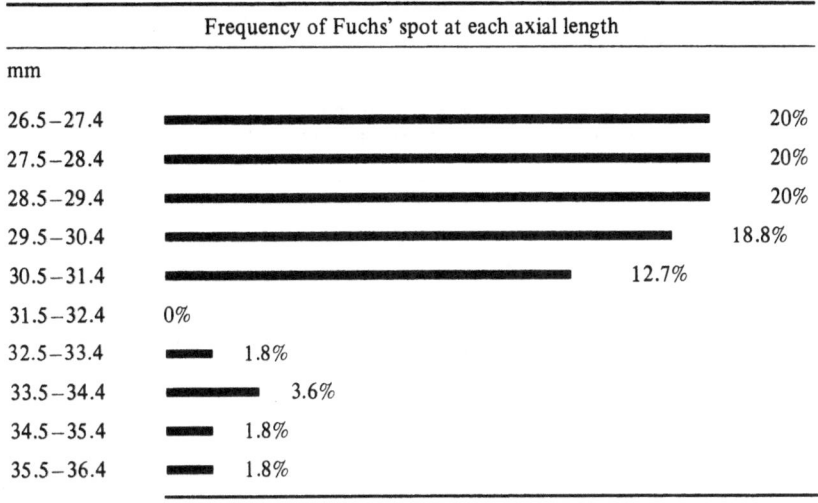

Frequency of Fuchs' spot at each axial length

mm	
26.5–27.4	20%
27.5–28.4	20%
28.5–29.4	20%
29.5–30.4	18.8%
30.5–31.4	12.7%
31.5–32.4	0%
32.5–33.4	1.8%
33.5–34.4	3.6%
34.5–35.4	1.8%
35.5–36.4	1.8%

Fuchs' spot in our sample. Above 31.5 mm of axial length Fuchs' spot becomes infrequent. This study corroborates therefore that Fuchs' spot affects mainly moderately high myopes with a moderate elongation of axial length corresponding to refractive values around − 12.0 D. By the way axial length and refraction were highly correlated in this study, the correlation coefficient being 0.7 ($p < 0.001$). However, considering the refraction curve of Betsch (1929) we know that the incidence of myopia decreases as the degree of myopia increases. In other words, excessive high myopes with excessive axial elongation are infrequent and so are Fuchs' spot in such eyes.

(5) Table 3 When axial length in eyes with Fuchs' spot was analyzed according to sex the difference between axial length in women (29.42 ± 1.95 mm) and in men (28.76 ± 2.68 mm) was not significant. On the other hand, women were at least twice as often affected as men in our material, corroborating other studies. Nevertheless, when Fuchs' spot occurs in men and women it does so at the same degrees of axial elongation.

Table 3. Comparison of axial length of eyes with Fuchs' spot in men and in women. The difference was not significant ($p > 0.05$).

	Axial length in eyes with Fuchs' spot Men *vs.* Women	
	N	Mean ± SD
Women	35	29.42 ± 1.95
Men	20	28.76 ± 2.68
		N.S.

(6) We wanted to know if eyes with Fuchs' spot differ from eyes without this lesion in anterior chamber depth, lens thickness, vitreous length and axial

length. We therefore compared the Fuchs' spot eyes with the non-affected fellow-eyes, as shown in Table 4. No significant differences were found. This might be expected from the well established strong right-left correlation of refraction and axial length.

Table 4. Comparison of axial length and its components in eyes with Fuchs' spot with the non-affected fellow-eyes of the same study group. Differences were not significant (p > 0.05).

| | *Fuchs' spot eyes compared to non-affected fellow eyes* | | | |
	ACD	LT	VL	AL
Fuchs' spot eyes	3.76 ± 0.36	4.27 ± 0.35	21.17 ± 2.01	29.11 ± 2.19
Non-affected fellow-eyes	3.76 ± 0.29	4.33 ± 0.56	21.30 ± 2.30	29.22 ± 2.35
	n.s	n.s	n.s	n.s

ACD = Anterior chamber depth
LT = Lens thickness
VL = Vitreous length
AL = Axial length

(7) Considering the prognosis we tested the correlation between the age of onset of Fuchs' spot and the degree of axial elongation. As is shown in Fig. 1 when age of onset is plotted against axial length a soft correlation becomes apparent, the correlation coefficient being − 0.33, which proofs significant. Thus manifestation tends to occur earlier with rising axial elongation.

(8) Finally we found no definite correlation between final visual acuity and axial length. Visual prognosis was determined by morphologic features, such as foveal involvement, recurrent hemorrhage and persistence of subretinal neovascularization. These morphologic features did not depend on increase in axial length or myopia. Therefore neither axial length nor the degree of myopia as such are completely reliable prognostic indicators for the degree of associated complications in pathological myopia. Nevertheless excessive axial elongation is the cardinal factor in the pathogenesis of Fuchs' spot.

SUMMARY

We reported the oculometric findings in 55 eyes with Fuchs' spot. Vitreous and axial length were grossly enlarged, while anterior chamber depth and lens thickness were normal compared to the emmetropic eye. The increased equatorial diameter revealed that axial elongation and equatorial expansion are combined. The great majority of eyes (91.5%) had an axial length between 26.5 and 31.4 mm. No oculometric differences between the sexes were detected. Manifestation of Fuchs' spot tends to occur earlier in life with rising axial elongation. No definite correlation was found between visual prognosis and axial length. Visual prognosis was determined primarily by morphologic features. Therefore neither axial length nor the degree of

Axial length and age of onset

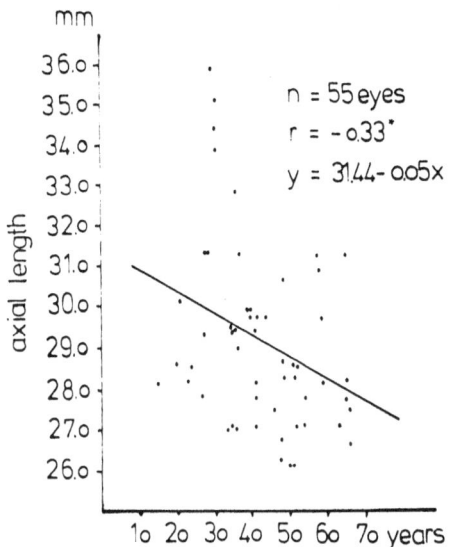

Fig. 1. Correlation of axial length and age at manifestation of Fuchs' spot in 55 eyes, which proofs to be significant (P < 0.05). Manifestation of Fuchs' spot tends to occur earlier in life with rising axial length.

myopia are completely reliable prognostic indicators for the degree of associated complications, such as Fuchs' spot, in pathological myopia. Excessive axial length is the cardinal factor in the pathogenesis of Fuchs' spot.

REFERENCES

Aiello, J.S. & Master, S. Fuchs' spot in the macula. A rare lesion in myopic patients. Am. J. Ophthalmol. 36: 1126 (1953).

Campos. R. La tache de Fuchs. Mod. Probl. Ophthalmol. 1: 364 (1957).

Curtin, B.J. & Karlin, D.B. Axial length measurements and fundus changes of the myopic eye. Am. J. Ophthalmol. 71: 42 (1971).

D'Hoine, G., Turut, P., François, P. & Hacke, J. Cl. L'atteinte maculaire des myopes. Bull. Soc. Ophthalmol. Fr. 74: 821 (1974).

Dominguez, A. Ultrasonic control of ocular dimensions and surgical indentation in retinal detachment. Mod. Probl. Ophthalmol. 18: 77 (1977).

Duke-Elder, S. System of Ophthalmology. Vol. V. Ophthalmic optics and refraction. London: Henry Kimpton (1970) p. 300.

Fried, M., Siebert, A., Meyer-Schwickerath, G. & Wessing, A. Natural history of Fuchs' spot: a long-term follow-up study. Presented at the Third Int. Conf. Myopia, Copenhagen, Denmark, August 24–27, 1980 (in press).

Förster, R. Ophthalmologische Beiträge. T.C.F. Berlin: Enslin (1862) p. 55.

Fuchs, E. Der zentrale schwarze Fleck bei Myopie. Zschr. f. Augenheilk. 5: 171 (1901).

Gass, J.D.M. Pathogenesis of disciform detachment of the neuroepithelium. VI. Disciform detachment secondary to heredodegenerative neoplastic and traumatic lesions of the choroid. Am. J. Ophthalmol. 63: 689 (1967).

Gerke, E. Dimensionen des Bulbus bei Ablatio retinae. Ber. Dtsch. Ophthalmol. Ges. 76: 549 (1979).

Gernet, H. Biometrische Befunde bei Rissamotio im kurzsichtigen Auge. Beitrag zur Pathogenese. Ophthalmologica 150: 386 (1965).

Jansson, F. Measurement of the intraocular distances by ultrasound. Acta Ophthalmol. Suppl. 74: 1 (1963).

Klein, R.M. & Curtin, B.J. Laquer crack lesions in pathological myopia: Am. J. Opthalmol. 79: 380 (1975).

Lehmus,   Die Erkrankungen der macula lutea bei progressiver Myopie. Inaug. Diss. Zürich (1875).

Lloyd, R.I. Clinical studies of the myopic macula. Trans. Am. Acad. Ophthalmol. Otolaryngol. 51: 273 (1954).

Levy, J.H., Pollock, H.M. & Curtin, B.J. The Fuchs' spot: an opthalmoscopic and fluorescein angiographic study. In: (Shimizu, K., Ed.) 'Fluorescein angiography'. Tokyo: Igaku Shoin, Publ. (1974) p. 182.

Levy, J.H. Pollock, H.M. & Curtin, B.J. The Fuchs' spot: an ophthalmoscopic and fluorescein angiographic study. Ann. Ophthalmol. 9: 1433 (1977).

Authors' Address:

Essen University Eye Hospital
Hufelandstrasse 55, D-4300 Essen 1
F.R.G.

ULTRASONIC STUDY OF AXIAL LENGTH CHANGES AFTER ENCIRCLING OPERATION

Y. BABA & A. SAWADA

(Miyazaki, Japan)

It has been reported previously that changes in the refractive state develop after an operation for retinal detachment and the quality of change varies according to the kind of the procedure used.

Axial length and the length of ocular dimensions were ultrasonically measured for six months in adult pigmented rabbit eyes after the encircling operation with different strength of tightness was performed. Ultrasonic ocular biometry was done with the Digital Biometric Ruler 300 (Sonometries). The propagation velocity of ultrasound in the Digital Biometric Ruler 300 was set at 1639 m/sec for the cornea, at 1532 m/sec for the anterior chamber and the vitreous, and at 1641 m/sec for the lens. Changes in refractive state were measured with Rodenstock's refractometer.

To affirm the accuracy and stability of the procedures of measurement, ocular biometry was performed and the radius of corneal curvature was measured ten times for a week in one rabbit. The values were constant and standard deviation was very minute (Table 1). Table 2 shows the average of the axial length and its components in all twenty five rabbits used for experiments. No significant difference was found between the two eyes. These measurements were done before the operation. The result confirmed that the contralateral eyes could be used as controls.

Table 1. Average of refractive power, radius of corneal curvature and components of axial length measured ten times in one untreated rabbit.

	Right eye $\bar{X} \pm$ S.E.	Left eye $\bar{X} \pm$ S.E.
Refractive power (D)	+ 1.18 ± 0.06	+ 1.14 ± 0.05
Radius of corneal curvature (mm)	7.28 ± 0.03	7.26 ± 0.03
Corneal thickness (mm)	0.41 ± 0.01	0.41 ± 0.01
Anterior chamber depth (mm)	2.20 ± 0.01	2.20 ± 0.01
Lens thickness (mm)	7.13 ± 0.01	7.09 ± 0.01
Vitreous length (mm)	6.53 ± 0.02	6.58 ± 0.02
Axial length (mm)	16.27 ± 0.02	16.28 ± 0.02

The strength of encircling was decided by the length of a silicone rod fixed on the sclera at the equator and tightened. Three kinds of strength of encirclement were adopted. They were 10%, 15% and 20% tightness. For

Table 2. Average and statistical analysis of refractive power and components of axial length in 25 normal rabbits used in experiments and observed for six months.

	Right eye $\bar{X} \pm$ S.E.	Left eye $\bar{X} \pm$ S.E.
Refractive power (D)	+ 1.40 ± 0.13	+ 1.37 ± 0.13
Radius of corneal curvature (mm)	7.44 ± 0.05	7.42 ± 0.05
Corneal thickness (mm)	0.43 ± 0.01	0.43 ± 0.01
Anterior chamber depth (mm)	2.11 ± 0.02	2.10 ± 0.02
Lens thickness (mm)	7.14 ± 0.07	7.16 ± 0.07
Vitreous length (mm)	6.68 ± 0.05	6.68 ± 0.05
Axial length (mm)	16.36 ± 0.09	16.37 ± 0.09

example, in 10% tightness, the eye ball was encircled with 90% of the length of the total circumference. The encircling operation was done in the right eyes in all rabbits. The left eyes were used as controls. Encirclement with 10% tightness was done in nine rabbits, with 15% tightness in nine rabbits, and with 20% tightness in seven rabbits. A total of 25 rabbits were used in the experiments.

Changes in refractive state after encirclement with three kinds of strength in tightening is shown in Fig. 1. Immediately after encirclement a marked degree of myopia developed in all the eyes fo three groups. The degree of myopia had a harmonious relation to the tightness of encirclement. During the first two weeks the degree of myopia decreased with a relative rapidity. After that, in groups of mild and strong tightness, the degree of myopia began to increase again. At two months after encircling the degree of myopia ceased to vary. At six months myopia in proportion to the strength of tightness in encircling was left.

It is very interesting to study the relation of changes in the total axial length and/or those in individual components of the total axial length to changes in the refractive state, although the problem should be discussed in more detail in the field of myopia research. Elongation in axial length after encircling is shown in Fig. 2. Marked elongation occurred immediately after the operation. The variation from controls was in proportion to the degree of tightening, as was the refractive change. The variation was 0.75 ± 0.04 mm in 10% tightness, 1.13 ± 0.23 mm in 15% tightness and 1.55 ± 0.06 mm in 20% tightness. These degrees of elongation tended to decrease during the first two weeks in all groups. Thereafter, in the groups in 10% and 15% tightness, axial length stopped to vary. Only in the group with tightness of 20%, axial length began to increase again. At two months axial length continued to increase, although variation was slight. At six months elongation of axial length was left significantly in proportion to the tightness of encirclement.

Axial length is composed of thickness of the cornea, depth of the anterior .chamber, thickness of the lens and length of the vitreous. Changes in any of these dimensions have an important relation to axial length. The cornea thickened in all groups with different tightnesses of encirclement immediately after encircling as shown in Fig. 3. However, after four days thickness of the cornea returned to the preoperative value. After that any significant difference in three groups with different tightness was not produced. And any significant difference from controls was not found.

198

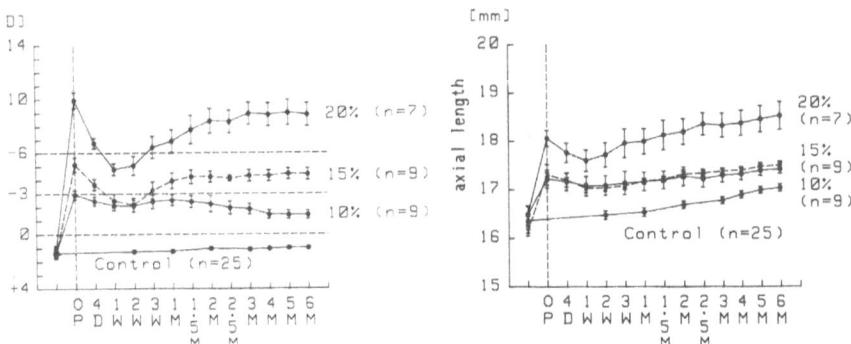

Fig. 1. Changes in refractive power after encircling operations with different tightnesses.

Fig. 2. Changes in axial length after encircling operations with different tightnesses.

Changes in depth of the anterior chamber are shown in Fig. 4. Immediately after encircling, depth of the anterior chamber was reduced in all three groups with different tightnesses. Thereafter in groups with weak and mild tightness (10% and 15%), reduction in depth of the anterior chamber became small. However, depth of the anterior chamber was kept reduced even at three and six months after encircling. On the other hand, in some eyes with strong tightness (20%), depth of the anterior chamber increased at two months after encircling. Three of seven rabbits showed remarkable increase in depth of the anterior chamber. They were those eyes in which strong myopia was produced. The fact is worthy of note in considering the mechanism of muopia developed after encircling.

Change in thickness of the lens are shown in Fig. 5. Immediately after encircling, thickness of the lens did not change in any groups with different tightnesses. At four days after encircling, thickness of the lens started to increase in all three groups. At two weeks, increase of lens thickness was in proportion to the tightness of encirclement. Variation from controls was 0.20 ± 0.04 mm in 10% tightness, 0.27 ± 0.07 mm in 15% tightness, 0.39 ± 0.04 mm in 20% tightness. After that the variation tended to reduce. In a group of weak tightness (10%) a significant difference from controls had disappeared at six months. In groups of mild and strong tightness (15% and 20%) a slight increase in thickness of the lens was still kept.

Vitreous length is the most important component of axial length. The changes after encircling are shown in Fig. 6. Immediately after the operation, vitreous length markedly elongated in all three groups in proportion to the tightness of encirclement. Variation from controls was 0.83 ± 0.06 mm in 10% tightness, 1.19 ± 0.21 mm in 15% tightness and 1.50 ± 0.04 mm in 20% tightness. The degree of elongation in vitreous length tended to reduce during the first two weeks in all three groups, as in the refractive state and in axial length. Thereafter the degree of elongation tended to increase slightly again up to two months after encirclement. After two months the variation was minimized. At six months vitreous length continued to be elongated in proportion to the tightness of encirclement. The variation was 0.52 ± 0.07 mm

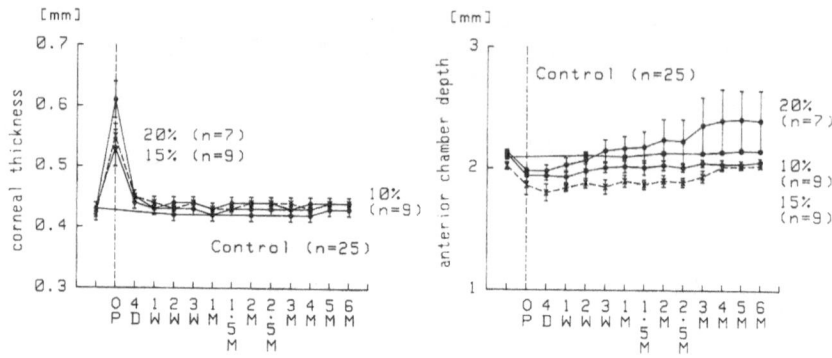

Fig. 3. Changes in corneal thickness after encircling operations with different tightnesses.

Fig. 4. Changes in anterior chamber depth after encircling operations with different tightnesses.

in 10% tightness, 0.66 ± 0.07 mm in 15% tightness and 0.94 ± 0.08 mm in 15% tightness.

We will now discuss the correlation of the range of fluctuation from the controls between several important factors — immediately after and at six months after the encircling.

Between refractive changes and elongation of axial length, a strong correlation was found immediately after the encircling as shown in Fig. 7. The coefficient was -0.7131. At six months the correlation was more close. The coefficient was -0.9128.

As shown in Fig. 8, a close correlation was also found between refractive changes and elongation of vitreous length. The coefficient immediately and at six months after encircling was -0.7467 and -0.7395, respectively.

It is important to study the correlation between fluctuation in axial length and that in individual components of axial length. As shown in Fig. 9, a strong correlation was found between fluctuation from controls in axial length and that in vitreous length. The coefficient immediately after encircling was 0.9407. The strong correlation was kept still at six months. The coefficient was 0.6145. Thus, it was proved that changes in vitreous length had a great influence on those in axial length.

In the study of refractive changes after encircling operation for retinal detachment of refractive factors, for example — the radius of corneal curvature and the lens position should be considered. Definite similarity between the variation curve in the refractive state and that in the radius of corneal curvature — except for immediately after encircling — was proved. As to the lens position, forward shift of the lens was suggested. Details of these results have been reported in other occasions.

DISCUSSION

It is well known that different kinds of refractive change develop after an operation for retinal detachment. The kind of refractive change is dependent

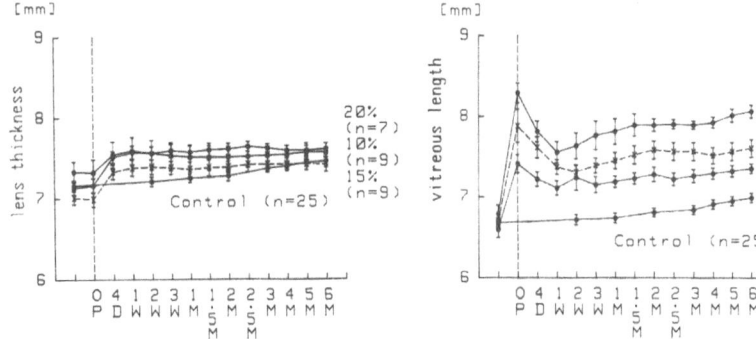

Fig. 5. Changes in lens thickness after encircling operations with different tightnesses.

Fig. 6. Changes in vitreous length after encircling operations with different tightnesses.

upon the kind of the operation performed. Hyperopia or hyperopic astigmatism can be explained by shortening of axial length. Myopia developed after encircling operation can be explained by elongation of axial length caused by the indentation of the wall of the eye at the site of encircling.

Encircling with three different tightnesses was done in enucleated human eyes. (Rubin 1975) Axial length elongation of 0.44 mm developed with weak tightness and that of 1.09 mm developed with medium tightness. With strong tightness, on the other hand, axial length was shortened by 0.35 mm.

Burton, *et al.* (1977) detected changes in the depth of the anterior chamber, lens thickness and vitreous length after hard silicone explants and hard silicone implants under scleral flaps. Significant alternation in axial length were found in approximately 60% of the eyes. Some eyes had axial lengthening and other eyes had axial reduction.

Larsen & Syrdalen (1979) found a significant increase in axial length from 0.62 to 1.24 mm in ten phakic eyes treated with encircling silicone rubber band for retinal detachment. The mean difference between the pre- and postoperative refractive power was − 2.4 D. These results cannot be precisely evaluated, because the strength of tightening was not definte. It is necessary to decide the strength of tightening in the encircling operation and to study the effect of difference in strength of tightness on changes in refractive power and changes in axial length and its components.

In the present study, encircling with different tightnesses, which was regulated by the length of the silicone rod sutured on the sclera, was done in three groups of rabbits.

Based on results in pigmented rabbit eyes after encircling with different tightnesses, the following conclusions can be drawn.

(1) The degree of myopia which developed immediately after the encircling operation at the equator was in proportion to the degree of tightness of encircling.

(2) At six months after encircling, myopia − in proportion to the degree of tightness − was still present.

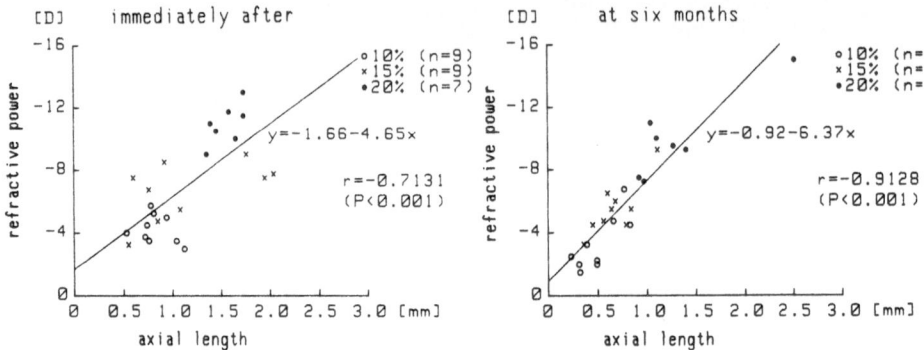

Fig. 7. Correlation between changes in refractive power and those in axial length immediately after encircling operations with different tightnesses and at six months later.

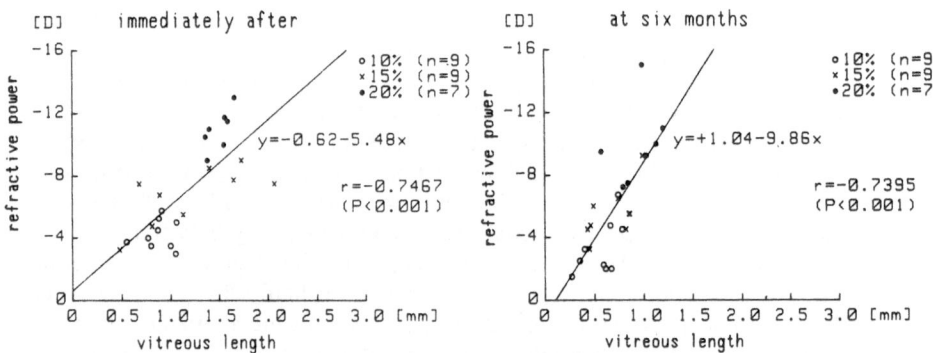

Fig. 8. Correlation between changes in refractive power and those in vitreous length immediately after encircling operations with different tightnesses and at six months later.

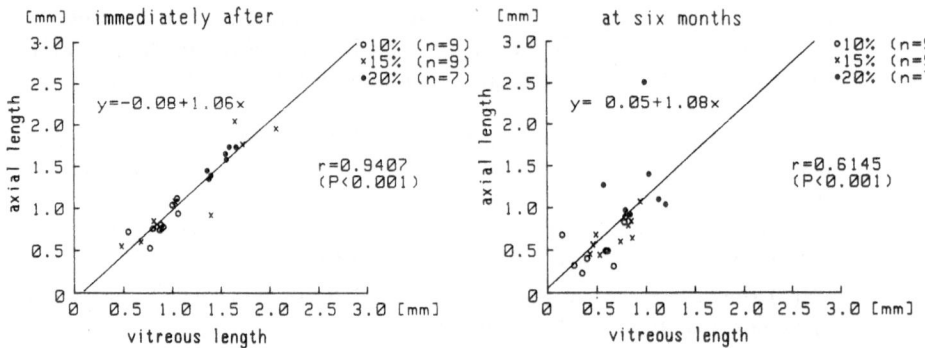

Fig. 9. Correlation between changes in axial length and those in vitreous length immediately after encircling operations with different tightnesses and at six months later.

202

(3) Variation in the degree of myopia was influenced by elongation of vitreous length as an axial factor, and by decrease in the radius of corneal curvature as a refractive factor.

REFERENCES

Burton, T.C., Herron, B.E. & Ossoinig, K.C. Axial length changes after retinal detachment surgery. Am. J. Ophthalmol. 83: 59 (1977).

Fiore, J.V. Jr. & Newton, J.C. Anterior segment changes following the scleral buckling procedure. Arch. Ophthalmol. 84: 284 (1970).

Hartley, R.E., & Marsh, R.J. Anterior chamber depth changes after retinal detachment. Br. J. Ophthalmol. 57: 546 (1973).

Jansson, F. Measurements of intraocular distances by ultrasound. Acta Ophthalmol. (Suppl). 74: 1 (1963).

Larsen, J.S. & Syrdalen, P. Ultrasonographic study on changes in axial eye dimensions after encircling procedure in retinal detachment surgery. Acta Ophthalmol. 57: 337 (1979).

Rosenthal, M.L., in discussion of Pischel, D.K. A method of scleral resection for retinal detachment. In: Importance of vitreous body in retina surgery (C.L. Schepens, ed.) St. Louis: C.V. Mosby Co. (1960) p. 165.

Rubin, M.L. The induction of refractive errors by retinal detachment surgery. Trans. Am. Ophthalmol. Soc. 73: 452 (1975).

Vanysek, J., Treisva, J. & Obraz, J. Measurements of the distances in the eye. In: Ultrasonography in ophthalmology. London: Butterworths (1969) p. 203.

Authors' Address:
Department of Ophthalmology
Miyazaki Medical College
Kihara, Kiyotake, Miyazaki 889- 16
Japan

AN IDEA FOR MEASUREMENT OF THE AXIAL LENGTH OF THE EYE WITH LASER AS VISUAL TARGET

The correlation between the refraction error and the shape of the eye

H. OKAMOTO

(*Tokorozawa, Japan*)

INTRODUCTION

Nowadays, the ultrasonic method is recognized as being the best for measuring the axial length of the eye in terms of safety and convenience, in the clinical field. However, the ultrasonic method is not accurate according to the method of measurement. We used a special contact lens for examination which rests on the sclera, fixing a probe perpendicular to the eyeball and used a weak He-Ne Laser as a visual target for the other eye, so that the position of the eyeball could be monitored objectively by a laser spot on the cornea.

With this method we measured the axial length of the eye in 69 male and 56 female of medical students, aged 19–21 years of the National Defense Medical College. We studied the correlation between the refraction and the axial length of the eye and compared the refractive factors between male and female.

METHODS AND SUBJECTS

Sixty-nine of the subjects used were male students and 56 were female. Their ages ranged from 19 to 21 years. Their refraction values were mainly with emetropia, but five cases of high myopia were also included (Fig. 1). In measuring the axial length of the eye, 0.4% procaine hydrochloride was applied to the conjunctival sac and measurement was made by the water immersion method with the subject in supine position.

Apparatus: Ultrasonic diagnostic apparatus was used in the experiment, (Model **AB 60 NS** of the Canada Ultrasonic Co). The values were recorded by the interval counter (General ZD 294 PS).

Transducer: A flat tip probe with a frequency of 8 MHz was used in measuring the axial length of the eye. The crystal was quartz, having a diameter of 6.25 mm.

A special contact lens was used which made it possible to adjust and hold the probe: Fig. 2 is a contact lens, the surface of which touches the sclera. It has a tube to house the probe in the center and is provided with a container to hold water. One must first confirm that the distance between the probe and the top of the cornea, has reached 10 mm on the oscilloscope.

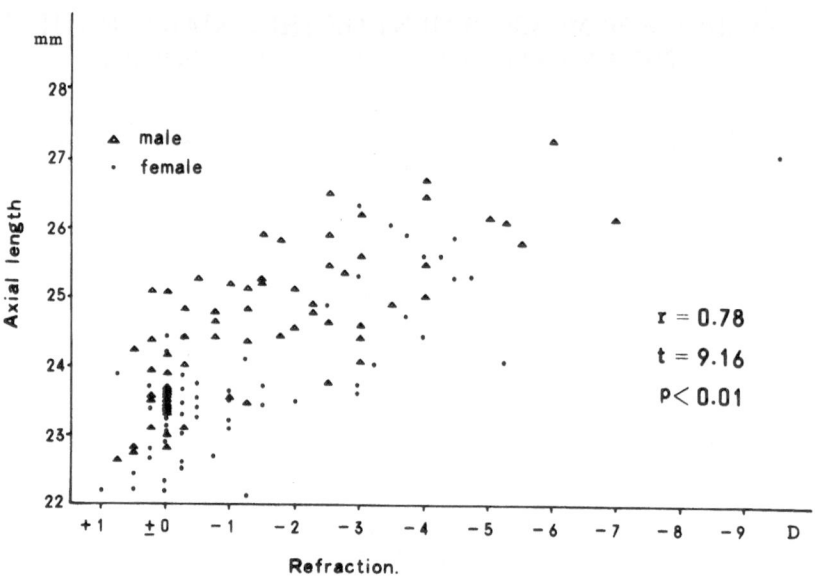

Fig. 1. Refraction value and axial length of the 125 eyes under study.

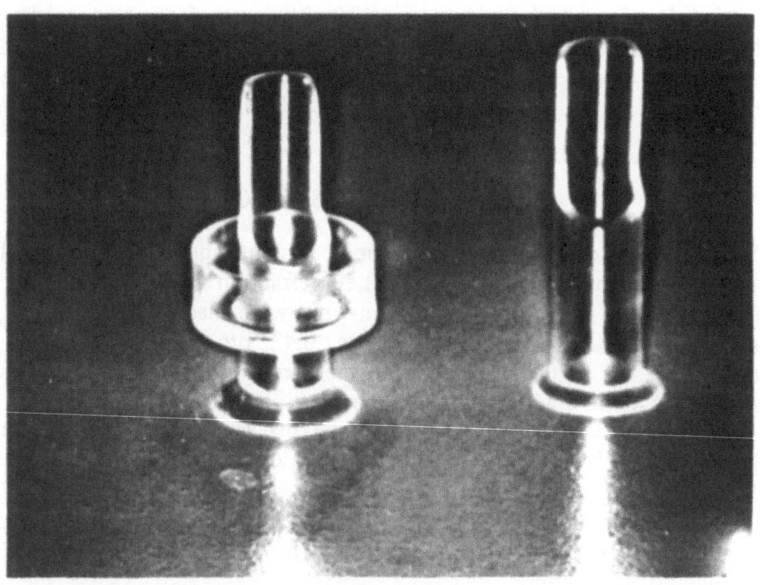

Fig. 2. Special contact lens for fixing the eye objectively.

Visual target for fixation: As shown in Fig. 3 the weak He-Ne laser (a commercially available laser pointer was used) was directed toward the mirror that is attached to the ceiling and which is inclined at about 20°. The position

206

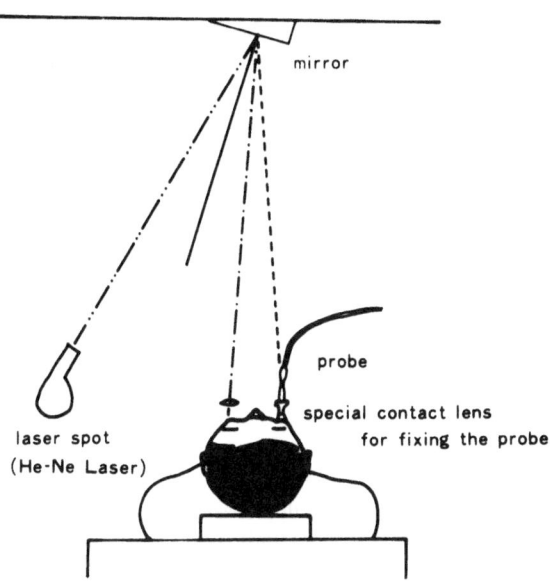

Fig. 3. Laser beam as visual target for fixing the eye objectively.

and the direction of the laser pointer was corrected so that a laser beam would hit the cornea properly. The beam of the laser pointer is a red light of 6323 Å with a diameter of 0.8 mm and angle of about 0.06°.

RESULTS

Accuracy

In order to confirm the accuracy of the method, we examined the difference between the laser and the finger tip as a visual target. Subjects were seven healthy female (11 eyes) with emmetropia and mild myopia. Measurements were made with subjects in supine position and five readings for each eye were recorded.

The sample means and standard deviations are listed in Table 1. There was not much difference in the absolute value of the axial length of the eye between the cases in which a laser was used as visual target and in cases where it was not $(0.1 > P > 0.05)$. However, better results were obtained when the laser was used $(P < 0.05)$ in the mean value for standard deviation.

The axial length of the right eye of 69 healthy male students and 56 female of the National Defense Medical College was measured and the correlation of refraction and other optical elements investigated using this method.

The correlation between the optical refraction and the optical elements

The length and other optical elements of the right eyes appear to be the same as those of the left eyes. We therefore studied the right eyes for the present

207

Table 1. Difference of accuracy of two methods.

	Visual Targets			
	Laser		Fingertip	
	mean	SD	mean	SD
Anterior chamber depth (mm)	3.83	0.027	3.80	0.034
Lens thickness (mm)	3.48	0.013	3.54	0.048
Vitreous length (mm)	16.61	0.026	16.57	0.058
Axis length (mm)	23.93*	0.026	23.91	0.069

SD: Standard Deviation
Each value is calculated 15 32 m/sec as the velocity for anterior chamber and vitreous, 1641 m/sec for lens. *: P > 0.05: P < 0.05

study. The correlation between the optical refraction and corneal curvature was -0.003 in 69 eyes of males, and -0.11 in 56 female. It has been confirmed that there is a tendency for corneal refraction to decrease in diopters when the refractive value decreases.

All the values of correlation are indicated in Table 2. The mean values of axial length (from corneal surface to the front surface of retina) of each diopter are shown in Fig. 4. The values of the axial length of males were longer than those of females at the range of $+1.0$ D to -2.0 D. ($P > 0.05$).

Table 2. The correlation between the refraction value and the optical elements.

	male (69 eyes)	female (56 eyes)
Anterior chamber depth	-0.32**	-0.38**
Lens thickness	0.26***	0.28***
Vitreous length	-0.76*	-0.78*
Axial length	-0.79*	-0.78*
Corneal curvature	-0.003***	-0.11***

*: P < 0.01   **: P < 0.05   ***: P > 0.05

DISCUSSION

The laser visual target

Since 1960, the methods for measuring the axial length of the eye using ultra-sound have been improved by many investigators (viz. araki 1961: 'the water immersion method; Coleman 1969: 'the interval counter method'; and Thijssen et al. 1979: 'the computer assisted method'.) Another way of improving axial length measurement is by monitoring the position of the eye at a stand still position.

We used a laser as a visual target for monitoring the fixation of the opposite eye. The advantages of using a laser as a visual target are:

(1) the visual target is small and clear;

(2) the visual target can be used at any refractive error;

(3) the laser spot on the cornea can be used as a monitor to help control the eye objectively.

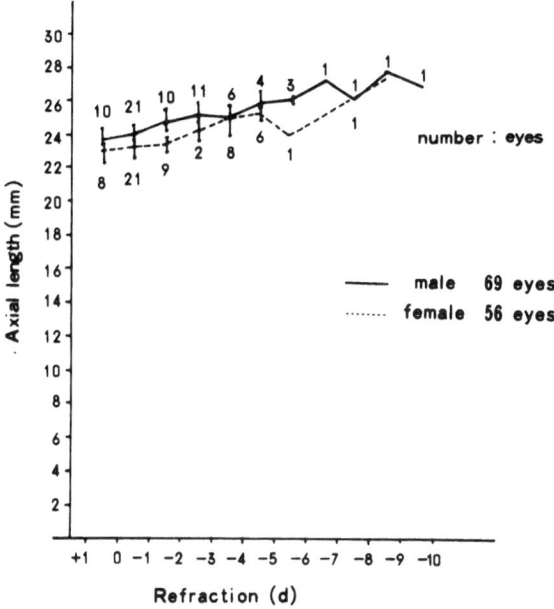

Fig. 4. Axial length of the eye at each refraction error.

The shape of the eyeball at refractive change

It is well known that there is a difference in the axial length of the eye between sexes (Kimura 1965). This also appears to be true of individuals.

We studied other refractive elements constituting the axial length of the eye. There was no difference in the ratio of corneal curvature to axial length between the sexes and between individuals in the range of + 1.0 — + 10.0 D of refraction error (see Fig. 5).

CONCLUSION

We have discussed a simple method using a laser as a visual target in measuring the axial length of the eye with ultrasound (A-mode).

As more accuracy was obtained using this method, we also studied the correlation between the refraction and the axial length of the eye (including anterior chamber depth, thickness of lens, axial length of the vitreous), using this optic-ultrasonic method.

Our subjects were 69 male and 56 female students from the National Defense Medical College.

Conclusions are as follows.

(1) The laser is useful as a visual target, to help control the ocular position objectively. Better accuracy was obtained than when a finger tip was used as the visual target (P < 0.05).

(2) The optical refraction is dependent on the ratio of the axial length to the corneal curvature despite the differences that may exist in eyeball size between individuals and sexes.

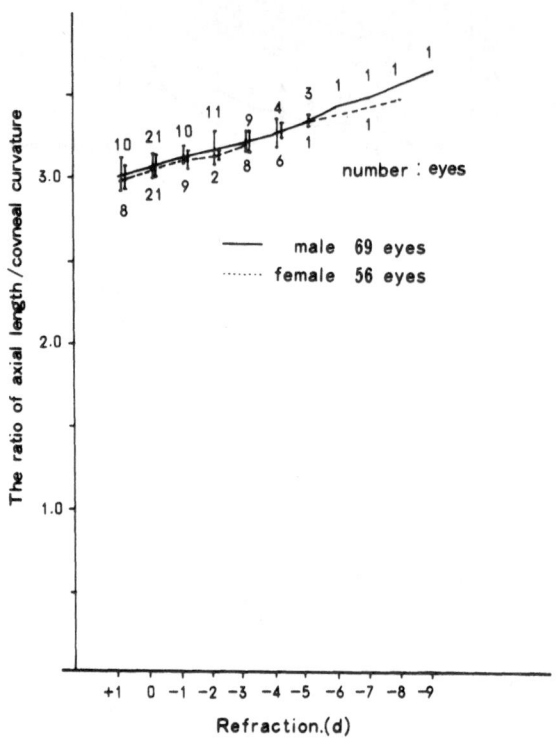

Fig. 5. The ratio of the axial length to the corneal curvature vs refraction error.

REFERENCES

Araki, M. Studies on refractive components of human eye by ultrasonic wave. Part 1. Accuracy of the measurement of ocular axial length by ultrasonic echography. Jap. J. Clin. Ophthalmol. 15: 111 (1961).

Coleman, D.J. Ophthalmic biometry using ultrasound. Int. Ophthalmol. Clin. 9 (3): 667 (1969).

Thijssen, J.M. Verbeek, A.M. & Bayer, A.L. Computer assisted echo-ophthalmolography, 2nd meeting of WFUMB at Miyazaki, (1979).

Kimura, T. Developmental change of the optical components in twins. Acta. Soc. Ophthalmol. Jap. 69: 963 (1963).

Author's Address:
Dept. of Ophthalmology
National Defense Medical College
Tokorozawa, Japan

THE GROWTH OF THE EYE
FROM THE AGE OF 10 TO 18 YEARS

A longitudinal study including ultrasound oculometry

H.C. FLEDELIUS
(Copenhagen, Denmark)

The growth pattern of the human eye has been clarified mainly *indirectly*, with conclusions based on *cross-sectional* studies covering various age groups.

Direct information, as derived from truly *longitudinal* series, is limited in ophthalmic literature. The exception is in the classical studies by Sorsby and co-workers (1961, 1970, 1973). Their statements on the subject are widely accepted, and generally supported regarding the *first* part of the growth curve (with a high 'cerebral' growth rate during the first 2–3 years of life).

The final part of the growth curve may, however, be questioned. Sorsby's view is that ocular growth rate is minimal after the age of about ten years, and at 13 the eye is considered fully grown – except for the *minor* fraction with progressive juvenile myopia.

Analysing longitudinal data from the age levels of ten and 18 years, the present report deals with this final phase of eye development. In brief, the question is: Will the findings imply *a pubertal growth phase*, or has ocular growth by and large stopped at the supposed Sorsby-level of 11 to 13 years?

MATERIAL AND METHODS

Material and methods are described in more detail in another paper given at the SIDUO VIII Symposium, dealing with myopia of prematurity (Fledelius 1981).

Out of 539 examined ophthalmologically around the age of ten years (Fledelius 1976), 137 were recalled for follow-up at the age of 18 years. With an initial aim of assessing the all-over ophthalmic risk associated with a low birth weight ($<$ 2000 g), the sample of re-examined may be divided by birth weight, into ex-prematures (LBW, n = 70) and full-terms (FT, n = 67).

At follow-up, myopes are (deliberately) over-represented due to selection criteria (Fledelius 1980, 1981).

I personally examined all who joined, at both age levels. The data relevant for this study were obtained by (a) determination of refraction after cycloplegia, given as spherical equivalent, (b) keratometry, and (c) ultrasound oculometry (Kretztechnik 7000, Fledelius 1976).

RESULTS

Concerning refraction, most persons showed the expected shift towards lower dioptric values, a so-called *increase* in refraction (127 out of 137). The remaining 10 were either static, or showed a slight *decrease* in refraction (not exceeding 0.5 D). Refractive change ranged from $-0.5\,D$ to 6.25 D in the total sample.

Except for the small subgroup of 'myopia of prematurity' (20 eyes, n = 13), there was no significant difference between birth weight groups regarding refractive value and refractive change (Fledelius 1980). In the following, the data will therefore on several occasions be pooled, irrespectively of birth weight class.

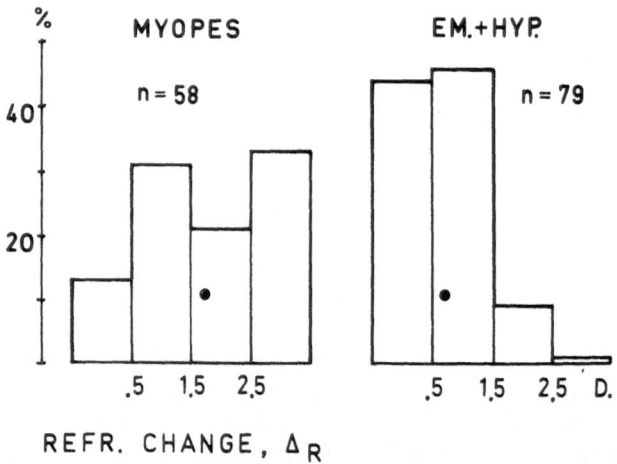

Fig. 1. Refractive change from age of 10 to 18 in myopes (left and in emmetropes + hypermetropes (right). Percentage distribution on four refractive change classes, as divided by the Δ R values of 0.5 D, 1.5 D, and 2.5 D. Median value is indicated by black dot.

Fig. 1 shows percentage distribution on various refractive *change* classes, in myopes and in emmetropes + hypermetropes. The latter are characterized by changes of a low order (median Δ R value 0.7 D, from age of 10 to 18), while refractive increase of myopic eyes ranks markedly higher (median value 1.7 D). The difference between the two patterns of the graph is significant ($p < 0.01$, χ^2-test).

The myopic skewing of the sample (and its apparent effect on refractive change) is to be kept in mind when assessing the *oculometric* results. In particular, this applies to the estimate of ocular growth (axial elongation) because of the strong correlation between refractive value and axial length. *Mean* values of axial length increase, from age of 10 to 18, thus will *not* reflect the 'growth norm' of the population during that period. Table 1 shows some such mean values from the sample. The table is given, partly to describe the material, and partly to signify the refractive skewing (towards myopia) due to selection for follow-up.

A better indication of the *basic* (or obligate) growth of the eye during adolescence is probably given by data from the refractively more *static* eyes of the sample. This is shown in Table 2, with the sample divided (as in Fig. 1) by *degree* of refractive change from the age of 10 to 18. The *static* eyes show an axial length increase of 0.4–0.5 mm, most of which is accounted for by the *posterior* eye segment. About 0.1 mm appears to be due to increase of anterior chamber depth, that is 20% of the actual increase.

Finally, conclusions may be drawn from the optically most 'normal' eyes, those with *emmetropia*. Axial length and corneal curvature radius (the two strongest determining refractive components) are shown in Table 3, which is based on available data from emmetropic eyes at the two age levels under study.

Reading Table 3 *horizontally*, it is evident that the ocular *size deficit of prematurity* at age of ten is *not* compensated for during adolescence. Ex-prematures thus do not catch up.

Reading the table *vertically*, an emmetropic eye elongation of 0.29 mm seems to signify the growth of the eye during adolescence. This conclusion is, however, not valid, because Table 3 is 'longitudinal' only for part of the individuals – namely those who remained emmetropic during the period. Some 10-year emmetropes (with relatively long axes) have developed myopia in the meantime and are consequently excluded from the 18-year

Table 1. Refractive value and axial eye length at the age of 18. The material is subdivided by sex and birth weight (LBW = ex-prematures, FT = full-terms). Further, refractive change (Δ Refr.) and axial elongation (Δ Axial length) from age of 10 to 18 are shown, all given as mean values. In addition, the range is shown for Δ axial length. Only right eyes are included.

	Refr. value at 18, (D)	Δ Refr. 10 to 18 (D)	Axial length at 18, (mm)	Δ Axial length 10 to 18 (mm)	Δ Axial length 10 to 18 (range, mm)
LBW ♂ (n = 36)	− 2.2	1.75	24.23	0.90	− 0.17 to 2.67
FT ♂ (n = 36)	− 0.2	1.26	24.19	0.73	− 0.22 to 2.19
LBW ♀ (n = 34)	− 0.9	1.29	23.38	0.64	− 0.29 to 1.92
FT ♀ (n = 31)	− 0.6	1.07	23.73	0.48	− 0.11 to 1.99

Table 2. Oculometric changes from the age of 10 to 18 concerning anterior chamber depth (ACD), lens thickness (LT), vitreous length (Vitr.) and axial length (AL), in four refractive *change* classes. These classes range from the very static eyes (Δ Refr. ≤ 0.5 D from 10 to 18) to those with most marked refractive change (> 2.5 D from 10 to 18). One hundred and thirty seven right eyes and 20 left eyes (from anisometropic eye pairs) are included. Mean values.

	Δ ACD (mm)	Δ LT (mm)	Δ Vitr. (mm)	Δ AL (mm)
Δ Refr. ≤ 0.5 D. (n = 49 eyes)	0.10	0	0.35	0.45
Δ Refr. 0.6–1.5 D. (n = 61 eyes)	0.09	0	0.40	0.49
Δ Refr. 1.6–2.5 D. (n = 24 eyes)	0.13	− 0.04	1.07	1.15
Δ Refr. > 2.5 D. (n = 23 eyes)	0.13	0.04	1.44	1.61

213

Table 3. Oculometric features of the emmetropic eye, at ages of ten and 18. Axial length and corneal curvature radius are given by their mean values. Further, the size deficit of prematurity (Δ LBW) is shown (right). The results are longitudinal only in part, cf. text.

		LBW	F-T	Δ LBW
Emmetropia at age of 10 (n = 47)	Axial length (mm)	23.0	23.47	0.47
	corn. curv. r. (mm)	7.60	7.86	0.26
Emmetropia at age of 18 (n = 56)	Axial length (mm)	23.29	23.76	0.47
	corn. curv. r. (mm)	7.67	7.90	0.23

emmetropes. Being replaced by formerly hypermetropic persons – with relatively short eyes – it is clear that the reported axial increase of 0.29 mm is to be found lower than the 0.4–0.5 mm growth estimate already given (based on longitudinal data and *static* eyes).

DISCUSSION

Part of the discussion is given above in relation to presenting the results. This applies for instance to the comments on refractive results of the sample, and to the (deliberate) skewing towards myopes, with its apparent effect on the assessment of ocular growth rate during adolescence.

The latter being the theme of the present study, it is concluded that there *is* a significant ocular growth in relation to puberty. The finding is at variance with the statements made by Sorsby and co-workers (cf. introduction), but seems reasonable from a general biological view. It would indeed be unique, if the eye be the only organ *not* to be influenced by the pubertal growth spurt. Considering the usual correlations between refractive components, it is no wonder either, that most eyes by and large retain their refractive value during this late growth phase.

Indirect support for the pubertal growth phase of the eye may be gained from measurements of cranial circumference. This parameter is presumed to follow the growth pattern of the brain, and their *is* a late increase in head circumference (Fledelius 1979).

Finally some short comments on Tables 1–3. Concerning axial elongation, the ranges (Table 1) suggest that a few eyes are getting *smaller* during adolescence. This is probably explained by ultrasound measuring error, taken in its broadest sense. Thus it is often difficult in the 10-year-old to obtain the ideal of a really calm measuring situation.

A remarkable feature of my 10-year-olds (reflected by Table 3) was the *very curved corneae* of ex-premature emmetropes (relatively low values of corneal curvature radius). This LBW-feature applied to the whole refractive range and, in particular to 'myopia of prematurity'. Concerning the latter, it was concluded (Fledelius 1976) that the anterior eye segment seems to be especially 'vulnerable' as related to the 'trauma of prematurity'. The conclusion may be valid also for the bulk of apparently quite healthy eyes of the LBW-group. Otherwise it is hard to explain the (permanent) difference between birth weight groups.

SUMMARY AND CONCLUSIONS

Eye growth during adolescence is analysed using *longitudinal* ophthalmic data (including ultrasound oculometry) obtained at the age levels of about ten years and of 18 years. The sample comprises 137 young Danes, divided into 70 with a birth weight below 2000 g and 67 full-terms.

Being skewed towards myopia, the sample does not give the true picture of population norms. The obligate growth of the eye, as related to the years around puberty, is better assessed from the refractively most *static* eyes of the sample, giving figures of 0.4–0.5 mm for axial elongation during adolescence. The result is at variance with classical statements (Sorsby, *et al.*) concerning an *earlier* arrest of ocular growth.

In my initial 10-year study an ocular growth deficit of ex-prematures was obvious. The deficit is not merely a delay, but a permanent feature, as proven by *adult* measurements. The emmetropic 18-year axial length mean value is 23.29 mm in ex-prematures, and 23.76 in full terms. The corresponding corneal curvature radius mean values are 7.67 and 7.90 mm.

The latter results indicate a *general* (arresting) influence of a low birth weight also on the anterior eye segment, in addition to the more obvious posterior eye segment changes (as evident from vitreous and axial length elongation).

REFERENCES

Fledelius, H.C. Prematurity and the Eye (thesis). Ophthalmic follow-up of children of low and normal birth weight. Acta Ophthalmol. (Kbh.), suppl. 128 (1976).

Fledelius, H.C. Prematurity and the eye. Some results from two follow-up studies of children from the longitudinal Copenhagen University Project 1959–61. Paper read in Dan. Paed. Soc. (1979).

Fledelius, H.C. Ophthalmic changes from age of 10 to 18 years. A longitudinal study of sequels to low birth weight. I., Refraction. Acta Ophthal. (Kbh.), 58: 889–898 (1980).

Fledelius, H.C. Myopia of prematurity, changes during adolescence. Paper read at SIDUO VIII Symposium, Nijmegen. Sept. 1980. (This book 225–231).

Sorsby, A., Benjamin, B. & Sheridan, M. Refraction and its components during growth of the eye from the age of three. Medical Research Council SRS 301, London, H.M.S.O. (1961).

Sorsby, A. & Leary, G.A. A longitudinal study of refraction and its components during growth. Medical Research Council SRS 309, London, H.M.S.O. (1970).

Sorsby, A. Growth of the eye in relation to refraction. In: Modern Trends in Ophthalmology 5. (A. Sorsby & S. Miller, eds.), London: Butterworth (1973) p. 100.

Author's address:
Bukkeballevej 38
DK-2960 Rungsted Kyst
Denmark

MYOPIA OF PREMATURITY – CHANGES DURING ADOLESCENCE

A longitudinal study including ultrasound oculometry

H.C. FLEDELIUS

(Copenhagen, Denmark)

'Myopia of prematurity' is almost obligatory in cases of incomplete cicatricial retrolental fibroplasia, but it occurs also in eyes where apparently the low birth weight has left no other changes.

In a previous study, the incidence of 'myopia of prematurity' was found to be 4.6% of all eyes (n = 604), in a truly consecutive series of children with a birth weight below 2000 g (Fledelius 1976). The children were examined ophthalmologically around the age of ten years.

Part of the material is now subject for ophthalmic follow-up at the age of 18. The aim of this presentation is to give some longitudinal data about eye changes during adolescence, a period which has a solid bearing on at least some categories of myopia. In the following, eye changes in 'myopia of prematurity' from the age of 10 to 18, will be compared with those of ordinary juvenile myopia.

MATERIAL

The ophthalmic study is a sidebranch to a prospective paediatric investigation, the 'University of Copenhagen Project 1959–61 on the Significance of Gestation and Delivery for the Health and Development of the Child'. Thorough descriptions of this project are given in three Danish theses (Villumsen 1970, Zachau-Christiansen 1972, Fledelius 1976), of which the latest deals with an ophthalmic 10-year status comprising 302 exprematures (LBW) and 237 full-term controls (FT).

In selection for follow-up, the ideal of representativity was sacrificed in order to include a disproportionate amount of myopes. In particular, cases of 'myopia of prematurity' were encouraged to attend for re-examination.

More details about the ophthalmic follow-up are given in a recent report on refractive changes during adolescence (Fledelius 1980). In brief, the follow-up comprised 138 young adults, 71 being low-birth-weighters and 67 controls.

One case of 'myopia of prematurity' had, however, to be excluded, due to (further) involutive eye changes since the 10-year examination, thus reducing the LBW-group of this presentation to 70.

All considered, the eyes being subject for follow-up were in a state where fundus evaluation and determination of visual acuity and refractive value could be performed.

A 'load' by advanced cases of retrolental fibroplasia (or other gross malformations) is thus avoided from the outset.

METHODS

Refractive values were determined in cycloplegia and axial ultrasound measurements performed with a Kretz technique 7000 equipment and an Ultrasonolux 10 Mc transducer. Central corneal curvature radius was measured by Javal Schiøtz Keratometry.

All measurements were performed by myself on both occasions. The ultrasonic method was described in detail elsewhere (Fledelius 1976).

In general, calculations and tabulations are based on *right* eye values only, due to the usually high correlation between the two eyes. In 'myopia of prematurity', however, the two eyes often differ in their degree of involvement, and the same may apply to other cases of anisometropia. In some cases, therefore, both eyes have been included, in order to gain more information from the measurements actually performed.

RESULTS

Myopia occurred in 45% of those re-examined at the age of 18. This skewing of the sample is on purpose, cf. Material. Analysing the results, the myopes will be subdivided as follows:

(a) 'Myopia of prematurity', 20 eyes (from 13 individuals, cf. Methods).

(b) Juvenile myopia of ex-prematures, 26 eyes (n = 22).

(c) Juvenile myopia of full-terms, 26 eyes (n = 26).

In several instances, (b) and (c) will be pooled as (d) juvenile myopia, 52 eyes.

Fig. 1 shows the myopic eyes under study, given by 18-year refractive value (abscissa) and refractive change from age 10 to 18 (ordinate), with 'myopia of prematurity' (top) separated from juvenile myopia (bottom).

Juvenile myopia is characterized by low or medium grade myopia; only 8 out of 52 eyes (15%) have (numerical) values above − 5 D., contrasting with 60% of eyes with 'myopia of prematurity' (12 out of 20).

Next, the graph (bottom) dealing with juvenile myopia shows an obvious association between final refractive value and refractive change during adolescence. The higher the myopia, the greater the refractive change from 10 to 18. Expressed by a linear regression, the correlation coefficient is rather high, r = 0.67.

Conversely, this association is weak in 'myopia of prematurity' (r = 0.28), a fact that is also apparent from the less orderly scatter of points in Fig. 1 (top). Moreover, *small* changes are a feature of 'myopia of prematurity'. ΔR is thus below 0.5 D. in 7/20 eyes (35%), compared with a share of only 2/52 (4%) in juvenile myopia.

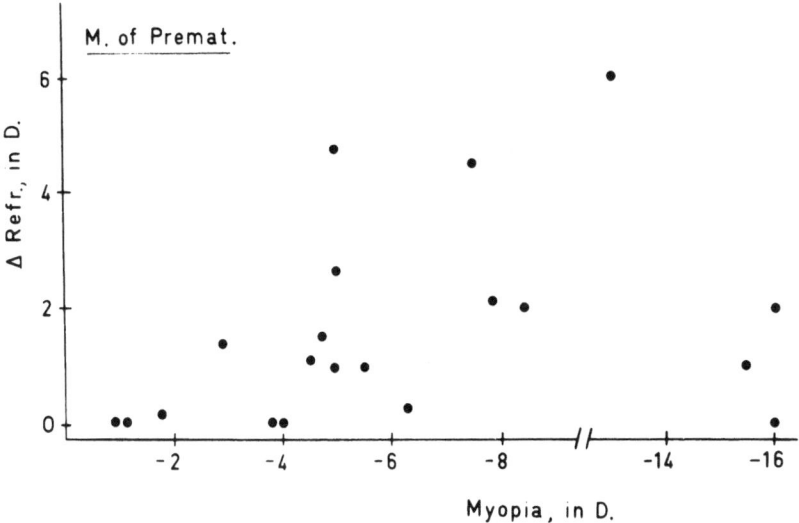

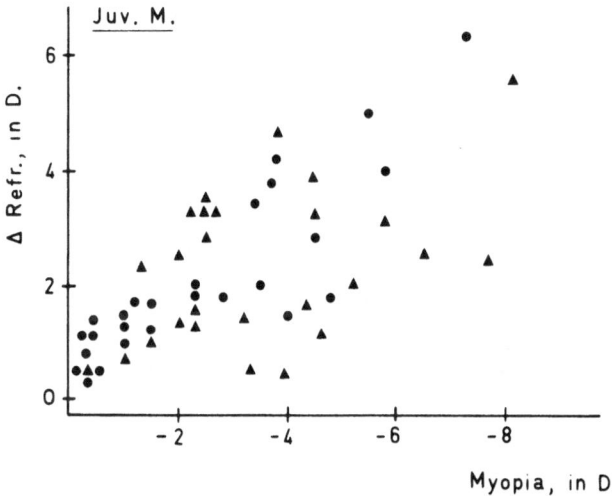

Fig. 1. Graphical presentation of the myopic eyes of the sample, with 'myopia of prematurity' (20 eyes, top) separated from juvenile myopia (52 eyes, after pooling of LBW and controls; bottom). On abscissa, the 18-year refractive *value*, in dioptres. On ordinate, refractive *change* from age of 10 to 18 (in dioptres, given a positive sign when denoting increase in refraction i.e. change towards higher myopia).

The same features are expressed in the block diagrams of Fig. 2. Percentage distributions are shown, on four refractive *value* classes (top), and on four refractive *change* categories (bottom).

Finally, Table 1 gives mean values and standard deviations concerning ultrasound oculometry and keratometric measurements. The sample is divided by birthweight and by type of myopia.

219

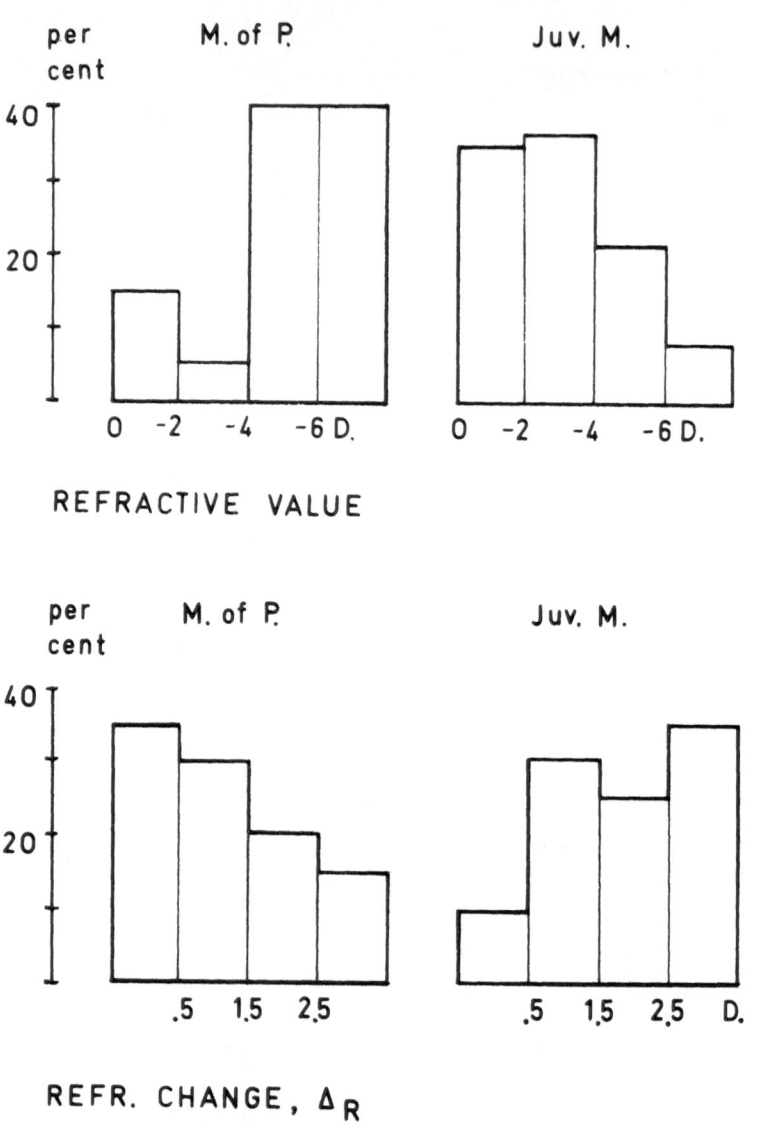

Fig. 2. Percentage distribution of 18-year refractive values (top) and of refractive change from age of 10 to 18 (bottom) in 'myopia of prematurity' (left, 20 eyes) and juvenile myopia (right, 52 eyes).

DISCUSSION

'Myopia of prematurity' appeared in ophthalmic literature about 25 years ago (Birge 1956, Alfano 1958), as a rather benign sequel to premature birth. A recent review of this truly *acquired* type of myopia was given in my 1976-thesis.

My own 10-year observations (n = 26 eyes) by and large confirmed the concept appearing from previous clinical reports by other authors: 'Myopia of

Table 1. Refractive values, keratometric readings and axial ultrasound eye measurements (mean values +/− SD) in 'myopia of prematurity' and juvenile myopia, the latter being divided by birth weight (into low-birth-weighters and full-terms). Refractive change from age of 10 to 18 is given with a positive sign cf. legend to Fig. 1. Δ Ax. length (in mm) denotes axial eye elongation from age of 10 to 18.

	Myopia of prematurity (n = 20 eyes)	Juvenile myopia of LBW'ers (n = 26 eyes)	Juvenile myopia of full-terms (n = 26 eyes)
Refractive value (D.)	− 6.76 ± 4.77	− 2.43 ± 2.03	− 3.50 ± 2.00
Δ Refr. (10 to 18)	1.61 ± 1.77	2.10 ± 1.49	2.34 ± 1.32
Axial length (mm)	25.65 ± 1.98	24.26 ± 1.37	25.27 ± 0.98
Δ Axial length (10 to 18)	1.01 ± 0.65	1.00 ± 0.73	1.24 ± 0.67
Ant. ch. depth (mm)	3.84 ± 0.21	4.02 ± 0.27	4.14 ± 0.19
Lens thickness (mm)	3.77 ± 0.19	3.60 ± 0.18	3.58 ± 0.21
Corneal curv. rad. (mm)	7.58 ± 0.31	7.58 ± 0.29	7.86 ± 0.23

prematurity' is of *early onset* (diagnosed in infancy or pre-school age), it is rather *high*, and rather *static* too.

This contrasts to the ordinary juvenile myopia, which is so labelled due to its usual *onset* around the age of 8–15. Almost constantly, there is a *progression* in relation to the pubertal growth phase, however, with *low and medium grade* myopia to prevail among the final values. To this may be added that − even in the light of current myopia pathogenesis theories − a strong hereditary basis seems probable.

Prospective *longitudinal* studies in refraction are rare, and the present one is the first to encompass the subgroup yet in focus, 'myopia of prematurity', in addition to the major refractive groups. In the present context, however, emmetropia and hypermetropia are let out. Focus is put on myopia, because such eyes seem most susceptible to the various stresses laid upon them around puberty.

Figs. 1 and 2 depicted the features of 'myopia of prematurity' as compared with those of juvenile myopia. The differences between the two are most clearly seen from Fig. 2. The profiles of the two sets of column-diagrams appear almost as mirror-images around an imaginary vertical midline.

The message of Fig. 1 is the predominance of rather *static* eyes in 'myopia of prematurity' also where high dioptric values are concerned. One might even question, whether the three eyes deviating by their *marked* refractive change (4–6 D.) be correctly labelled as having 'myopia of prematurity'. It is to be kept in mind, that my *initial* classification of ex-prematures' myopia was based on the *time of onset* (= diagnosis) of the myopic state. The three eyes in question *might* be very early cases of ordinary juvenile myopia. A hypothetical transfer of the three eyes into the group of LBW-juvenile myopia would consequently influence the mean values of Table 1. 'Myopia of prematurity' would thus appear even more static, with a marked lowering of Δ R., from 1.61 to 0.97 D., and the same would be obvious from a 'corrected' Fig. 1. The other possibility is that the 'pubertal impetus' to eyes with myopia (and myopia to be) is so strong, that even some eyes with the arrested growth-pattern of 'myopia of prematurity' are forced into the usual direction. Most such eyes, however, remain rather static.

The *oculometric* features of 'myopia of prematurity', as we know them today, derive from eye measurements in children, who had not yet reached puberty (Fledelius 1976, Tane *et al.* 1978): First, axial lengths are shorter than expected from dioptric values. Further, the anterior eye segment seems to be arrested during its *infantile* growth-phase, resulting in small and curved corneae and a relatively shallow anterior chamber.

In a recent report, also based on the present 18-year material (Fledelius 1981), a *basic* 'pubertal' elongation of *static* eyes is given as 0.4 — 0.5 mm. With their greater refractive change (from age of 10 to 18), eyes with myopia are found to elongate *more*, cf. the mean value of 1.24 mm for juvenile myopia of full-terms (Table 1).

The myopic low-birth-weighters show a slightly smaller increase in axial length (1.0 mm), and with no difference between the ordinary juvenile and the pathological type 'myopia of prematurity'. Low-birth-weighters' corneae remain more curved than those of the full-terms.

Finally, the slight differences between anterior chamber depth values and between lens thickness values, as demonstrated around the age of ten, are retained according to Table 1. In 'myopia of prematurity' lenses are relatively thick and anterior chambers relatively shallow.

SUMMARY AND CONCLUSIONS

A report is given on 137 young adults, followed ophthalmologically from age of 10 to 18. Seventy had a birth weight < 2000 g, while 67 served as full-term controls.

Focus is put on features of 'myopia of prematurity' (20 eyes) and of ordinary juvenile myopia (52 eyes). The former is of early onset, and proves to be rather high and static. Conversely, juvenile myopia starts later and shows a characteristic progression in relation to the also otherwise marked growth-phase around puberty.

Mean values are given for refractive values, ocular ultrasound measurements, and keratometric readings. Emphasis is laid on refractive change and axial elongation during adolescence.

The changes are most obvious in juvenile myopia, but 'myopia of prematurity' might appear less static during adolescence than expected. Theoretically, this may be due to inclusion of some 'juvenile' eyes into the group of 'myopia of prematurity'.

The anterior eye segment in 'myopia of prematurity' remains somewhat arrested in development. The cornea is more curved, the anterior chamber more shallow, and the lens relatively thicker than in eyes with juvenile myopia.

222

REFERENCES

Alfano, J.E. Myopia of prematurity. Am. J. Ophthal. 46: 45. (1958).

Birge, H.L. Myopia caused by prematurity. Am. J. Ophthal. 41: 292. (1956).

Fledelius, H.C. Prematurity and the eye (thesis). Ophthalmic follow-up of children of low and normal birth weight. Acta Ophthalmol. (Kbh.), suppl. 128 (1976).

Fledelius, H.C. Ophthalmic changes from age of 10 to 18 years. A longitudinal study of sequels to low birth weight. I., Refraction. Acta Ophthalmol (Kbh.), 58, 889–898 (1980).

Fledelius, H.C. Changes in refraction and eye size during adolescence. With special reference to the influence of low birth weight. Paper read at the Third Int. Conf. Myopia, Copenhagen 1980. To appear in conference report (1981).

Tane, S., Ito, S., Kushiro, H. & Kohno, J. Echographic biometry in myopia of prematurity in Japan. SIDUO VII Symposium, Münster (1978). Diagnostica Ultrasonica in Ophthalmologia, (H. Gernet ed.) Münster: Remy Verlag (1979).

Villumsen, Aa.L. Environmental factors in congenital malformations (thesis) Copenhagen: F.A.D.L. (1970).

Zachau-Christiansen, B. The influence of prenatal and perinatal factors on development during the first year of life (thesis). Elsinore, Denmark: P.A. Andersens Forlag, (1972).

Author's Address:
Ultrasound Lab
University Eye Clinic of Rigshospitalet
DK-2100 Copenhagen, Denmark

INTRAOCULAR LENS INSERTION MADE
TO ULTRASONIC MEASURE

H. GERNET

(Münster, F.R.G.)

ABSTRACT

An uniocular implantation of a lens of standard dioptric power may cause considerable discomfort to a patient by postoperatively producing a high ametropia and consequently a non-acceptable aniseikonia when adequately corrected. This remark has been confirmed by recent literature on problems with lens implantations. It is, therefore, evident that prior to implantation accurate echographic biometry should be performed. The techniques and the accuracy obtainable will be given and the results of 'implantations to measure' will be shown elsewhere.

Author's Address:
University Eye Clinic
Münster, F.R.G.

SOURCES OF ERROR IN THE CALCULATION OF INTRAOCULAR LENS POWER

JEFFREY S. HILLMAN & F.T. de DOMBAL

(*Leeds, United Kingdom*)

INTRODUCTION

The introduction of the intraocular lens (IOL) is one of the major advances in modern ophthalmology. The improved quality of vision over the aphakic spectacle lens is considered by many to justify the slight increase in surgical hazard. Most surgeons implant IOLs of standard power and prescribe a thin spectacle lens to correct the residual refractive error. The current availability of IOLs in a wide range of powers allows the surgeon to exercise control over the postoperative refraction. A number of formulae and nomograms have been developed for the calculation of IOL power including those of C.D. Binkhorst (1972, 1973), Colenbrander (1973), Gernet & Osterholt (1973), R.D. Binkhorst, R.D. Binkhorst (1975), Fyodorov, Galin & Linksz (1975), van der Heijde (1975), Thijssen (1975) & Drews (1977b). Calculators with IOL programs are commercially available and the necessary program data has been published by R.D. Binkhorst (1976), Drews (1977a, 1977c) Hoffer & Allen (1978), Kollarits, Kollarits & Torchia (1979) & Thijssen (1980). This paper considers some of the problems and limitations of the methods of axial length measurement by ultrasound for such calculations and considers the benefits of calculation over the use of IOLs of standard power.

MATERIAL & METHOD

This prospective study was made upon 160 eyes undergoing routine cataract extraction with insertion of an IOL. 100 eyes in 95 patients (mean age 66 ± 17 years) received an IOL of standard power + 19.0 D in aqueous and this group served as controls. The Calculated group consisted of 60 eyes in 59 patients (mean age 70 ± 10 years) which received an IOL of calculated power.

Three methods were used for axial length measurement in the Calculated group. In all 60 eyes measurement was made after pupil dilation using a Kretz 7200MA ophthalmic A-scan instrument with a 10 MHz transducer coupled to the eye by 5% methylcellulose in a scleral contact lens water bath (Fig. 1). Polaroid photographs were taken when the ultrasound was aligned along the optic axis as shown by high echo peaks from the cornea, both lens surfaces and the vitreoretinal interface (Fig. 2). Axial length was measured firstly

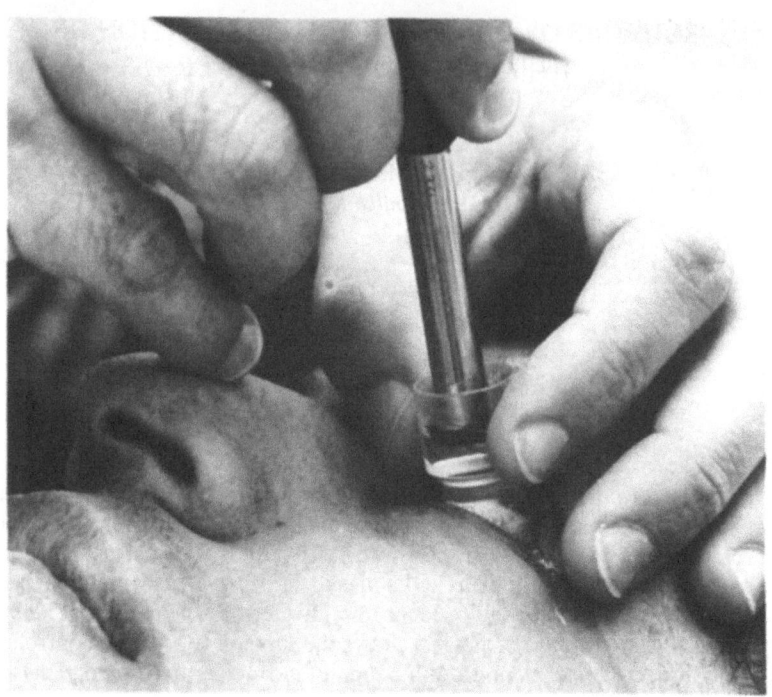

Fig. 1. Kretz transducer coupled to the patient's eye with 5% methylcellulose in a scleral contact lens water bath.

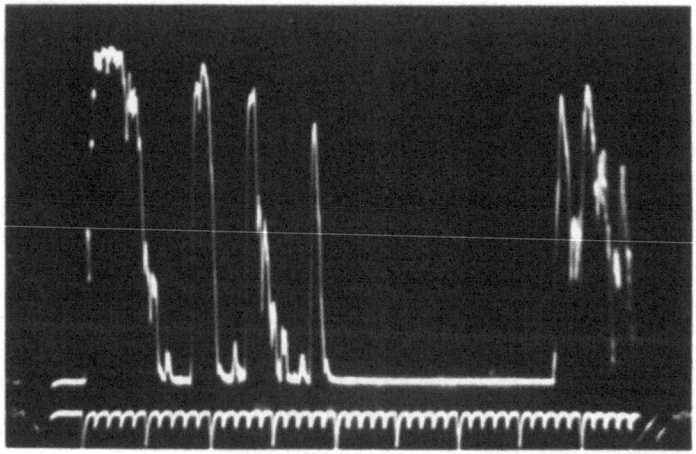

Fig. 2. Transducer alignment along the optic axis is shown by high echo peaks. From Left to Right echoes are from main bang, cornea, anterior lens surface, posterior lens surface and vitreoretinal interface.

using a scale calibrated in mm (mm technique) assuming a hypothetical common speed of 1550 m/s for ultrasound in ocular tissues. Measurement was determined secondly using a scale calibrated in microseconds (μs/technique) from which the thickness of each ocular component was calculated independently using ultrasound speeds of 1642 m/s for lens and 1532 m/s for aqueous and vitreous. The sum of these distances was taken as the axial length. Instrument calibration was checked for each measurement.

In addition to these two methods, in the last 27 eyes axial length was also measured using the Sonometrics Ocuscan 400 instrument with a Digital Biometric Ruler (DBR) using a 15 MHz transducer and assuming a hypothetical common speed of 1548 m/s for ultrasound in ocular tissues.

Central corneal keratometry was performed in two meridia using a Haag-Streit keratometer and the values were averaged. Calibration of the instrument was verified throughout the study.

The formulae of R.D. Binkhorst (1976) using data of axial length, corneal curvature and distance from corneal apex to anterior surface of IOL (taken as 3.19 mm) were programmed (F.T. de D) into a Wang 2200T computer. The first formula for the calculation of IOL power for emmetropia was:

$$D = \frac{1336\,(4\,r - a)}{(a - d)\,(4\,r - d)}$$

D = Dioptre power of IOL in aqueous
r = Corneal curvature radius in mm
a = Axial length of eye in mm
d = Postop. a/c depth plus corneal thickness in mm

The second formula for the prediction of postoperative refraction with the power of IOL implanted was:

$$Rs = \frac{1336\,(4\,r - a) - D\,(a - d)\,(4\,r - d)}{1336\,[v\,(4\,r - a) + 0.003\,ar] - D\,(a - d)\,[v\,(4\,r - d) + 0.003\,dr]}$$

Rs = Spectacle refraction in Dioptres
v = Vertex distance in metres

Surgery was performed by the same surgeon (J.S.H.) in each case using a standard microsurgical technique under general anaesthesia with hyperventilation and a Rayner Binkhorst pattern 4-loop IOL inserted and sutured to the iris after cataract extraction. The postoperative refraction was recorded as spherical equivalent at about the sixth postoperative week when it had stabilised sufficiently for spectacle prescription. The success in achieving emmetropia in the Control group was compared with the accuracy of refraction prediction in the Calculated group. The axial length measurements using the different techniques were compared and the accuracy of the predictions of postoperative refraction from each measurement technique compared.

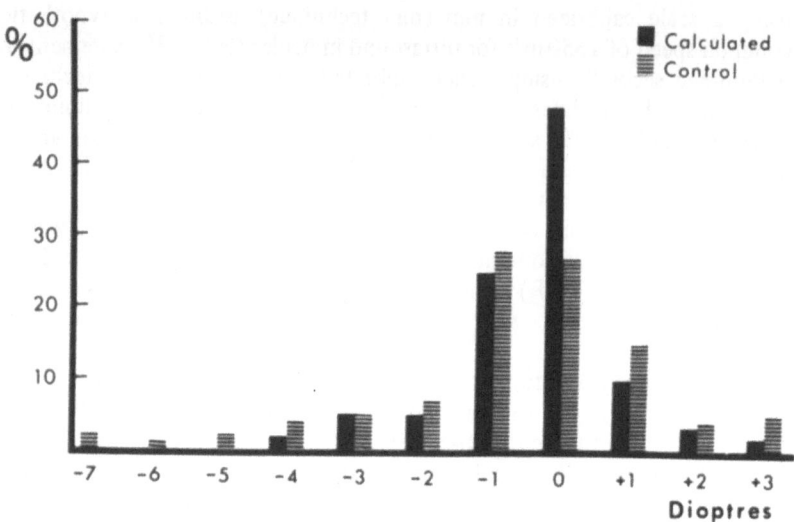

Fig. 3. The difference between the postoperative refraction and emmetropia for the control group compared with the difference between the postoperative refraction and the predicted refraction (mm technique) for the calculated group.

RESULTS

A comparison between the success in achieving emmetropia in the control group and the accuracy of prediction of postoperative refraction in the calculated group (using the mm technique) is shown in Fig. 3. A greater percentage have an accurate result in the calculated group and using simple nonparametric statistics one would expect these findings by chance in < 1 in 100 series and this is of statistical significance. Fig. 4 compares the accuracy of prediction of postoperative refraction for the different techniques of axial length measurement. Table 1 presents the mean postoperative refraction in

Table 1. Comparison between the mean postoperative refraction for the control group and the mean error of prediction of postoperative refraction for the three techniques of axial length measurement.

Controls	Calculated		
	mm	μs	DBR
− 0.7 ± 2.2 D	− 0.4 ± 1.4 D	− 0.6 ± 1.7 D	− 0.9 ± 1.9

Table 2. Comparison between the 'error' rates in achieving emmetropia in the control group and in predicting the postoperative refraction in the calculated group for the three techniques of axial length measurement.

	Controls	Calculated		
		mm	μs	DBR
> 1.0 D	30.0%	16.7%	28.4%	33.3%
> 2.0 D	19.0%	8.4%	6.7%	11.1%

228

Table 3. The mean differences in axial length measurement for the μs and DBR techniques compared with the mm technique as standard.

μs	DBR
-- 0.26 ± 0.26 mm	+ 0.26 ± 0.62 mm

the control group and the mean errors of postoperative refraction predictions by the three techniques of measurement used in the calculated group. Table 2 compares numerically the 'error' rates in achieving emmetropia in the control group with the prediction 'error' rates for the different axial length measurement techniques. This 'error' rate is most favourable in the mm technique rather than in the control group or in the other calculated groups. Table 3 compares the differences between the axial length measurements using the mm, μs and DBR techniques using the mm technique as standard. The μs technique measured shorter with a mean difference (± S.D.) of − 0.26 ± 0.26 mm whilst the DBR measured longer with a mean difference (± S.D.) of + 0.26 ± 0.62 mm.

DISCUSSION

The use of a standard + 19.0 D IOL gives postoperative refraction results which are clinically acceptable in a large percentage of cases and which give the desired quality of vision. There are, however, occasional surprises when a postoperative high myopic or high hypermetropic result occurs. The particular value of the use of IOLs of calculated power is not so much in results which are closer to emmetropia but in the elimination of these extreme postoperative refractions. It is also of value to be able to select a postoperative refractive state and to seek iseikonia.

All formulae for IOL power calculations are limited by the quality of the data presented. The theoretical limitation to accuracy of biometry by ultrasound is the width of a quarter wavelength and this is 0.04 mm for a 10 MHz transducer but in practice this accuracy is never achieved. The system has a number of limitations which vary from one instrument and operator to another. With a sound beam of finite width the peripheral waves are reflected before the central ones (in this study the Kretz transducer had a 5 mm beam width and the DBR a 2 mm beam width). Off-axis measurement either angular or linear induces error. The end-wall echo returns from the vitreoretinal interface and not from the neuro-retina where the optical image is to be formed. These several factors tend to give under-measurement. Axis alignment by echo peaks gives measurement along the optic axis which is approx. 0.1 mm longer than the visual axis. In practice, the actual amounts of these errors are fairly constant and compensation for them may be made by the ophthalmologist who is familiar with his equipment and techniques. In this study a correction factor of + 0.25 mm was added to each axial length measurement by the computer before calculation.

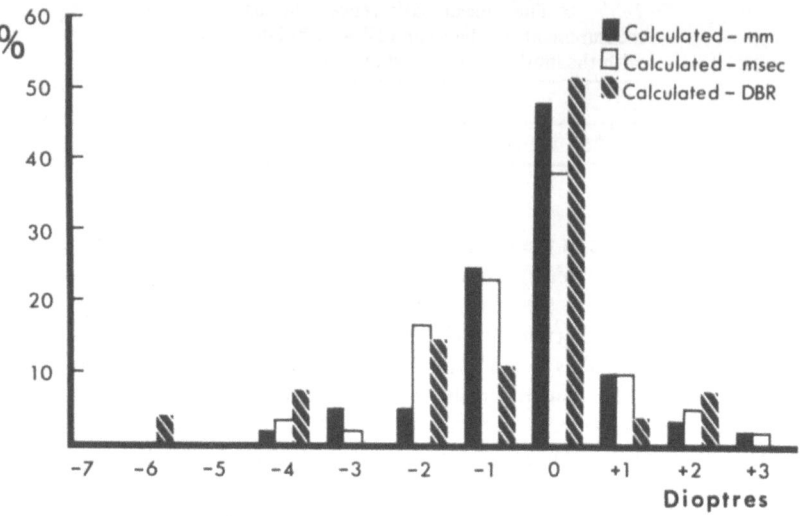

Fig. 4. The difference between the postoperative refraction and the predicted refraction compared for axial length measurements by the mm technique (60 eyes), msec technique (60 eyes) and the DBR (27 eyes) for the calculated group.

The accuracy of the system will depend heavily upon the particular characteristics of the ultrasound equipment. The modification of the signal by suppression of low amplitude echoes will reduce sensitivity and accuracy and so this should be kept to a minimum. The method used to determine measurements from the trace is very important. The mm technique has theoretically the greater error by the assumption of a hypothetical common tissue speed for ultrasound. The μs technique is theoretically more accurate whilst only slightly more complicated. The DBR used in this study used a common ultrasound speed but had the benefit of electronic measurement to reduce observer error. Accuracy of measurement is dependent upon the calibration system of the instrument and when measurements are read off Polaroid photographs there is a limitation in excess of 0.1 unit (mm or μs). Setting up the calibration scale on the Kretz instrument is not without error and on comparing μs calibration against a 63.94 μs delay line on ten calibration attempts, a mean error of $0.2 \pm 0.5\,\mu s$ was found and this is equivalent to 0.15 mm on measuring eye axial length. The value of calculating IOL power will be reduced by postoperative astigmatism and surgical technique of suture placement and tension must minimise surgically-induced astigmatism. For the 160 eyes in this study the mean postoperative astigmatism ($\pm$ S.D.) was 1.8 ± 1.2 D. The accuracy of the IOL stated powers is of basic importance and several studies have shown unacceptable variations from the stated powers in IOLs from a wide range of manufacturers (McReynolds & Snider (1978), Olson, Kolodner & Kaufman (1979) & Lloyd, Montgomery & Gills (1979). A recent study by Olson (1980) indicates an improvement in the optical quality of IOLs and most manufacturers now claim a tolerance of ± 0.5 D in aqueous.

230

The different axial length measurements obtained from the same eyes using three different systems in this study are of interest and in accord with the findings of Fledelius (1975) who used earlier model instruments. It has been assumed in this study from the greater accuracy of postoperative refraction prediction that the mm technique gave the most accurate measurement. On comparison of the axial length measurements, the μs technique gave axial lengths 0.26 ± 0.26 mm shorter and the DBR axial lengths 0.26 ± 0.62 mm longer than the mm technique. These findings stress the importance of using a delay line or calibration block to check each measurement system.

On considering the accuracy of prediction of postoperative refraction, the different mean results of -0.4 D for the mm technique, -0.6 D for the μs technique and -0.9 D for the DBR are all clinically acceptable. The standard deviations of these refraction means are more important; for they ultimately determine the ability to eliminate high postoperative ametropia. In this respect the mm technique proved the most consistent with S.D. of ± 1.4 D, the μs technique having S.D. ± 1.7 D and the DBR S.D. of ± 1.9 D. There were no benefits from the added complexity of calculation of axial length by the μs technique and the only benefit of the DBR (in the small series studied) was simplicity of operation.

Some companies manufacturing IOLs are now producing IOLs in steps of 0.25 D. A consideration of the effects of measurement errors shows that a 0.1 mm change in axial length measurement changes the postoperative refraction by c 0.25 D, a 0.1 mm change in keratometry changes it by c 0.5 D, a 0.1 mm change in anterior chamber depth changes it by c 0.25 D and a 1.0 D change in IOL power changes the postoperative refraction by c 0.75 D. The amount of astigmatism will vary with the individual surgeon. Taking these effects into account together with the variations shown in this paper in the measurement of axial length, there appears little justification for the use of IOLs in steps of less than 1.0 D despite the apparent accuracy of the calculations.

CONCLUSIONS

The three different techniques used in this study for measuring axial length gave different results of which the simpler mm technique gave the most accurate prediction of postoperative refraction with the smallest standard deviation. One cannot assume system accuracy and it is important to use a delay line or standard calibration block to check each system of measurement. Each operator should determine which technique gives the most consistent results and should consider the application of a correction factor for that system. The use of IOLs of calculated power increases the percentage of eyes which achieve emmetropia and reduces the incidence of high postoperative ametropia. Despite the apparent accuracy of calculations of IOL power there does not appear to be a justification for using IOLs in power steps of less than 1.0 D.

REFERENCES

Binkhorst, C.D. 'Power of the prepupillary pseudophakos', Brit. J. Ophthalmol. 56: 332 (1972).

Binkhorst, C.D. 'The iridocapsular (two loop) lens and the iris clip (four loop) lens in pseudophakia'. Trans.Am. Acad. Ophthal. Otolaryng. 77, OP-589 (1973).

Binkhorst, R.D. 'The optical design of intraocular lens implants'. Ophthalmol. Surg. 6 (3): 17 (1975).

Binkhorst, R.D. 'Pitfalls in the determination of intraocular lens power without ultrasound', Ophthalmol Surg. 7 (3): 69 (1976).

Colenbrander, M.C. 'Calculation of the power of an iris clip lens for distant vision', Brit. J. Ophthalmol. 57: 735 (1973).

Drews, R.C. 'Programs for the HP-25/C calculator for lens implant powers', Am. Intra-Ocular Implant Soc. J. 3: 48 (1977a).

Drews, R.C. 'A practical approach to lens implant power', Am. Intra-Ocular Implant Soc. J. 3: 170 (1977b).

Drews, R.C. 'Calculation of intraocular power – a program for the Hewlett Packard 97 calculator', Am. Intra-Ocular Implant Soc. J. 3: 209 (1977c).

Fledelius, H. & Alsbirk, P.H. 'Comparative ultrasound oculometry', Ultrasonography in Ophthalmology – Bibl. ophthal. No 83: 263. Basel: Karger (1975).

Fyodorov, S.N., Galin, M.A. & Linksz, A. 'Calculation of the optical power of intraocular lenses', Invest. Ophthalmol. 14: 625 (1975).

Gernet, H. & Osterholt, H. 'Augenseitige Optik', Ophthalmologica 166: 120 (1973).

van der Heijde, G.L. 'A nomogram for calculating the power of the prepupillary lens in the aphakic eye', Ultrasonography in Ophthalmology – Bibl. ophthal., No 83: 273. Basel: Karger (1975).

Hoffer, K.J. & Allen, D.R. 'A simple lens power calculation program for the HP-67 and H P-97 calculators', Am. Intra-Ocular Implant Soc. J. IV, 197 (1978).

Kollarits, F.J., Kollarits, C.R. & Torchia, R.T. 'A Fortran IV program for intraocular lens power calculation', Am. Intra-Ocular Implant Soc. J. V, 330 (1979).

Lloyd, T., Montgomery, D. & Gills, J.P. 'Deviation from labeled dioptric power for 400 lenses' Am. Intra-Ocular Implant Soc. J. V, 229 (1979).

McReynolds, W.U. & Snider, N.L. 'The quick simple measurement of intraocular lens power and lens resolution at surgery', Am. Intra-Ocular Implant Soc. J. IV, 15 (1978).

Olson, R.J., Kolodner, H. & Kaufman, H.E. 'The optical quality of currently manufactured intraocular lenses', Am. J. Ophthalmol. 88: 548 (1979).

Olson, R.J. 'Intraocular lens optical quality: update 1979', Am. Intra-Ocular Implant Soc. J. 6: 16 (1980).

Thijssen, J.M. 'The emmetropic and iseikonic implant lens: computer calculation of the refractive power and its accuracy', Ophthalmologica 171: 467 (1975).

Thijssen, J.M. Computation of emmetropizing and iseikonizing implant lenses by means of a pocket calculator, Int. Ophtholmol. 2: 39 (1980).

Authors' Address:
Dept of Ophthalmology (J.S. Hillman)
Dept. of Surgery (F.T. de Dombal)
St. James's University Hospital
Leeds LS9 7TF, United Kingdom

DETERMINATION OF INTRAOCULAR LENSES
BY ULTRASOUND

J. STROBEL

(*Giessen, F.R.G.*)

The implantation of intra ocular lenses (IOL) began in November, 1949. Ridley implanted two acrylate lenses into the posterior chamber after planed extracapsular cataract extractions (Ridley 1951). Twenty-one and 15 D myopic eyes were the result. Since that time methods of calculating the power of IOL and the means to check the calculations have been developed. In order to test these we must compare the supposed refractive error with the real one. An often employed preoperative estimation of IOL-power is based on the basic refraction of the eye. A 9 D-surprise after the operation is then possible. It is therefore better to make sophisticated measurements to get the data necessary for use in a calculation scheme. Colenbrander, Fyodorov, R. Binkhorst, Gernet and other authors have developed such calculations (Colenbrander 1973, Fyodorov 1975, R. Binkhorst 1975, Gernet 1978), and Lepper and coauthors have developed a new system for measurement (Lepper, *et al.* 1980). Binkhorst uses a programmable calculator (Binkhorst 1975). We tested this last method in the period between 1976 and 1978 (Strobel 1979). Meanwhile, we have also developed a more practical, easier to handle way of doing these calculations. Our material includes information on all of our patients who underwent IOL implantation.

From 1975 to April 1980 we inserted IOL of different types into our patients (Table 1). The number of implants performed each year are to be found in Table 2. Most of these lenses were calculated using Binkhorst's formulas (Fig. 1). The figure shows the percentage of calculated and uncalculated lenses. The reasons that we carried out implants without using calculations are also given. These are:
(1) in 1975 the method was not available,
(2) in 1976 we did not trust the method,
(3) in 1977, after having had deviations of up to 10 D, we tried R.D. Binkhorst's method
(4) from 1978 we were hindered from doing the required measurements for various reasons e.g. patients were confined to bed or, there were no possibilities for doing the keratometer readings because of high, irregular astigmatism.

The age of the patients involved is shown in Fig. 2. This diagram is similar to that showing the dependence of cataract development on age. The list of indications for implants includes macula diseases.

Table 1. Calculated and implanted IOL-types.

Binkhorst 4 loop	420
Binkhorst 2 loop	29
Worst	3
Fyodorov	5
Pearce	21
Shearing	17
Boberg-Ans	17
Little-Arnott	5
Choyce	2
Harris	1

Table 2. Numbers of implants, calculated and not calculated, from 1975 to 1980.

Implants	4	38	81	122	232	118
Year	1975	1976	1977	1978	1979	1980 (– April)
Calculated	0 (0%)	2 (5%)	65 (80%)	108 (89%)	232 (100%)	113 (96%)
Not calculated	4 (100%)	36 (95%)	16 (20%)	14 (11%)	0 (0%)	5 (4%)

Axial length measurements currently employ ultrasonography. All our measurements were made using a Kretz 7200 MA. We took seven polaroid pictures and chose the best ones for measurements (Buschmann 1974). The time required to traverse the eye was measured. The units are in μs. The two keratometer readings were carried out using a Javal-keratometer. The units are in m.

We have developed a new computer method using the measured or well known parameters to calculate the diopters of the IOL. We use a simple mini computer with screen, typewriter and printer (old name PET, new name Cbm). The programming language is BASIC (abbreviation for beginners all purpose symbolic instruction code) and is easy to learn. It is possible for us to write our own programs for the IOL-calculations. Our first program uses the computer without printer. Mathematical calculations such as calculating the mean of keratometer readings are performed by the program. In contrast to the pocket computers it is not necessary to remember what the meanings of the keys A, B, C, D, E, F etc are. The time the computer needs for calculation is only about 1 s; the results then are found on the screen. These results are: the correlation between IOL-power and refractive error, the IOL-power for emmetropia and the calculation of refractive error without IOL. This latter point is essential before starting implantation, especially with myopic eyes. In the case of an iseikonic calculation it is possible to see the IOL-power which will make the eye iseikonic. The screen shows the diopters of IOL with one estimated anterior chamber depth. To compare the refractive error of lenses within the anterior chamber (e.g. Choyce) with iris-supported lenses (Binkhorst 4 loop lenses) or posterior chamber lenses (e.g. Pearce) one has to start the program again using another value for the estimated anterior

234

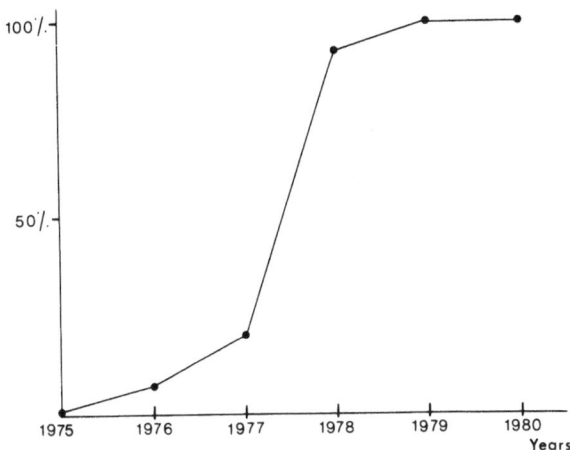

Fig. 1. Calculated IOL in % of implants from 1975 to 1980.

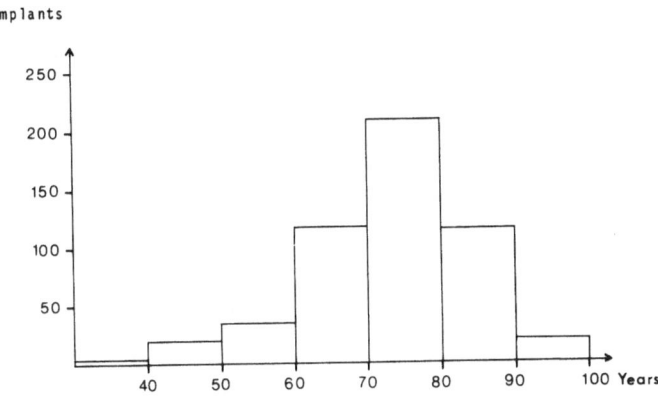

Fig. 2. Age of patients with implants.

chamber depth. We have developed a second program to use in combination with a printer. The same input is required. The results are printed out. Table 3 shows the print of an iseikonic calculation.

The head first shows the refractive error without IOL, then the iris-supported IOL-power for emmetropia and finally for iseikonia. The first column shows the IOL-power. The headlines divide anterior chamber lenses, iris-supported and posterior chamber lenses. For each lens type the refractive error in the column below can be found. The calculation of anterior chamber lenses is based on an expected anterior chamber depth of 3 mm, iris-supported lenses of 3.5 mm and posterior chamber lenses of 4 mm. The computer marks the important area for implants. With the same program one

Table 3.

Universitaets Augenklinik Giessen
  Leiter Prof. Dr. K.W. Jacobi

Date: 10.9. 1980
Signatur: Str
Eye to be operated: left

Calculation of IOL-power

Program Dr. J. Strobel

Without IOL there will be 8.11 diopters in glass.
Emmetropia with iris-supported IOL of 10.84 diopters.
Iseikonia with 16.23 diopters in iris-supported IOL.

Dioptric power of IOL	Calculated glasses to be add to IOL in diopters		
	Anterior Chamber lenses	Iris-supported Lenses	Posterior chamber lenses
4.5	4.71	4.85	4.99
5	4.32	4.48	4.63
5.5	3.93	4.1	4.27
6	3.54	3.73	3.91
6.5	3.15	3.35	3.55
7	2.75	2.97	3.19
7.5	2.36	2.59	2.82
8	1.96	2.21	2.46
8.5	1.56	1.83	2.09
9	1.16	1.44	1.72
9.5	.75	1.05	1.34
10	.35	.66	.97
10.5	− .06	.27	.59
11	− .47	− .13	.21
11.5	− .89	− .52	− .17
12	− 1.3	− .92	− .55
12.5	− 1.72	− 1.32	− .94
13	− 2.14	− 1.73	− 1.32
13.5	− 2.56	− 2.13	− 1.71
14	− 2.98	− 2.54	− 2.1
14.5	− 3.4	− 2.95	− 2.5
15	− 3.83	− 3.36	− 2.89
15.5	− 4.26	− 3.77	− 3.29
16	− 4.69	− 4.19	− 3.69
16.5	− 5.12	− 4.6	− 4.09
17	− 5.56	− 5.02	− 4.49
17.5	− 6	− 5.45	− 4.9
18	− 6.44	− 5.87	− 5.31
18.5	− 6.88	− 6.3	− 5.72

also gets a second print-out. The upper part looks like the first print-out. The lower portion shows the input data and some special calculations, e.g. the eye length in mm and the mean of the keratometer readings. A third print shows the function between the refractive error and IOL-power for three IOL-types. There is no constant correlation between the refractive deviation of the three IOL-types. The first print is taken to the operation theatre. During the operation the required IOL-type and the IOL-power are decided upon.

It was necessary to implant IOL with a power of 11 to 31 D (Table 4). The mean is 19.7 D IOL-power. This is a little bit more than the IOL-power for emmetropia for an emmetropic normal eye. The reason for this is that we feel it is better to make the eyes myopic rather than hypermetropic.

Table 4. Power of calculated and implanted IOL.

Diopters of implant lenses	Number of implant lenses				
10–11.9	3	x			
12–13.9	6	x			
14–15.9	10	x			
		x			
16–17.9	54	xxx			
		xxx			
18–19.9	259	xxxxx	xxxxx	xxxxx	xxx
		xxxxx	xxxxx	xxxxx	xx
20–21.9	123	xxxxx	xx		
		xxxxx	x		
22–23.9	47	xxx			
		xx			
24–26.9	13	x			
		x			
27–28.9	3	x			
29–31	2	x			

We divided the lenses into four groups (Table 5). We calculated the mean, number of cases and the standard deviation of error between estimated diopters in glasses and the real spherical equivalent before dismissal. We found that there is a difference between the estimated and the real refractive error. This error is different in all four groups. It should be mentioned that the number of cases in the posterior chamber group is not high. The standard deviation is about 1.5 D.

Table 5. Refractive errors in diopters.

IOL-type	Mean	Number	Standard deviation
Iris-supported ic	− 0.79	184	1.5
Iris-supported ex	− 0.9	240	1.4
Posterior chamber lens ic	− 1.6	11	2.6
Posterior chamber lens ex	− 0.3	38	1.7
Total	− 0.8	473	

In the Binkhorst formula there are several variables. We tested the influence of each variable and calculated the regression line. We found no correlation either between the error in determination of the eye length and keratometer reading, or lens thickness, or refractive error at the time of dismissal, or vision or IOL-type. However we found a correlation between the error in the estimated refractive error and the eye length and power of IOL. The factor is 0.17.

It is possible that we have a constant error. For a better estimated correction we have to add about $-0.8\,D$ to the calculated refractive error, depending on the type of implanted IOL. We also have an inconstant deviation. We have seen the factor in the regression line. This correction is included in our program. This is easy to do using a computer. In conclusion, one can say that the formula is good, but it is necessary to control the results and to make the necessary corrections.

REFERENCES

Binkhorst, R.D. The optical design of intraocular lens implant. Ophthalmic Surg. 6: 17 (1975).

Buschmann, W. & Bluth, K. Eine echographische Methode zur Verlaufskontrolle angeborener Glaukome. Albrecht von Graefes Arch. Klin. Ophthalmol. 192: 313 (1974).

Colenbrander, M.C. Calculation of the power of an iris clip lens for distance vision. Br. J. Ophthalmol. 57: 735 (1973).

Fyodorov, S.N., Galin, M.A. & Linksz, A. Calculation of the optical power of intraocular lenses. Invest. Ophthalmol. 14: 625 (1975).

Gernet, H., Ostholt, H. & Werner, H. Intraoculare Optik in Klinik and Praxis. München: Rothacker (1978).

Lepper, R.D., Trier, H.G. & Reuter, R. Neuartige Ultra-schallbiometrie. Klin. Mbl. Augenheilk. 177: 101 (1980).

Ridley, H. Intra-ocular acrylic lenses. Trans. Ophthalmol. Soc. U.K. 71: 617 (1951).

Strobel, J. & Jacobi, K.W. Zur Brechkraft der intraocularen Linsen. Ber. Dtsch. Ophthalmol. Ges. 75: 603 (1978).

Author's Address:
University Eye Clinic
Giessen, F.R.G.

PREDICTIVE VALUE OF CALCULATED DIOPTRIC POWER OF PREPUPILLARY IMPLANT LENSES

J.M. THIJSSEN & A.F. DEUTMAN

(*Nijmegen, The Netherlands*)

1. INTRODUCTION

The calculation of the power of implant lenses has an intuitive importance, because of the large spread in ametropia occuring in a population. Many studies have been published about optical calculations to obtain emmetropizing lenses (cf. Troutman 1962, Binkhorst 1972, Colenbrander 1973, Binkhorst 1973, Gernet & Ostholt 1973, Oguchi & Van Balen 1974, Thijssen 1973, 1975, 1980, Heyde 1975). But only very few have been devoted to computer calculation of iseikonizing implant lenses (cf. Thijssen 1975, Binkhorst 1976). The introduction of pocket calculators (Binkhorst 1976. Thijssen 1980) decreases the distance of theory to clinical practice considerably.

The relative lack of retrospective knowledge concerning the value of the ultrasonic biometry and the subsequent calculations has forced us to get some clear answers to questions like: which is the most probable postoperative location of the implant lens, how reliable is the predicted emmetropic lens power, which strategy is followed by our surgeons when confronted with the choice between induced emmetropia, iseikonia and isometropia. A clear bias in the presented data has to be mentioned beforehand. A preliminary study showed us that the emmetropizing values that were calculated were systematically too low. So the reaction of the surgeons has been to take more the iseikonizing side of the region of choice than the emmetropizing.

2. METHODS

The equipment we are using for the biometry is a Kretztechnik 7200 MA A-mode apparatus with a 8 MHz transducer (Krautkrämer). The biometry is performed while using a waterbath sclera lens (cf. Thijssen 1975). The echograms are recorded on a polaroid photograph together with a 50 kHz square wave. Two pictures at least are taken from each eye. The magnification of the photographs is determined from the square wave and the time between echo-peaks is measured from the pictures as well. The echographic data (axial length, anterior chamber, lens) are complemented by keratometric data (Gambs) and the spectacle refraction of both eyes. The computer program calculated the real dimensions of the eyes, taking into account the different sound velocities of the anterior chamber, the vitreous and the lens (cf. Thijssen 1975). The program for the pocket calculator (Thijssen 1980) only uses the axial lengths, the corneal dioptric powers, as well as the spectacle refraction of the healthy eye. This means that sometimes a minor correction to the axial length is necessary in case an extremely thick lens is present (see 3.1 Results, Eye lens).

3. RESULTS

3.1 Eye Lens

Thickness of eye lenses is examined because we wanted to ensure that a simplified calculation scheme which takes into account a standard value of 4 mm is useful. As can be seen in Fig. 1. The extreme values differ considerably. If the additional correction for the actual lens thickness is omitted an error of -0.3 D to $+1$.D may be introduced. When the 90% boundaries of the distribution are taken the deviation range becomes -0.2 D to $+0.3$ D, which may be neglected as compared to the overall postoperative accuracy.

The range of thickness values is considerable larger than given by Oguchi & Van Balen (1974), which may be due to the larger number of cases involved in our study (82 as compared to 217). Delmarcell et al. (1969) found a negative correlation between lens thickness and anterior chamber depth and Oguchi & Van Balen (1974) observed a negative correlation between the pre-operative and post-operative depths of the anterior chamber. In other words a tendency of the anterior chamber to normalize after lens removal is present, which reverses the changes due to a cateract (correlation coefficient -0.76). We may conclude that the preoperative anterior chamber depth should not be used in the calculations of the power of implant lenses.

We have adopted a postoperative value of 3.5 mm in our computer calculations, and, additionally, in our calculation scheme developed for a pocket calculator we take into account a lens thickness of 4 mm (Thijssen 1980).

3.2 Calculated Lenses

The results of our calculations are shown in Fig. 2. The data display a large spread, expressed by a standard deviation of 5 D. A 75% of the cases is found in the region of ± 2.5 D around the average. The distribution of iseikonizing lenses is skewed towards higher powers, but a $+3$ D shift can be observed to a first approximation. As has been reported before (Thijssen 1980) the spread of the calculated aniseikonia of the emmetropizing lenses is also considerable: from -4% to $+17\%$ in a group of 50 patients.

3.3 Postoperative Results

The postoperative refraction, while taking into account the average astigmatism, is used to estimate the emmetropizing implant power. This power

240

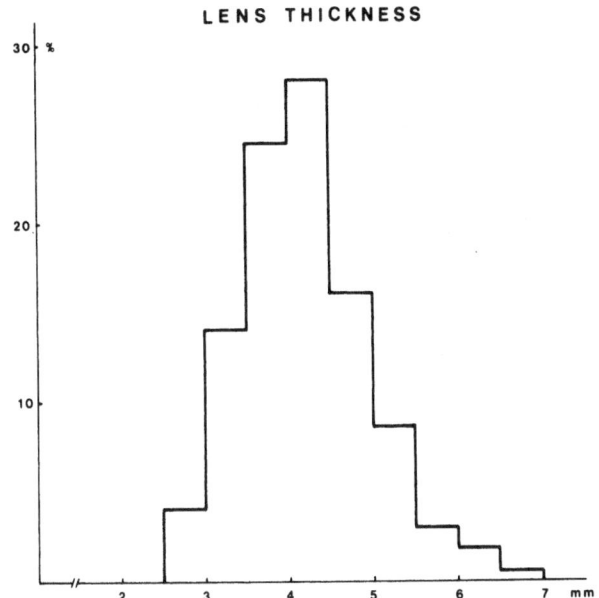

Fig. 1. Ultrasonically measured thickness of lenses (n = 217).

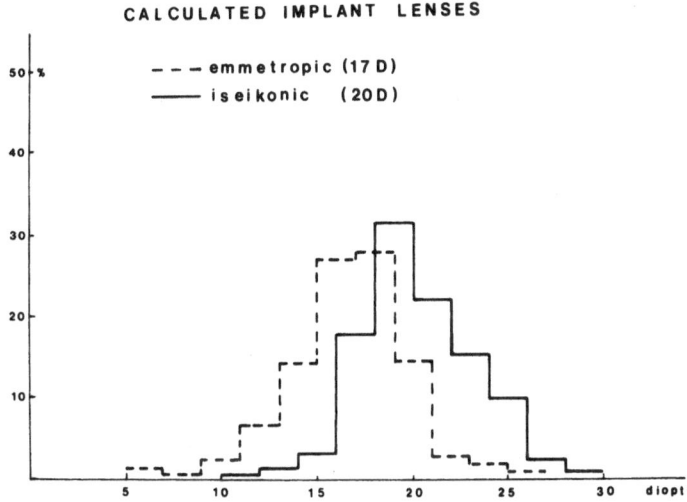

Fig. 2. Power of implant lenses producing emmetropia, or iseikonia (n = 217), difference of the mean values: 3 D.

must be considered an approximate value since it is obtained by simple subtraction of the refraction from the implanted lens power. As can be seen from Fig. 3, the retrospectively calculated lenses are almost exactly 2 D higher than the prospective ones, which indicated a good predictive value except for a systematic deviation of 2 D. The actually implanted lenses are

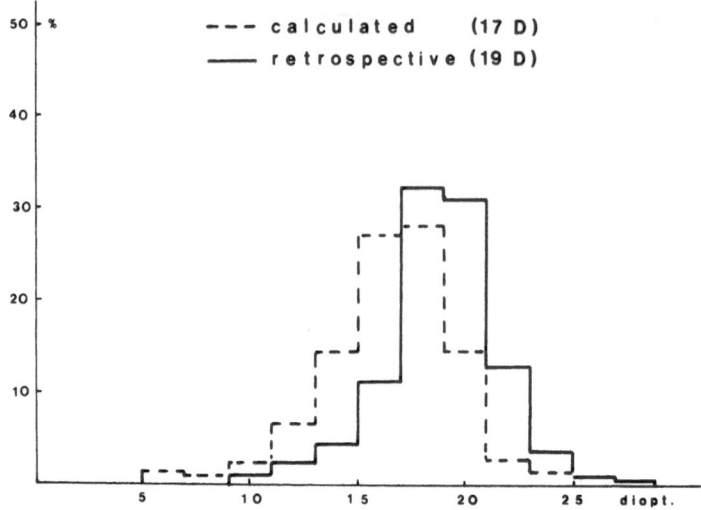

Fig. 3. Power of preoperatively calculated emmetropizing lenses compared to retrospectively calculated emmetropizing lenses, difference of the mean values: 2 D.

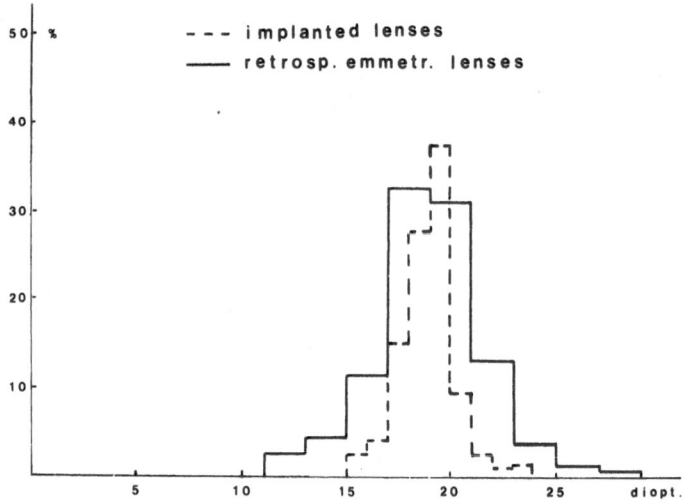

Fig. 4. Actually implanted lenses compared to retrospectively emmetropizing lenses.

shown in Fig. 4 together with the retrospectively obtained emmetropizing values. It may be clear that the implanted lenses are narrowly distributed around the mean value of 19 D. The spread is restricted on both sides by the decision to take 15 D as the lowest value for implantation and 25 D as the highest. The average of 19 D is higher than the average predicted emmetropizing value for reasons as mentioned in the introduction.

4. DISCUSSION

The value of ultrasonic biometry, keratometry and subsequent calculation of implant lenses has proven to be significant for the prediction of emmetropizing lenses. It is shown in this paper that 25% of the eyes would have obtained a refraction error of more than ± 2.5 D if a standard lens of 19 D was implanted. This observation was also found by Kraff *et al.* (1978), who postoperatively examined the emmetropizing power of 450 patients. A further factor to be considered is the aniseikonia occuring in cases with extreme keratometric and axial length values. An intriguing result of the present study is the systematic deviation of the pre- and postoperatively found emmetropizing lenses. Possible causes for this error may be:

(1) The assumed thickness of the retina of 0.4 mm is too large and should be reduced to 0.2 mm (cf. Oguchi & Van Balen 1974) which will result in a decrease of the deviation by 0.6 D.

(2) The axial length is actually shorter than measured by ultrasound. This is not unrealistic with the Kretztechnik 7200 MA equipment. As shown in Fig. 5 a 20 dB decrease in (apparent) reflectivity of the posterior pole, which may be caused by the increased attenuation of a cataracteous lens, will result in an increased eye length measurement. This of course applies only when the length is obtained from the echoes at the base line level (leading edge measurement). A more reliable measurement is performed by taking the distance of the peak values. In our clinical routine we have taken the first procedure and most probably introduced a systematic error of the order of 1 D.

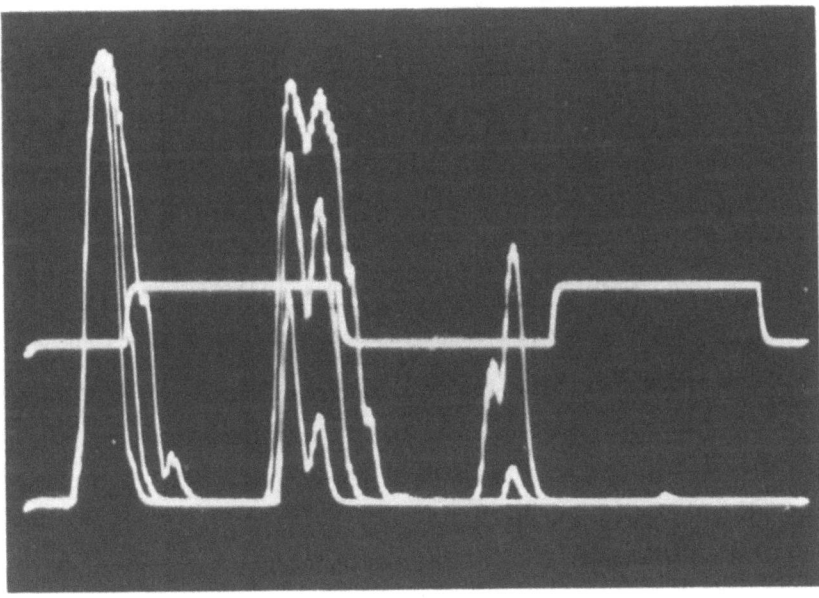

Fig. 5. Influence of reflectivity on base-line measurement of distances from an echogram. Three superimposed echograms with 10 dB mutual reflectivity differences. Note the exact alignment of the peaks.

(3) Postoperative changes of the corneal curvature also add to the systematic deviation (cf. Binkhorst 1976) because both the corneal and the axial length will decrease accordingly, and another 0.4 D may be explained.

An actual question as to whether the preoperative calculation of lens implant is a necessary routine may be answered partly by the data presented in this paper. Further information regarding the relation of preoperative ametropia to aniseikonia is to be considered as well. It may be concluded that implantation of a standard lens of 19 D will produce emmetropia on the average and a refraction error of more than 2.5 D is to be expected in 25% of cases, which may be considered to be an unacceptable fraction.

ACKNOWLEDGEMENT

The authors are very much indebted to J.W. Boonenburg, M.D. who made the data available.

REFERENCES

Binkhorst, C.D. Power of the prepupillary pseudophakos. Brit. J. Ophthalmol. 56: 332 (1972).

Binkhorst, R.D. The optical design of intraocular lens implants. Ophthalmol. Surg. 6: 17 (1975).

Binkhorst, R.D. Pitfalls in the determination of intraocular lens power without ultrasound. Ophthalmol. Surg. 7 (3): 69 (1976).

Colenbrander, M.C. Calculation of the power of an iris clip lens for distant vision. Br. J. Ophthalmol. 57: 735 (1973).

Delmarcelle, Y., Collignon, J., & Luyckx, J. La profondeur de la chambre anterieure de l'oeil et ses facteur constituants. Bull. Soc. Belge Ophtalmol. 152: 447 (1969).

Gernet, H., & Ostholt, H. Augenseitige Optik: ein neues Gebiet der klinischen Okulometrie. Ophthalmologica 166: 120 (1973).

Heyde, G.L. van der. A nomogram for calculating the power of the prepupillary lens in the aphakic eye. Bibl. Ophthalmol. 83: 273 (1975).

Kraff, M.C., Sanders, D.R., & Lieberman, H.L. Biometric analysis of intraocular lens power required to produce emmetropia: results of 450 implants. Am. Intraoc. Impl. Soc. J. 4: 45 (1978).

Oguchi, Y., & Van Balen, A.Th.M. Ultrasonic study of the refraction of patients with pseudophakos. Ultrasound Med. Biol. 1: 267 (1974).

Thijssen, J.M. The emmetropic and the iseikonic implant lens: computer calculation of the refractive power and its accuracy. Ophthalmologica (Basel) 171: 467 (1975).

Thijssen, J.M. Computation of emmetropizing and iseikonizing implant lenses by means of a pocket calculator. Int. Ophthalmol. 2: 39 (1980).

Troutman, R.C. Artipkakia and aniseikonia. Trans. Am Ophthalmol. Soc. 60: 590 (1962).

Authors' Address:
Institute of Ophthalmology
University of Nijmegen,
6500 HB Nijmegen, The Netherlands

A COMPUTERIZED METHOD TO ANALYSE ECHOGRAMS FOR THE CALCULATION OF INTRAOCULAR LENSES

B. PRAHS

(Würzburg, F.R.G.)

By the calculation of intraocular lenses postoperative disturbances of binocular vision – caused by aniseikonia and uncomfortable glasses – can be avoided. The precision in calculating intraocular lenses depends, apart from the calculation hypotheses, on the accuracy of oculometry.

The highest achievable precision in oculometry is one-half of the used wavelength. A measurement frequency of 10 MHz corresponds to a wavelength of about 0.16 mm in the globe – with this frequency an error of ± 0.08 mm is unavoidable. Random errors can occur from effects such as small movements of the transducer or the subject's eye. The transducer unit must be aligned so that the amplitudes of the anterior and posterior lens echoes are maximized while the distance from the vitroretinal spike is simultaneously maximized. It requires skill to meet this criterion for axial measurement. Jansson (1963) found out that an error of five degrees in the transducer orientation can result in an error of 0.1 mm in the measurement of the length of the visual axis. When there are no proper echoes for the anterior and posterior lens surface – which is rather often in cataractous eyes – variations in the axial length of 0.4 mm and more may occur. These errors can be reduced by averaging a large number of repeated measurements. This is time consuming but the only way to reduce random errors. To shorten this statistical evaluation we designed a computerized method to analyse the echograms with regard to different sound velocities and average the results.

METHOD

The measurement is done with a 10 MHz transducer unit. Transducers of higher frequencies can improve the axial resolution. The tissue absorption, however, is also increased with the frequency so that the sensitivity is degraded. To avoid flattening of the cornea and misalignment of the transducer beam we use a contact eyecup as proposed by Gernet (1963). The transducer unit is aligned so that the amplitudes of the anterior and posterior lens echoes are maximized. In this position, with small variations caused by eye movements and small movements of the transducer, a series of photos is taken from the display system of the ultrasonograph apparatus. By using a camera with winder a large number of photos can be taken in short time.

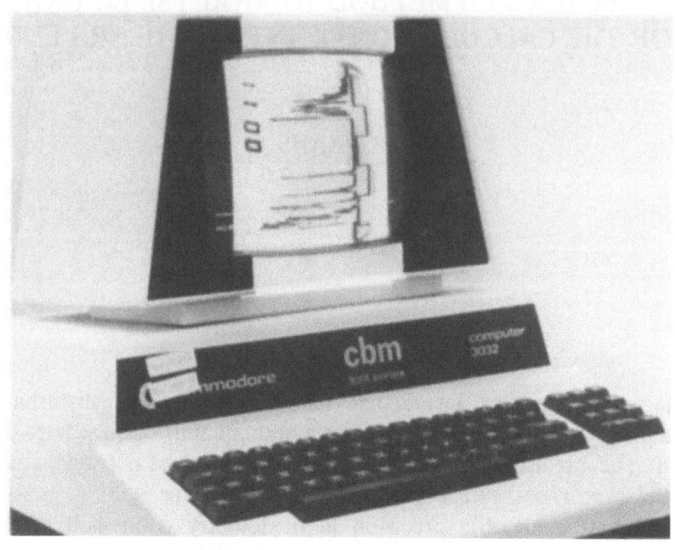

Fig. 1. Projection of an echogram on the computer screen. A programmed pointer is displayed on the screen simultaneously.

The photonegatives are projected on a computer screen (Fig. 1). A programmed pointer which is simultaneously displayed on the screen is successively adjusted to the echoes of the cornea, to the anterior lens surface, to the posterior lens surface and to the retina. All these positions are recorded by pressing a key.

The calibration is done by measuring a fixed distance on the photographed calibration scale in the same way.

The calculations of the axial length and the intraocular distances are done automatically by the computer using different sound velocities. At the end of the analysis of a series of echograms the results are averaged. Giving additional information about corneal radii and the spectacle refraction, the corresponding refractive power of the lens to implant and the resulting aniseikonia are displayed on the computer screen immediately.

ADVANTAGES OF THE METHOD

(1) The advantage of a statistical analysis is obvious.
(2) Short examination times are reached by using a camera with winder.
(3) The enlargement of the echograms during the projection improves the reading.
(4) No calculation has to be done, so no calculation errors can occur.
(5) The handling of the computer and the adjustment of the pointer to the echoes of interest are simple tasks that can be delegated.

(6) The different speed of ultrasound in the anterior chamber, lens, and vitreous body is taken into account.

REFERENCES

Gernet, H. Measurement of the eye in vivo. Graeve. Arch. Ophthalmol. 166: 402 (1963).
Jansson, F. Measurements of intraocular distances by ultrasound. Acta Ophthalmol. (Suppl.) 74: (1963).

Author's Address:
University Eye Hospital
Würzburg, F.R.G.

NOONAN'S SYNDROME, ECHOGRAPHIC STUDY

H.M. SORIANO & J.B. LAMARCHE

(Buenos Aires, Argentina)

The Noonan's syndrome, a Turner like phenotype with normal sex chromosomal pattern, is characterized by the presence of multiple congenital defects like hypertelorism, pterygium coli, hypogonadism, pulmonar and intestinal lymphangiectasia (Baltaxe 1975, Herzog 1976), congenital cardiopathy and ocular abnormalities. The ophthalmic alterations found in the literature are: obliquity of the palpebral fissure downward and laterally (antimongoloid), hypertelorism, epicantus, ptosis, myopia, iris coloboma, keratoconus and cataracts. Exophthalmus is also described in the literature (Foucaul 1971, Noonan 1968) but in our opinion this deformity results from malar hypoplasia which produces a pseudoexophthalmus. Three cases of cavernous angioma in the frontal region were described by Noonan (1968).

PERSONAL CASE

A 17-year-old male patient with a Noonans syndrome presented: pterigium coli, hypogonadism, aortic stenosis, mitral insufficiency, small atrial septal defect, mild mental retardation and normal sex chromosomal pattern.

The following ocular abnormalities were found in the first examination: obliquity of the palpebral fissure, ptosis, pseudoexophthalmus. Visual acuity of the right eye was 20/40 and of the left eye 20/50 with hyperopic correction. The right fundus showed persistence of the hyaloid artery and vitreous opacities. The left eye was normal. A second examination was performed six years later. The patient's complaints were poor vision and pain in the right eye that showed a cataract, and a secondary glaucoma with a very shallow anterior chamber. Gonioscopy showed a closure of the angle in the right eye and an open angle in the left. The right fundus showed a hazy vitreous with withish exsudates. The left fundus a fibrous proliferation from the optic nerve to the macular region.

The visual fields were constricted by an inferior excavation in the right eye and an enlargement of the blind spot, in the left eye. An echographic examination was performed with a 7200 MA Kretztechnik equipment and a tumor pattern was found in the inferior region. The echogram showed a solid tumor with very high reflectivity in all directions. The echographic diagnosis was a choroidal angioma, which occupied the inferior and temporal quadrant

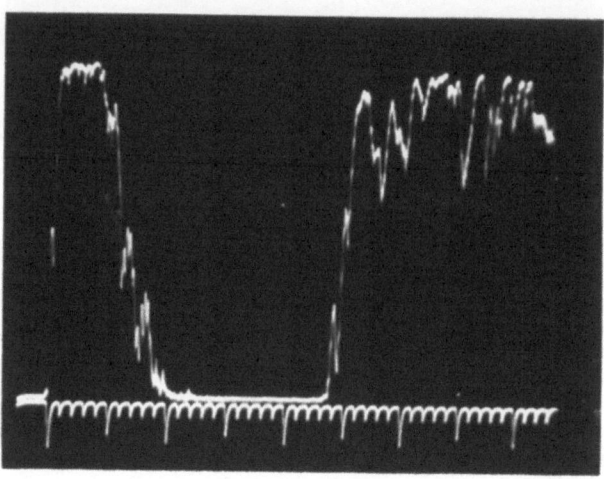

Fig. 1. Ecographic pattern of the retinal angioma. Notice the very high reflectivity of the tumor-probe 8 MHz.

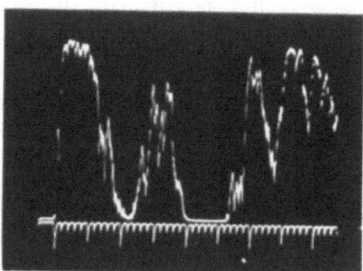

Fig. 2. Ecographic pattern of the vitreous organisation and the retinal angioma.

(Figs. 1 & 2). The enucleation was performed because the eye became painful and blind, in spite of treatment.

The histopathologic examination demonstrated the presence of cataract, inflammatory cells and exsudates in the vitreous, subretinal serous exsudates, atrophy of the pigment epithelium and drusen. The retina showed segmental atrophy, gliosis, fibrosis, calcium deposits and microcistic degeneration. The inferior region presented a vascular tumor with gliosis, fibrosis, capillaris and vessels with hialinized wall (Figs. 3 & 4). The final diagnosis was: Retinal Angioma, with gliosis and fibrosis, diffuse retinal degeneration with gliosis, subretinal and vitreous exsudates, and cataract.

DISCUSSION

In the Noonan's syndrome the ocular anomalies are more present than in the Turner syndrome but of minor importance. An intraocular tumor was never

250

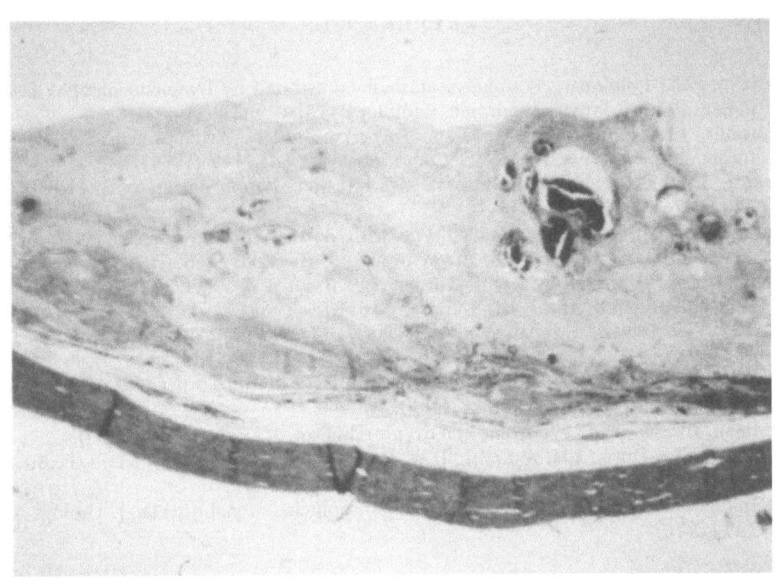

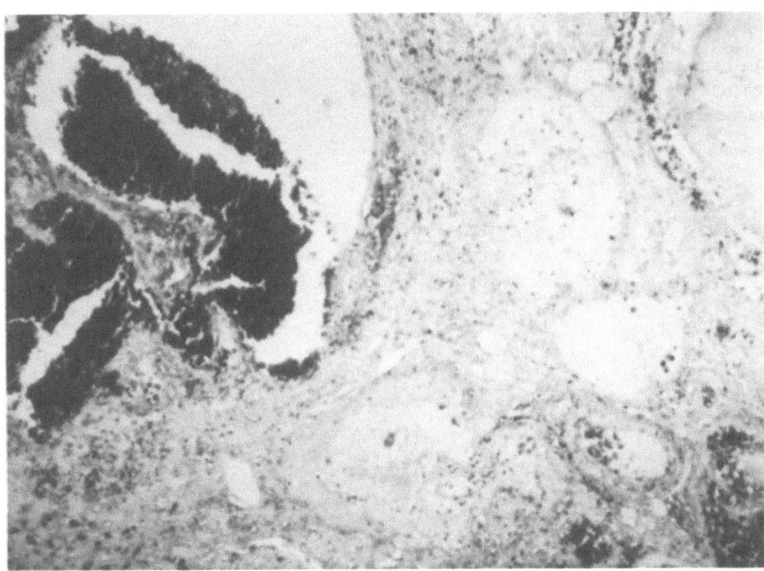

Fig. 4. Microscopic picture of tumor history.

described before. Our case also presents other important alterations, like vitreous organization and secondary glaucoma. We also intend to emphasise the importance and reliability of the echographic examination that permit us not only to detect an unsuspected lesion but also to make the exact diagnosis.

REFERENCES

Baltaxe, H.A. Pulmonary lymphangiectasia demonstrated by lymphangiography in two patients with Noonan's syndrome. Radiology 115: 149 (1975).

Foucault, J.P. Noonan's syndrome and Turnerian mosaics. Attemps at classification of turnerian phenotypes. Arch. Mal. Coeur Vaisseaux 64: 1142 (1971).

Herzog, D.B. The Noonan's syndrome with intestinal lymphangiectasia. J. Pediatr. 88: 270 (1976).

Horst, R.L. Van der. Turner phenotype with normal sex chromosomal pattern and congenital heart disease (Noonan's synrome), S.Afr. Med. J. 48: 219 (1974).

Noonan, J.A. Hypertelorism with Turner phenotype: a new syndome with associated congenital disease. Am. J. Dis. Children 116: 373 (1968).

Nora, J.J. The Ullrich-Noonan syndrome (Turner phenotype). Am. J. Dis. Children 127: 48 (1974).

Nora, J.J. & Sintra, A.K. Direct familial transmission of the Turner phenotype. Am. J. Dis. Children 116: 343 (1968).

Redman, J.F. Noonan's syndrome and oryptorchidism. J. Urology 109 (1970).

Summit, R.L., Optiz, J.M. & Smith, D.W. Noonan's syndrome in the male. J. Peditr. 67: 936 (1965).

Tejani, A. Noonan's syndrome associated with polycistic renal disease. J. Urology 115: 209 (1976).

Authors' Address:
H.M. Soriano
Centro Oftalmológico de Alta Complejidad
Alsina 174
Avellaneda Pcia. de Buenos Aires
Argentina

J.B. Lamarche
Centre Hospitalier Universitaire de Sherbrooke
Québec, Canadá

FIVE YEARS ULTRASONOGRAPHIC EYE EXAMINATION IN CHILDREN

P.A.M. GOMMERS & A.TH.M. VAN BALEN

(Rotterdam, The Netherlands)

The purpose of this paper is to give a survey of ultrasonographic examination of the eyes of children up to 15 years of age. The sample of 105 patients was taken in the period 1974–1979. Only the A-scan method was used (unit 7200 MA Kretz-technik). General anesthesia was used in 11 cases. The sex distribution (70 male, 31 female, Table 1) is totally incidental as far as we know. Eleven patients had a second examination to check eventual progression or regression of a process. Table 2 gives four different indication groups, that are analysed separately in the next tables. The diagnostic score in the first group (i.e. eye pathology, Table 3) is quite high. One false negative echogram (homogeneous vitreous) was a persistent hyaloid artery. In the ultrasonographic diagnosis group of persistent hyperplastic primary vitreous (PHPV) and retrolental fibroplasia (RLF) the ultimate diagnosis was PHPV once and RLF six times.

Table 1.

	Number of patients	♂	♀	Number of examinations
Total	101	70	31	112
No follow-up	7	5	2	7
In the survey	94	65	29	105

Table 2.

Pathology of the eye	40 examinations
Pathology of the orbit	24 examinations
Trauma of the eye	35 examinations
Biometric examination of the eye	6 examinations
Total	*105* examinations

Table 3. Pathology of the eye.

Ultrasonographic diagnosis		Confirmation	
Retinal detachment	3	3	
Hemorrhage	2	2	
Non-homogeneous vitreous	7	7	
Homogeneous vitreous	10	8	no follow-up 1/false negative 1
Retinoblastoma	5	5	
Coats	5	5	
PHPV and RLF	7	7	

Table 4. Pathology of the orbit.

tumor 13

Ultrasonographic diagnosis	Confirmed	Not confirmed
dermoid cyst	dermoid cyst	
cyst	arachnoidea cyst	
granuloma	chronic inflamed lacrimal gland	
lymphoma/sarcoma		lipoma
lymphoma/sarcoma		cavernous hemangioma
hemorrhage in cyst		lymphangioma
glioma		rhabdomyosarcoma
haemangioma cavernosum		dermoid cyst
no diagnosis		histiocytosis
no diagnosis		histiocytosis
no diagnosis		lipogranuloma
no diagnosis		cyst with fibrosis
no diagnosis		chronic inflamed lacrimal gland

no tumor 11

Table 5. Trauma of the eye.

Ultrasonographic diagnosis		Confirmed
retinal detachment	7	7
hemorrhage	5	5
non-homogeneous vitreous	4	2*
homogenous vitreous	15	15
luxated lenses and aphakia	3	3
no foreign body	1	1

*2 × old hemorrhage.

The results of ultrasonographic examination in the 'pathology of the orbit' group are presented in Table 4. The results of examinations of trauma of the eye are given in Table 5. In more than 50% of the cases pathology of the posterior part of the eye could be demonstrated. Biometry of the eye for calculations of the dioptric power of an artificial lens is seldom indicated in children. Biometry in cases of anisometropia to calculate the aniseikonia that will result in contact lens correction and correction with glasses will probably be a frequent indication in the near future.

CONCLUSION

Ultrasonographic examination in pathology of the eye is of high diagnostic value in our clinic. The same applies for trauma of the eye. The ultrasonographic diagnosis of orbital pathology is reliable as far as the differentiation tumor versus no tumor is concerned. The differentiation of the structure and therefore of the nature of the orbital processes was not so good, with the exception of the differentiation cyst versus solid tumor. Ossoinig's diagnostic score (98%) could not be equaled in our series. The combination of A- and B-scan methods will probably enhance our results.

CASE HISTORY

A.K.M., born 1969
1971 Extreme proptosis on both sides.
      Restricted eye movements in all directions (Fig. 1).
1974 Fundoscopy: on both sides coloboma of the optic disc (Fig. 2).
1977 VA RE 0.05, VA LE 0.
      X-ray of the orbits: no abnormality.
      CT-scan: retrobulbar circumscripted tumor (Fig. 3).
      Ultrasonography gave the typical pattern of a cyst, situated directly behind the eye (Fig. 4).
      During lateral orbitotomy (left) a cyst near the optic nerve was found. By punction 6 cc clear fluid could be evacuated. The cyst was excised. Proptosis disappeared. The fundus did not change.

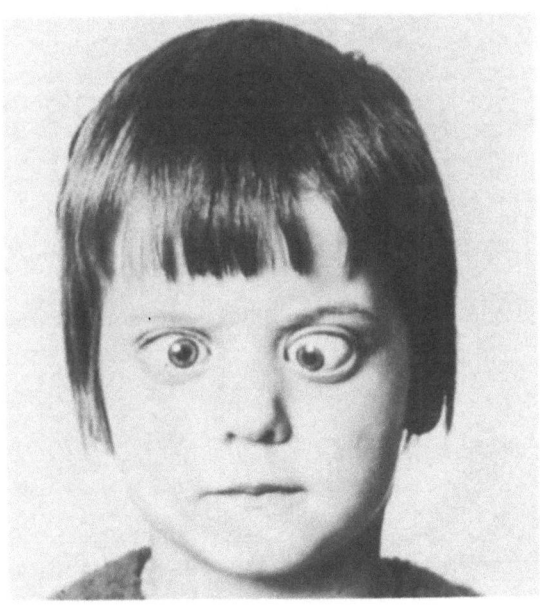

Fig. 1. Extreme proptosis on both sides.

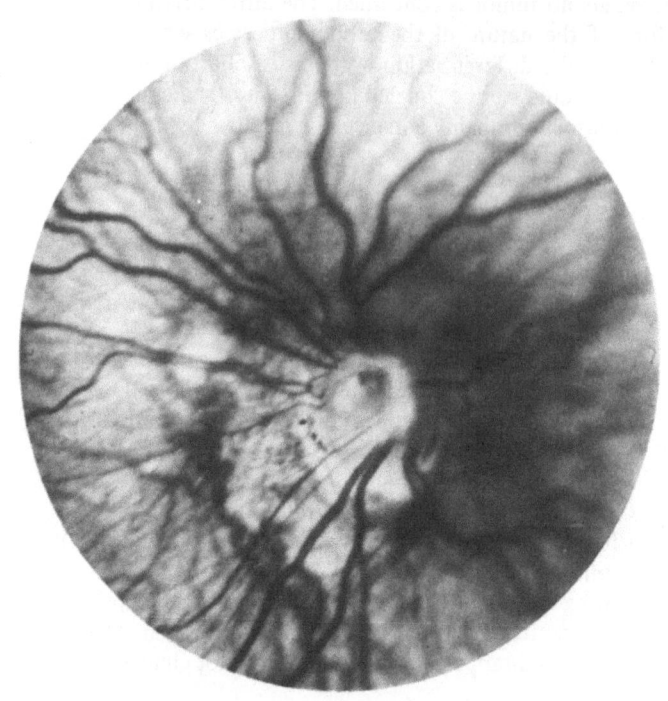

Fig. 2. Coloboma of the optic disc.

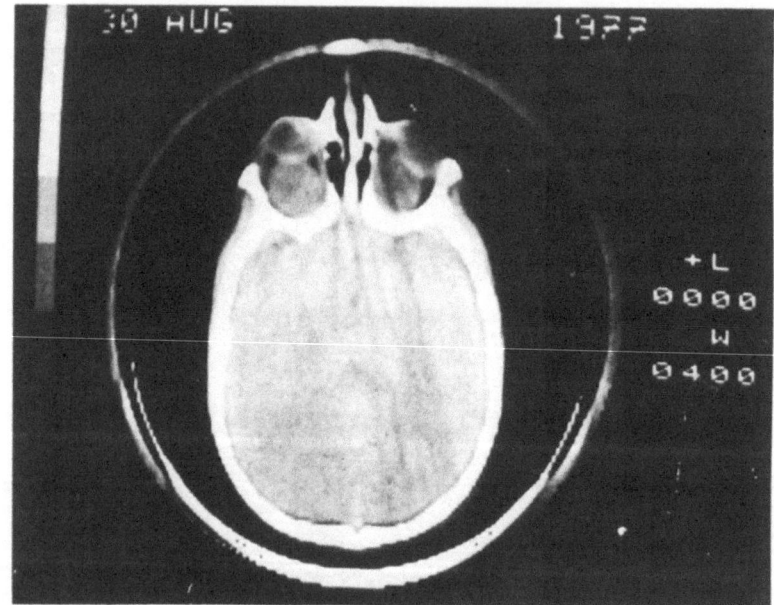

Fig. 3. CT-scan: retrobulbar circumscripted tumors.

256

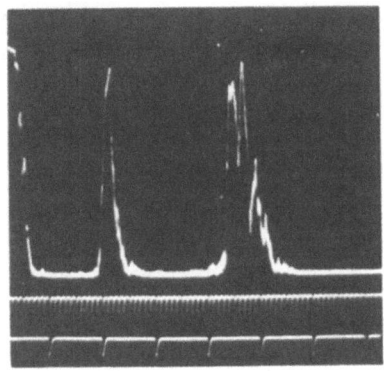

Fig. 4. Ultrasonography: typical pattern of a cyst, situated directly behind the eye (both sides).

REFERENCES

Gitter, K.A. The use of diagnostic ultrasonography in pediatric ophthalmology. In: Ultrasonographia Medica, Vol II (1971) pp. 321–332.

Ossoinig, K.C. & Till, P. Ten-year study on clinical echography in orbital disease. In: Ultrasonography in Ophthalmology, Bibl. Ophthalmol. 83: 200–216 (1975).

Authors' Address:
Eye Department
Erasmus University Rotterdam
Eye Hospital
Schiedamsevest 180
3011 BH Rotterdam
The Netherlands

257

COMPUTER ASSISTED ACOUSTIC MEASUREMENTS OF THE POSTERIOR OCULAR COATS

M.E. SMITH, D.J. COLEMAN & F.L. LIZZI

(*New York, U.S.A.*)

ABSTRACT

The thickness of the posterior ocular coats of the eye (the retina, choroid, and sclera) has only been evaluable by indirect methods such as histologic examination, which allow extrapolation to the *in vivo* thickness. Many functional and aging processes are related to the integrity and thickness of these structures, thus the ability to provide an *in vivo* measurement would be valuable in studying both normal variations and disease states.

We have devised a system for such measurements, using computer-assisted ultrasonic evaluation. Samples obtained with a high-resolution, combined B- and A-scan instrument can be analysed and thin boundary layers can be delineated to an accuracy of 10 microns, by analysis of the resonant reflectance from the front and rear surfaces of the retina, choroid, and sclera.

We have studied a series of patients to determine the normal values for thickness of the posterior ocular coats in various locations within the eye. Specifically, comparison of these structures in the macular area to more peripheral areas are presented.

The range of normal thickness to those observed in pathologic studies such as macular degeneration, trauma, inflammatory conditions, and myopia will be discussed.

Authors' Addresses:
The New York Hospital – Cornell Medical Center (Dr. Smith, Dr. Coleman)
New York, U.S.A.

Riverside Research Institute (Dr. Lizzi)
New York, U.S.A.

A COMPARATIVE ECHOGRAPHIC AND BIOCHEMICAL STUDY OF THE SUBRETINAL FLUID (S.R.F.) IN IDIOPATHIC RETINAL DETACHMENT

G. CENNAMO, A. LOFFREDO, A. SAMMARTINO & A. DE LELLIS

(Naples, Italy)

The study of subretinal fluid (S.R.F.) composition may provide useful information about the pathogenesis and behavior of idiopathic retinal detachment. It is generally believed that S.R.F. initially consists of degenerated fluidified vitreous passing through a retinal break into to the space between the neurosensorial and neuroepithelial layers. Later S.R.F. becomes richer in proteins, probably because of leakage from choroidal vessels (Akhmeteli, *et al.* 1977, Chignell, *et al.* 1977). S.R.F. has been the object of much research, but its study presents a great deal of difficulty for various reasons: (a) the easy contamination of the sample with blood on extraction; (b) the small quantity of extractable material; (c) the variety of separation techniques employed by different authors, which hinders comparison of the results. Moreover, the study of S.R.F. alone provides us with data relative to its composition, but not with data comparable to the structure of the vitreous, from which the S.R.F. is originally derived. A-scan echography, on the other hand, allows us to study the S.R.F. and the vitreous as a whole at the same time thus enabling us to discover any meshwork changes in the vitreous or reflectivity modifications in the S.R.F. (Gallenga 1973, Ossoinig 1966).

The aim of the present study is therefore to detect echographic changes — both in the vitreous and in S.R.F. — in idiopathic retinal detachment which is different in age and clinical properties, and to compare these results with the electrophoretic findings in S.R.F. protein composition. Eighteen cases of idiopathic retinal detachment were studied.

A-SCAN Echography was carried out by a Kretz 7200 MA apparatus with an 8 MHz probe calibrated on a synthetic tissue model, following Till & Ossoinig (1977). Data were collected both at the tissue (T) and vitreous levels (T + 6 dB) of amplification. Samples of S.R.F. were obtained during idiopathic retinal detachment surgery by opening the sclera and by choroid puncture without the use of diathermy. The fluid was aspirated directly at the level of the scleral wound using a needle cannula in order to avoid blood contamination. Moreover, samples in which such contamination was evident, were discarded. The sample were stored at + 4°C for 36–48 hours before analysis. A serum sample extracted at the same time, from the same subject, underwent a similar examination. The analyses were performed by electrophoretic tracing on polyacrylamide gel, following the technique of Ornstein &

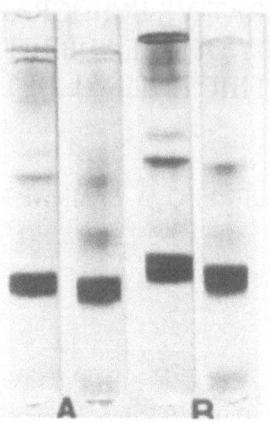

Fig. 1.

Davis, 1964. The separated protein bands, dyed with Black Starch, appeared like dark discs in a transparent gel and were read at 520 nm on the Beckmann CDS 100 for graphic registration (Fig. 1).

RESULTS

Echographic examination confirmed the knowledge that S.R.F. is acoustically homogeneous (Witold, *et al.* 1977) in a large number of cases (Fig. 2).

On the basis of the age of detachment, acoustically homogeneous S.R.F. nearly always belonged to more recent cases of detachment. In contrast to this, there was an almost constant lack of homogeneity of different degree in older detachments (of over three months old). Some correlation always existed between vitreous and S.R.F. modification in detachments of the same age. A more marked vitreal change corresponded to a greater lack of S.R.E: echographic homogeneity (Fig. 3). In two cases out of 18 there was an obvious difference in the vitreous and S.R.F. echographic data: although detachment was recent, there was a marked change in S.R.F. without any significant change in the vitreous. (Figs. 4, 5). An assessment of the echographic findings concerning S.R.F. belonging to older detachments stressed a

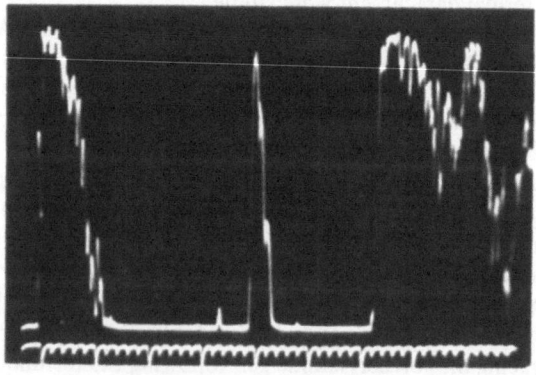

Fig. 2.

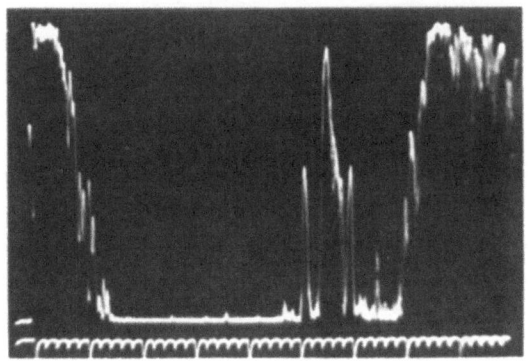

Fig. 3.

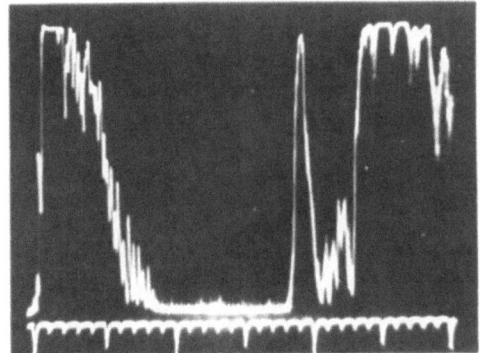

Fig. 4.

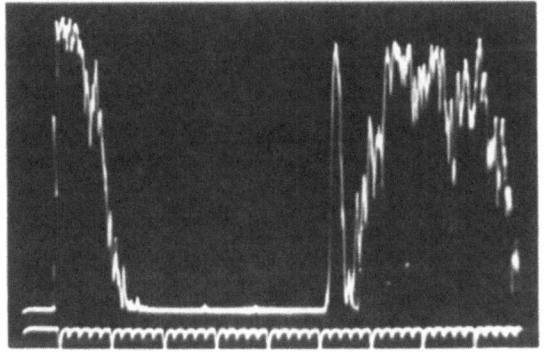

Fig. 5.

261

262

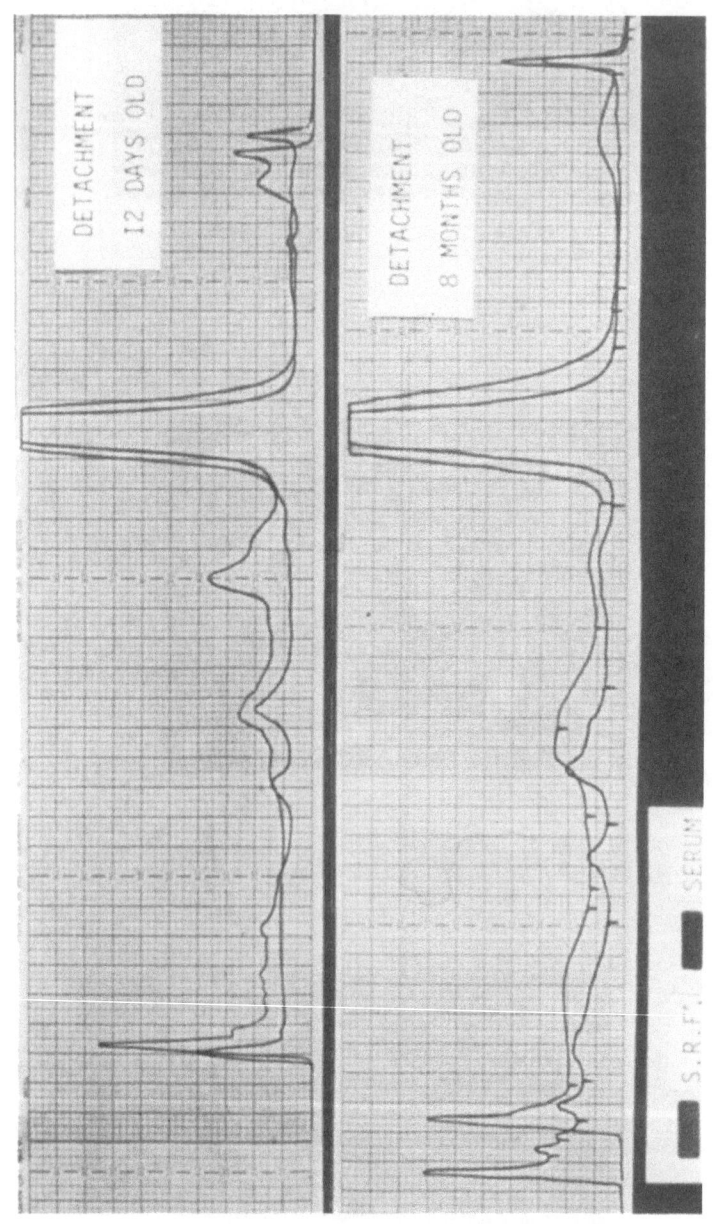

Fig. 6.

correlation between the lack of homogeneity found and this fluid's high protein content (Fig. 6). In these two cases – belonging to the set of recent detachments and with a marked echographic modification in S.R.F. as compared to the vitreous – there were also clinical uveal signs of inflammation. The results of S.R.F. electrophoretic examination revealed an early appearance of more mobile electrophoretic fractions (prealbumin, albumin and transferin) in recent retinal detachment. On the contrary, the slower polyglobuline fractions, on the other hand, appeared later in older detachments. (Loffredo, *et al.* 1977, Loffredo, *et al.* 1978). Moreover, an increase in total protein content was confirmed in older detachments. In the two cases characterized by clinical signs of inflammation, the presence of slower polyglobulin fractions was found, as well as an increase in total SRF protein content, even though these detachments were recent.

DISCUSSION

The examination of vitreous and S.R.F. echographic data and their comparison with S.R.F. protein content allowed us to draw the following conclusions:

(1) S.R.F. echographic homogeneity usually corresponds to its low protein content, and to an absence of slower polyglobulin fractions which also present a larger molecular size. We observed that recent detachments belonged to this group.

(2) In older detachments, on the other hand, the most evident vitreous and S.R.F. changes correspond to a higher S.R.F. protein content, with a marked presence of polyglobulin fractions. This may lead to the assumption that S.R.F. polyglobulin fraction increase causes a greater lack of echographic homogeneity.

(3) Vitreous echographic change is generally less evident than that in S.R.F. but always proportionate to this. This may imply that vitreous change is subordinate to that in S.R.F. which leads to the hypothesis that with the aging of detachment an inverse process occurs in which the S.R.F. influences vitreous structure, while initially the vitreous influenced S.R.F. composition. The echographic and biochemical data relative to recent detachments, moreover would favour the hypothesis that S.R.F. is of vitreous origin.

The presence of evident S.R.F. echographic change, with a corresponding increase in total protein content in inflammatory detachments given value to the hypothesis of direct participation of the choroidal vessels in S.R.F. composition; this may be the result of inflammation initially altering the blood barrier.

REFERENCES

Akhmeteli, L.M. Kasavina, B.S. & Petropavlovslaja,   Biochemical investigation of the subretinal fluid. Brit. J. Ophthalmol. 59: 70 (1975).

Bonavolonta, A., Loffredo, A., Sammartino, A. & De Luca, M. Protein composition of the subretinal fluid (S.R.F.) before and after treatment by diathermy. 3rd Int. Cong. Eye Res. Osaka, Japan, (1978).

Chignell, A.H., Carruthers, M. & Rahi, A.S.H. Clinical, biochemical and immunoelectrophoretic study of subretinal fluid. Brit. J. Ophthalmol. 55: 525 (1971).

Gallenga, P.E. In: Diagnostica ultrasonica in Ophtalmologia, Siduo IV (M. Massin & J. Poujol, eds.) Paris: Centre National d'Ophtalmologie (1973) p. 163.

Loffredo, A. De Luca, M. & Sammartino, A. Studio comparativo clinico e biochimico del liquido sottoretinico nel distacco di retina. Atti LVIII Congr. S.O.I., Roma (1977).

Ornstein, L. & Davis, B.J. Disc electrophoresis. Method and application to human serum protein. Ann. N.Y. Acad. Sc. 121: 404 (1964).

Ossoinig, K. Ultrasonics in Ophthalmology. Basel: Karger (1967) p. 116.

Witold, J. & Orlowski-Szczypinski, J. Ultrasonography of Subretinal Space in Rhegmatogenous Retinal Detachment. Mod. probl. ophthalmol. 18: 40 (1976).

Till, P. & Ossoinig, K.C. First experiences with a solid tissue model for standardization of A- and B-scan instruments in tissue diagnosis. In: Ultrasound in Medicine (D. White, ed.) New York: Plenum Press (1977) p. 2167.

Author's Address:
A. Loffredo
Istituto di Clinica Oculistica
2nd School of Medicine
University of Naples
Naples, Italy

A CHARACTERISTIC ECHOGRAPHIC SIGN OF CHOROIDAL DETACHMENT – THE APPEARANCE OF THE ANGLE OF JUNCTION WITH THE OCULAR WALL

Aspect échographique de l'angle de raccordement à la paroi oculaire dans le décollement choroïdien

J. POUJOL

(Paris, France)

SUMMARY

In addition to the other well-known characteristic signs of a choroidal detachment (bifid echo visible in A mode and lateral location easily seen in B mode), another characteristic sign is described: the appearance of the angle of junction with the ocular wall.

A decrease of more than two thirds of the choroidal thickness after the image of a swelling indicates the choroidal nature of the latter, whereas a retinal detachment causes little change in the choroido-retinal thickness measured by echographic means.

Le diagnostic échographique de décollement de la choroïde peut être moins simple qu'il n'est habituel de le considérer. Des signes classiques permettent de le reconnaitre: en mode A, l'aspect bifide de l'écho du soulèvement, en mode B, sa localisation latérale (Coleman, *et al.* 1977) et, de manière moins constante, son départ abrupt, presque perpendiculaire à la paroi oculaire. L'aspect échographique de la choroïde est mieux connu actuellement (Coleman 1979, Poujol 1979), et un autre signe caractéristique peut être décrit: c'est l'aspect de l'angle de raccordement à la paroi oculaire, de la choroïde décollée, où l'on observe une quasi-disparition de cette membrane au niveau du soulèvement.

Ce signe n'est facilement observable qu'en mode B. Il apparait à condition que le pouvoir de résolution soit suffisant: pouvoir de résolution en profondeur pour la chorio-rétine en place et pouvoir de résolution latéral pour la chorio-rétine soulevée, qui est située à peu près perpendiculairement à la première. Nous avons pu mettre ce signe en évidence avec les appareils de Bronson-Turner, Biophysic Médical EO2, Sonometrics Ocuscan et Biophysic Médical Triscan.

On peut considérer que la nature d'un décollement est choroïdienne lorsqu'on observe un amincissement de plus des deux tiers de l'épaisseur de la chorio-rétine après le début d'un soulèvement intra-oculaire et que l'image de la membrane soulevée garde une épaisseur correspondant à ce qui fait défaut

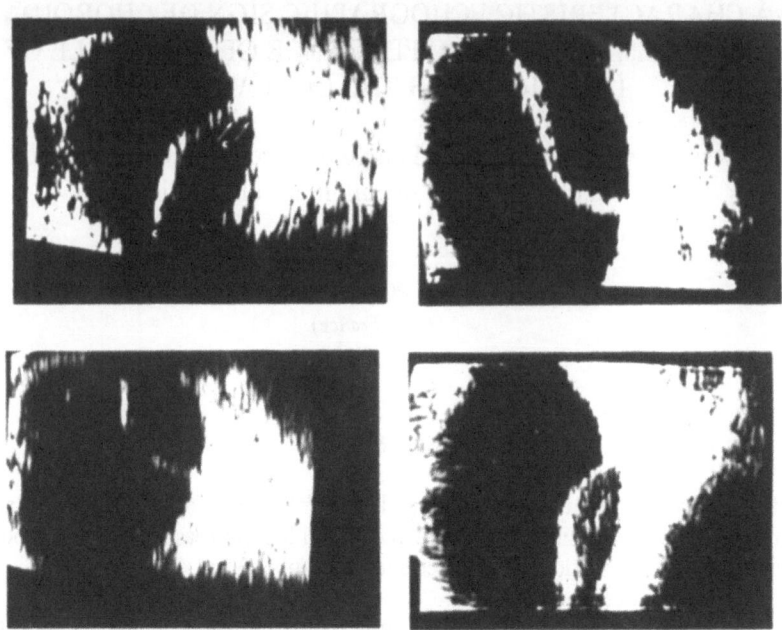

Fig. 1. Angle de jonction de décollements choroïdiens avec la paroi oculaire. Echo-grammes enregistrés avec trois appareils différents. C = choroïde.

au niveau de la paroi du globe (Fig. 1). La fréquence selon laquelle cet aspect de l'angle de jonction entre le soulèvement et la paroi oculaire peut être observé dans le décollement choroïdien, dépend essentiellement de la possibilité d'orienter correctement la sonde sur l'oeil pour trouver un plan de coupe convenable. Ceci est parfois difficile sur des yeux blessés ou récemment opérés. Nous avons pu mettre ce signe en évidence dans environ 70% des décollements choroïdiens.

Cet aspect caractéristique de l'angle de raccordement d'un soulèvement peut-il être observé dans d'autres affections que le décollement choroïdien? — Un décollement de rétine ou un rétinoschisis n'entrainent qu'une très faible diminution de l'épaisseur de la chorio-rétine.

— L'excavation choroïdienne d'un mélanome de la choroïde est bien différente: si la choroïde disparait sur une courte distance au niveau de la tumeur, l'image de la rétine soulevée apparait très mince. Inversement, dans les faux mélanomes par décollement choroïdien spontané, l'aspect caractéristique de l'angle de raccordement aide, ainsi que d'autres signes, à reconnaitre la nature non tumorale du décollement (Brachet, *et al.* 1980).

L'aspect particulier de l'angle de raccordement du soulèvement avec la paroi oculaire, dans le décollement choroïdien, nous parait spécifique et semble être un signe utile, à rechercher.

BIBLIOGRAPHIE

Brachet, A. Peyre, C. Poujol, J. & Terrassier J. Les décollements spontanés de la choroïde. Bull. Soc. Ophtalmol. France 1981, 3, 249–253.

Coleman, D.J. Lizzie, F.L. & Jack, R.L. Ultrasonography of the Eye and Orbit. Philadelphia: Lea & Febiger (1977).

Coleman, D.J. Lizzi, F.L. & Smith, M.E. In vivo measurements of chorio-retinal thickness with ultrasound. 2nd Meeting of the World Federation for Ultrasound in Medicine and Biology (4th World Congress on Ultrasonics in Medicine) Miyazaki, 22–27 July 1979. Abstract p. 166.

Poujol, J. Ultrasonographic measurement and clinical value of choroidal thickening. 2nd Meeting of the World Federation for Ultrasound in Medicine and Biology (4th World Congress on Ultrasonics in Medicine) Miyazaki, 22–27 July 1979 (T. Wagai & R. Omoto, eds.) Amsterdam: Excerpta Medica, (1980) p. 101.

Author's Address:
Centre National d'Opthalmolologie des
Quinze-Vingts
Paris, France

A-SCAN ECHOGRAPHY OF THE EYE AND ORBIT —
A TRAINING FILM
FOR MEDICAL STUDENTS AND DOCTORS

F. DAXECKER

(*Innsbruck, Austria*)

ABSTRACT

This film serves as material for the teaching of students and for further information to doctors. It is a report about the physical bases of ultrasonography, the origin of echoes in tissues, the A- and B-scan mode and the obtainable results. Furthermore, the technique of examination of eye and orbit is shown and a case is demonstrated. Duration: 8 min, 16 mm colour, magnetic film, in English.

Author's Address:
University Eye Clinic
Innsbruck, Austria

RETINAL TEAR ON B-SCANNING

A.M. VERBEEK

(Nijmegen, The Netherlands)

After examining the eye with the Kretztechnik 7200 MA apparatus and after quantitative membrane differentiation (Ossoinig 1972) we use the Bronson-Turner unit for supplementary information (especially topographic) (Bronson *et al.* 1976). Special attention is then paid to the relation between membrane structures and the ora serrata and the optic disc, to the optic disc itself (cupping, edema, drusen), to signs of proliferative disease, to signs of traction of vitreous structures on the retina and to structures in the subretinal space in case of a retinal detachment. Sometimes we found it possible to detect retinal tears with this unit. When a discontinuity in a membrane structure quantitatively qualified as being retina, is seen, there are three possibilities:

(1) it results from an acoustic artefact caused by retinal folding,

(2) it results from an acoustic artefact by shadowing of a structure anterior to the retina, or

(3) it is a real retinal tear.

So after detection of a possible retinal tear the same area is investigated from different angles and from different positions to exclude the possibilities (1) and (2). (Fig. 1a, b; Fig. 2, a, b, c). With the grid (Fig. 3) it is possible to give the surgeon information of the maximal diameter of the tear.

REFERENCES

Bronson, N.R., Fisher, Y.L., Pickering, N.C., Trayner, E.M. Ophthalmic Contact B-Scan Ultrasonography for the clinician (1976). Inc. Westport Conn.: Intercontinental Publication.

Ossoinig, K.C. Clinical Echo-Ophthalmography (1972). Current concepts in ophthalmology (F.C. Blodi, ed.) Saint-Louis: C.V. Mosby Co. (1972), p. 101 ev.

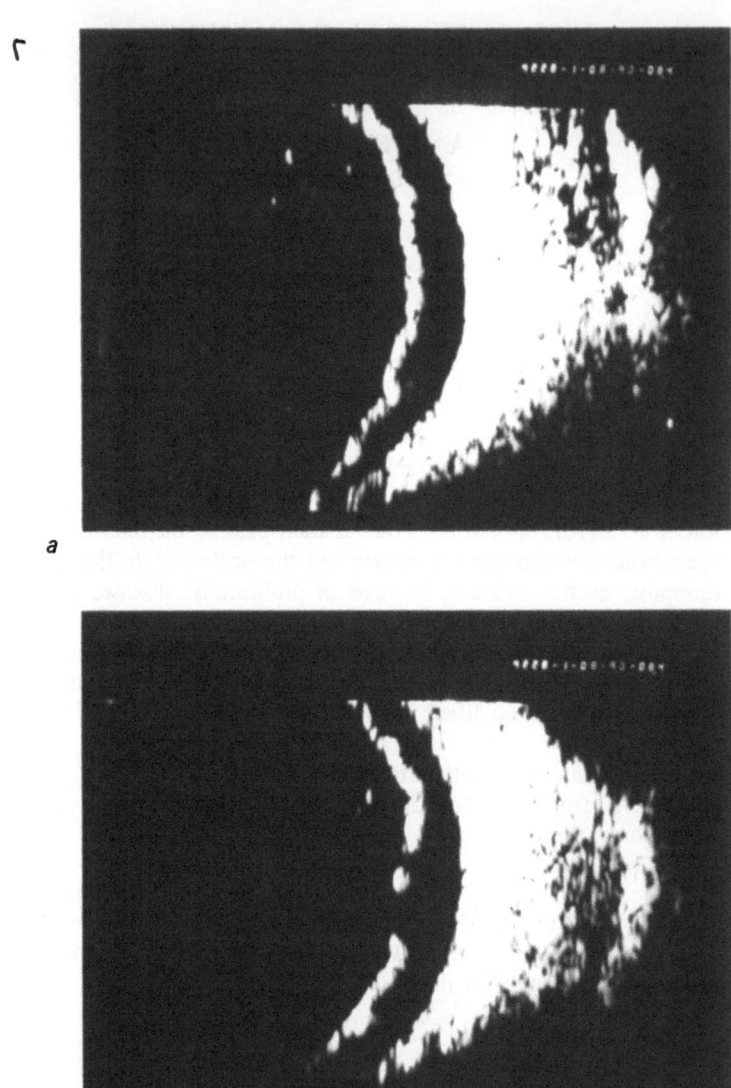

Fig. 1a. De

1b. The same patient. A retinal tear with operculum in the upper temporal quadrant.

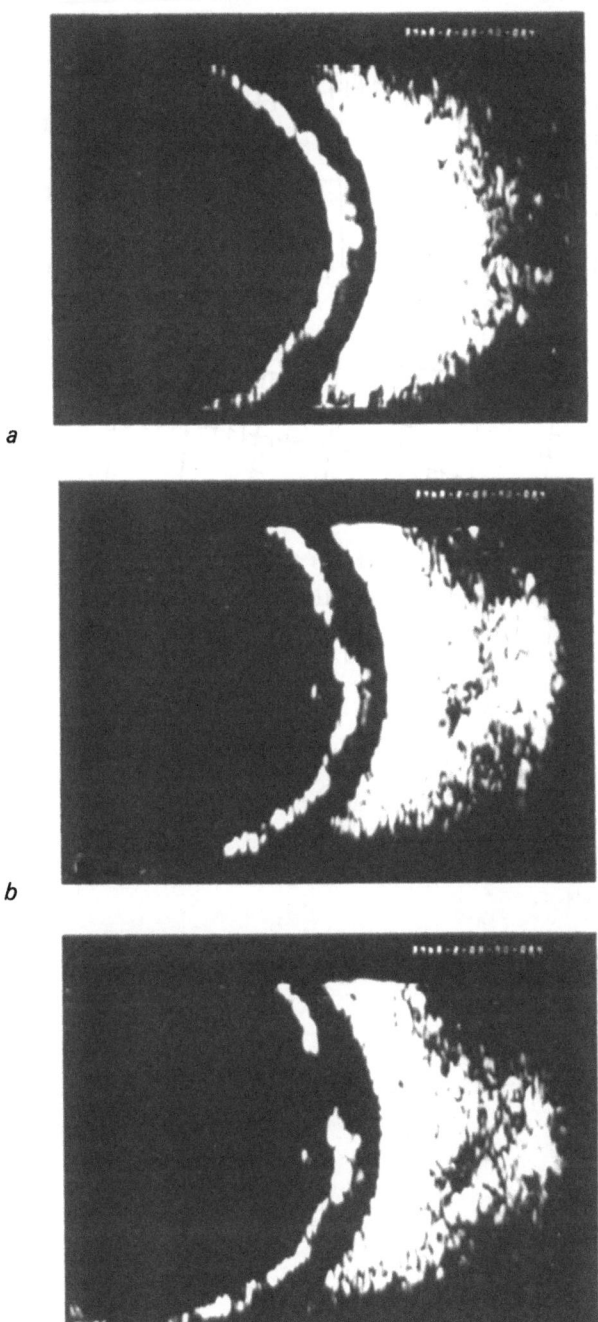

Fig. 2a. Detached retina in a patient with homogeneous vitreous opacities; fundus poorly visible in detail.
2b, c. Scanning over a 4 mm maximal diameter retinal tear.

271

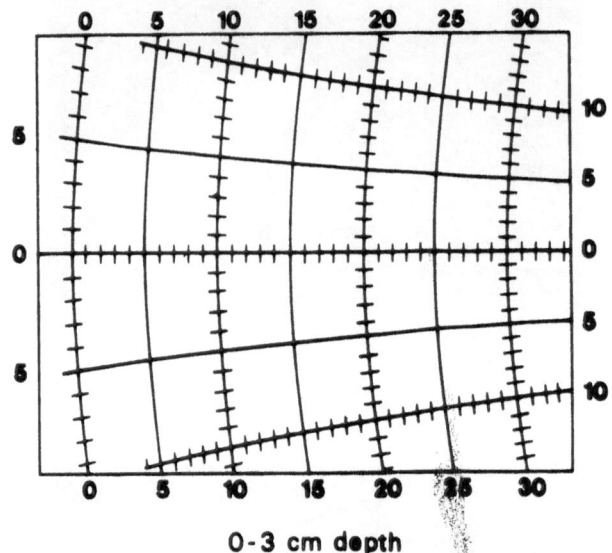

0 - 3 cm depth

Fig. 3. from: Ophthalmic contact B-scan Ultrasonografy for the clinician (Bronson *et al.* 1976).

Author's Address:
Institute of Ophthalmology
(Head: Prof. Dr. A.F. Deutman)
University of Nijmegen
Philips van Leydenlaan 15,
6500 HB Nijmegen
The Netherlands

THE ROLE OF ULTRASOUND IN THE INVESTIGATION AND MANAGEMENT OF ORBITAL DISEASE

Introductory Lecture

J.E. WRIGHT

(*London, United Kingdom*)

During the past eight years there has been a rapid change in the type of investigative technique which can be used to define abnormal tissue within the orbit. The development of the CT scanner by Hounsfield was a milestone in medical science and his discovery has had a tremendous impact on the investigation and management of orbital disease. CT scans have enabled the clinician to define the position and extent of orbital lesions with great accuracy. The role of ultrasound has in my view, been changed by this development and I hope that by discussing the various investigative techniques available to the orbital surgeon, I can show where ultrasound can help in the assessment of a patient with an orbital problem.

For the past eight years, ultrasonic scans have been a routine part of the assessment of patients attending the Orbital Clinic. The apparatus used at Moorfields was designed by scientists at the Atomic Energy Research Establishment at Harwell, working in collaboration with myself and Dr. Glyn Lloyd. I was able to obtain sufficient funds to start the Ultrasonic Department at Moorfields and we were fortunate to be joined by Miss Marie Restori whose publications are well known. She is a graduate physicist and has worked in close collaboration with myself and later, Mr. David McLeod, concentrating on a variety of clinical problems within the eye and the orbit. I have therefore been closely connected with the application of ultrasonic examination in ophthalmology for a number of years. During that time we have endeavoured to critically assess the usefulness and correct role of each of the investigative techniques comparing conventional radiography, tomography, CT scanning, and ultrasound.

During the past 12 years I have seen a large number of patients with orbital disease. Table 1 shows how frequently various orbital lesions have occurred. Dysthyroid eye disease is the most common cause of unilateral proptosis closely followed by vascular abnormalities, and the pseudo tumour/lymphoma group.

There are a number of investigative techniques which the ophthalmic surgeon can use to try to define the likely nature, the site, and extent of an orbital lesion. It is most important that the patient is examined thoroughly and a detailed clinical history must be obtained. Failure to pay attention to these preliminaries can result in a number of mistakes being made in the interpretation of the results of various investigations. The position of the globe in relation to the surrounding bone should be assessed and the amount of proptosis measured. Any vertical or horizontal displacement of the eye

Table 1.

Thyroid dysfunction	178	Neurofibromatosis	14
Fractures and trauma	68	Optic nerve gliomas	13
Vascular anomalies	148	Neurilemmomas	10
Pseudotumours	87	E.N.T.	69
Neoplasm (excluding lacrimal gland	82	Normal	43
Inflammatory	82	Others	100
Dermoid cyst and other cysts	46	Bone Changes	10
Lacrimal gland	53		
Meningiomas	38		

Total = 1041

should be noted for this may give a clue to the position of an orbital tumour. The cranial nerves must be thoroughly examined, including assessment of the visual fields and visual acuity. Routine examination with the slit lamp and examination of the fundus must always be performed together with palpation of the orbit and measurement of the range of ocular movement. Once this has been done the clinician should have a very good idea of the likely position and extent of an orbital mass, and in many cases the patient will have given the clinician excellent clues to the likely nature of the lesion. In particular, the length of history, presence of pain or tenderness, and of course the age of the patient, are important in assessing the likely nature of the orbital process. Once the clinician has completed his examination and assessment of the patient, he can decide which investigations are most suitable to the patient's assessment.

Conventional radiographs should be obtained in all patients. These should include an under-tilted occipitomental view, a lateral view, and oblique views, to demonstrate the optic canals. Tomography may be required to demonstrate certain areas in more detail. The surgeon who contemplates orbital surgery must be sure of the integrity of the walls of the orbit. These radiographs will show him if the walls are intact or have been breached. It is our experience that all the E.N.T. causes of proptosis can be diagnosed with these radiographs. The same is true of the changes produced by fractures to the facial bones, and in particular blow-out fractures of the floor and medial wall. I do not think that ultrasonic scans have any part to play in the assessment of the cases I have alluded to.

Contrast radiography should be confined to the investigation of certain vascular lesions within the orbit. Some years ago, orbital venography was used to show the presence of orbital tumours but it's use is now confined to the delineation of primary orbital varices. Selective external and internal carotid angiography is useful to define arteries supplying very vascular tumours within the orbit and this technique is an essential preliminary prior to their removal. Carotid angiography should also be used to demonstrate the site of any arteriovenous shunts either within the orbit or within the region of the cavernous sinus. The diagnosis in these cases is usually made on clinical grounds but if embolization of the feeder vessels is contemplated, highly detailed angiographs are an essential prerequisite.

The advent of computerized tomography has had a profound effect on the investigation of orbital disease. The high resolution scans which can be obtained in both the axial and coronal plane enable the clinician to define the position and extent of orbital lesions with great accuracy. Ultrasonic examination cannot do this as accurately, nor can the posterior part of the orbit be examined with conventional ultrasonic apparatus. I find it somewhat distressing to read and hear papers which seem to ignore the role that CT scanning now plays in the investigation of orbital disease. Indeed, it does a disservice to the ultrasonographer and ophthalmic ultrasound in general for ultrasound to be used for tasks which can be done far better and more accurately, by CT scans.

Ultrasound has a definite part to play in the diagnosis and management of orbital lesions, but the efforts of the ultrasonographer should be directed to the recognition of echo patterns which will enable the clinician to make a more accurate pre-operative diagnosis. CT scanning is widely used and there are few ophthalmic departments in the developed countries which do not have access to a CT scanner. It is logical that computerized tomography should be used in conjunction with ultrasound, thus providing the clinician with a more comprehensive picture of the patient's orbital problem.

The commonest cause of unilateral proptosis is dysthyroid eye disease. The diagnosis is based on the recognition of clinical signs which in my experience is much more reliable than any biochemical tests so far devised. In nearly all cases, there is some degree of lid retraction often combined with lid lag and restriction of upward movement of the globe. Investigations should include an assessment of the activity of the thyroid gland, measurement of thyroid antibodies and the TRH test. The TRH test is a very sensitive indication of thyroid dysfunction in the absence of frank hyper or hypo-thyroidism. It measures the response of the pituitary to the injection of a synthetic dose of Thyrotrophin releasing hormone. The blood levels of thyroid stimulating hormone are assessed during a 30 min period after the injection of the synthetic TRH. We have found it a most useful test for it provides supportive evidence of thyroid abnormality in 75–80% of cases. There remains a group of patients in whom the diagnosis is based on clinical signs unsupported by the most sophisticated biochemical tests. CT scanning can be particularly helpful in these cases for the size of the extraocular muscles can be assessed in the axial and coronal planes. The ultrasonic assessment of the size of the extraocular muscles provides results which are much inferior to those produced with high resolution CT scans. There are anatomical reasons for this discrepancy. They will be discussed more fully in the section on optic nerve tumours.

The vascular group of lesions are the most frequent cause of proptosis. The commonest abnormality is the primary orbital varix. They are present from early childhood and these hugely dilated channels are often in direct communication with the internal jugular vein, so that any rise in the jugular venous pressure will cause enlargement of the abnormal veins within the orbit producing a variable proptosis. Some ophthalmologists and pathologists confuse these lesions with lymphangiomas of the orbit. In my experience lymphangiomas are relatively rare. Ultrasonic scans will demonstrate the variable size of the veins within the orbit, but the best way to delineate these lesions, is by frontal venography.

Capillary haemangiomas are almost as common as varices. The orbital mass is usually associated with a strawberry patch on the overlying skin or conjunctiva. The diagnosis is therefore obvious. In most cases the mass disappears by the time the child is four or five years old and the majority require no treatment whatsoever.

Cavernous haemangiomas are relatively uncommon, frequently the patient is over the age of 25 years. Cases have been recorded under this age. These are comparatively rare. The lesions are discrete and well encapsulated. They grow slowly and have a typical ultrasonic picture giving rise to high amplitude echoes with well demarcated borders and low attenuation of the sound. The site and extent can be well demonstrated with the CT scanner, but it is ultrasound which differentiates these lesions from neurilemmomas, which ultrasonically can be completely empty or filled with echoes of medium amplitude. Again there is poor attenuation but this is not as poor as that seen in cavernous haemangiomas, and the amplitude of the echoes is much lower than that seen in cavernous haemangiomas.

The vascular tumours must be correctly classified both by the clinician and the ultrasonographer. Some reports detail a quite bizarre variety of vascular lesions which on histological and other grounds cannot be recognised by the experienced clinician.

Tumours arising from the optic nerve are fairly rare. The clinical features of these tumours are well recognised and CT scans can show their size and extent very accurately. Ultrasonic techniques can detect the presence of these tumours, but cannot define their extent as accurately as CT scans. We have used C-scans of the optic nerve to provide a coronal view of the nerve surrounded by the tumour. Some authors have advocated the use of A-scans to measure the optic nerve diameter. The accuracy of this method is dependant on the beam of ultrasound striking the optic nerve at right angles. Any slight obliquity of the beam to the nerve will produce measurements which are very inaccurate. CT scans show that the optic nerve has a fairly straight course within the orbit. Adduction of the globe produces a slight sinuosity but it is difficult to see how any ultrasonic probe can direct the beam of ultrasound at right angles to the nerve unless bone is removed from the lateral wall of the orbit before the probe is introduced. This is true of the normal orbit, but also in patients where there is a considerable degree of proptosis. The anatomy of the orbit precludes similar attempts if the transducer is placed in the upper or lower parts of the orbit.

Ultrasonic examination of the orbit will play an increasing role in the investigation and management of the various disease processes which affect the retro-ocular tissues. Coleman and others are already assessing the potential of spectral analysis. Our efforts should be directed towards tissue recognition, correlating our findings with the morphological characteristics seen with CT scans. It is important that we do not continue to use ultrasound for tasks which are better performed by computerized scanning. Ophthalmic ultrasound has already proved itself invaluable in the investigation and management of certain intraocular conditions. Its role in relation to orbital disease is assured, but we will have to be selective in its application.

Author's Address:
Moorfields Eye Hospital
London, United Kingdom

276

DIFFERENTIAL DIAGNOSTIC RESULTS OF CLINICAL ECHOGRAPHY IN ORBITAL TUMORS

P. TILL & W. HAUFF

(*Vienna, Austria*)

Since 1973 the echographic department of 2nd University – Eye Clinic in Vienna performed 7980 orbital examinations. 422 orbital and periorbital tumors and pseudotumors were detected from four different examiners of our laboratory. 358 of these lesions were differentiated with standardized echography, based on a combination of standardized A-scan (7200 MA unit Kretztechnik), contact B-scan (Bronson-Turner unit) and Doppler ultrasound (Minivason 9 Kretztechnik). With standardized echography more than 99% of orbital lesions causing signs or symptoms can be detected. 85% (358 lesions) of the detected lesions (422) were differentiated into 28 different tumors or groups of abnormalities with a sensitivity of the method of 94%: 290 of the 316 verified cases were correct and 26 incorrect differentiated. Table 1 demonstrates the echographic differential diagnoses; 316 lesions were verified by operations with histology, biopsies, carotisangiographies, clinically or echographically follow up examinations etc. Twenty-six incorrect false positive cases are on the other side identical with the 26 false negative cases in the table; if a diagnostic test is false positive in a certain disease, the test on the other side does not diagnose this lesion and is present as one false negative case in this group of lesion. Six false negative cases until now are not to classify echographically and their histologic correlations see Table 2.

Vecchio (1966) pointed out that, dispite apparent high efficiency of a diagnostic test in preliminary evaluation in groups of known diseased and nondiseased subjects, care must be taken when applying the results to unselected groups because of the magnification of false positive errors by a relative low prevalence of disease in the general population. He suggests the use of a predictive value. Russel (1966) extended Vecchio's predictive value concept to provide an index of the reliability of a clinical diagnosis (L.B. Lusted 1968). Predictive Value (PV) is defined as:

$$PV(\%) = \frac{\text{number of correct cases}}{\text{no. of corr.} + \text{no. of false pos. cases}} \times 100$$

and Sensitivity

$$(S)\% = \frac{\text{no. of correct cases}}{\text{no. of corr.} + \text{no. of false neg. cases}} \times 100$$

Table 1. Results of echographic differential diagnosis in orbital tumors.

Total	Echographical differential Diagnoses	Unverified	Verified Correct	Incorrect + false	−	S.	P.V.
24	Dermoid & epidermoid	5	15	4	1	94%	79%
15	Dermolipoma	0	15	0	0	100%	100%
4	Conjunctival cyst	0	4	0	0		
42	Muco-pyocele	5	36	1	0	100%	97%
21	Cav. hemang. adult	9	11	1	2	85%	92%
1	Sclerosing cav. hem.	0	1	0	0		
10	Infantile hemangioma	2	8	0	0		
1	Lymphangioma	1	0	0	0		
4	Neurofibroma	0	4	0	0		
33	Sphenoid wing mening.	5	21	7	1	95%	75%
91	Lymhoma/pseudotumor	9	74	8	3	96%	90%
3	Mixed tumor of lacr. gl.	0	1	2	0		
17	Metastatic carcinoma	0	17	0	4	81%	100%
1	Scirrhose metast. carc.	0	1	0	0		
1	Metast. carc. of rect. musc.	0	1	0	0		
26	Periorbital malignancy	3	23	0	5	82%	100%
7	Orbital hematoma	1	6	0	0		
1	Subperiost. hematoma	0	1	0	0		
2	Hematoma of musc. sheaths	0	2	0	0		
1	Hematoma of opt. n. sheath	0	1	0	0		
6	Glioma of optic nerve	1	4	1	0		
3	Meningioma of opt. nerve	0	2	1	0		
1	Neurinoma	0	0	1	2		
13	Carotid-cav. fistula	0	13	0	0	100%	100%
3	Orbital varix	0	3	0	0		
2	Racemose angioma	0	2	0	2		
12	Ectatic lacrimal sacc.	0	12	0	0	100%	100%
13	Orbital abscess	1	12	0	0	100%	100%
358		42	290	26	20	94%	92%
64	Without echogr. diff. diag.)				+ 6*		
			316		26		
422					26		

*History of six additional false negative cases (see Table 2)
S.: Sensitivity of method, P.V.: Predictive Value of method.

Table 2. Histologic diagnoses of the six additional false negative cases from Table 1 (Until now acoustic differention not performed).

1. Angiolipoma
2. Hemangioma of venous type
3. Capillary and venous hemangioma
4. Chron. tuberculoid inflammation of lacrimal gland
5. Granulomatous inflamation of lacrimal gland
6. Fibrolipoma

In Table 3 is demonstrated the matrix of possible outcomes which result from deciding between two diseases. In Table 1 sensitivity and predictive value were only calculated in more than ten correct diagnosed and verified cases.

The degree of sensitivity in standardized echography for the differential

Table 3. Matrix for possible outcomes which result from deciding between two diseases.

	Test result Positive	Negative	
Disease 1	Correct (truly pos.)	False neg. (error of 1st kind)	Total diseased patients tested ↓
		↘ etc.	
Disease 2	False pos. (error of 2nd kind)	Sensitivity (%) = $\dfrac{\text{correct cases}}{\text{corr.} + \text{false neg.}} \times 100$	
	total pos. tests ↓ Predictive value (%) = $\dfrac{\text{correct cases}}{\text{corr.} + \text{false pos.}} \times 100$		

diagnoses of orbital conditions depends largely on the type of lesion: arteriovenous fistulas, for instance, produce pathognomonic A-scan pattern that are identifiable in every single case. Sphenoid wing meningiomas are diagnosed with a sensitivity of 95%, whereas metastatic carcinomas, with only 81%, are often difficult to distinguish from a few other lesions. Table 4 shows the histologic diagnosis of the 26 false positive echographic differentiations.

Fig. 1 demonstrates typical A-scan echograms from different kinds of lesions. All echograms are obtained with the 7200 MA unit (Kretzechnik) at tissue sensitivity. Standardized A-scan determines during the *quantitative echography* reflectivity and internal structure of a lesion; using tissue sensitivity, the sound beam is aimed perpendicular to the lesion surface. The amplitude of the inner lesion spikes (i.e., spikes between anterior and posterior surface signals) is evaluated. Such perpendicular echograms are obtained in several different sound-beam directions. Reflectivity is now measured and depends from spike height at tissue sensitivity as percentage of display height. Cavernous hemangiomas of the adult type (Fig. 1b) show high reflectivity with spike height 80–95% of display height; the honeycomb-like structure is indicated by a chain of alternatively higher (longer) and lower (shorter) echo spikes that represent the large, smooth, highly reflective surfaces of the cavernous spaces, and the weakly scattering stagnant blood within the spaces. In contrast the reflectivity of the group of lymphoma/pseudotumors is low (spike height 5–40% of display height) as can be seen in Fig. 1c.

The most important step in *topographic echography* is to determine the borders of a lesion with standardized A-scan echography. The borders of an orbital mass lesion can be distinguished in: (1) diffuse extension of the lesion without surface signals; (2) a poorly outlined lesion has wide, multipeaked, indistinct surface signals (Fig. 1d); (3) a well-delineated lesion has a single-peaked, high, distinct surface spike and (4) a thick capsule of solid lesion or cystic wall has a very distinct, steeply rising, high, double-peaked surface spike (Fig. 1g). By combining transocular and paraocular approaches, the meridians involved, the relation of the lesion to normal structures and the

279

Table 4. Histologic diagnoses of the 26 false positive echographic tumor diagnoses.

Echographic diagnoses	False +	Histologic diagnoses
Dermoid & epidermoid	4	1. A-v. racemose angioma 2. Angiolipoma 3. Rhabdomyosarcoma 4. Rhabdomyosarcoma
Muco-pyocele	1	1. Lymphoepithelial carcin.
Cav. hemangioma adult	1	1. Dermoid (choesterol cont.)
Sphenoid wing meningioma	7	1. Racemose angioma 2. Metastat. carcinoma 3. Cavernous hemangioma 4. Metastat. hypernephroma 5. Chron. inflamm. pseudotu. 6. Hemang. of venous type 7. Cavernous hemangioma
Lymphoma/pseudotumor	8	1. Neurinoma (fasc. type A) 2. Polymorph. solid carcin. 3. Epipharynx carcinoma 4. Meningioma 5. Hepatocell. metast. carc. 6. Lymphoepithel. carcin. 7. Invasive epithelioma 8. Capillary and ven. hemang.
Mixed tumor	2	1. Chron. tuberculoid inflamm. of lacr. gland 2. Granulomatous inflamm. of of of lacrimal gland
Glioma of of opt. nerve	1	1. Cystic degen. neurinoma of N. VI.
Meningioma of opt. nerve	1	1. Fibrolipoma
Neurinoma	1	1. Metastat. carcinoma
	26	26

shape of the lesion is determined. In the next step of topographic examination maximum width and depth of the tumor is measured. With *kinetic echography* consistency and vascularity of a lesion can be evaluated. If blood flow is present, spontaneous and continuous movement is seen as it is pathognomonic in arteriovenous fistulas (Fig. 1i).

Periorbital malignancies are characterized by irregular internal structures, shapes and borders. Although these tumors are low-reflective, bony remnants within the tumor tissue causes a sufficient number of high, irregulary distributed spikes to differentiate these tumors from mucoceles and other regularly structured masses. Since echography does not indicate the cell type, a number of lesions that destroy bone fall into this category: carcinomas, sarcomas, histiocytomas and sphenoid wing meningiomas. Although such

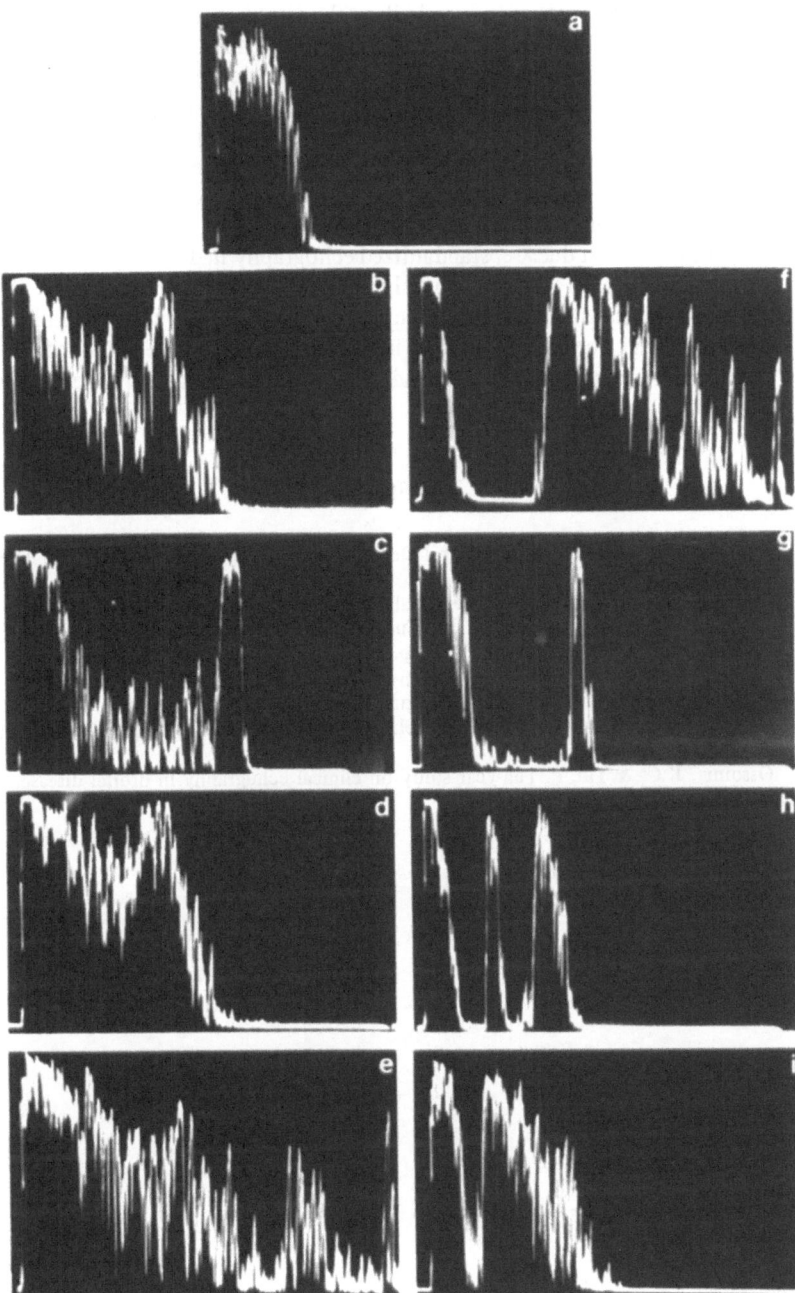

Fig. 1. A-scan echograms from various orbital tumors obtained with 7200 MA (Kretztechnik) at tissue sensitivity: (a) normal orbital tissue (b) cavernous hemangioma of adult type (c) lymphoma (d) metastatic carcinoma (e) periorbital malignancy (f) sphenoid wing meningioma (g) mucocele (h) dermoid (with septum) (i) arteriovenous fistula

281

meningiomas and cancer create similar echographic patterns, they can usually be differentiated on the basis of their location and the relationship of their size to the proptosis of the eye: meningiomas are located superiorly, often even more laterally (Fig. 1f), whereas cancer most often originates from ethmoidal and maxillary sinuses (Fig. 1e). Meningiomas usually produce a high degree of proptosis while they are still relatively small, whereas periorbital malignancies grow to extensive size before causing noticeable proptosis (Ossoinig 1979).

During the past decade, standardized echography had become an important diagnostic tool in clinical opthalmology. The applicability, success and clinical usefulness of echography depend on the experience and skill of the examiner and the design of the instrument used; we recommend to use standardized A-scan unit and standardized examination techniques as were created by Ossoinig.

REFERENCES

Lusted, L.B. Introduction to Medical Decision Making. Springfield: Charles C. Thomas (1968.)

Ossoinig, K.C. Preoperative Differential Diagnosis of Tumors with Echography: IV. Diagnosis of Orbital Tumors. In: Current Concepts in Opthalmology, Vol. 4 (F.C. Blodi, ed.) St. Louis: Mosby (1974) p. 313.

Ossoinig, K.C. Standardized Echography: Basic Principles, Clinical Applications, and Results. In: Opthalmic Ultrasonography: Comparative Techniques (R.L. Dallow, ed.) Int Opthalmology Clinics, Vol. 19(4) Boston: Little, Brown & Co. (1979) p. 127.

Ossoinig, K.C. & Till, P. Ten-year study on clinical echography in orbital disease. Bibl. Opthalmol. 83:200 (1975).

Authors' Address:
II Universität-Augenklinik
Alserstrasse 4
A-1090 Wien, Austria

282

ECHOGRAPHIC DIFFERENTIATION OF
VASCULAR TUMORS IN THE ORBIT

K.C. OSSOINIG

(Iowa City, Iowa, U.S.A.)

With standardized echography, based on the standardized A-scan method and aided by contact B-scan and Doppler techniques, all orbital lesions causing symptoms or signs can be detected reliably and accurately. With standardized echography, orbital lesions can be differentiated into 70 types of lesions or groups of conditions; the sensitivity of standardized echography in this differential diagnosis exceeds 90%, and its accuracy is more than 80%. Vascular orbital tumors (both neoplasms and malformations) are among the most thoroughly studied lesions in echographic differential diagnosis. With standardized echography, they can be subdivided into ten individual types or groups of lesions. They are: typical cavernous hemangiomas occurring in adults; highly sclerosed cavernous hemangiomas in adults; hemangiomas of the mixed (capillary and cavernous) type occurring in infants; cavernous hemangiomas in infants; the group of capillary hemangiomas hemangio-endotheliomas, hemangio-pericytomas, angiofibromas and angiosarcomas (which cannot be further differentiated into individual lesions); lymph-angiomas; A-V malformations (arteriovenous aneurysms of the orbit); varices; large 'high-flow' A-V fistulas of the brain that drain through the orbit and produce pathognomonic echographic patterns; and small 'low-flow' A-V fistulas of the brain that congest the orbit and produce characteristic echo-graphic signs which differ from the high-flow fistulas.

The echographic differential diagnosis is mainly based on nine acoustic criteria, three of which are evaluated by quantitative, topographic and kinetic echography each (Table 1). Rarely, one or two of these acoustic criteria provide the diagnosis (e.g., in high-flow A-V fistulas where a dilated superior ophthalmic vein with arterialized blood flow clinches the diagnosis). Usually, the nine differential criteria together make the echographic diagnosis. Tables 2–6 list the acoustic differential criteria typically found in the more frequently encountered vascular orbital tumors, i.e., cavernous hemangiomas of the adult type, mixed type hemangiomas in infants, varices, high-flow A-V fistulas and lymphangiomas. As can be seen from the tables, the two hemangioma types occurring in adults versus infants or children are two entirely different lesions.

Figs. 1–5 illustrate A-scan echograms typically seen in these different vascular lesions, except for low-flow fistulas, whose orbital echographic findings are illustrated in Fig. 6. Fig. 7 demonstrates the value of B-scan in

© 1981. Dr W. Junk Publishers, The Hague

Table 1. Basic acoustic differential criteria for echographic diagnosis of orbital lesions.

I. Quantitative echography* (A)	(1) *Internal Structure* (length and height of lesion spikes)
	(2) *Reflectivity* (spike height in % of display height at tissue sensitivity)
	(3) *Sound Attenuation* (angle kappa at medium spike height or height of normal orbital signals following lesion spikes)
II. Topographic echography (A, B)	(4) *Borders*
	(5) *Shape*
	(6) *Location*
III. Kinetic echography (A)	(7) *Bloodflow* (vascularity)
	(8) *Mobility*
	(9) *Consistency*

*Surface spikes are excluded from quantitation.

Table 2. Acoustic differential criteria found in typical *Cavernous Hemangiomas of the adult.*

(1) regular heterogenous (honeycomb-like) internal structure: higher as well as longer spikes (septa) alternate with lower as well as shorter spikes (stagnant blood)

(2) high reflectivity (80%–95% at first 10 μs)

(3) medium sound attenuation (angle kappa $\simeq 45°$; stagnant blood is very absorbent)

(4) well outlined, encapsulated (bumpy surface)

(5) roundish/oval shape (globe often causes dell)

(6) location within muscle cone (more temporal)

(7) no detectable bloodflow (stagnant blood)

(8) mobile

(9) hard, but gets smaller upon prolonged pressure of 30 to 60 s duration (delayed compressibility)

topographic evaluations showing the optic nerve riding along the superonasal surface of a cavernous hemangioma, clarifying the spatial relationship between a dilated superior ophthalmic vein (high-flow A-V fistula) and the optic nerve, and showing the winding course of the dilated vein throughout the superior orbit. The A-scan echograms of a high-flow A-V fistula of the brain (draining through the orbit), and of the normal fellow orbit, in Fig. 4, were obtained from a 12-year-old boy who was thought to have congenital hemangioma of the face and orbit. The echographic diagnosis was established after only 20 s of A-scan examination, on the basis of the pathognomonic

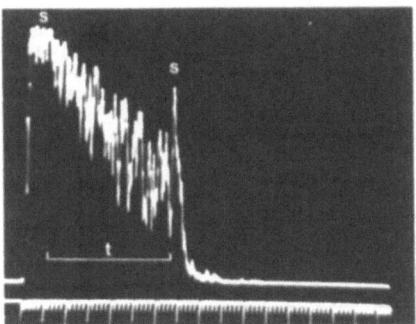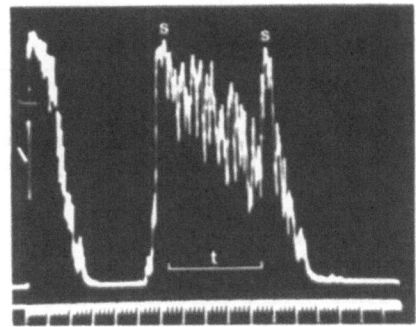

Fig. 1. Paraocular (left) and transocular (right) echograms of cavernous hemangioma (adult type). t tumor pattern; s surface spikes.

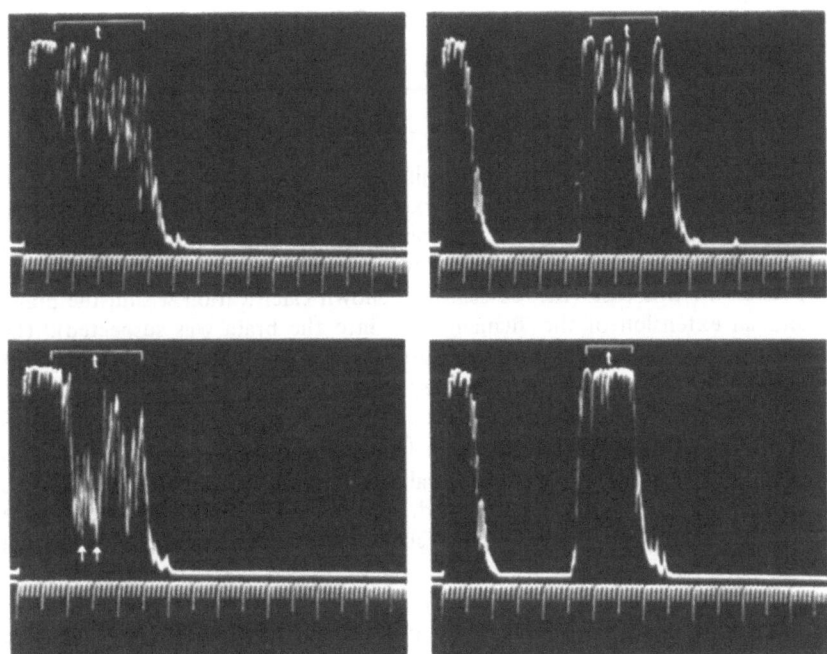

Fig. 2. Paraocular and transocular echograms of hemangioma (infant type). Top left pattern from cavernous portion; bottom left echogram from mixed cavernous higher spikes)/capillary (lower spikes) portion of the same tumor. Top right echogram obtained prior to, bottom right pattern obtained during, pressure with probe (which results in barrowing of tumor pattern because of softness of hemangioma). t tumor echogram; → spikes blurred due to blood flow in capillary portion of hemangioma.

Table 3. Acoustic differential criteria found in typical *Mixed* (capillary and cavernous) *Hemangiomas in infants and children.*

(1) irregular internal structure (echogram also changes significantly with beam direction)
(2) irregular reflectivity (ranging from 10% to 100%)
(3) weak sound attenuation (flowing blood absorbs less energy)
(4) variable, often irregular or diffuse borders
(5) irregular shape
(6) location in superior anterior orbit (rarely in muscle cone)
(7) marked blood flow (mixed arterial and venous)
(8) immobile
(9) partially soft

Table 4. Acoustic differential criteria found in typical *Varices.*

(1)   regular homogeneous internal structure
(2)   low reflectivity (5%–20%)
(3)   weak sound attenuation (angle kappa < 30°)
(4)   sharply outlined (vessel wall)
(5)   shape of tortuous vessel
(6)   superior orbit (most frequently)
(7)   no blood flow (except during initial phase of Valsalva and upon pressure with probe)
(8)   mobile
(9)   extremely soft (often collapsible)
(10) highly positive Valsalva (see (Fig. 3)

findings of a dilated superior ophthalmic vein with fast, arterial blood flow in it. It is interesting to note that an extensive clinical and radiological workup (including tomographies and CT-scans) had been performed prior to the echographic diagnosis in order to evaluate whether cosmetic surgery was possible in this case (the CT-scan had shown calcification within the brain, and an extension of the 'hemangioma' into the brain was suspected). The conclusion of this extensive workup was that the 'hemangioma' did not extend into the brain, and surgery was therefore possible. The carotid angiogram which confirmed the echographic diagnosis was only performed after the correct diagnosis of A-V fistula had been made by echography, which of course ruled out any surgical intervention for cosmetic reasons. This is one of many cases we experienced, which illustrate the clinical importance and central role of standardized echography in the evaluation of orbital lesions.

Because of its high sensitivity and accuracy in detection, differentiation, localization and measurement of orbital structures, and because of its complete harmlessness, standardized echography is an ideal method for screening orbits with suspected orbital lesions. Echography also indicates the usefulness or necessity of further diagnostic tests and aids in the planning of surgery (excisional biopsies versus diagnostic biopsies). And because it is harmless, echography is the ideal tool for following up the course of orbital disease (e.g., development of an orbital abscess in orbital cellulitis) and the effectiveness of chemotherapy or radiation. The echographic localization and

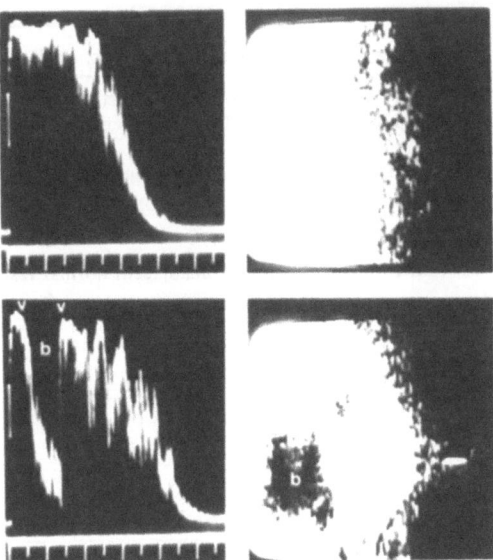

Fig. 3. A-scan and B-scan echograms of orbital varix displayed prior to (top), and during Valsalva (bottom). While the top patterns are normal in appearance, the bottom echograms clearly show the varix. The varix filled up within 5 s of the Valsalva procedure. b blood in varix; v surface spikes from vessel wall.

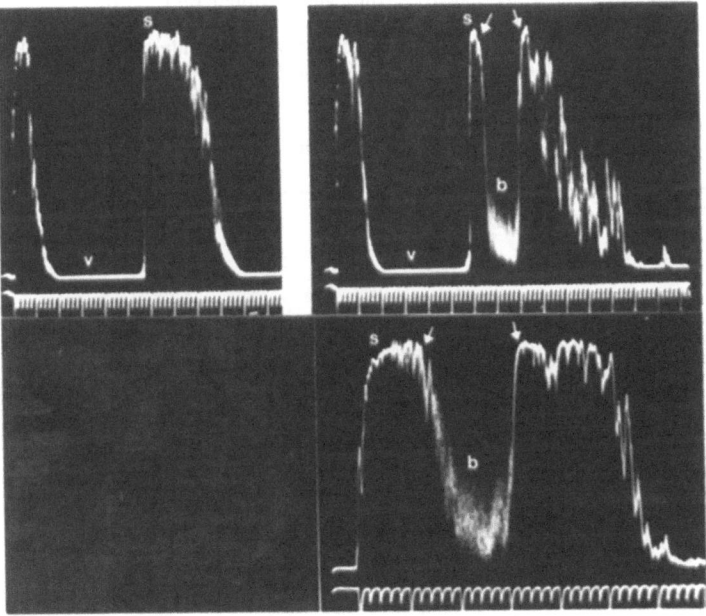

Fig. 4. A-scan echograms of normal orbit (left) and dilated superior ophthalmic vein (right) from case of high-flow A-V fistula (draining through orbit). Top echograms are shown with regular horizontal screen expansion. The lower echogram is shown with maximal horizontal expansion (following *P. Till*) to stress the display of the fast blood flow within the vessel. v vitreous; s sclera; b fast flowing blood in dilated vein; → vessel walls.

Table 6. Acoustic differential criteria found in typical *Lymphangiomas.*

(1)	regular, highly heterogeneous (cavernous) internal structure
(2)	alternately very high (septa) and very low (homogeneous fluid in spaces) reflectivity
(3)	weak sound attenuation
(4)	irregular borders
(5)	irregular shape
(6)	location often in retrobulbar orbit
(7)	no bloodflow (but Doppler response from adjacent normal vessels frequently enhanced)
(8)	often immobile
(9)	soft (firm when bleeding into lesion occurred)
(10)	negative Valsalva

Table 5. Acoustic differential criteria found in *High-flow A-V fistulas.*.

(1)	regular homogeneous internal structure
(2)	low to extremely low reflectivity (2%–15%)
(3)	weak sound attenuation (angle kappa < 30°)
(4)	sharply outlined (vessel wall)
(5)	shape of winding vessel
(6)	location in superior orbit (courses from anterior nasal aspect of orbit to posterior, more temporal location of superior orbital fissure)
(7)	fast (often pulsating) bloodflow throughout entire lesion
(8)	mobile (shifts with eye movement)
(9)	firm, but compressible with increased pressure overcoming arterialized blood pressure in vein (with early collapse during diastolic phases)
(10)	dilatation and arterialized blood flow in anastomosing angular and facial veins often detectable
(11)	thickened extraocular muscles neighbouring the superior ophthalmic vein (medial rectus, superior oblique, superior rectus, lateral rectus)

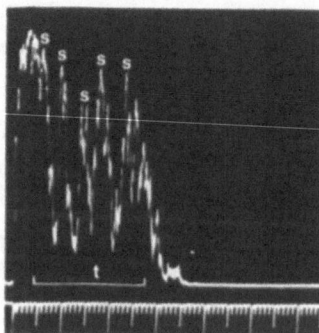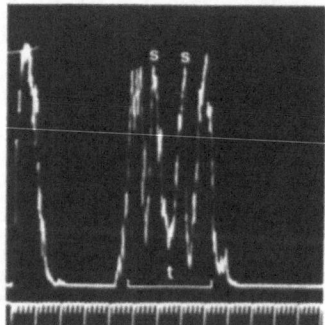

Fig. 5. Paraocular (left) and transocular (right) echograms of lymphangioma. t tumor pattern; s septa.

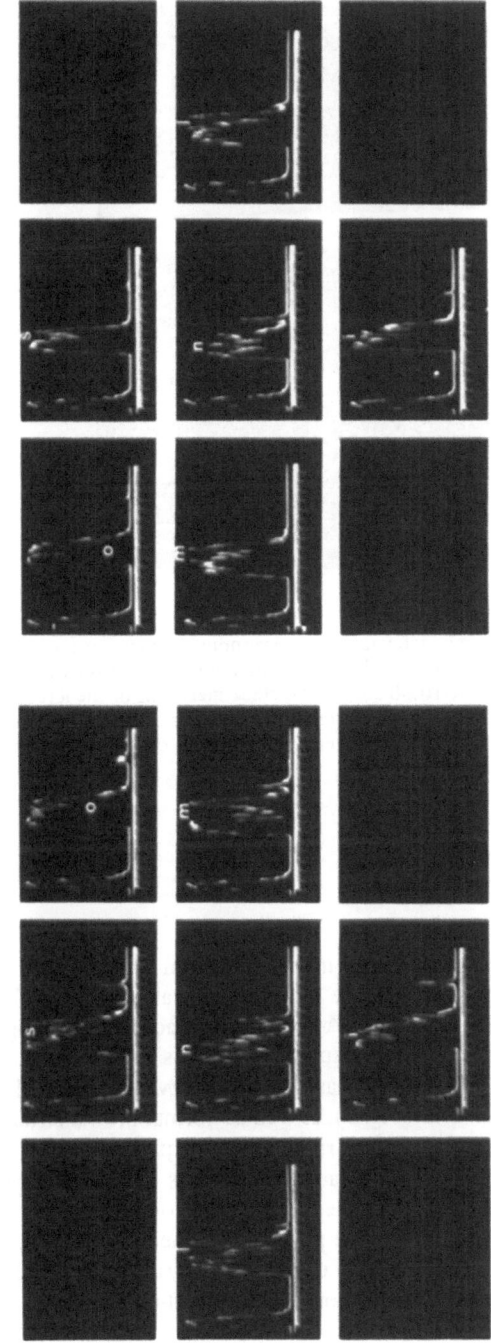

Fig. 6a. Documentation of maximal diameters of the optic nerve (n), the medial rectus (m), the lateral rectus (l), the superior rectus (s), and the inferior rectus (i) muscles, as well as the thickness of anterior superonasal orbital fat tissues (o), in right orbit of patient with right low-flow A-V fistula (congesting the orbit). Note the increase in size of all these structures as compared to left orbit (Fig. 6b).

Fig. 6b. Documentation of size of optic nerve and extraocular muscles as well as orbital fat tissues in left (normal) orbit of patient with right low-flow A-V fistula (compare with Fig. 6a). Note that the various structures are located in the figure as examiner sees them when looking at patient from the front.

289

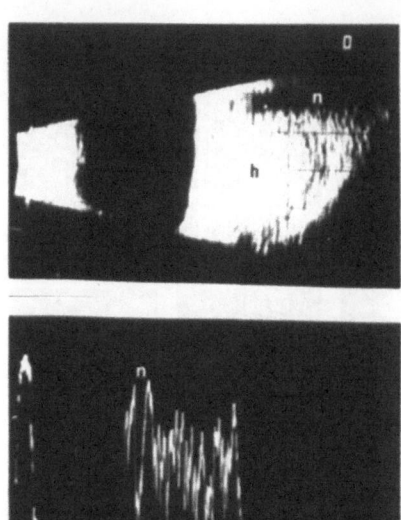

Fig. 7a. A-scan and B-scan echograms of cavernous hemangioma of the adult type showing the close spatial relationship of the tumor and optic nerve. The sagittal acoustic plane was aligned with the 10:00 and 4:00 o'clock meridians of the left orbit, indicating that the optic nerve was riding on the superonasal surface of the hemangioma. h hemangioma; n optic nerve; the upper end of the B-scan corresponds with the nasal end of the acoustic section.

the projection of the borders of a malignant tumor toward the surface of the skin can be very important for the optimal application of radiotherapy. One of the great assets of standardized A-scan and contact B-scan echography is its dynamic nature and 'real time' display that allows the direct observation of patho-physiological changes, such as the blood flow in abnormal vessels and the enlargement of a varix (Fig. 3), as well as normal orbital structures (optic nerve and extraocular muscles) during a Valsalva procedure, the thinning of the optic nerve or of the extraocular muscles during changes of gaze direction, the adherence of a lesion to the ocular wall, etc. Finally, standardized echography offers the possibility of being totally integrated into the opthalmological service, and is under full control of the ophthalmologist, who can use it in an optimal fashion tailored to the needs of each particular case.

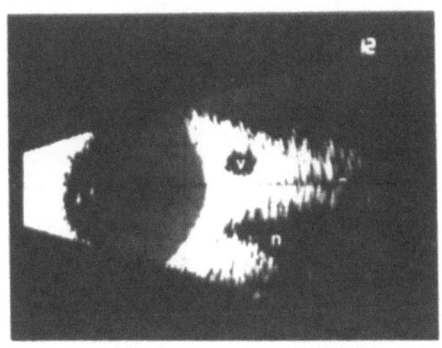

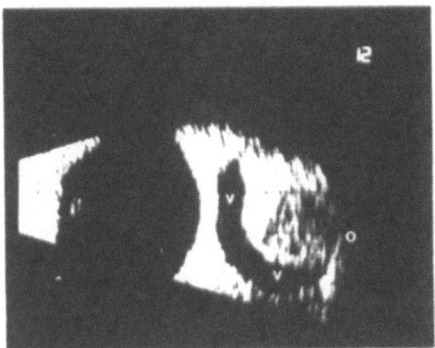

Fig. 7b. B-scan echograms of high-flow A-V Fistula of brain (draining through orbit) obtained along a vertical sagittal plane (top) and along a superior horizontal plane (bottom). v dilated superior ophthalmic vein; n optic nerve; o area of superior orbital fissure. The upper ends of the B-scans correspond with the superior (top pattern) and nasal (bottom echogram) ends of the acoustic planes.

Author's Address:
Dept. of Ophthalmology
University of Iowa
Iowa City, IA 55242 U.S.A.

COMPARISON OF
ECHOGRAPHIC AND COMPUTERTOMOGRAPHIC EXAMINATIONS IN ORBITAL DISEASES

K. BLUTH & J. PLANITZER

(Berlin, G.D.R.)

Echography of the orbit has become a routine method since Ossoinig's 1963 report on sucessful A-scan echography and Baum and Greenwood's earlier 1958 report on B-scan echography in the detection of orbital disease.

Computerized tomography which has been used in the GDR since 1979 is a relatively new method for investigating diagnosis of orbital diseases.

The aim of this work is to demonstrate and evaluate the reliability of echography and computerized tomography according to the results obtained in findings of orbital lesions and differentiation of tissue.

MATERIALS AND METHODS

Last year 75 patients with suspected orbital lesions were examined by echography and axial computerized tomography.

The ultrasound examinations were performed using the 7100 MA from Kretztechnik. In addition the Bronson-Turner apparatus was used for real-time scanning.

The computerized tomography was carried out with a body-scanner, the Somatom SD using 256 detectors and placed in the position used for orbit examinations. The density scale differed from -1000 (air) to $+1000$ (bone). The retrobulbar fat is represented by minus-units, whereas tumor tissue has density-units from 50 to 80 Hounsfield units. Verification of the diagnosis was obtained by comparing it with histological examinations follow-ups made up to now.

RESULTS

Orbital lesions were detected by ultrasonic examination in 69 cases. One case was false-negative. Five cases were tumor-negative, verified by the clinical follow-up.

The results obtained by computerized tomography were positive in findings of pathological orbital lesions in 65 cases. Five cases were false-negative.

Of the 70 cases suffering from orbital changes, 42 cases were verified by

Table 1. Results of detection of orbital lesions with echography and computertomography.

	Lesion	No lesion	Correct
Echography	69	1	99%
CT	65	5	93%
Both methods	70		100%

Table 2. Histological results of 42 cases of orbital tumors (70 cases examined).

Pseudotumor	8
Meningeoma	6
Lymphoma	5
Haemangioma	5
Metastasis	4
Mucoceles	2
Lymphangioma	2
Adenoma of lacrimal gland	2
Paraganglioma	1
Cholesteatoma	1
Boeck's sarcoid	1
Epidermiscyst	1
Neurofibroma	1
Lymphogranuloma	1
Wegner's granuloma	1

histopathological examination. There is no doubt that the reliability and accuracy of both methods together is nearly 100% in the detection of orbital lesions.

The task of tissue differentiation involves further difficulties. Both methods, ultrasonography and computerized tomography allow further differentiation of changes. Orbital lesions can be classified by ultrasonography — naturally dependent upon the equipment being used — into acoustic homogenous lesions with a solid or cystic character and inhomogenous lesions, e.g. metastatic tumors. In addition we distinguished inflammatory changes as endocrine exophthalmos. We tried to find some characteristic subdivisions for each of these categories, for tumors with a high number of cells or a certain cellulose density.

The reliability of computerized tomography consists in detection of exact location, size and shape, delineation from surrounding tissue and associated changes, and, of course, in analysis of density. The characterization of computertomographic criteria allows one to distinguish homogenous hypodense orbit tumors, as lipomas and homogenous hyperdense orbit tumors, as meningeomas, or as inhomogeneous changes. The contrast enhancement enables further differentiation, an increasing density was noticed in cases of metastatic lesions, haemangiomas and meningeomas. In contrast to this is lipomas which showed no reaction to the contrast enhancement. The radiation dose amounts to about 3 R/slice. The tissue differentiation was carried out with ultrasound in 24 cases, with computerized tomography in

294

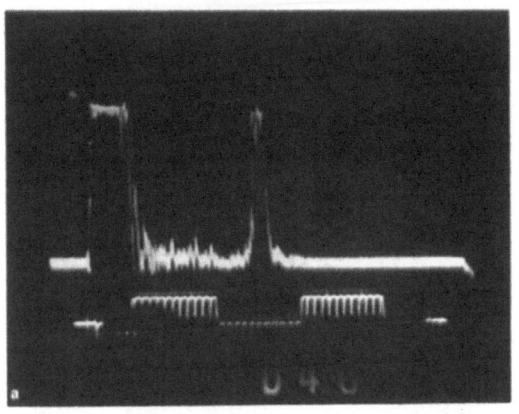

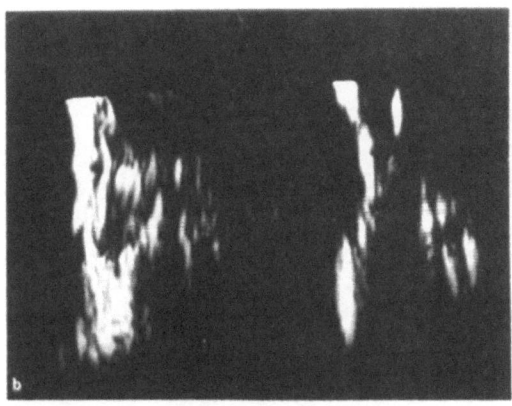

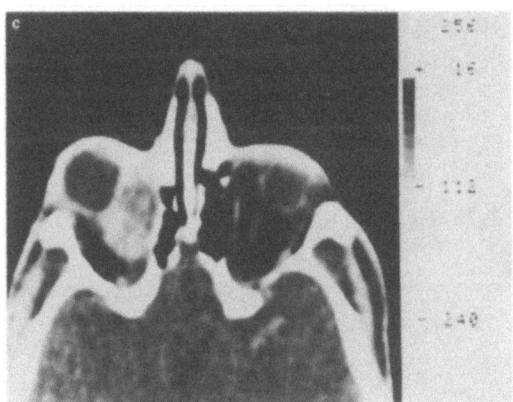

Fig. 1. A-scan, B-scan and CT of an orbital metastasis.

295

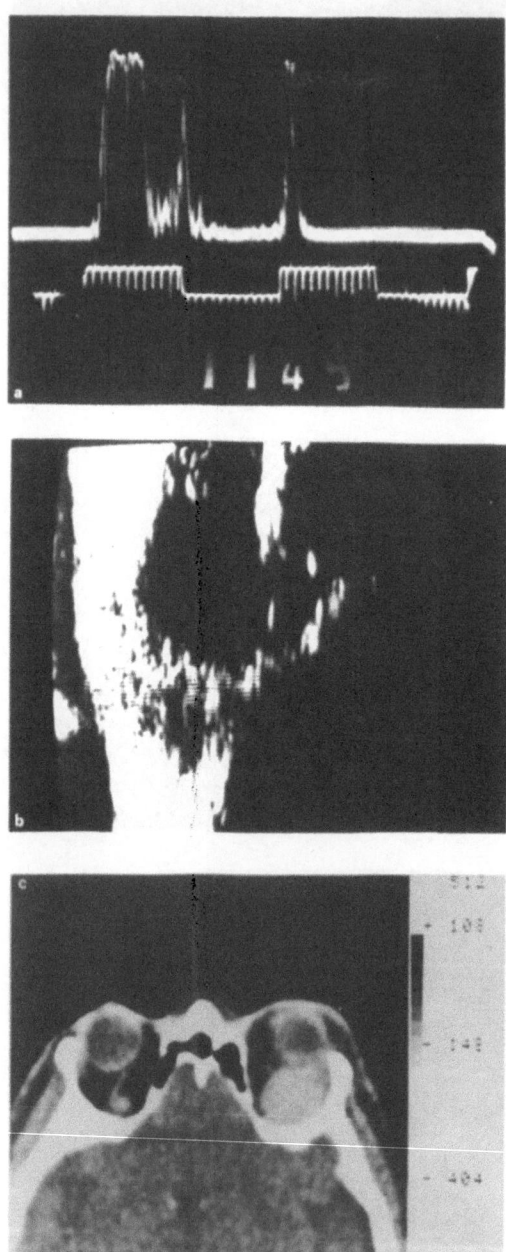

Fig. 2. A-scan, B-scan and CT of an lymphoma.

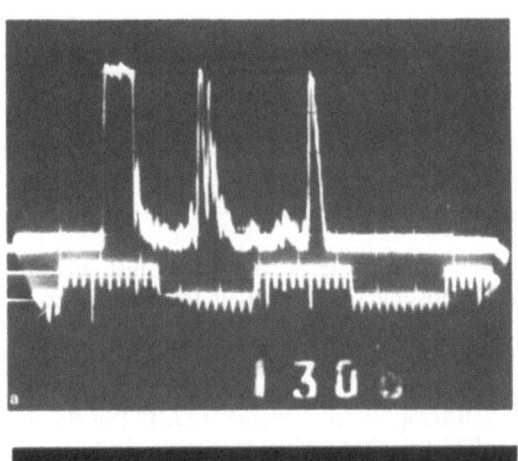

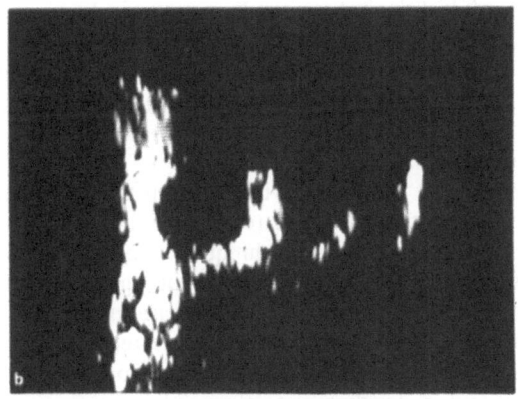

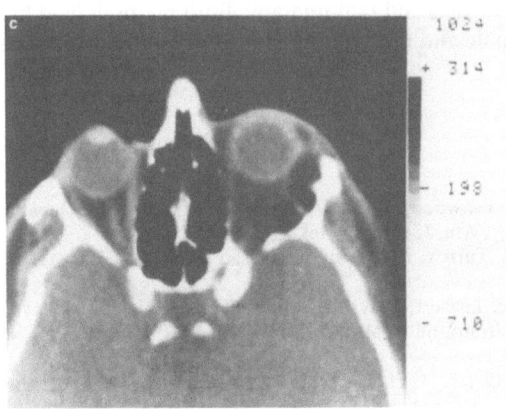

Fig. 3. A-scan, B-scan and CT of 2 dermoidcysts lateral.

Table 3. Results of echographic and computer-tomographic differential diagnosis (70 cases).

	Differentiation	
Echography	24	35%
CT	29	41%
Both methods	38 cases	56%

29 cases, in common 38 (= 56%), verified by histological examination or follow-up. It was impossible to differentiate the other 22 cases.

Critical analysis of the foregoing results shows the impossibility of exact differentiation between various types of similar tissue variations. Our average in echographic differentiation of tissue is below normal in comparison to other statistics (Ossoinig 1970, Gallenga 1972). The polymorphy alone in the few cases of histological diagnosis examined shows the difficulty of exact differentiation. In spite of this, both methods combined have improved the diagnosis of orbit lesions. Computerized tomography is especially helpful in detection of apical lesions and associated changes in the bony wall of the orbit. The results obtained prove the reliability of ultrasound demonstration in subtle tissue variations.

An improvement in the differentiation of soft tissue variations could be achieved above all by using standardized and optimized instrumentation (Ossoinig 1975), high resolutions techniques, improved gray scale, spectral-analysis and mechanical processing of ultrasound signals.

Orbital echography should be one of the basic means of examinations in diagnosis of orbital disorders. It should be preferred especially when dealing with children where damage due to radiation should be avoided wherever possible. It is useful in deciding upon the need and time of surgical therapy, for control of medical and radiotherapy. Both methods lend high level support to the topographic and morphological information of orbital changes.

REFERENCES

Baum, G. & Greenwood, I. The application of ultrasonic locating techniques to ophthalmology. Am. J. Ophthalmol. 46: 319 (1956).

Bronson, N.R. & Turner, F.T. A simple B-scan ultrasonoscope. Arch. Ophthalmol. 83: 18 (1977).

Buschmann, W. & Linnert, D. Visualization of orbital tissues using various echographic techniques. Ultrasound in Med. a. Biol., Vol. 2 (D.N. White, ed.) New York: Plenum (1976) p. 295.

Coleman, D.J., Lizzie, L.F. & Jack, R.L. Ultrasonography of the eye and orbit. Philadelphia: Lea & Febinger (1977).

Coleman, D.J. Reliability of ocular and orbital diagnosis with B-scan ultrasound. II. Orbital diagnosis. Am. J. Ophthalmol. 74(4): 704 (1972).

Gallenga, R. Ecografia dell'orbita. Arch. Rass. Ital. Ottal. 7: 81 (1972).

Nover, A. Schmitt, J., Wende, S. & Aulich, A. Computertomography in der Ophthalmology. Klin. Mbl. Augenheilk. 168: 461 (1976).

Nover, A., Schmitt, J. & Brodehl, D. Echographie und Computer-Tomographie bei Orbitaprozessen. Klin. Mbl. Augenheilk. 172: 187 (1978).

Purnell, E.W. Ultrasonic interpretation of orbital diseases. Proc. Int. Congr. Ultrasonography in Ophthalmol. St. Louis: Mosby (1968).

Ossoinig, K.C. A-scan echography and orbital disease In.: Proc. 2nd. Int. Symp. on Orbital Disorders. Med. Probl. Ophthalmol. 14: 203 (1975).

Ossoinig, K. & Till, P. Ten year study on clinical echography in orbital diseases. Ultrasonography in Ophthalmology, Bilbl. Ophthalmol. Basel: Karger (1975) p. 200.

Trier, H.G. Gewebsdifferenzierung mit Ultraschall. Bibl. Ophthalmol. No. 86, Basel: Karger (1977).

Author's Address:
Dept. of Ophthalmology (Dr. Bluth)
Dept. of Neurology (Charité) of the Humboldt University (Dr. Planitzer)
Berlin, G.D.R.

ECHOGRAPHY IN ORBITAL RHABDOMYOSARCOMA

R. ROCHELS & G. REIS

(Mainz, F.R.G.)

ABSTRACT

Report on the echographical findings in four children suffering from orbital rhabdomyosarcoma.

(A) Quantitative echography (A-scan):
 − irregular structure, poorly outlined borders
 − very low reflectivity, weak sound attenuation

(B) Kinetic echography (A- B-scan):
 − hard consistency
 − little mobility

(C) Topographic echography (A- B-scan):
 − no relation to the striated outer ocular muscles
 − localisation in the temporal-upper (2), temporal-lower (1), nasal-upper (1) quadrant of the orbit

(D) Tissue differentiation (A-scan):
 − no correlation between echographical findings and the histological type of rhabdomyosarcoma

(Published in great detail in Ophthalmologica, Basel 180: 274−276, 1980)

Author's Address:
University Eye Clinic
Langenbeckstrasse 1
D-65 Mainz, F.R.G.

COMBINATION OF ECHOGRAPHY WITH CORONAL CT
IN THE DIAGNOSIS OF ORBITAL DISORDERS

Y. NISHIMOTO, Y. BABA, H. SHIBATA & A. SAWADA
(Miyazaki, Japan)

Since the introduction of computerized tomography in 1972, many papers on the comparison of this newly developed technique of imaging with echography in the diagnosis of orbital disorders have been published.

The essentials in imaging of orbital disorders are anatomical localization and tissue differentiation of the lesion. On anatomical localization of orbital lesions, the results in axial computerized tomography have been tremendously successful, except that orbital lesions along the superior or inferior wall have sometimes been missed (Sawada & Cornell 1976).

Many authors have the opinion that both echography and computerized tomography should be used in combination in the diagnosis of orbital and periorbital lesions, because both of them have their own advantages. Bigar, *et al.* (1979) divided the orbit into three parts, and evaluated standardized A-scan echography and computerized tomography for the diagnosis of lesions in each part of the orbit. They advocated echography combined with conventional radiology as the first step. When these procedures found and differentiated a lesion in the anterior third of the orbit, computerized tomography was not necessary. When a lesion was found in the middle third of the orbit, computerized tomography was as desirable as echography. When a lesion was found within the apex of the orbit and extending into the adjacent structures, computerized tomography had a great advantage.

Recently coronal computerized tomography has been popularized (Grove, *et al.* 1978, Dallow, *et al.* 1978, Nishimoto, *et al.* to be published). Coronal computerized tomography is said to cover up faults of axial computerized tomography in displaying anatomical structures. It is the aim of the present paper to compare the usefulness of coronal computerized tomography and echography in 21 cases with various kinds of orbital lesions in Miyazaki Medical College Hospital.

The equipment used for coronal computerized tomography was the whole body scanner, CT/T-X-2 made by GE in USA. The equipment used for echography was Kretztechnik 7200 MA and Bronson-Turner Ophthalmic B-scan.

CASE REPORTS

The Twenty-one cases reported here were divided into several groups based on the location of the lesion (Table 1).

Table 1. Results of echography and computerized tomography in 21 cases of orbital disorders.

Case	Age and Sex	Diagnosis/Symptoms	Detection Echo.	CT	Differentiation Echo.	CT
1	36, M.	L. dermoid cyst	+	+	+	+
2	31, M.	R. malignant lymphoma	+	+	+	−
3	75, M.	L. pleomorphic adenoma	+	+	+	−
4	38, M.	R. inflammatory granuloma	+	+	+	−
5	69, W.	R. lymphoid pseudotumor	+	+	+	−
6	67, M.	L. lymphoid pseudotumor	+	+	+	−
7	55, W.	L. mucocele	+	+	+	+
8	51, W.	B. mucocele	+	+	+	+
9	16, M.	R. hematoma	+	+	+	+
10	14, W.	L. blow-out fracture	+	+	+	+
11	54, W.	B. orbital myositis	+	+	+	+
12	75, W.	R. orbital myositis	+	+	+	+
13	62, M.	R. orbital myositis	+	+	+	+
14	56, W.	L. orbital myositis	+	+	+	+
15	52, M.	R. squamous cell carcinoma	+	+	+	+
16	43, M.	L. hyperthyroidism	+	+	+	+
17	54, M.	L. exophthalmos	−	−		
18	50, M.	B. exophthalmos	−	−		
19	49, M.	L. blepharoptosis	−	−		
20	77, W.	L. superior orbital fissure syndrome	−	−		
21	6, M.	L. traumatic disorder of ocular motility	−	−		
		total +	16	16	16	11
		−	5	5	0	5

Anterior Third of the Orbit

Lesions located in the anterior part of the orbit were dermoid cyst and metastatic malignant lymphoma in the orbital rim.

Case 1: The patient with dermoid cyst was a 36-year-old man. Since childhood, a small lump had existed under the medial part of the left upper lid. After the lump was accidently struck three weeks prior to consultation, it increased in size. A small soft tumor was palpable on the upper medial rim of the left orbit. Inward movement of the left eye was slightly impaired. Otherwise, no abnormality was found. In A-scan echography with water bath, the lesion was sharply outlined with a distinct wall structure and was obviously hard. The inner reflectivity was extremely low (Fig. 1). It was pathognomonic for dermoid cyst. Axial computerized tomography showed a round, very low density area anterior and medial to the eye ball surrounded by a capsule-like structure. Coronal computerized tomography showed clearly that the low density area was not connected to the bony wall of the orbit and the paranasal cavity (Fig. 2). The tumor was histopathologically dermoid cyst.

Case 2: Another case with the lesion in the anterior part of the orbit was a metastatic malignant lymphoma in the upper medial rim of the right orbit in

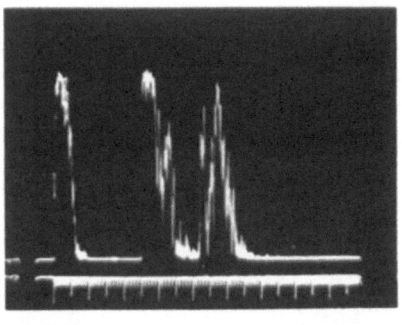

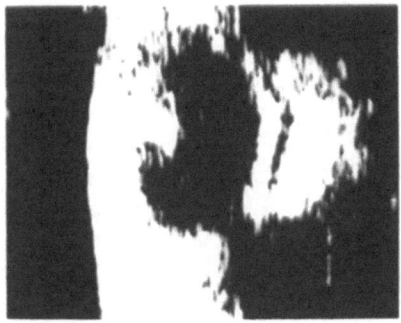

Fig. 1. A- and B-scan echography of dermoid cyst (Case 1).

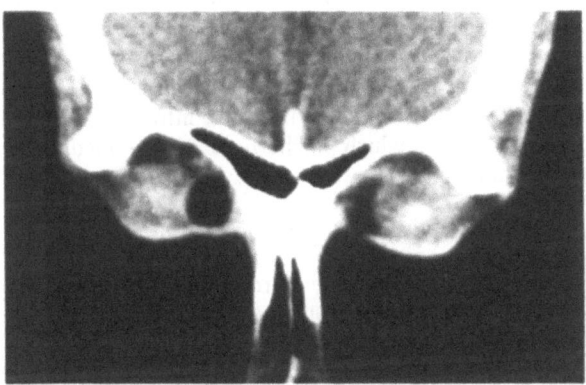

Fig. 2. Coronal CT of dermoid cyst (Case 1).

a 31-year-old man. One year before consultation a malignant lymphoma in the right frontal and temporal area extending into the cranial cavity had been surgically removed. A-scan echography showed that the new tumor was located in the anterior part of the orbit and that inner reflectivity was medium or high (Fig. 3). It was not consistent with lymphoma/sarcoma/ pseudotumor group. Axial computerized tomography showed a relatively

303

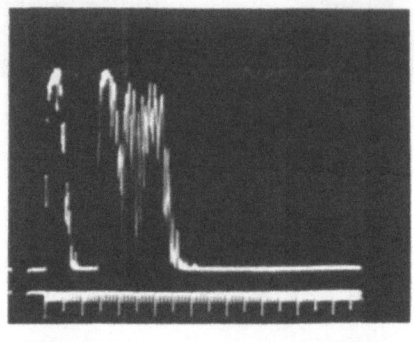

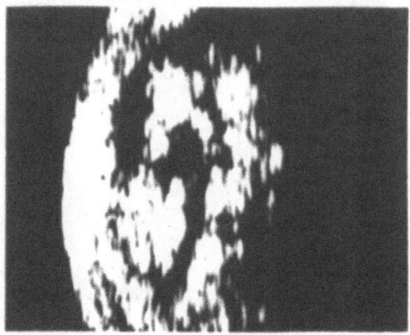

Fig. 3. A- and B-scan echography of metastatic malignant lymphoma (Case 2).

sharply outlined, high density mass located superomedial to the eye ball in the section slightly above the optic nerve. Coronal computerized tomography showed a flat high density area located superomedial to the eye ball. Invasion to the orbital wall was not seen. The tumor was histopathologically malignant lymphoma (Fig. 4). Tumor cells infiltrated into adipose tissues forming a small net-like structure, which might have caused medium or high inner reflectivity in echography.

Middle Third of the Orbit

Lesions were found in the middle third of the orbit in 12 out of 21 cases. These cases were made up as follows: pleomorphic adenoma (1), inflammatory granuloma (1), lymphoid pseudotumor (2), mucocele (2), orbital hemorrhage (1), muscle hypertrophy (4) and orbital wall fracture (1).

Case 3: A 75-year-old man noticed diplopia and protrusion of the left eye two months before the consultation. The left eye protruded by 5 mm compared with the right eye. Movement of the left eye was moderately restricted upward and laterally, and slightly restricted medially and downward. The optic disc was slightly blurred and the choroidal folds were seen superolateral to the optic disc. In A-scan echography a sharply outlined lesion with medium inner reflectivity and mixed high and low spikes was found superolateral to the left eye ball. The echographic finding suggested a mixed

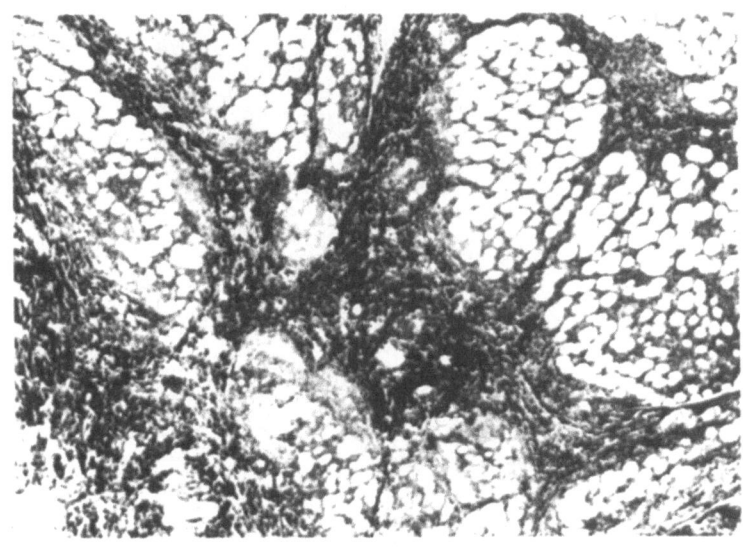

Fig. 4. Histopathological section of metastatic malignant lymphoma (Case 2).

tumor of rich tubular structure (Fig. 5). Axial computerized tomography showed that the left eye ball was pushed anteriorly, and that a sharply outlined mass with relatively high density (CT number: 34.6) was located behind the eye ball, extending laterally (Fig. 6A). Coronal computerized tomography showed that the mass was above the eye ball, pushing it downward. However, invasion of the mass to the orbital wall was not found (Fig. 6B). Histopathologically the lesion was pleomorphic adenoma (Fig. 7). Irregularity of cell arrangement and abundance of interfaces produced a peculiar finding on the A-scan echogram.

Of the 12 cases with the lesion in the middle third of the orbit, three cases were inflammatory pseudotumor.

Case 4: A 38-year-old man noticed protrusion of the right eye. One year earlier he had been operated on for inflammatory granuloma in the right frontal and ethmoidal sinuses. The tumor had extended into the orbit. At the present consultation the right eye protruded by 2.5 mm compared with the left eye. Movement of the right eye was slightly restricted in all directions. The optic disc was slightly pale and retinochoroidal degeneration around the optic disc was seen. In A-scan echography bone defect was seen and inner reflectivity was low. The finding was consistent with lymphoma/sarcoma/pseudotumor group. Axial computerized tomography showed that a high density mass occupied totally the medial part of the orbit and extended into the ethomidal sinus. Although the contour of the medial wall of the orbit was relatively clearly kept, the invasion of the mass into the nasal cavity was seen. In coronal computerized tomography at a level slightly posterior to the eye ball, a high density mass was seen in the medial part of the orbit, with a part of the mass extending into the ethmoidal and maxillary sinuses. The mass was

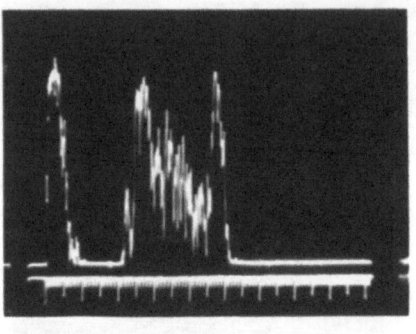

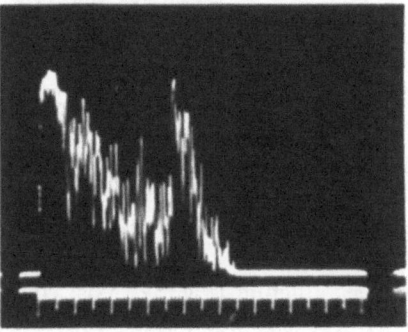

Fig. 5. A-scan echography of pleomorphic adenoma (Case 3).

not enhanced with contrast agent. The lesion was suspected to be inflammatory granuloma of the same type as that previously removed. Systemic corticosteroid and local irradiation were given.

Case 5: Two years prior to consultation, a 69-year-old woman noticed swelling of the right lower lid and was operated on for a small tumor. Shortly before consultation the right eye began to protrude. At consultation it protruded by 6 mm compared with the left eye, and was turned laterally. Movement was moderately limited in all directions. A- and B-scan echography showed a regular and well-outlined lesion with low inner reflectivity. The echographic finding was consistent with lymphoma/sarcoma/pseudotumor group (Fig. 8). In axial computerized tomography at a level slightly below the optic nerve, a high density mass (CT number: 54.0) was found behind the eye ball, extending laterally (Fig. 9A). In coronal computerized tomography the mass extended inferiorly and laterally, and reached to the inferior wall of the orbit. The bone was not destroyed (Fig. 9B). The CT number was increased up to 82.6 with contrast enhancement. The lesion was removed surgically and proved histopathologically to be lymphoid pseudotumor.

Another case of lymphoid pseudotumor was seen in a 67-year-old man. With A-scan echography the localization and tissue differentiation was available. Axial and coronal computerized tomography could demonstrate the location but could not differentiate the lesion.

306

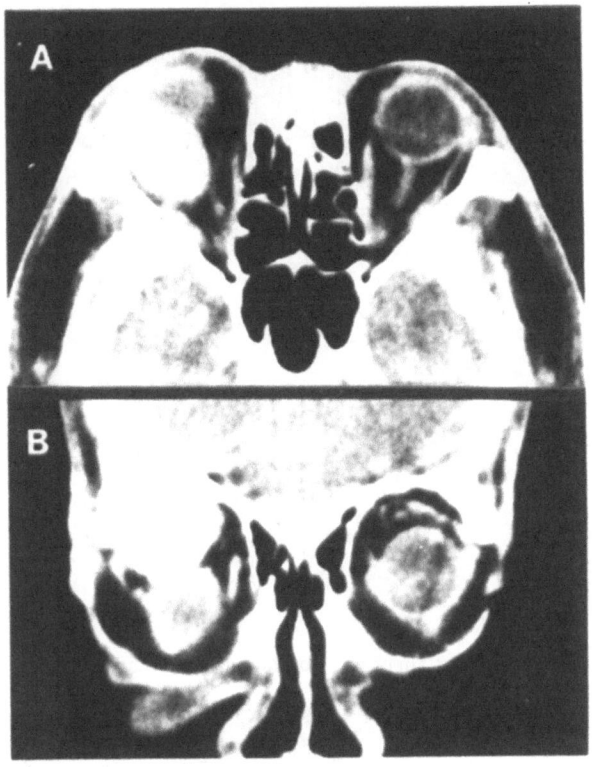

Fig. 6. Axial (A) and coronal (B) CT of pleomorphic adenoma (Case 3).

Case 7: A 55-year-old woman felt a painful lump in the superior area of the left orbit for three months before consultation. During this time the lump gradually increased in size and diplopia was noticed. At consultation, the left upper lid was hanging down slightly. Eye movement was limited upward and medially. The left eye protruded by 2 mm compared with the right eye. A hard tumor along the superomedial rim of the orbit was palpated. A- and B-scan echography revealed a well-outlined tumor with extremely low inner reflectivity (Fig. 10). Bone defect was demonstrated. The echographic finding was pathognomonic for mucocele. Axial computerized tomography showed that an encapsulated soft mass (CT number: 21.6) was located along the orbital wall, partly extending into the nasal cavity. Coronal computerized tomography revealed that the tumor had a strong relation with the ethmoidal sinus. The density within the capsule was barely enhanced with the contrast agent (Fig. 11). At the operation the diagnosis of mucocele was established.

Another case of mucocele was seen in a 51-year-old woman. With A-scan echography the localization and tissue differentiation were available. Axial and coronal computerized tomography could demonstrate the location and differentiate the lesion.

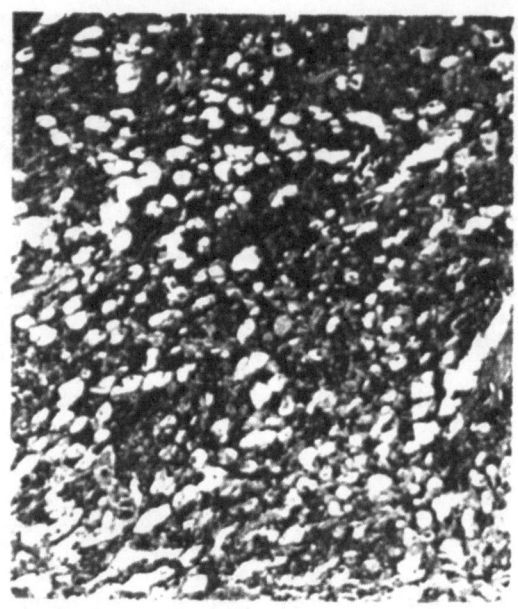

Fig. 7. Histopathological section of pleomorphic adenoma (Case 3).

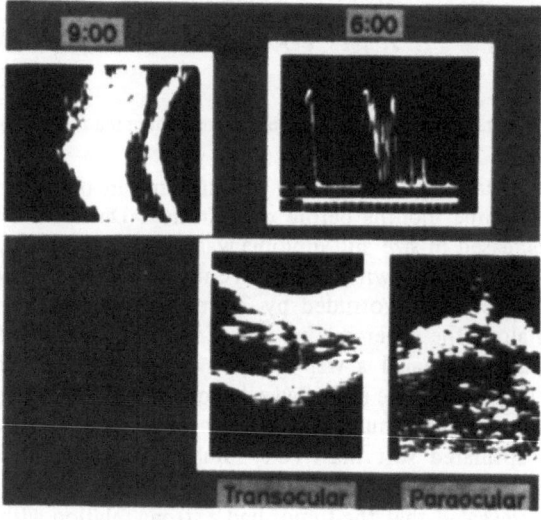

Fig. 8. A- and B-scan echography of lymphoid pseudotumor (Case 5).

Case 9: A 16-year-old boy was struck in the right eye one week prior to consultation. Two days after the accident the right eye began to be pushed out. At consultation the right eye was pushed forward by 8 mm compared with the left eye. Upward movement was strongly limited. With the forced duction test strong resistance was found. In A- and B-scan echography,

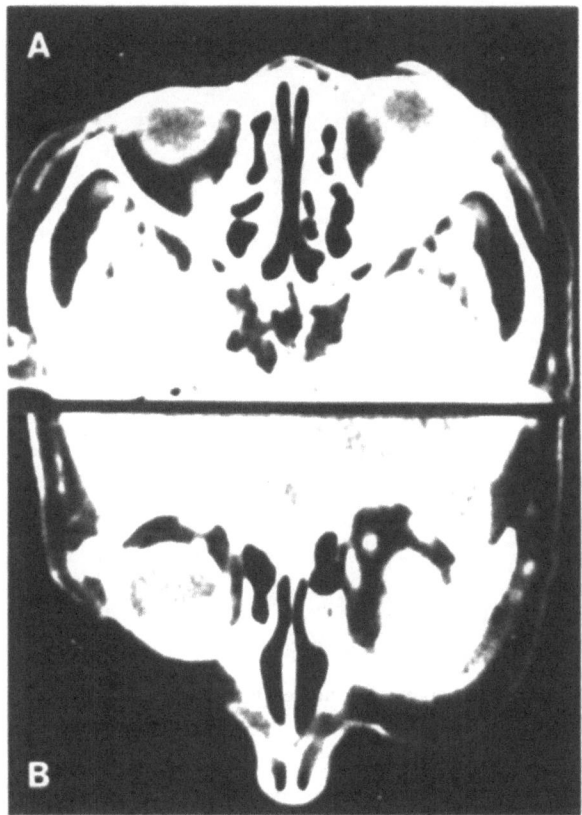

Fig. 9. Axial (A) and coronal (B) CT of lymphoid pseudotumor (Case 5).

a well-outlined lesion with medium inner reflectivity (60%) was found in the area between the posterior wall of the eye and the orbital wall. Thickness of the lesion was 13.5 mm (Fig. 12). Axial computerized tomography showed a homogeneous high density mass (CT number: 70.7) occupying almost the whole of the right orbit (Fig. 13A). Coronal computerized tomography showed a high density mass above the right eye ball, stretching backward and pushing the eye ball downward (Fig. 13B). One week later, A-scan echography showed that thickness of the lesion was markedly reduced to 7 mm. Inner reflectivity became low (15%) (Fig. 14). In computerized tomography the mass was shown to be decreased in size. Based on the history of trauma, sudden onset and rapid reduction of the size and inner reflectivity, a hematoma was highly suspected.

Case 10: A 14-year-old girl was struck in the left eye one week prior to consultation. After that the left eye was turned laterally and diplopia was noticed. Inward movement of the left eye was strongly limited. Upward and lateral movements were moderately limited. With the forced duction test

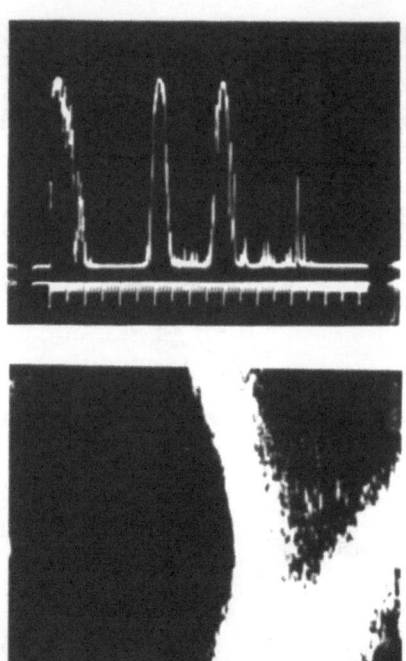

Fig. 10. A- and B-scan echography of mucocele (Case 7).

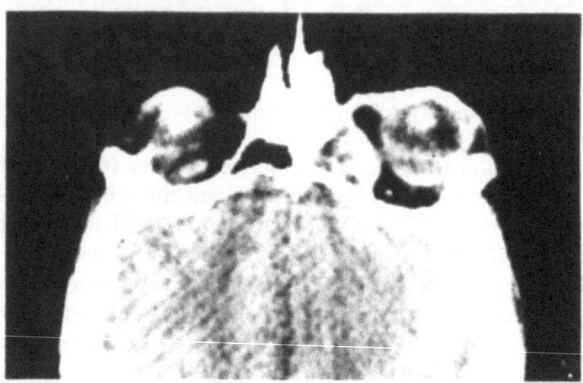

Fig. 11. Coronal CT of mucocele (Case 7).

strong resistance in the horizontal direction was found. Vertical movement was moderately resisted. A-scan echography revealed destruction of the medial wall of the orbit. Axial computerized tomography at the level of the optic nerve showed a high density mass within the ethmoidal sinus connecting to the medial wall of the orbit (Fig. 15A). In coronal computerized tomography in the section just behind the eye ball, a high density mass protruding from the inside of the orbit into the ethmoidal sinus was shown.

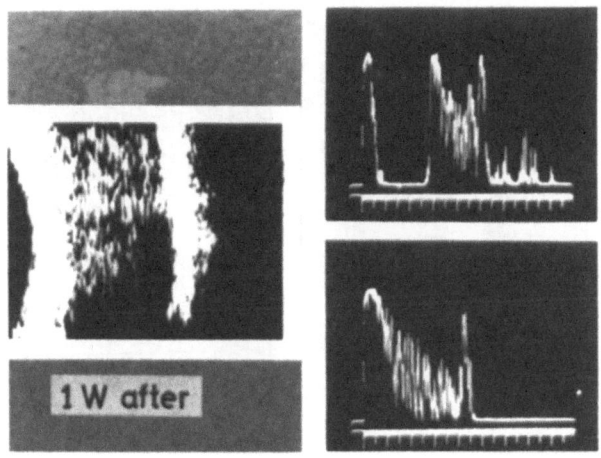

Fig. 12. B- and A-scan echography of orbital hematoma one week after trauma (Case 9).

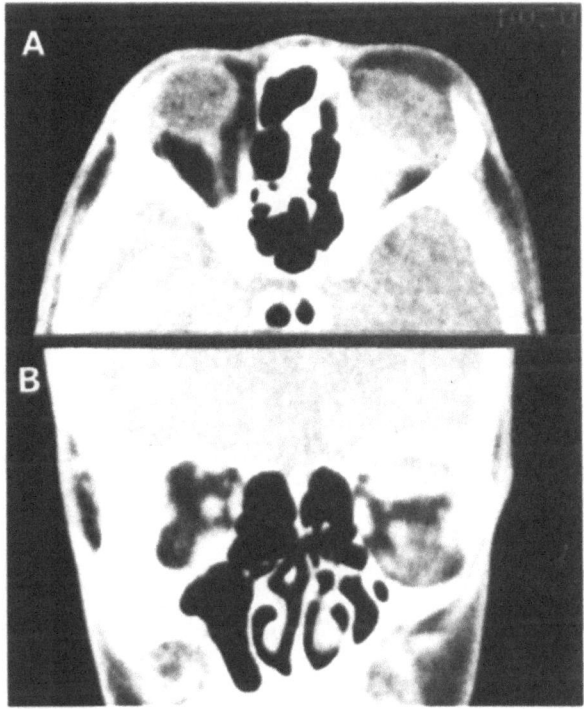

Fig. 13. Axial (A) and coronal (B) CT of orbital hematoma (Case 9).

The optic nerve was slightly shifted medially. The medial rectus muscle was not seen in the orbital cavity and was incarcerated into the ethmoidal sinus (Fig. 15B). In such a case, computerized tomography, particularly coronal, was very useful in demonstrating incarceration of horizontal extraocular muscles.

311

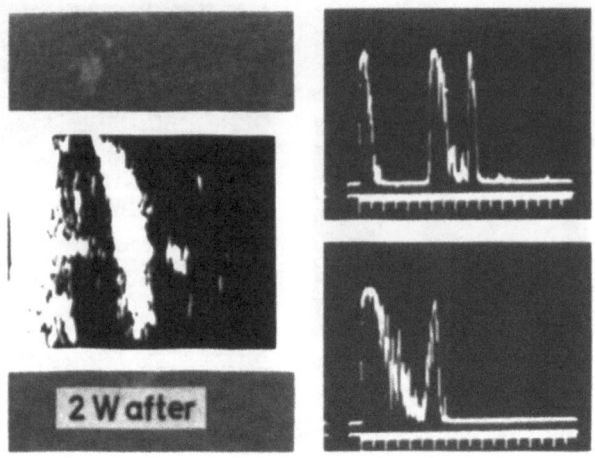

Fig. 14. B- and A-scan echography of orbital hematoma two weeks after trauma (Case 9).

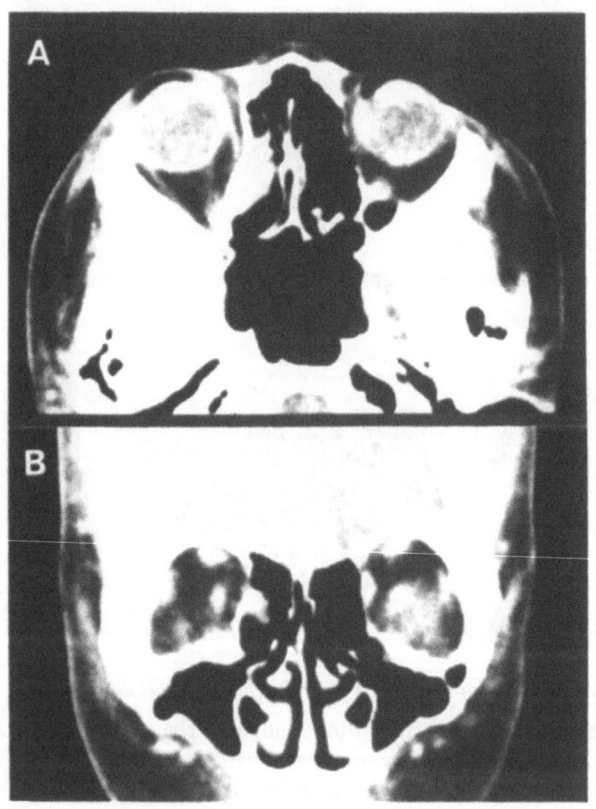

Fig. 15. Axial (A) and coronal (B) CT of blow-out fracture (Case 10).

In the 12 cases with the lesion in the middle third of the orbit, four cases with muscle hypertrophy were included. All of them were orbital myositis without thyroid dysfunction. Details of these cases were presented in another paper (Shibata *et al.* to be published).

Posterior Third of the Orbit

Two cases were included in the present study, in which the lesion was located from the middle to the posterior third of the orbit.

Case 15: A 52-year-old man noticed swelling and pain in the right lower lid and protrusion of the right eye. The right eye protruded by 6 mm compared with the left eye. Lateral eye movement was moderately limited. The lower lid and the buccal area on the right side was swollen. A-scan echography revealed that a lesion of irregular acoustic structure was located in the lower half of the right orbit (Fig. 16), and the bone of the medial and inferior wall of the orbit was destroyed. Axial computerized tomography showed that the right orbit was totally occupied except for the temporal part, by a high density mass, which was not enhanced with contrast agent. The medial wall of the orbit was completely destroyed and the nasal cavity and the ethmoidal sinus on the right side were occupied with the mass which was continuous to the mass in the orbit (Fig. 17A). Coronal computerized tomography showed that the optic nerve, and medial and inferior rectus muscles were pushed

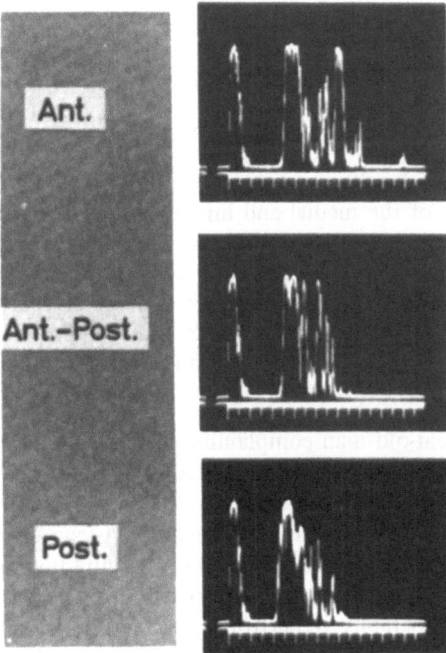

Fig. 16. A-scan echography in Case 15.

313

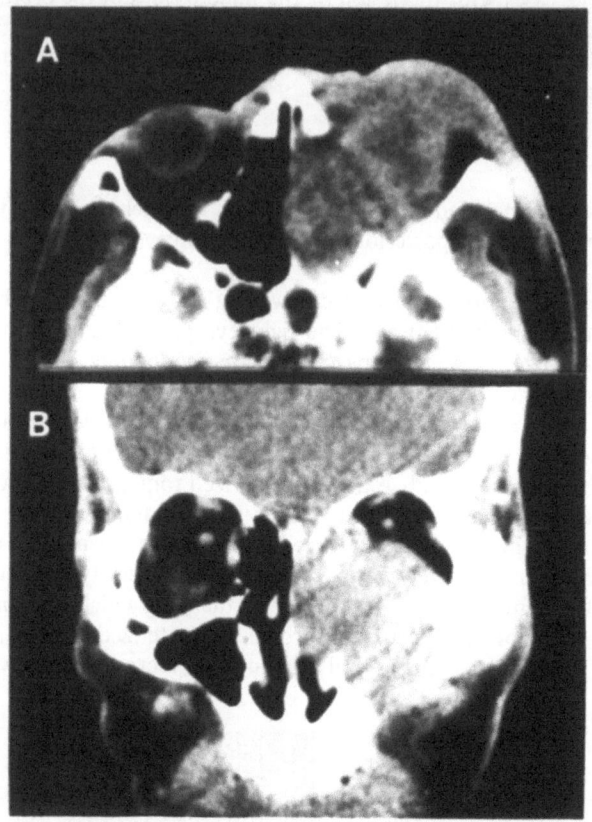

Fig. 17. Axial (A) and coronal (B) CT in Case 15.

upward by a high density mass occupying the lower half of the right orbit. Wide destruction of the medial and inferior wall of the orbit, and invasion of the mass to the nasal cavity, the ethmoidal and maxillary sinuses were clearly demonstrated (Fig. 17B). The specimen at biopsy from the nasal cavity was diagnosed to be squamous cell carcinoma. Irregular acoustic structures and irregular inner reflectivity, often low is characteristic of periorbital malignancies (Ossoinig & Till 1975). This might explain the finding in A-scan echography.

Case 16: A 43-year-old man complaining of slight protrusion of the left eye was examined. At consultation the left eye was found to be pushed forward by 2.5 mm compared with the right eye. Movement was slightly limited in all directions. Visual function was not impaired. A-scan echography suggested abnormality in the rectus muscles, although definite findings were not clearly shown, possibly due to the lesion's far posterior location. In axial and coronal computerized tomography hypertrophy of the inferior rectus muscle in the left eye was found. After systemic survey primary hyperfunction of the thyroid gland of slight or moderate degree was proved.

314

In the remaining five cases, no abnormality was found by echography nor by computerized tomography. These cases were exophthalmos (2), blepharoptosis (1), superior orbital fissure syndrome (1) and traumatic disorder of ocular motility (1).

SUMMARY

Results of detection and differentiation with echography and computerized tomography (axial and coronal) in 21 cases of orbital disorders are summarized in Table 1.

In 16 out of 21 cases, some abnormality was found by echography as well as by computerized tomography. It should be noted that coronal computerized tomography was always combined with axial computerized tomography in the present study. When axial and coronal computerized tomography were done in combination, the efficiency in detecting abnormality in the orbit was quite equal to that of echography, because lesions along or within the superior or inferior wall of the orbit, which had sometimes been missed in axial computerized tomography, was clearly demonstrated in coronal computerized tomography.

Concerning to tissue differentiation, echography, particularly A-scan echography was definitely superior to computerized tomography.

REFERENCES

Ambrose, J. Computerized transverse axial scanning (tomography) 2. Clinical application. Br. J. Radiol. 46: 1023 (1973).

Bigar, F., Spiess, H. & Gruber, H.U. Kombinierte Anwendung der Computertomographie und Echographie in der Ophthalmologie. Klin. Mbl. Augenheilk. 174: 806 (1979).

Buschmann, W. & Linnert, D. Zusammenwirken von Ultraschalldiagnostik und Röntgen-Computertomographie bei raumfordernden Orbitaprozessen. Klin. Mbl. Augenheilk. 173: 155 (1978).

Buschmann, W., Linnert, D., von Rostkron, G. & Haigts, W. Indikationsstellung für echographische und röntgenologische Untersuchungsverfahren in der Ophthalmologie. Ber. Dtsch. Ophthalmol. 76: 85 (1979).

Dallow, R.L., Momose, K.J., Weber, A.L. & Wray, S.H. Comparison of ultrasonography, computerized tomography (Emi scan), and radiographic techniques in evaluation of exophthalmos. Trans. Am. Acad. Ophthalmol. and Otolaryng. 81: OP-305 (1976).

Dallow, R.L. & Weber, A.L. Combined ultrasonography, computerized tomography, and radiology in evaluation of orbital disease. Proc. of the 3rd Int. Symp. Orbital Disorders, Amsterdam 1977. The Hague: Dr. W. Junk bv Publishers (1978) p. 15.

Fledelius, H.C. & Gylensted, C. Ultrasonography and computer tomography in orbital diagnosis with special reference to dysthyroid ophthalmopathy. Acta Ophthalmol. 56: 751 (1978).

Grove, A.S., Tadmor, R., New, P.F.J. & Momose, K.J. Orbital fracture evaluation by coronal computed tomography. Am. J. Ophthalmol. 85: 679 (1978).

Hodes, B.L. & Weinberg. P. A combined approach for the diagnosis of orbital disease. A.M.A. Arch. Ophthalmol. 95: 781 (1977).

Kaneko, A., Hiroe, Y. & Inoue, H. Comparison of ultrasonography and computerized tomography in ophthalmology. Rinsho Ganka 31: 119 (1977).

Nishimoto, Y., Shibata, H., Ishii, F., Sawada, A., & Fujimoto, T. Coronal CT of orbital disorders. Folia Ophthalmol. Jpn. (to be published).

Nover, A., Schmitt, J. & Brodehl, D. Echographie und Computertomographie bei Orbita-prozessen. Klin. Mbl. Augenheilk. 172: 187 (1978).

Ossoinig, K.C. & Till, P. Ten-Year Study on clinical echography in orbital disease. Ultra-sonography in ophthalmology Basel: S. Karger (1975) p. 200.

Ossoinig, K.C. Echographie und Computer-Tomographie in der Diagnostik orbitaler und periorbitaler Läsionen. Ber. Dtsch. Ophthalmol. Ges. 76: 59 (1979).

Sawada, A. & Cornell, H. Computerized tomography compared with A-scan echography in detection of orbital disorders (preliminary report). Acta Soc. Ophthalmol. Jpn. 80: 1090 (1976).

Shibata, H., Masuyama, Y., Nishimoto, Y. & Sawada, A. Echography in orbital myositis. (to be published).

Wright, J.E., Lloyd, G.A.S. & Ambrose, J. Computerized axial tomography in the detection of orbital space-occupying lesions. Am. J. Ophthalmol. 80: 78 (1975).

Authors' Address:
Department of Ophthalmology
Miyazaki Medical College
Kihara, Kiyotake, Miyazaki 889-16
Japan

ECHOGRAPHY IN UNUSUAL ORBITAL COMPLICATIONS OF PARASINUSAL DISEASES

W. HAUFF & P. TILL

(Vienna, Austria)

With the help of standardized echography the acoustic differentiation of abscesses from other echographically similar lesions such as hematomas or lymphomas/sarcomas/pseudotumors usually does not present great difficulties. The history of (1) acute orbital cellulitis (2) the presence of inflammatory signs and pain as well as (3) the evidence of a periorbital sinusitis is usually reason enough to suggest that the low to medium reflective circumscribed, poorly outlined lesion is an abscess. The evaluation of the consistency of abscesses and its changes during a following period naturally do not represent important diagnostic help. A decrease in reflectivity and an improvement of the demarcation of the lesion during the follow-up period, however, are helpful (Ossoinig 1977–1978, 1979).

CASE REPORTS

Case 1

In one patient the absence of inflammatory signs and pain – with sudden onset of hematoma of the lids, proptosis within minutes and secondary glaucoma (Fig. 1) – made the echographic differentiation difficult. A-scan echography detected a large, poorly outlined mass lesion with low to medium reflectivity (Fig. 2) in this healthy 50-year-old male. It was diagnosed as circumscribed, spontaneous orbital hematoma. Echographically no defect in the bony orbital wall was found. During the following period of twenty-four hours consistency and reflectivity decreased, as in hematomas. Because of the therapy–resistent acute glaucoma, a transfrontal decompression of the orbit in the neuro-surgical department was performed. During operation we discovered an empyema of the frontal sinus, which had broken into the orbit. Clinical signs of hematoma of the lids and the sudden onset of the proptosis in this healthy male who had no history of sinusitis were the main reasons for the echographic diagnosis of 'hematoma'.

Case 2

An 11-year-old boy developed a painless swelling of the upper lid and increasing proptosis of the right eye within a week. He had no fever and there

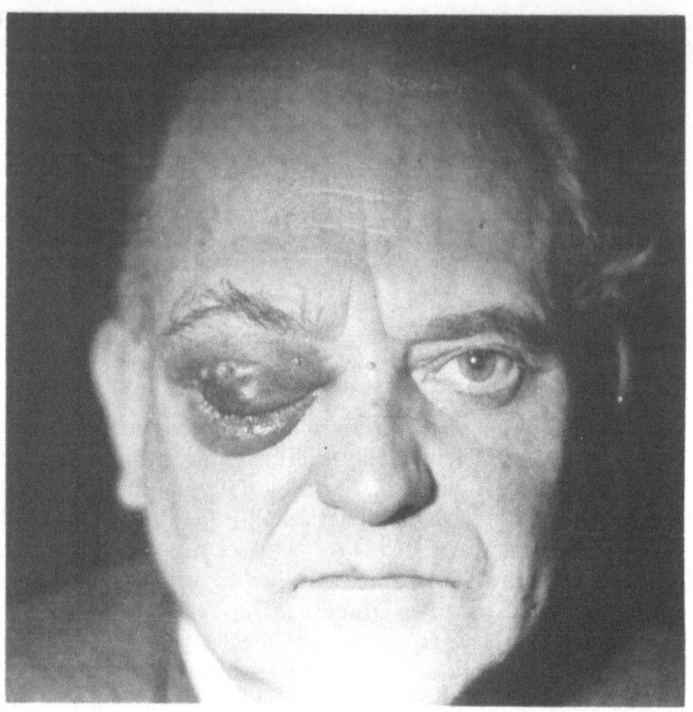

Fig. 1. 50-year-old, healthy male with sudden onset of lid hematoma, proptosis, and secundary acute glaucoma of the right eye.

were no signs of inflammation. A-scan echography showed a circumscribed, poorly outlined, low reflective lesion in the nasal retrobulbar region of the right orbit (Fig. 3) and a large bone defect in the nasal posterior orbital wall. X-ray and rhinological examinations revealed a purulent pansinusitis. Because of these findings the echographically detected orbital mass lesion was distinguished as an abscess. This was confirmed by the fact that local and general treatment with antibiotics healed the sinusitis and the orbital abscess disappeared (echographically proved). The primary cause of the sinusitis was a throat-nose fibroma, which extended into the ethmoidal sinuses; CT gave reason to suspect this fact. Two weeks later it was confirmed by rhinological operation. The histological section showed a fibroma with cystic regressive transformation. This case demonstrates that it is possible to differentiate an orbital abscess with A-scan echography in spite of the absence of local or general inflammatory signs.

Case 3

A 38-year-old female suffering from an antibody deficiency-syndrom noticed a swelling of the right upper lid without inflammatory signs; ten days later she complained of intermittend diplopia and came to our eye-department. At

318

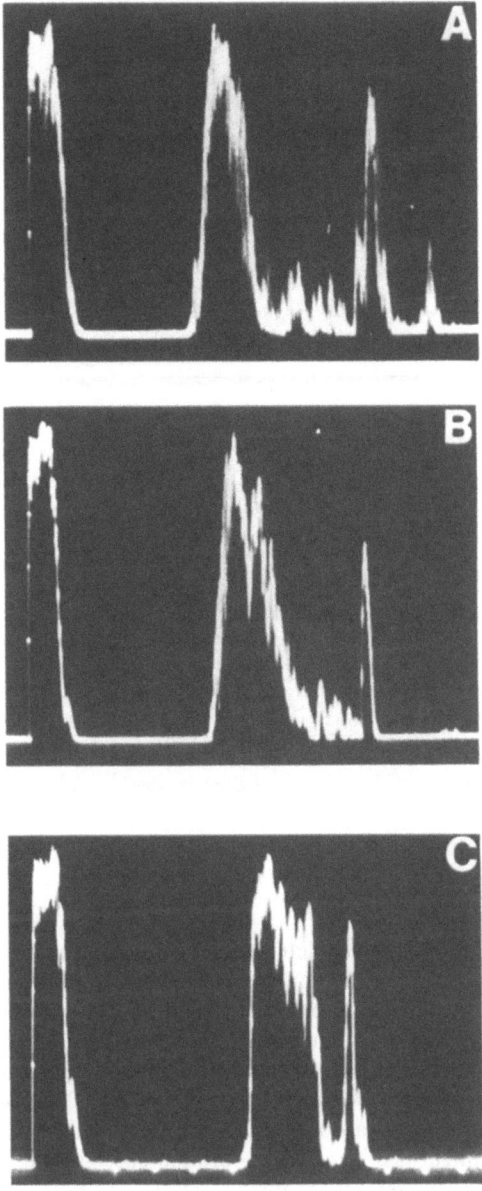

Fig. 2. Transocular A-scan echograms of low reflective, circumscribed and poorly outlined lesion of the right orbit (A) Decrease of consistency, size and reflectivity within 24 h (B) and small residuum three weeks after operation. (C) Examination was performed (1971) with Kretz-unit 7000.

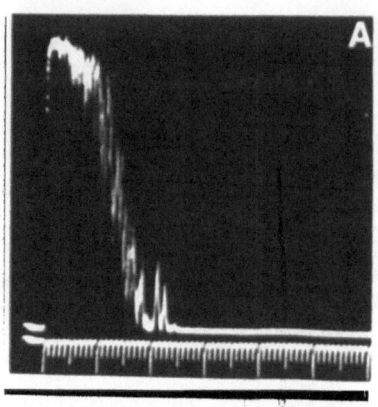

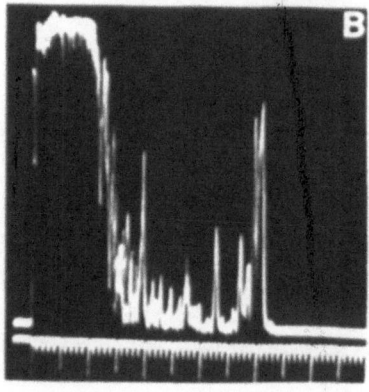

Fig. 3. Paraocular A-scan echograms of a 11-year-old boy with throat-nose fibroma:
A : normal orbit.
B : orbital abscess.

this time A-scan echography detected pathological penetrance through the orbital bony wall in the direction of the parasinuses. X-ray examination confirmed the echographic diagnosis of pansinusitis. In spite of treatment with antibiotics and antibody-concentrates by the intern department, the fevered patient now developed signs of inflammation of the lids, increasing proptosis with manifest diplopia and edema of the optic disc. A-scan echography now detected a poorly outlined, low reflective orbital mass lesion, which was distinguished as a large orbital abscess (Fig. 4A). Additional general therapy with steroids for three weeks healed the orbital inflammation and the orbital abscess disappeared (Fig. 4B & C). Up now there have been no complaints from the patient or relapses.

Clinical A-scan echography of the orbit is an important aid in identifying unusual orbital complications of parasinusal diseases when even clinical symptoms are absent. The standardized A-scan unit 7200 MA (Kretztechnik) can be applied under almost any circumstances: in the clinic, the operating-room or at patient's bedside. The use of echography is limited neither by the patient's age nor his general health.

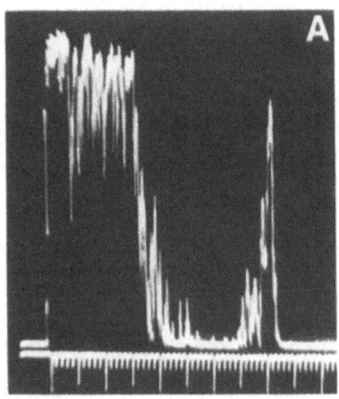

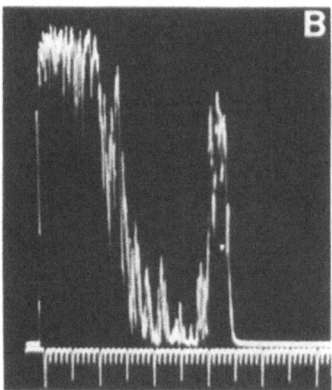

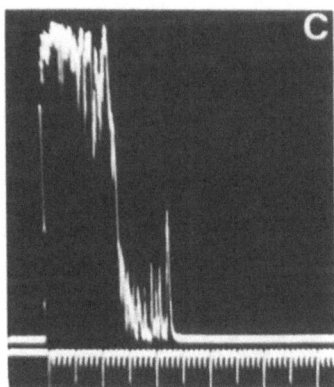

Fig. 4. Paraocular A-scan echograms of a 38-year old female with antibody deficiency-syndrome:

A: orbital abscess at the beginning of inflammatory lid signs.

B: decrease of size two weeks after beginning with steroid therapy.

C: small residuum of the abscess three weeks later.

REFERENCES

Ossoinig, K.C. Echography of Orbital Disorders. In: Clinical Handbook of Ultrasound (M. de Vlieger, ed.) New York: Wiley (1978) p. 881.

Ossoinig, K.C. Echography of the Eye, Orbit and Periorbital Region. In: Orbit Roentgenology (P.H. Arger d.) New York: Wiley (1977) p. 224.

Ossoinig, K.C. The Role of Clinical Echography in Modern Diagnosis of Periorbital and Orbital Lesions. In: Proc. 3rd Int. Symp. on Orbital Disorders (C. Bleeker, ed.) The Hague: Junk (1978) p. 496

Ossoinig, K.C. Standardized Echography: Basic Principles, Clinical Applications, and Results. In: Ophthalmic Ultrasonography: Comparative Techniques (R.L. Dallow ed.) International Ophthalmology Clinics Vol. 19(4) Boston: Little, Brown & Company (1979) p. 127.

Till, P. Echography of retrobulbar hematomas. (Ger.) Klin. Mbl. Augenheilk. 158: 723 (1971).

Till, P. Echography in Rhinogenic Orbital Conditions. In: Modern Problems in Ophthalmology: Orbital Disorders. (G.M. Bleeker, et al., eds.) Vol. 14 Basel: Karger (1975) p. 273.

Authors' Address:
II. Univ.-Augen Klinik
Alserstrasse 4
A-1090 Vienna, Austria

EIGHT YEARS OF A- and B-SCAN ULTRASONOGRAPHY IN TUMOURAL DIAGNOSTICS OF THE GLOBE AND ORBIT

A. REIBALDI, V.V. LORUSSO & N. DELLE NOCI

(Bari, Italy)

INTRODUCTION

The use of ultrasonography in the diagnosis of eye tumours, both endobulbar and orbital, is arousing more and more interest and rapidly gaining recognition as an efficient means of examination, as it is quick, reliable, innocuous and easily repeated.

Our aim in this paper is to report the results obtained with ultrasonography in our studies into eye tumour pathology at Bari General Infirmary over the past eight years, using both A-scan (Kretz 7200) and B-scan (Bronson-Turner unit).

BULBAR DIAGNOSTICS

Between 1972 and 1979 we examined 109 patients echographically for suspected endobulbar growths – a total of 114 eyes in all.

In 29 of these cases ultrasonography gave us a negative result: in 18 opacity of the optic media prevented thorough examination of the fundus; in six we were able to examine by means of fluorescienangiography and transillumination. Both confirmed the findings of the ultrasonographic test. In the other five cases – all of which were out-patients sent to our Ultrasonography Centre for diagnosis – we used only ophthalmoscopy alongside of echography (Reibaldi, *et al.* 1979).

We diagnosed endobulbar tumors in 85 cases, of which 49 were malignant melanomas of the choroid, 26 retinoblastomas and ten other types of tumours.

Malignant Melanomas of the Choroid

Out of the 49 cases of suspected malignant melanomas of the choroid diagnosed, 36 were hospitalized and enucleated. Of these, the opacity of the optic media of nine prevented even us from conducting an accurate ophthalmoscopic test. In the other 27 cases we combined ultrasonography with ophthalmoscopy and, fluorescien angiography with transillumination, even though the fluorescien angiography gave us very unreliable results in five cases out of the 27. In one case only we were able to conduct all the different tests which confirmed the ultrasonographic diagnosis of melanoma. The histological report, however, revealed only an intense vascular congestion of the choroid. Finally, the 13 out-patients which we examined at the clinic and who refused to be operated upon were later enucleated in other centres and the histological report always confirmed our findings.

Retinoblastoma

Retinoblastoma is the most common malignant tumor in children. With the aid of ultrasonography we diagnosed the tumor in 26 patients, two of them could not be examined in any other way because of the opacity of the media. In the other 24 cases, however, we were able to use ophthalmoscopy and echography. The diagnoses, however, was rather uncertain in three cases. Apart from this, we gave six patients, five of whom had an aqua-serum ratio greater than 1, a dose of aqua-serum GPT. Finally, we examined in another four cases using X-rays. This gave us negative results due to a total lack of calcification. We did not get histological confirmation in three cases because enucleation was refused.

Other Tumours

In 1972 we were confronted with a case of melanocytoma of the optic nerve which was confirmed first with ultrasonography and later histologically, even though in the light of recent developments in pathological anatomy we could have avoided enucleation.

In one patient with secondary detachment of the retina, ultrasonography, together with fluorescien angiography helped us to diagnose an 'angioma of the choroid', a relatively rare tumour, found at the posterior pole of the globe, next to the head of optic nerve. We diagnosed eight metastatic tumours of the choroid, in four cases due to cancer of the breast, in two cases cancer of the stomach, one case due to cancer of the bladder and one case due to cancer of the parathyroid.

Because of the opacity of the media, ultrasonography was the most important test in the two cases of stomach cancer and the cancer of the parathyroid. In addition to the other means of analysis it helped us to localize a metastatic carcinoma of the choroid in the other six patients.

ORBITAL DIAGNOSTICS

During the past eight years we have observed 175 cases of unilateral exophthalmus either in hospitalised patients or in out-patients referred to our Clinic for suspect orbital growths. In 30 cases analysis was negative (with ultrasonography 12 turned out to be cases of retrobulbar hematoma) and the ultrasonographic findings were confirmed by other tests and follow-up. In the other 145 cases, however, we diagnosed the following endo-orbital growths: 126 solid tumours, 11 angiomatous tumours, eight cystic tumours.

Solid Tumours

These are generally divided into (a) sarcomas and (b) metastatic carcinomas, mostly due to the spread of tumours from contiguous anatomic structures (malignant melanomae of the choroid and retinoblastoma, tumours of the eyelids or of the conjuctiva).

In our 126 cases of solid orbital tumours, 102 were confirmed by other means of examination. For the most part they were also confirmed first by the surgical findings and then by the histological report. In the following cases we did not have a subsequent confirmation of our echographical analysis: one case of myositis; two cases of bony malformation; and 14 cases of pseudotumours.*

Cistic Tumours

We had eight cases of exophthalmus in which we diagnosed cystic tumours: three were meningoceles, two mucoceles, one dermatoid cyst and one hydatideic cyst. These analyses were later confirmed, first by surgical intervention, and then by the histological report (with the exception of one case where the CT findings ruled out the presence of a tumour).

Angiomatous Tumours

Under this heading we have grouped all the 'cavernous hemangiomas'. In adults these are considered the most frequent type of primary tumours and are most found in the vicinity or inside of the muscle cone. We saw 11 cases of these tumours which are the most paradigmatic kind of angiomatous tumours and are distinguishable from LDH because they show growth at successive check-ups. In nine cases surgical intervention and histological reports confirmed our ultrasonographic diagnosis, while in two cases solid-tumours-type echoes led us to incorrectly diagnosing one carinoma and one inflammatory pseudotumour.

Having studied the results obtained with echographical diagnostics of endobulbar tumours we would like to draw attention to the following points:

—the remarkable reliability of ultrasonography both in detecting the presence of tumours and in proving their absence;

—the extreme usefulness of this means of diagnosis especially where opacity of the media is concerned: in the cases we examined, out a total of 114 eyes 31 had opaque media.

When we are dealing with clear media, we regard ultrasonography as complementary to the following other means of diagnosis: *ophthalmoscopy*, especially indirect binocular and contact-glass ophthalmoscopy. In our opinion, this should remain the fundamental test for tumour diagnosis.

Transillumination, however, has two notable limitations: it cannot localize certain types of lesions accurately and it gives incorrect results in certain cases.

Fluorescien angiography also has two disadvantages: first, it involves the injection of contrast into the blood and second, it does not always differentiate between different types of tumours.

Similarly, *scintigraphy* is still a rather unreliable test since it relies upon the evaluation of tissual radioactivity on successive days. On how to interpret the results of the administration of doses of GPT, GOT or LDH, the various schools have still not managed to agree; and X-rays, retinoscopy and electroretinography are only useful in particular cases.

In orbital diagnostics, ultrasonography, too, has also proved to be very reliable: out of 175 cases it allowed us to rule out the presence of tumour in 30 cases, while out of 145 ultrasonographically positive cases, our first diagnosis was correct in 118 cases. The arrival of CT has proved to be of enormous help in cases with a positive echographical diagnosis. If necessary it can be used in addition to arteriography, phlebography, thermography and scintigraphy.

Echography, for both bulbar and orbital complaints plays a part not only in choosing the right therapeutic approach, but also in conducting periodical checks throughout therapy.

Summarizing then, we affirm very strongly the extraordinary reliability of ultrasonography, specially when A-scan and B-scan are used together: where B-scan gives a more precise topography of a tumor, A-scan is more exact in the diagnosis of tissue. Other advantages to bear in mind are its repeatability (as often as once a day), its innocuity, the case of examination and its low cost.

We still think it is advisable, however, and, even necessary in spite of the usability of echography, that it be used in addition to whatever other diagnostic procedures are available that are not dangerous to the patient, to provide us with a correct diagnosis, and that this diagnosis always be confirmed by the histology.

REFERENCES

Reibaldi A., Capotorto B. & Delle Noci N. Utilità dell'Ecografia nella Diagnosi e Terapia dei Tumori dell'Apparato Oculare. Com. XXX Congr. Naz. Soc. Ital. di Chirurgia Oncologica, Roma 8–10 novembre 1979.

Authors' Address:
Institute of Ophthalmology
University of Bari
Bari, Italy

ECHOGRAPHIC DIFFERENTIAL DIAGNOSIS OF OPTIC-NERVE LESIONS

K.C. OSSOINIG, G. CENNAMO & S. FRAZIER-BYRNE

(Iowa City, Iowa, U.S.A.)

With B-scan echography, the normal optic nerve can be traced along its anterior course within the orbit, the optic disc can be located and large lesions of the optic nerve can be detected.

Standardized A-scan, however, is the most sensitive method for detecting optic-nerve lesions within the orbit and the most accurate means to measure optic-nerve width (accuracy is 0.5 mm). With this method, optic-nerve lesions may frequently be differentiated: (1) Neural swelling can be distinguished from widening or separation of the optic-nerve sheaths (Figs. 3, 4). (2) Solid thickening of the sheaths can be differentiated from increased sub-arachnoidal fluid separating the sheaths from the nerve (Fig. 5). (3) Optic-nerve gliomas can be called once their thickness becomes more than twice the diameter of the normal optic nerve in the fellow orbit (Fig. 7). (4) Similarly, optic-nerve meningiomas can be called when the overall thickness of the nerve structures exceeds their normal size by more than 100% (Fig. 6); other non-neoplastic

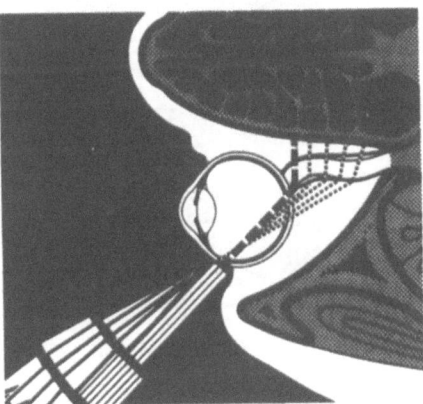

Fig. 1. Horizontal schematic section through eye and orbit illustrates dynamic scanning of optic nerve showing its maximal thickness along different sections behind the globe. Refraction of the sound beam toward the nerve surface allows the display of true acoustic cross sections. Note that sound propagation is just schematically drawn, which – between posterior ocular wall and optic nerve – may not correspond to real propagation (see text). Usually probe is placed at temporal ocular surface as shown in picture; occasionally, optic nerve winds behind globe in such a way that probe placement on nasal side is more effective.

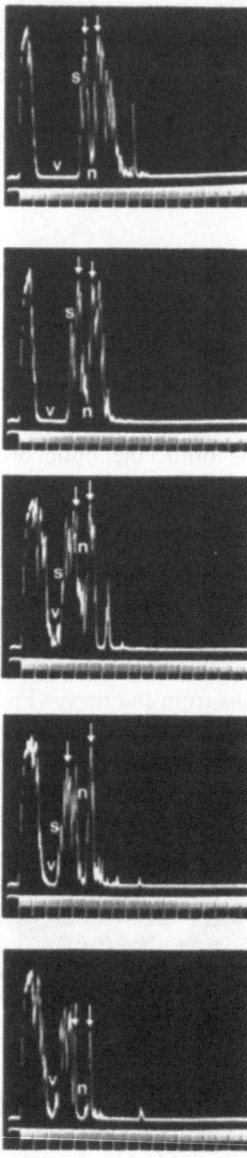

Fig. 2. Series of A-scans corresponding (top to bottom) to beam paths indicated in Fig. 1 (left to right). Note the decreasing width of the ocular pattern as more posterior segments of the optic nerve are displayed. v vitreous; s sclera (low spike because of oblique sound-beam incidence); → temporal (left) and nasal (right) arachnoidal surfaces outlining maximal thickness of nerve (n). Note the steep fall and rise of these arachnoidal spikes (perpendicular sound-beam incidence).

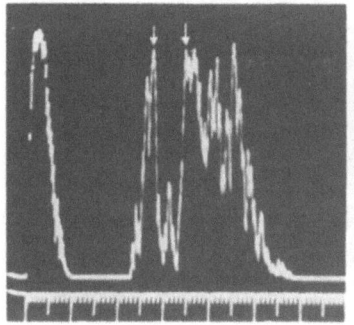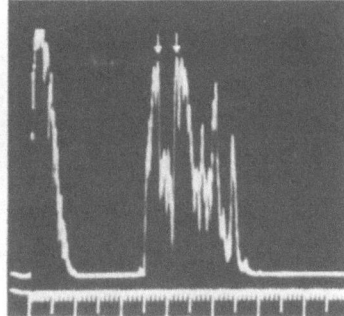

Fig. 3. Echograms showing moderate swelling of right optic nerve (left) and normal left optic nerve (right echogram). → arachnoidal surfaces.

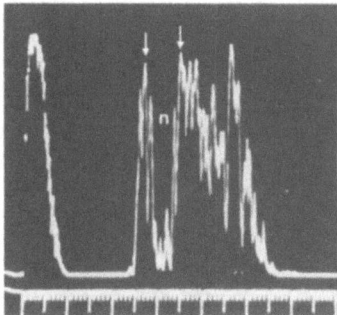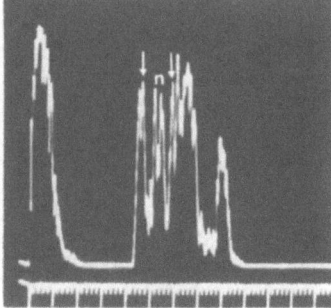

Fig. 4. Echograms displaying sheathing phenomenon: swelling of optic nerve and its sheaths (left) and atrophic nerve with wide distension of optic-nerve sheaths due to pseudo-tumor cerebri (right). → arachnoidal surfaces; n optic nerve with pia mater (higher spikes outlining nerve).

lesions, for instance optic neuritis, may stretch the nerve sheaths to a maximum of twice the normal size only. Smaller tumors may be diagnosed when they cause asymmetric thickening of the nerve structures. (5) Optic-nerve gliomas can be distinguished from meningiomas. (6) Optic-nerve atrophy can also be demonstrated with standardized A-scan echography (Fig. 8).

Fig. 1 illustrates the dynamic A-scan procedure used to scan the optic nerve from the back of the eye toward the orbital apex. Refraction of the sound beam toward the optic nerve, which occurs somewhere between the posterior ocular wall and the optic-nerve surface, must be postulated in order to explain the fact that the beam can be directed in a perpendicular direction toward most of the surface of the orbital extension of the optic nerve. This perpendicular approach is proven in the A-scan echograms by steeply rising or falling surface spikes, as seen in Fig. 2. Using the parallel beam and signal processing provided by the standardized 7200 MA A-scan, it is impossible to obtain such steep echo signals with oblique sound-beam incidence. With the scanning method shown in Fig. 1, only the most posterior portion of the orbital optic nerve (within the orbital apex) cannot be measured accurately.

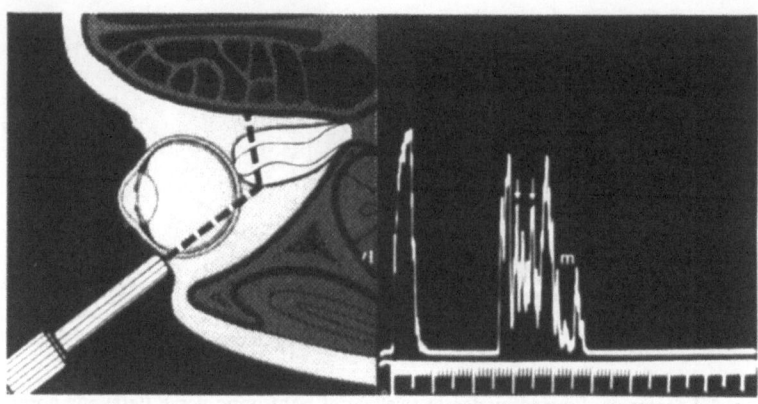

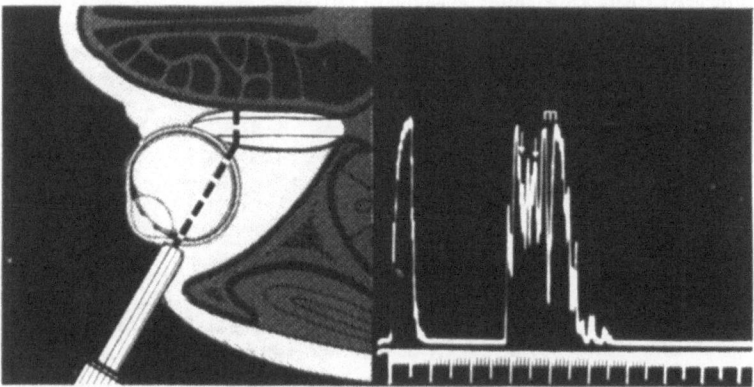

Fig. 5. Illustration of examination technique used to differentiate optic-nerve lesions (showing the sheathing phenomenon) into those with thickened sheaths and those with increased sub-arachnoidal fluid (this case); see also remark in legend to Fig. 1 about sound propagation. → surface of optic nerve (pia mater); the two highest spikes on either side of the nerve correspond with arachnoidal surfaces. Note the narrowing of the overall optic-nerve width (distance between arachnoidal surfaces). Also note the narrowing of the medial rectus muscle (m) that is also being stretched by this maneuver.

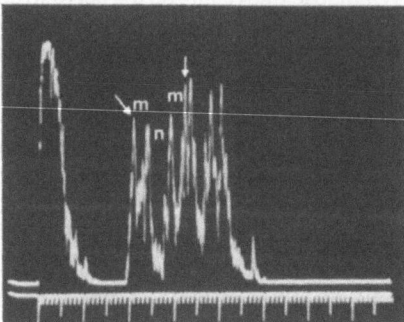

Fig. 6. A-scan echogram of ring meningioma of optic nerve. n optic nerve; m thickened sheaths (meningioma). Note that overall width of optic nerve as indicated by distance between the temporal (left) and nasal (right) surfaces of the tumor (arrows) is almost three times the normal optic-nerve size.

330

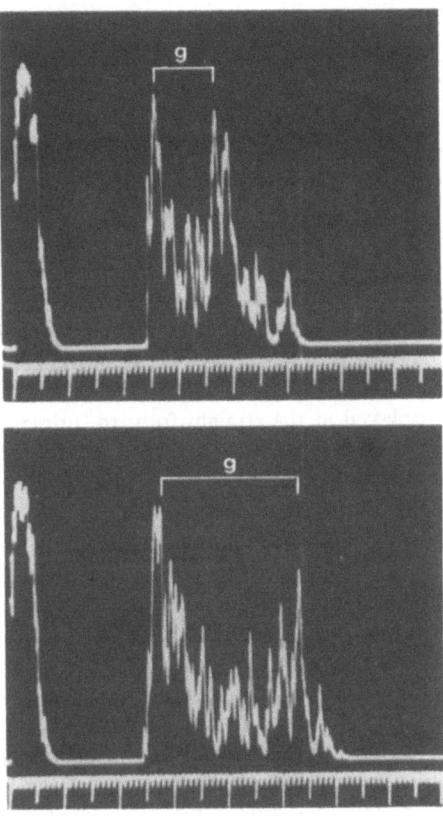

Fig. 7. Echographic cross section (top pattern) and long section (bottom echogram) of optic-nerve glioma (g).

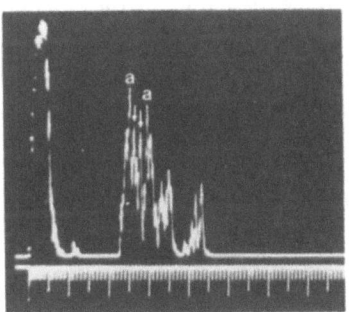 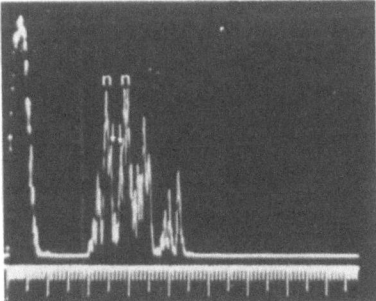

Fig. 8. Echograms of atrophic right optic nerve (left) and normal left optic nerve (right) in a patient. a arachnoidal surfaces; → optic-nerve surface (pia mater). Note the sheathing sign caused by increased amounts of sub-arachnoidal fluid surrounding the atrophic nerve. Also note the equal overall size (distance between arachnoidal surfaces) of both nerves and the fact that even the normal nerve (right echogram) may show some (minor) sheathing sign.

However, any thickening of that portion exceeding 0.75 mm can be clearly shown through a comparison of the two orbits.

The display of a maximally wide defect representing the lower-reflective optic nerve and, at the same time, steeply rising surface spikes (usually from the arachnoidal surfaces of the optic-nerve sheaths) indicates the maximum diameter of the optic nerve in the area scanned by the beam. Fig. 3 illustrates a slightly swollen optic nerve and the normal nerve thickness in the fellow orbit of this patient. Fig. 4 demonstrates the cross section of an optic nerve, which shows thickening of both the nerve itself and its sheaths (left), and the cross section of another optic nerve that displays distension of the sheaths of the nerve by increased sub-arachnoidal fluid (right). Fig. 5 illustrates the technique used to clearly differentiate between thickening of the optic-nerve sheaths and distension of the sheaths by increased fluid: First, the optic-nerve structures are displayed in the straight-forward, primary-gaze position. Then the patient is instructed to look toward the probe ($\simeq 30°$ from primary-gaze direction), thus stretching the optic nerve. If the sheaths are thickened, the cross diameter will not change significantly during this procedure. If, however, the optic-nerve sheaths are distended by increased sub-arachnoidal fluid (as illustrated in Fig. 5), this manoeuvre will decrease the width of the optic nerve in the echogram, since the fluid is distributed over a longer distance and the distension of the optic-nerve sheaths is thus decreased. Fig. 6 shows an acoustic cross section in a case of optic-nerve sheath meningioma. The fact that the overall thickening of the optic nerve in this case is much more than twice the thickness of the nerve in the fellow orbit proves that a neoplasm is present. The 'sheathing phenomenon' in the echogram indicates that the tumor is an optic-nerve ring meningioma. Fig. 7 shows an optic-nerve glioma. In this case, it is mainly the optic nerve itself which is thickened. Again, the thickening goes far beyond twice the size of the normal optic nerve in the fellow orbit, thus proving the presence of the tumor. Fig. 8 illustrates echographic findings in optic-nerve atrophy. The overall width of the nerve structures is still equal to the normal size; however, while the atrophic optic nerve itself is thinner, more fluid is found to be present in the sub-arachnoidal space. Thus, an atrophic optic nerve clearly displays the sheathing sign, while its width measured from arachnoid to arachnoid remains the same as the normal nerve.

Authors' Addresses:
Dept. of Ophthalmology (Dr. Ossoinig, Mrs. Frazier-Byrne)
University of Iowa
Iowa City, Iowa, U.S.A.

Istituto di Clinica Oculistica (Dr. Cennamo)
2nd School of Medicine
University of Naples
Naples, Italy

332

ECHOGRAPHIC FOLLOW-UP OF DYSTHYROID
EYE DISEASE

M. ZINGIRIAN, P. ROSSI & G.P. FAVA

(Genoa, Italy)

Since the works of Ossoinig (1977), echography has a well established place in the evaluation of a patient with dysthyroid eye disease. The measurement of the extraocular muscle thickness, particularly, appears a fairly exact and reproducible technique and is likely the most useful and widely used examination in these patients.

This work was designed to correlate the echographic measurements with the clinical and humoral findings and with the effects of medical or surgical therapy on Graves' disease.

MATERIAL AND METHODS

Fifty-eight patients with dysthyroid eye disease were examined. Twenty-seven showed an active Graves' disease: 31 appeared euthyroid (normal T3–T4 serum levels, without severe clinical manifestations), after medical (26) or surgical (5) management.

According to the severity of the involvement, the eye changes were clinically classified into the six classes recommended by the American Thyroid Association. Due to the different prognostic implications, the patients were divided into two groups: those falling into classes 0 and 1 (22 patients) and those falling into classes 2 through 6 (36 patients).

The immunological characteristics of the disease were evaluated assessing the presence of circulating thyroglobulin antibodies (TGA) and anti-mitochondria antibodies (TMA). The ophthalmological examination included:

Hertel's exophthalmometry.

Hess-Lancaster testing for medial rectus (M.R.) function.

Medial rectus thickness evaluation according to the A-Scan echographic criteria established by Ossoinig.

RESULTS AND DISCUSSION

The mean M.R. thickness was 5.72 ± 0.8 mm. Thirty-eight patients showed a M.R. thickness over the normal values or a side difference greater than 2 mm.

The muscle thickness evaluation was confined to the medial rectus because this is the one muscle most frequently involved in dysthyroid orbitopathy and because its measurement is the most accurate one (McNutt 1975, Ossoinig 1977, Schalka 1977, Shammas, *et al*. 1980). Therefore, this limitation should not greatly affect our results. The correlations between M.R. thickness and the other parameters can be summarized as follows: (Table 1).

(1) The *clinical features* (Table 1a) of dysthyroid eye disease correlate fairly, but not strictly with the M.R. thickness. In a consistent percentage of cases these parameters behave in an opposite way. While a normal M.R. thickness can be considered of little clinical significance, it should be stressed that in a rather large number of cases an increased M.R. thickness is associated with minimal clinical signs: a finding that may have a prognostic value, in the lack of other orbital symptoms.

(2) *Exophthalmometrical readings* concerned both the actual degree of proptosis and the side differences. A pathological exophthalmometry value (Table 1b) is generally associated with an increased M.R. thickness. Discrepancies are mainly due to pathological exophthalmometry values associated with a normal M.R. thickness; the opposite finding is much more uncommon. Asymmetry in the exophthalmometrical readings (Table 1c) associated with an increased side variation of the M.R. thickness in about 50% of cases.

(3) As can be expected, M.R. thickness and *adduction changes* (Table 1d) are strictly bound, the only important exception being that an enlarged M.R. can still induce a normal adduction.

(4) The *immunological characteristics* (Table 1e) of the disease, cannot be strictly correlated with the M.R. changes: a discrepancy that endocrinologists are well aware of with regard to the other clinical features of dysthyroid orbitopathy.

(5) A successful *management* (Table 1f) of the general disease, as suggested by normal thyroid function blood tests and by the decrease in the subjective complaints, does not seem to restore M.R. thickness to its normal value.

CONCLUSIONS

Three points can be stressed from these considerations: Echography is a fairly reliable investigation that can lead to an early diagnosis of dysthyroid orbitopathy in some 10% of otherwise normal cases, but a large number of false-negative cases are encountered.

M.R. thickness is commonly related to the immunological derangements of Graves' disease, more than to hormonal changes. Actually, our investigations show that circulating antibodies levels do not strictly correlate with M.R. thickness changes: other factors should be considered.

A M.R. thickness increase can be an early sign of orbit involvement in Graves' disease, but it generally does not subside after a successful management of the other signs and symptoms of Graves' disease. Therefore, it is of little value in the evaluation of the treatment effectiveness.

Table 1. Results.

	Normal	M.R. thickness side diff. ≤ 2 mm	Pathol.	M.R. thickness side diff. > 2 mm.
(a) Clinical features				
classes 1 − 2	7		15	
classes 3 − 6	13		23	
Exophthalmometry				
(b) absolute value				
19 mm.	5		7	
19 mm.	15		31	
(c) side difference				
2 mm.		21		14
2 mm.		11		12
(d) Adduction				
normal	15		17	
impaired	5		21	
(e) Immunological features				
TGA/TMA +	10		17	
TGA/TMA --	10		21	
(f) Treatment effect				
euthyroid	13		18	
dysthyroid	7		20	

REFERENCES

McNutt, L.C., Kaefring, S.L. & Ossoinig, K.C. Ecographic measurement of extraocular muscles In: Ultrasound in Medicine, Vol. 3A (D. White & R.E. Brown, eds.) New York: Plenum Press (1977) p. 932.

Ossoinig, K.C. Echography of the eye, orbit and periorbital region In: Orbit Roentgenology (P.H. Arger, ed.) New York: J. Wiley & Sons (1977) p. 224.

Skalka, H.W. Clinical presentation, extraocular muscle and perineural optic nerve changes in endocrine orbitopathy. Proc. of the VII Siduo, Münster, 1978.

Shammas, H.J.F. & Minckler, D.S. Ultrasound in early thyroid orbitopathy Arch. Ophthalmol. 98: 277 (1980).

Authors' Address:
University Eye Clinic
Genoa, Italy

SWOLLEN EXTRAOCULAR MUSCLES –
ULTRASONOGRAPHIC FINDINGS AND CLINICAL APPEARANCE

R.F. GUTHOFF & W. SCHROEDER

(Hamburg, F.R.G.)

Ossoinig (1966, 1971) was the first who described exact muscle measurements using the A-scan unit and Coleman (1972) & co-workers pointed out that enlargement of the extraocular muscles mainly in Graves' disease can be diagnosed with B-scan techniques. Since that time many invasive diagnostic manipulations have been avoidable. In Hamburg we are routinely using the Kretz 7200 MA and the Bronson Turner unit. To differentiate muscle enlargement from other space occupying lesions we found B-scan to be sufficient in most cases.

For this study we collected all ultrasonographic examinations with muscle thickening since 1977 and the pattern of muscle involvement was noted. During the last year the maximal distances of globe excursions in 32 patients were measured according to Kestenbaum (1961) in order to correlate muscle function and ultrasonographic results. Altogether 84 patients were examined – 47 with bilateral findings – so that the data of 131 orbits could be used.

Fifty-four patients had Graves' disease, 44 bilaterally, ten with muscle involvement in orbital lymphoma, seven with myositis, four with ocular cellulitis, three with muscle metastasis of breast cancer, one with orbital haemorrhage, one with neurofibromatosis, one with sarcoidosis, one with histiocytosis X, one with extra-ocular growth of a malignant melanoma of the choroid, which infiltrated the inf. rect. muscle.

The distribution of the muscles involved is listed in Table 1. Regarding the connection of motality and muscle enlargement there were quite different results in the various groups. In one early stage of *Graves' disease* the swollen sup. rect. muscles complex caused an isolated monolateral eye-lid retraction with downward gaze. In another patient the bigger sup. rect. muscle on the right side showed a poorer function than the less involved left one, which might indicate a negative correlation between muscle swelling and motor activity. But in a patient with Graves' disease shown in Fig. 1 where abduction was restricted on the left eye, the medial rectus muscle was enlarged. This seems to be a passive limitation to motility.

In mild cases of *myositis* we found no disturbances of ocular motility at all. In Fig. 2 an example of the involvement of sup. rect., oblique and med. rect. muscle is shown and again, no decrease of active motility. But we did,

Table 1. Distribution of muscle involvement in patients with extraocular swollen muscles.

	number of orbits	number of muscles involved						
		m. rect. med.	m. rect. sup.	m. lev. palp.	m. rect. lat.	m. rect. inf.	m. obl. sup.	m. obl. inf
graves disease	98	56 (50%)	71 (65%)	14 (13%)	19 (17%)	18 (17%)	8 (7%)	1
orbital lymphoma	13		7		6	3		
Myositis	7	3	3		12	1	1	
orbital cellulitis	4	3	2			1		
muscle metastasis of breast carcinoma	3	2	1				1	
orbital haemorrhage	1	1						
neurofibromatosis	1	1						
sarcoidosis	1						1	
histiocytosis X	1	1	1			1		
extraocular growth of a melignant melanoma of the choroid	1					1		

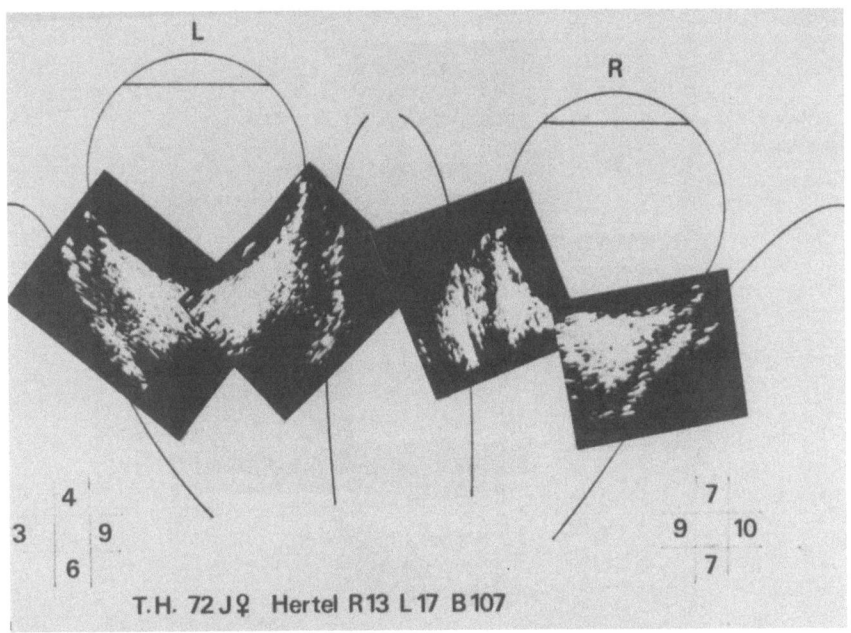

Fig. 1. Unilateral Graves' disease with a most involved medial rectus muscle. Adduction was nearly maximal (9 mm), but abduction markedly decreased (3 mm).

however, find a deficiency for elevation in adduction probably caused by Brown's phenomenon — the inability of the swollen sup. obl. muscle to slide through the trochlea. Only four days later, after two subconjunctival injections of dexamethason, the complaints disappeared and motility was almost fully restored. There was, however, only a slight reduction in ultrasonographic findings — three months later the orbit appeared to be normal.

In chronic and acute severe cases of myositis we found the eye almost completely fixated. In our cases of *lymphoma*, reduction of muscle function was a constant finding. In some cases after irradiation motility was partly recovered (nine patients); in 4 out of 13 in spite of a good remission of the tumor, muscle function remained poor.

We also found reduction of active muscle function in two cases of direct muscle *metastasis* of breast cancer. In the third patient (Fig. 3) not the motoractivity but the passive flexibility of the involved muscle seemed to be reduced, and retraction of the globe appeared while abduction was induced. This phenomenon is thought to be caused by a paramuscular mass, which is seen clearly in the frontal section, and it may exaggerate the muscle infiltration in the hortizontal picture.

In cases of *cellulitis*, the affected muscles always showed poor functioning. These improved sooner after treatment than the ultrasonographic findings. In Fig. 4 a 4 year old boy is demonstrated with a subperiostal infiltration and a slight swelling of the med. and sup. rect. muscle, three days later after surgical treatment when infiltration was still motility had returned to normal.

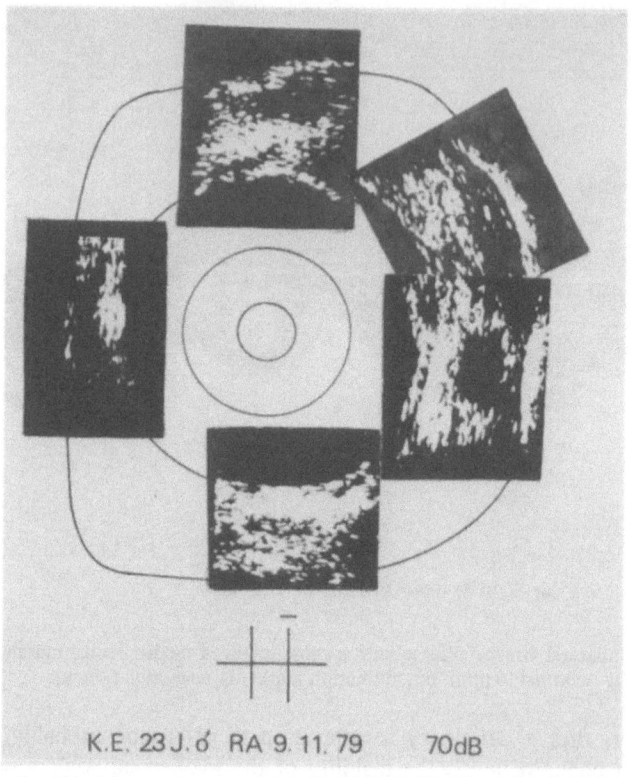

Fig. 2. Acute myositis with severe involvement of sup. rect., sup. oblique and medial rectus muscle. Motility according to Brown's phenomenon.

We found the pattern of muscle involvement in graves' disease similar to other authors (Ullerich & Horst 1956, Shammes, *et al.* 1980), the slightly lower number of enlarged inf. rect. muscles in our sample might be due to the larger B-scan transducer, which makes it more difficult to examine the lower part of the orbit. Our findings that there was no general correlation between muscle involvement and motility may be explained by the fact that the stage of histological muscle degeneration (Daiker 1979) as well as electromyographic (Jensen 1971, Esslen & Papst 1961) results are not correlated to the outer shape of the muscle. Endocrine orbitopathy is primarily a disease of all connective tissues so that the swelling of muscles alone cannot explain the disturbances of ocular motility. In all cases of lymphoma, regardless of their stage of malignancy, and in metastatic infiltration, the affected muscles showed a reduced motor activity. This fact might occasionally be helpful in differential diagnoses of Graves' disease. Concerning ocular myositis, we were surprised to see obviously swollen muscles in the ultrasonogram with no reduction of motor activity and we could find no previous reports of this phenomenon. We noticed that there are fluent borders between so-called episcleritis, tennonitis and ocular myositis, which only affects motility in

340

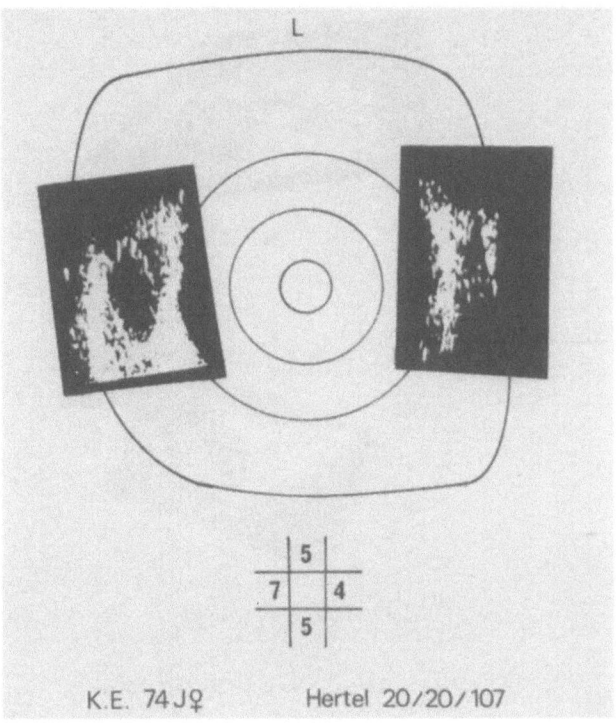

Fig. 3. Patient with orbital metastisis of breast cancer. Involvement of medial rectus. muscle and paramuscular tissue. Abduction was reduced to 4 mm.

severe cases. Because of the quick response to steroid therapy, it can be used as a diagnostic aid. Clinical symptoms quickly vanish but muscle swelling remains for several weeks.

Summarizing our results, we conclude that: there were no definite correlations of extraocular muscle enlargement and motor activity in Graves' disease, but a good correlation when lymphoma, orbital cellulitis or metastases had been the cause of muscle swelling. In doubtful cases of myositis we found ultrasonography to be a very sensitive method for diagnosing muscle swelling even before other clinical symptoms — especially disturbances of ocular motility — appear.

REFERENCES

Coleman, D.J. Rehability of ocular and orbital diagnosis with B-scan ultrasound: II Orbital diagnosis. Am. J. Ophthalmol. 74: 708 (1972).

Daiker, B. Das gewebliche Substrat der verdickten äuBeren Augenmuskeln bei der endokrinen Orbitopathie. Klin. Mbl. Augenheilk. 174: 843 (1979).

Esslen, E. & Papst, W. Die Bedeutung der Elektromyografie für die Analyse von Motilitätsstörungen der Augen. Bibl. Ophthalmol. Fasc. 57. Basel: S. Karger (1961).

Jensen, S.F. Endokrine Ophthalmoplegia. Is it due to myopathy or to mechanical immobilisation? Act. Ophthalmol. 49: 679 (1971).

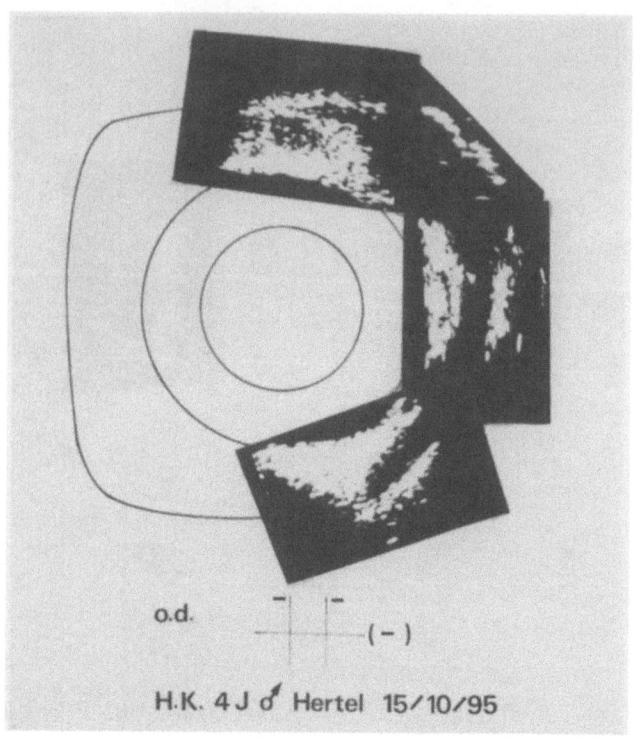

Fig. 4. Subperiostal infiltration in a case of orbital involvement in sinusitis. Elevation and adduction had been reduced.

Kestenbaum, A. Clinical methods of neuro-ophthalmologic examination. New York & London: Grune & Stratton 2. (1961) p.237.
Ossoinig, K. Die Ultraschalldiagnostik der Orbita. Klin. Nbl. Augenheilk. 149: 817 (1966).
Ossoining, K. Echo orbitography, a reliable method for the differential diagnosis of endokrine exophthalmos. in (L. Fellinger & R. Hofer, eds.) Further Advances in Thysoid Research, Wien, G. Gistel & Co., (1971) p. 871.
Shammas, H.J.F. Minckler, D.S. & Ogden, C. Ultrasound in early Thyroid Orbitopathy. Arch. Ophthalmol. 98: 277 (1980).
Ullerich, K. & Horst, W. Zur Typenlehre des endokrinen Exophthalmus. Klin. Mbl. Augenheilk. 128: 215 (1956).

Authors' Address:
R.F. Guthoff
Universitäts Augenklinik Eppendorf
Martinistr. 52
D-2000 Hamburg 20
BRD

W. Schroeder
AK Heidberg, Augen abteilung
Tangstedter Landstr. 4000
D-2000 Hamburg 62
BRD

ECHOGRAPHY IN ORBITAL MYOSITIS

H. SHIBATA, Y. MASUYAMA, Y. NISHIMOTO & A. SAWADA

(*Miyazaki, Japan*)

ABSTRACT

With the advance of diagnostic techniques in soft tissues, a great deal of information on orbital inflammation can be attained. Echography is one of the advanced approaches to orbital soft tissues. Myogenic lesions are a fruitful target for echographic orbital examination.

Results of A- and B-scan echography in five cases with suspected or established orbital myositis will be described. Differential diagnosis from other low-reflective lesions such as endocrine ophthalmopathy or lymphoma/ sarcoma/pseudotumor group will be discussed.

CASE REPORTS

Specific findings of these five cases of orbital myositis are summarized in Table 1.

Case 1: A 54-year-old woman had occasionally suffered from pain deep in the left orbit for four months prior to consultation. Each attack was of acute onset and continued for a week. One month prior to consultation she noticed double vision and protrusion of the left eye. At the first consultation on February 2, 1979, corrected visual acuity of the left eye was 0.8. The left eye protruded by 7 mm compared with the right eye. The upper lid of the left eye was slightly swollen. No tumor was palpated. The eye position was orthophoric. Lateral eye movement of the left eye was limited. Forced duction test showed a strong resistance in the horizontal direction. Tensilon test was negative. Lateral bulbar conjunctiva was slightly hyperemic and edematous. No distinct abnormality was found in the cornea, lens, vitreous and fundus. Plain x-ray of the orbital apex and the orbital canal did not reveal any abnormality.

In A- and B-scan echography, a poorly outlined low reflective lesion in the lateral side of the left orbit, corresponding to the lateral rectus muscle, was demonstrated (Fig. 1). The lesion extended superiorly to the area of superior rectus muscle and inferiorly as well as posteriorly to the area of inferior rectus muscle. Inner reflectivity was low. The echographic finding was consistent with that of lymphoma/sarcoma/pseudotumor.

Table 1. Specific findings of five cases of orbital myositis.

Case	Sex	Age	Onset	Laterality	Exophthalmos	Motility limitation	Echo.	CT	EMG	Thyroid dysfunction	Pathol. proved
1	W	54	Acute	L-R	8/15	L) Lateral	+	+	+	−	+
2	W	28	Acute	L	10/12	L) Lateral	+	+	−	−	
3	W	56	Chronic	L-R-L	7/11	L) Downwards	+	+	+	−	
4	M	64	Chronic	R	18/15	R) Upwards	+	+	−	−	
5	W	76	Chronic	L	17/17	L) Blepharoptosis	+	+			+

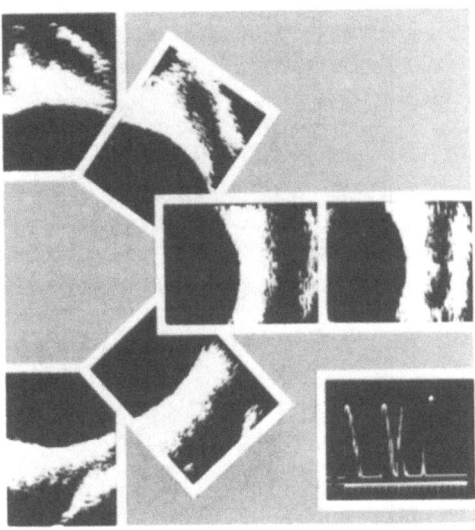

Fig. 1. A- and B-scan echograms of Case 1.

In axial computerized tomography an oval, relatively sharply outlined, dense mass was seen in the lateral portion of the left orbit. The mass was not enhanced with contrast agent. The size of the mass changed with eye movement. At outward gaze the mass thickened and at inward gaze it flattened. The mass proved to be an enlarged lateral rectus muscle.

In electromyography the lateral rectus muscle of the left eye showed a myopathic pattern. Erythrocyte sedimentation rate was elevated up to 66 mm at one hour and 108 mm at two hours. Thyroid function was within the normal range.

Despite intensive administration of corticosteriods, congestion of the lid and the conjunctiva, exophthalmos and ocular immobility intensified with recurrent exacerbation and remission for three months.

In July, 1979, in the remission stage, biopsy from the lateral rectus and inferior oblique muscle was done. In A- and B-scan echography at that time an area of low reflectivity – which had previously extended superiorly, inferiorly and posteriorly – disappeared. The lateral rectus muscle was relatively outlined and the inner reflectivity was medium (Fig. 2). At surgery, thickness of the lateral rectus muscle was within the normal range. But the muscle lost its colour completely and sclerotized. Under the light microscope (Fig. 3), marked hyalinization in the muscle and disappearance of the muscle fibers were observed. Slight small cell infiltration was seen in the perivascular space. B- and A-scan echograms at 6 o'clock meridian of the left eye showed a round, relatively well outlined lesion of low reflectivity (Fig. 4.). At surgery the inferior oblique muscle was purplish and remarkably thickened. The muscle was so weakened as to be torn very easily. Under the light microscope (Fig. 5), scattered degenerated muscle fibers of various sizes were seen. Small cell infiltration and moderate fibrosis were seen in the stroma. Under electron microscopy, intramuscular nerve fibers were not involved.

345

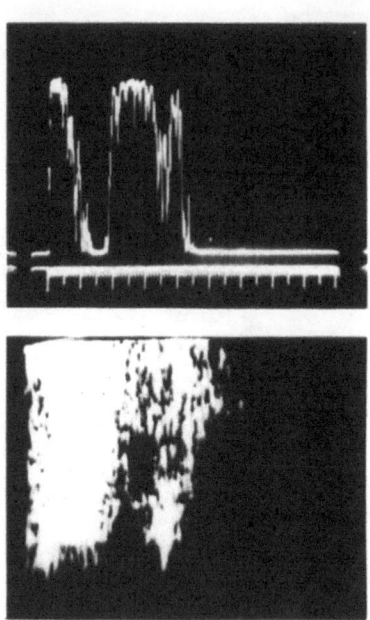

Fig. 2. A- and B-scan echograms of the lateral rectus muscle of the left eye at the time of biopsy.

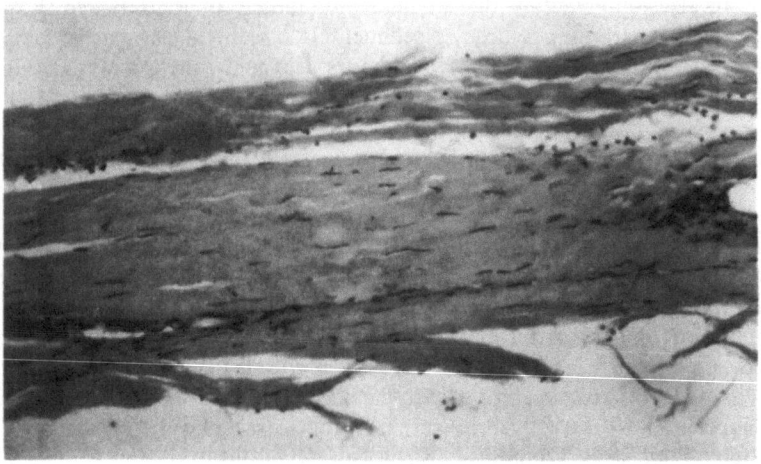

Fig. 3. Light micrograph of the lateral rectus muscle of the left eye.

Several weeks after the remission in the left eye, deep pain in the orbit was felt in the right eye. The right eye protruded 3 mm compared with the left eye. The anterior portion of the right eye was strongly congested to the same degree as the left eye had been previously. Eye movement was limited in all

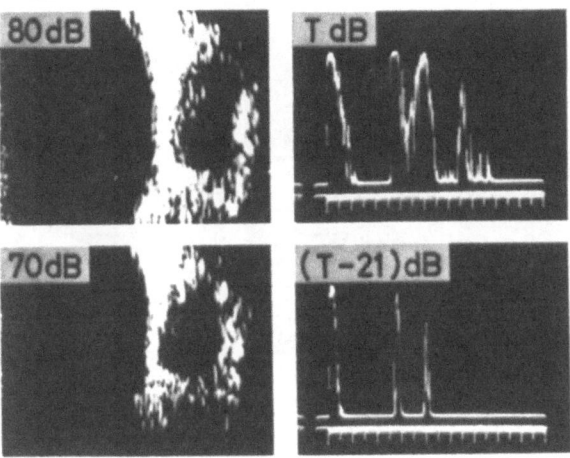

Fig. 4. B- and A-scan echograms of the left eye in 6 o'clock meridian.

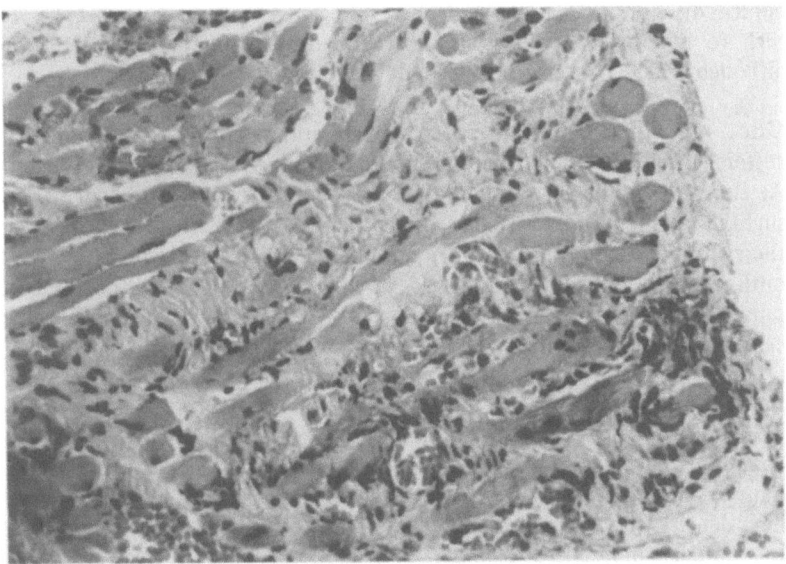

Fig. 5. Light micrograph of the inferior oblique muscle of the left eye.

directions. Echography and CT showed thickening of horizontal muscles. Ocular myositis was strongly suspected, although it is said to involve only a unilateral eye.

In the second, third and fourth case, thickening of extraocular muscles was shown in echography as well as in computerized tomography (Table 1). Clinical disorders in orbital myositis were responsive to corticosteroid treatment to more or less extent. Fig. 6 is the A-scan echograms and computerized

347

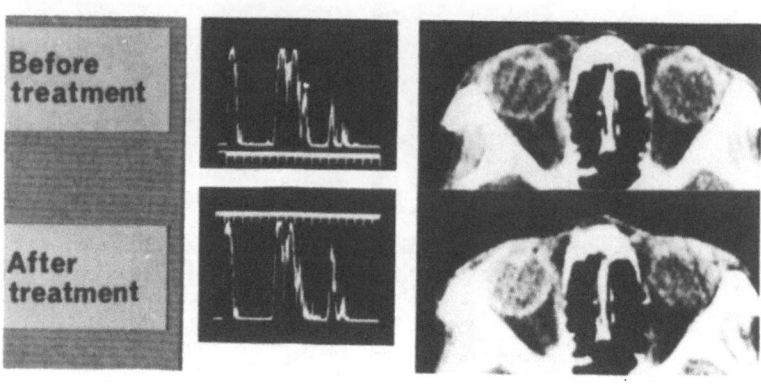

Fig. 6. A-scan echograms and computerized tomograms before and after corticosteroid treatment in Case 2.

tomograms before and after corticosteroid treatment in a 28-year-old woman (Case 2). It is worthy of note that the medial rectus muscle of the left eye was still thick despite the disappearance of motility limitation or other clinical discomfort. Variation of inner reflectivity in A-scan echography from high to medium might suggest structural changes in the muscular tissues, although the changes have not been determined.

Case 5: For three months prior to consultation, a 76-year-old woman had suffered from swelling of the right upper lid with exacerbation and remission. At consultation the right upper lid was moderately swollen and hanging down slightly. Position and movement of the right eye were normal. Protrusion of the right eye was not found. In A- and B-scan echography, a relatively poorly outlined, low reflective lesion was shown. The lesion in the posterior was separated into two portions by a steeply rising high spike on the A-scan echogram. The echographic findings were consistent with lymphoma/sarcoma/pseudotumor group (Fig. 7). Based on the location, the superior rectus and the levator muscle – mainly the latter – were diagnosed to be involved in the lesion. It was impossible to determine the exact site of involvement. In axial computerized tomography at the level of the optic nerve and horizontal muscles, no abnormality was found. However, at a level 5 mm higher, an oval, high density mass behind the eye extending to the apex, was shown (Fig. 8). In coronal computerized tomography, an elongated oval, sharply outlined, high density mass was shown. In successive sections, a mass extending posteriorly was identified with the entire course of the superior rectus and levator muscle. The diagnosis in computerized tomography was hypertrophy of the levator-superior rectus muscle complex. At surgery, a tumor the size of the little finger was found above the eye ball, extending backward. The tumor was dark reddish, and soft. It was easily separated from the adjacent tissues. The appearance was not like that of a normal muscle. Under the light microscope (Fig. 9), marked hyaline changes and swelling of muscle fibers were observed. Fibrosis and lymphocytic infiltration in the stroma were seen. Histopathological diagnosis was orbital myositis.

348

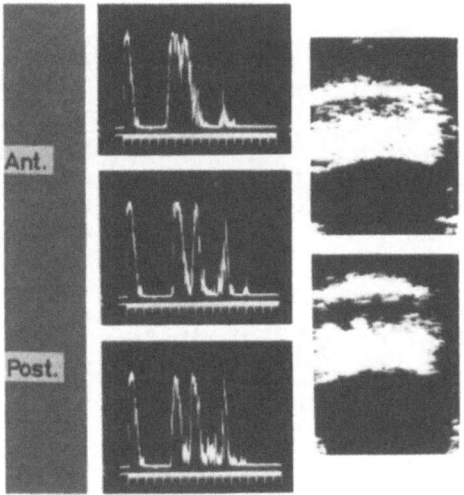

Fig. 7. A- and B-scan echograms in 12 o'clock meridian in Case 5.

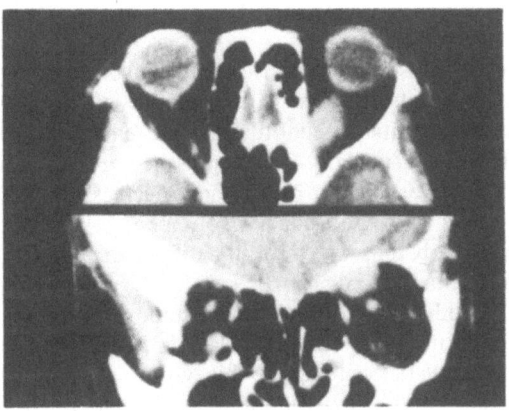

Fig. 8. Axial and coronal computerized tomograms.

DISCUSSION

Clinical manifestations, pathology and diagnosis of orbital pseudotumor have been reviewed by Jakobiec & Jones (1979). Orbital myositis has been proposed as a specific pseudotumor, because extraocular muscles are predominantly involved, although other orbital tissues are not free from the inflammatory process. Orbital myositis is believed to be a legitimate subtype of idiopathic inflammatory pseudotumor and to be not always due to Graves' disease. Orbital myositis tends to be unilateral. Bilaterality should cause one to suspect a systemic disease or endocrine exophthalmos. In orbital myositis

Fig. 9. Light micrograph of the levator muscle.

the inferior rectus muscle is most frequently involved, either alone or with other muscles. This is also the case with endocrine exophthalmos. Differential diagnosis between orbital pseudotumor and endocrine exophthalmos is frequently difficult, particularly in the presence of inflamatory signs in the anterior orbit. However, pain at onset, rapid decrease of vision, abnormality in the cerebrospinal fluid, occasional involvement of the first division of the trigeminal nerve, early onset of motility disturbance and rapid response to corticosteroid treatment are diagnostic keys.

Echographic findings in orbital pseudotumor have been discussed else-where. Pseudotumors form echographically a large group with lymphomas and sarcomas. Acoustic criteria of this group are low reflectivity, hard consistency, little sound attenuation and no vascularity. These malignant and benign lesions cannot be further differentiated with ultrasound (Ossoinig 1975). However, echographic findings specifically confined to orbital myositis, has been studied little.

Pattern of B-scan echography in orbital myositis of nonspecific etiology were described by Coleman (1972). Myositis was included in the same category as thyroid ophthalmopathy, pseudotumor and reactive lymphoid hyperplasia. Inflammatory changes could be diffuse or localized. The inflammatory tissue could form a discrete mass acoustically appearing to be a tumor, which was very difficult to be distinguished from a neoplastic tumor. In another paper, Coleman, *et al.* (1972) stressed that it was very important, and could be done only by echography, to demonstrate inflammatory edema in adjacent normal orbital structures in cases of myositis, sclerotenonitis and optic neuritis. In the B-scan echogram of Case 1 (Fig. 1) extremely low reflective area extending widely in the posterior of the eye ball is considered as a good presentation of marked enlargement of Tenon's space with edema fluid. Later Coleman, et al. (1977) suggested that misinterpretation of a rounded tumor for localized enlargement of a muscle would be avoided by serially delineating the exact extent of the target muscle. Ossoinig (1978) listed acute and chronic myositis as part of the conditions causing thickening of extraocular muscles without significant involvement in other orbital tissues in the unilateral eye. The exact cause of thickening of extraocular muscles could not be identified by echographic examination alone. Other symptoms and signs were to be considered. For example, in a case of acute myositis, echographic signs of episcleritis and clinical symptoms of pain or lid swelling were to be noted.

Based on findings in A- and B-scan echography in the present study, it is very interesting to investigate changes in the inner reflectivity of the target muscle as well as in its border, and compare the function and anatomical changes of the muscle with findings in echography.

Another approach to soft tissues – computerized tomography in orbital myositis – has been studied by Trokel & Hilal (1978), Jacobs, et al, (1980) and others. Trokel & Hilal showed axial computerized tomograms before and after corticosteroid treatment in a 22-year-old man with exophthalmos, local pain and injection, and mobility disturbance. The massively enlarged lateral rectus muscle before treatment was no longer present seven months later. For the analysis of muscle findings in computerized tomography, Jacobs, et al. divided orbital pseudotumor into myositic and nonmyositic groups. Further more, orbital myositis might be separated into two types, focal and diffuse. Casts on computerized tomograms were differently characteristic in both types of orbital myositis. The first case in the present paper corresponds to the diffuse type and the fifth case to the focal type of orbital myositis.

The conclusion drawn from the present five cases and the literature is that it is absolutely necessary to combine echography with axial and coronal computerized tomography in the diagnosis and in the evaluation of treatment of orbital myositis.

REFERENCES

Coleman, D.J. Reliability of ocular and orbital diagnosis with B-scan ultrasound. 2. orbital diagnosis. Am. J. Ophthalmol. 74: 704 (1972).

Coleman, D.J., Jack, R.L., Jones, I.S. & Franzen, L.A. High resolution B-scan ultrasonography of the orbit. VI. Pseudotumors of the orbit. A.M.A. Arch. Ophthalmol. 88: 472 (1972).

Coleman, D.J., Lizzi, F.L. & Jack, R.L. Ultrasonography of the eye and orbit. Philadelphia: Lea & Febiger (1977) p. 325.

Jacobs, L., Weisberg, L.A. & Kinkel, W.R. Computerized tomography of the orbit and sella turcica. New York: Raven Press (1980) p. 109.

Jakobiec, F.A. & Jones, I.S. Orbital inflammation. Clinical Ophthalmology: Vol. 2 (35) New York: Harper & Row (1979).

Ossoinig, K.C. A-scan echography and orbital disease. Orbital disorders. Basel: Karger (1975) p. 203.

Ossoinig, K.C. The role of clinical echography in modern diagnosis of periorbital and orbital lesions. Proc. 3rd Int. Symp. Orbital Disorders. The Hague: Dr. W. Junk bv Publishers (1978) p. 496.

Trokel, S.L. & Hilal, S.K. Thin section computerized tomography: analysis of 600 orbit studies. Proc. 3rd Int. Symp. Orbital Disorders. The Hague: Dr. W. Junk bv Publishers (1978) p. 107.

Authors' Address:
Department of Ophthalmology
Miyazaki Medical College
Kihara, Kiyotake, Miyazaki 889-16
Japan

B-SCAN ULTRASONOGRAPHY IN OPTIC NEUROPATHY

C.H. KERLEN

(*Utrecht, The Netherlands*)

INTRODUCTION

The purpose of this study has been an investigation of the reliability of ultrasonography in the diagnosis of retrobulbar neuritis. This type of optic neuropathy usually is diagnosed by means of subjective symptoms as there are:
  (1) A more or less sudden decrease of vision, mostly of one eye,
      accompanied by pain on ocular movements;
  (2) Development of a central scotoma;
  (3) Colour vision disturbances.
If the inflammation occurs in the trunk of the optic nerve it is likely that no
ophthalmoscopic changes are found and we may speak of a disease wherein
neither the patient nor the doctor sees anything. Therefore the diagnosis made
by means of these symptoms is almost completely patient-dependent.
Objective changes in the echographic pattern of the optic nerve could be produced in these cases by means of B-scan ultrasonography for the first time in
1972 (Coleman & Carroll 1972). They used the immersion type A and B mode
equipment developed earlier (Coleman, Konig & Katz 1969), commercially
available as the Ophthalmoscan. They described the pattern of the normal optic
nerve as a sonolucent (black) triangular notch in the (white) retrobulbar fat
tissue with smooth borders and an anterior angle of about 40 degrees (Fig. 1).
In retrobulbar neuritis (Fig. 2):
  (1) The outline is irregular in its anterior part;
  (2) There is an accentuation or even doubling of the optic nerve sheath;
  (3) Usually parallel to the posterior pole of the eye there is a group of
      echoes in the nerve.
It must now be emphasized that the findings with equipment other than
Coleman's could be different. Therefore, it is not justified that the results
should be compared with each other.

METHODS

In the University Eye Hospital at Utrecht we use the Ophthalmoscan 100
apparatus with the 10 MHz transducer because of the high resolution and
relatively good penetration of the ultrasound beam.

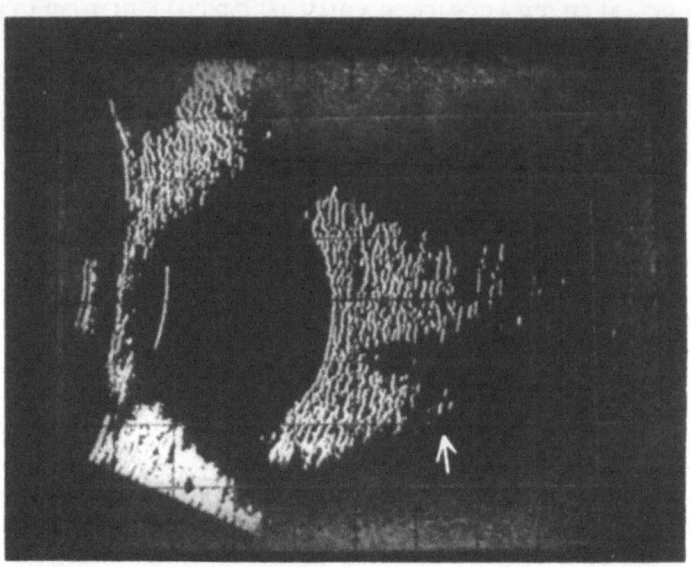

Fig. 1. Echographic pattern of normal optic nerve.

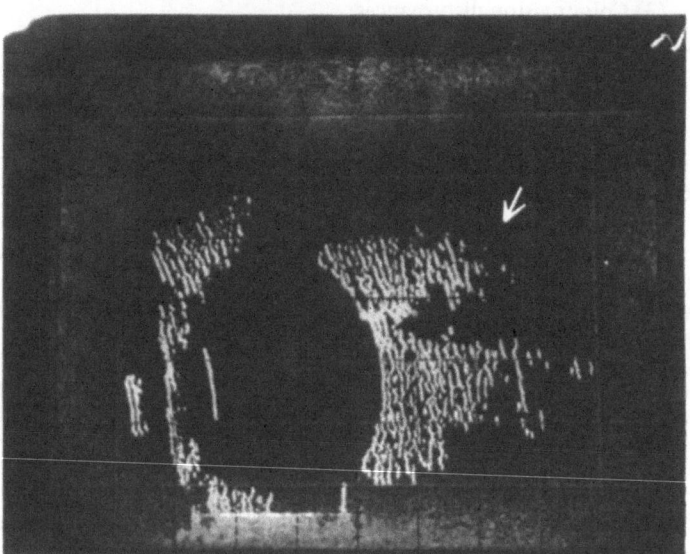

Fig. 2. Retrobulbar neuritis.

The patients were referred to us with the clinical diagnosis of suspected retrobulbar neuritis, with the question to confirm the diagnosis echographically or not. Later on, a complete neurological and internal examination was done, including cerebrospinal fluid analysis with special attention to the presence of subfraction of γ-globulin in it, as one of the characteristics of multiple sclerosis, which is the commonest cause of retrobulbar neuritis in our temperate climate. Therefore, the presence of multiple sclerosis could be used as a standard for establishing the echographic diagnosis of retrobulbar neuritis.

Table 1. Results in echographic diagnosis of retrobulbar neuritis.

		(44 patients)
32 (73%)	M.S.	neurological examination + CSF +
5 (11%)	M.S.	neurological examination + CSF − or unknown
4 (9%)	unknown	
3 (7%)	false,	2 false + 1 false −

RESULTS (Table 1)

Forty-four patients with 82 eyes were examined. Of these 44 patients one eye only was examined in six cases.

In 32 patients (73%) the diagnosis multiple sclerosis was neurologically established with positive CSF analysis.

In five patients (11%) the diagnosis was M.S. according to neurological examination notwithstanding negative CSF analysis.

In four cases (9%) the diagnosis remained uncertain neurologically: two patients refused lumbar puncture and two could not be traced further.

In three cases (7%) the diagnosis was false (two false positive and one false negative).

Therefore in 37 patients (84%) the echographic diagnosis of retrobulbar neuritis could be confirmed clinically by the presence of M.S. with a high degree of probability.

POSTSCRIPT

One case not really belonging to this series required our special attention: An 18-year-old boy was referred to us with a history of rapid decrease of vision with a central scotoma of the left eye, followed within a week by the same symptoms of the other eye, just resembling some cases of retrobulbar neuritis. However, the optic disc showed some congestion. The E.R.G. was normal, but the V.E.P. was negative. No neurological or internal disorder was found. There was no impairement of vision. It became apparent from pedigree study that this was a patient with Leber's optic atrophy. The ultrasonic nerve pattern of both eyes appeared to be different from that described above. The earlier affected left eye showed a small anterior angle with a smooth outline and a kind of bud at the extremity (Fig. 3 & 4). The

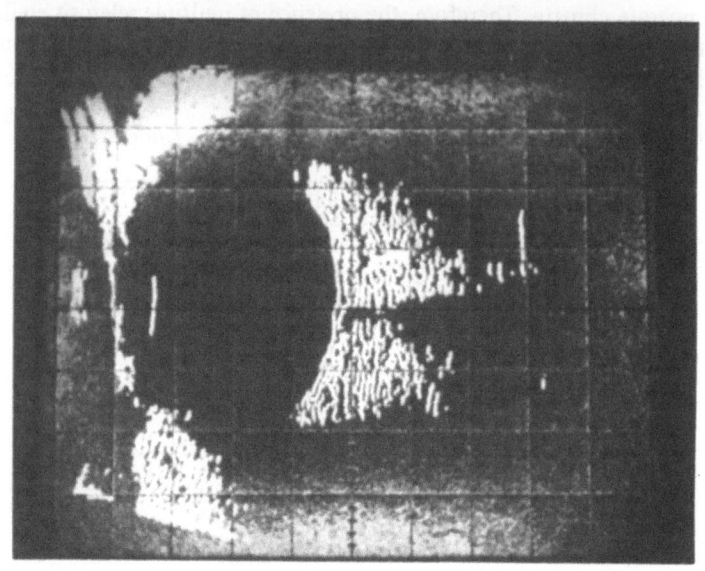

Fig. 3. Nerve pattern of earlier affected left eye in a case of **Leber's** optic atrophy.

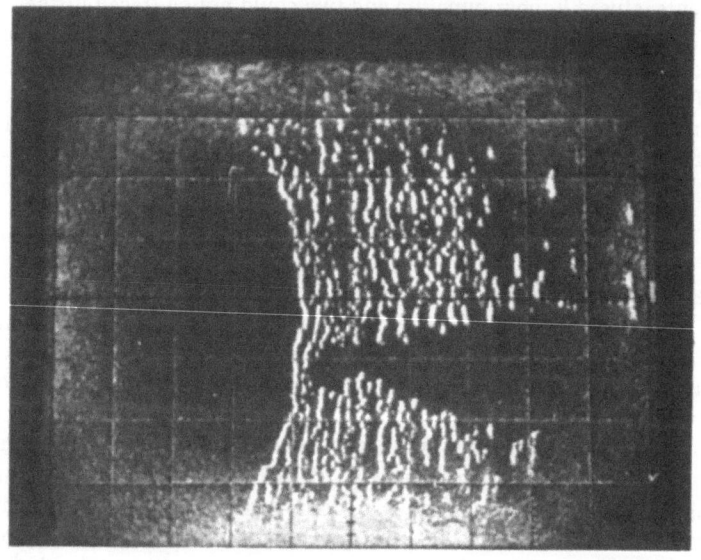

Fig. 4. Magnification of Fig. 3.

356

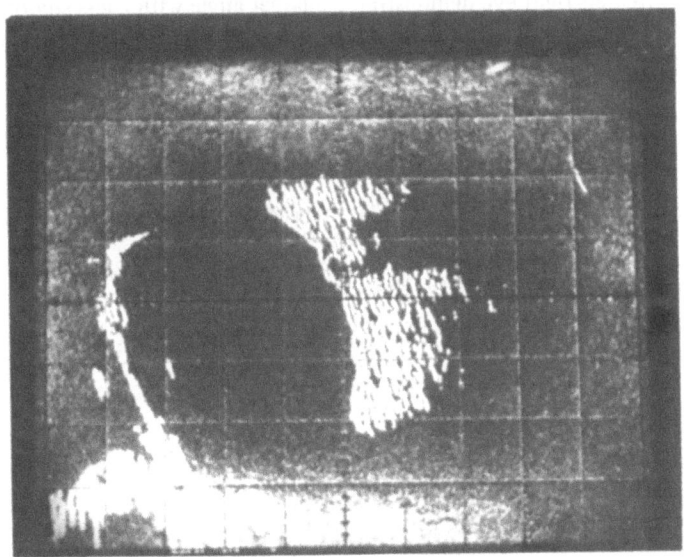

Fig. 5. Nerve pattern of later affected right eye in the same patient with Leber's optic atrophy.

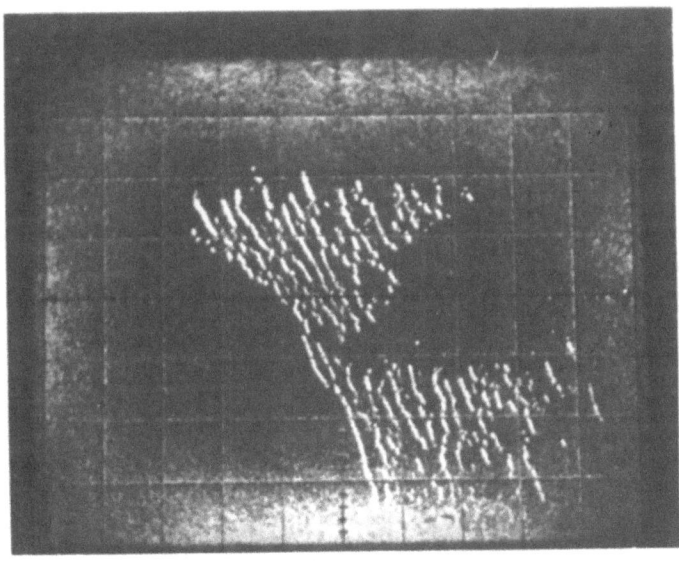

Fig. 6. Magnification of Fig. 5.

later affected right eye demonstrated a larger angle with a less smooth outline of the optic nerve but not as irregular as in retrobulbar neuritis (Fig. 5 & 6). As far as we know this picture has not been described before.

REFERENCES

Coleman, D.J., Konig, W.F. & Katz, L. A hand operated ultrasound scan system for ophthalmic evaluation. Am. J. Ophthalmol., 68: 256 (1969).

Coleman, D.J. & Carroll, F.D. A new technique for evaluation of optic neuropathy. Am. J. Ophthalmol., 74: 915 (1972).

Author's Address:
C.H. Kerlen
Oogleiders gasthuis
F.C. Dondersstraat 65
Utrecht, The Netherlands.

ULTRASONOGRAPHY OF THE OPTIC NERVE

Results of measuring the dural diameter

W. SCHROEDER & R. GUTHOFF

(Hamburg, F.R.G.)

INTRODUCTION

In the last ten years the following authors have written about ultrasonography of the optic nerve. Oksala's experimental results (1972) lead to the conclusion that the optic nerve could not be examined exactly by A-scan. Coleman (1972) & co-workers presented information about patterns in optic nerve lesions seen by B-scan. Ossoinig (at least in 1973) stated that the optic nerve could be determined exactly. Skalka (1976) — using Ossoinig's method — published the results of his measurement of the 'perineural space' of the optic nerve. Cohen & co-workers (1976) examined the cupping of the optic disc, and Fisher (1976) discovered, that drusen of the optic disc produce a characteristic spot of hyperreflectivity in contact B-scan. Mrs. Restori's C-scan (1977) enabled her to examine cross sections of the optic nerve. Our own technique of examination is deduced from Ossoinig's, but our experiences (7 years) seem to be different in some points. The results obtained in various optic nerve lesions will be presented in the following paper to evaluate their diagnostic help.

METHODS

Using the Kretz 7200 MA equipment we prefer to abduct the globe and place the transducer near the lateral corneal limbus in order to project the sound beam perpendicularly to the optic nerve. Our experiments using anatomical preparations have proved to us that in the cross-sectional ultrasonogram of the optic nerve the limiting echos are produced by the dura. Because the subarachnoidal space could rarely be demonstrated by us we have confined ourselves to the measurement of the dural diameter (DD). The average normal DD is 3.6 ($\pm$ 0.6) mm, which is based on a double running time of ultrasound of 4.7 ($\pm$ 0.9) μs. In practice the normal range is between 4 and 6 μs (six and more are pathologic). Comparing the right with the left optic nerve a difference of more than 0.5 μs is significant.

RESULTS

Congenital defects. In colobomata — especially in those which are hidden behind a cataract — B-scan shows the continuity between the vitreous cavity and the retrobulbar cystlike formation. This may be helpful if the foramen opticum is enlarged and the coloboma is to be differentiated from a glioma. By A-scan cystlike patterns and an increased DD can be found in both conditions. Drusen of the optic disc sometimes cause a swelling, which is to be differentiated from papilloedema (in intracranial hypertension). In these cases A-scan is helpful because it is the normal DD, which excludes intracranial hypertension. Drusen are directly detected by B-scan. Out of eight cases in which drusen were only suggested ophthalmoscopically, B-scan cleared up seven (Table 1).

Table 1. Optic Disc Drusen.

Drusen	Ophthalmoscopy	B-scan	A-scan (DD) [μs]
Clear	18	25	
Suggested	8	1	4.8 ± 0.6
n	26	26	

Table 2. Neuritis.

Neuritis	n	DD increased
Anterior	14	14
Posterior	25	17
	39	31

Inflammations. In anterior neuritis (that is, a neuritis with swelling of the disc) an increased DD is a constant finding during the first three weeks after onset of the illness. In posterior neuritis (that is, a neuritis without apparent disc symptoms) out of 25 cases 17 showed an increased DD (Table 2). During the course of neuritis the improvement of visual acuity runs nearly parallel to the normalizing of the DD.

Papillitis can be differentiated from anterior neuritis by a normal DD. The term papillitis could now be reserved to disc swelling caused by intraocular inflammations such as uveitis, retinochoroiditis etc.

Intradural compression. In intracranial hypertension papilloedema is strictly the intracranial pressure the DD becomes normal within a few days, whereas papilloedema ramains for several weeks (Table 3).

Another cause of intradural compression are the tumors of the optic nerve, in which the DD is permanently increased (Table 4). Monolateral gliomas showed an increased DD in all those cases in which the foramen opticum was enlarged. In two bilateral cases it failed on one side. In meningeomas of the optic nerve sheath, DD could be found to have increased, at least at the onset of visual loss. This persisted even though the initial papilloedema had turned

Table 3. Intracranial Hypertension.

	Papilloedema				DD increasing		
	n	monol.	bilat.	absent	monol.	bilat.	absent
Before treatment	22	2	20	0	4	18	0
After treatment	15	2	8	5	0	0	15

Table 4. Intradural Tumors.

Gliomas	11
for. opt. enlarged	13 (2 × bilat.)
DD increased	11
Meningeomas	8
optocil. veins	4
DD increased	8

Table 5. Extradural Compression.

Tumors	n	DD increased
of sinuses	18	
outside the muscle cone	16	
inside the muscle cone	23	3[†]
sphenoidal	14	12
Grave's Disease	80	4
Infiltrative Lesions	47	3

[†]In most cases DD could not be determined because of the dislocation of the optic nerve, which was demonstrated by B-scan.

to disc atrophy. The essential optociliary veins appear many years later. Leucemic infiltration may also occur intradurally. We observed one case: Visual acuity was counting fingers; there was a normal intracranial pressure, but the discs were pale and blurred. DD however was found to have increased markedly.

Extradural compression. It occurs mostly in orbital apex and sphenoidal tumors, seldom in swelling of the extraocular muscles in Graves' disease (Table 5). It regularly leads to an increasing of the DD, which can be noted before a swelling of the disc appears and which remains even when the optic disc becomes pale – provided the compression lasts.

Trauma. Indirect trauma caused an increase of DD in 3 of 8 cases, indicating a hematoma within the optic nerve sheath. In contrast to this, direct trauma in each case showed an enlarged DD.

Neuropathies. Acute neuropathies of ischemic, metabolic or hereditary origin do not change the dural diameter from normal.

Atrophy. The DD in optic atrophy of several types was compared. No significant decrease or increase of the DD was obtained, except under persisting compression.

CONCLUSIONS

Our results of our measurement of the dural diameter agree with the different patho-physiological conditions. The method is especially helpful in diseases with secundary changes of the optic disc, such as swelling or atrophy. It gives special information through follow-up in neuritis or optic nerve compression. Last, but not least, it completes the neuro-ophthalmological examination by adding quantitative results.

REFERENCES

Ossoinig, K.C. Echography of the eye. In: Radiology of the orbit (P.H. Arger, ed.) N.Y.: Wiley & Sons (1976).

Schroeder, W. Schallaufzeitmessung im distalen Sehnerfquerschnitt. Klin. Mbl. Augenheilk. 169: 743 (1976).

Schroeder, W. Ultrasonography of the optic nerve. Proc. 3rd Int. Symp. on orbital disorders (Amsterdam 1977), The Hague: Junk p.   (1978).

Schroeder, W. & Guthoff, R. Modellversuche zur Messung des Sehnerven. In: SIDUO VII (H. Gernet, ed.) Münster: Remy (1979) p.

Skalka, H.W. Ultrasonography of the optic nerve. In: Neuro-ophthalmology update (J.L. Smith, ed.) N.Y.: Masson (1977).

Authors' Address:
Eye Dept. Allgem. Krankenhaus Heidberg, (Dr. Schroeder)
Tangstedter Lstr. 400, D-2000 Hamburg 62
F.R.G.

University Eye Clinic (Dr. Guthoff)
Martinistr. 52, D-2000 Hamburg 20
F.R.G.

MOTILITY DISORDERS IN HIGH MYOPIA

I. PALLIKARIS, H. SPIESS, J. LANG & F. BIGAR

(*Zürich, Switzerland*)

Patients with high myopia can present motility disorders. Vertical imbalance with hypotropia and limitation of vertical excursion (HAEVY EYE, Donders 1864 Ward 1967) can be associated with horizontal deviations.

Echography and computerized tomography were used for the evaluation of the rectus muscles in six high myopic patients with motility disorders, and in 23 patients presenting no manifest motility abnormalities. Five of the six patients had previous unsuccessful surgery of the horizontal muscles. Computerized tomography gives information on the anatomical relationship between the shape of the globe, the rectus muscles and the orbital walls, whereas, A-scan echography (Ossoinig 1977) permits measurements of the rectus muscle thickness.

In all six patients with high myopia (minimum-11 D, maximum-22 D) with motility disorders the upper and lateral parocular space was found to be extremely narrow and the superior and lateral rectus thinned. In one patient the superior rectus muscle was nasally displaced. Examples of the two classes of patients are shown in Figs. 1 & 2.

DISCUSSION

The disproportion between the size of myopic globes and the orbital volume can cause firstly a mechanical dismotility of the eye and secondly a thinning of the muscle by abnormal pressure within the narrow parocular space. Squint surgery in such cases is therefore often disappointing. The chronic pressure leads to a fibrotic degeneration of the muscle as demonstrated by Hugonnier & Magnard (1960). Haevy eye syndrome and horizontal motility limitation in high myopic patients are caused by mechanical reasons.

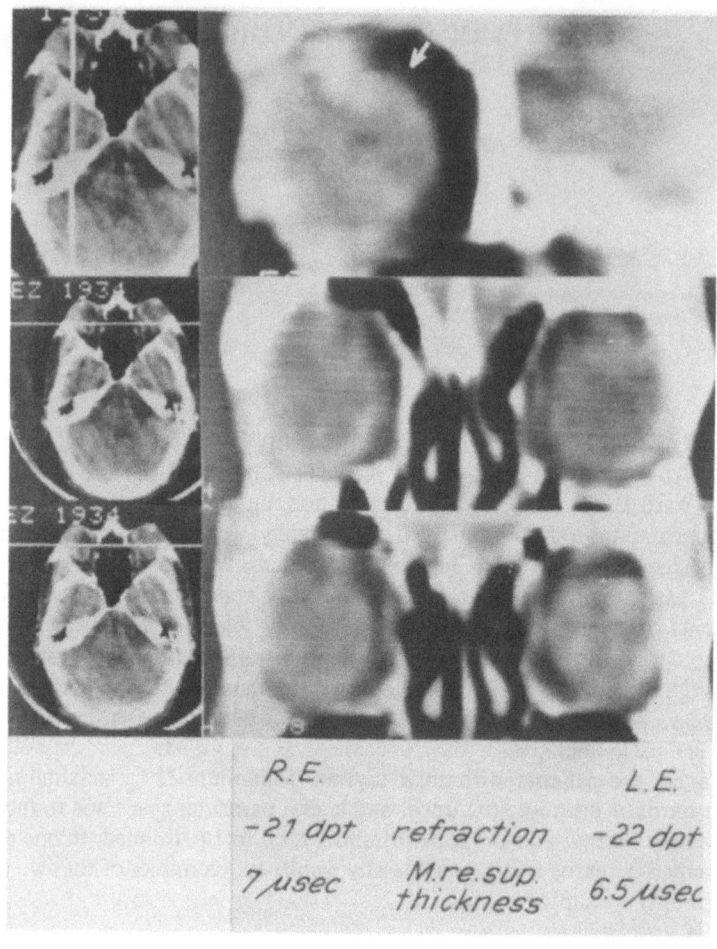

Fig. 1. High myopia without motility disorders

Arrow: Free space between
orbital upper-wall and sclera
for the Muscle Rectus-Superior.

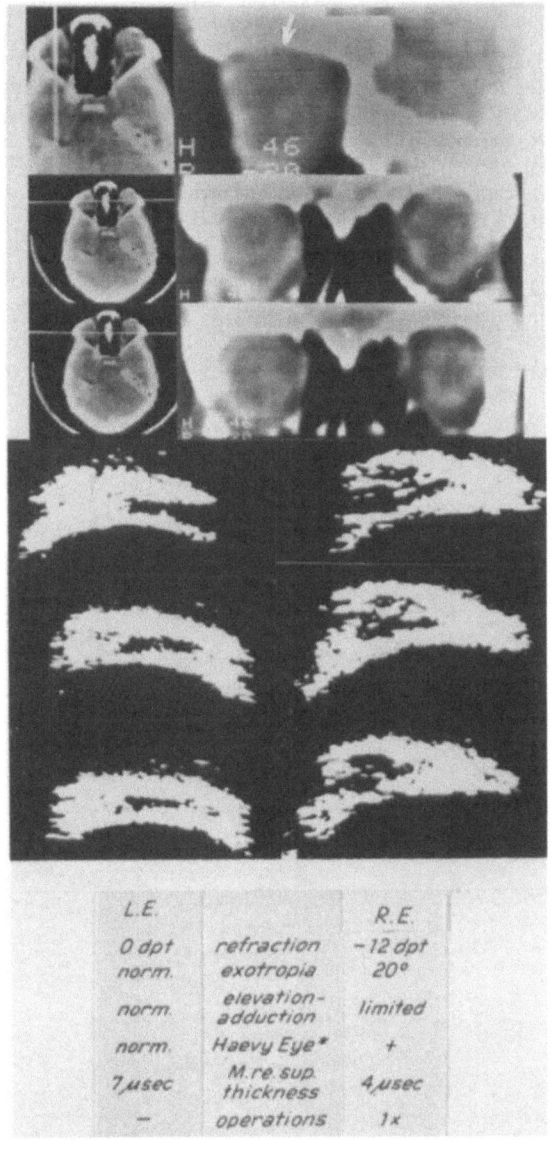

Fig. 2. Left eye highly myopic (Haevy Eye Syndrome), thin superior rectus muscle.

Arrow: No space between
orbital upper-wall and sclera.

REFERENCES

Ward. The Haevy Eye Syndrom, Trans. Ophthalmol. Soc. V.K. 87: 717 (1967).

Donders, On the Anomalies of accomodation and Refraction of the Eye. (bibl) London (1864).

Hugonnier, & Magnard. The nervous syndrome of high myopia. Bull. Soc. Franc. Ophthalmol. 73: 80 (1960).

Ossoinig, K.C. Echograph of the eye, orbit, and periorbital region In: Orbit Roetgenology (P.H. Arger, ed.) New York: Wiley (1977) p. 224

Authors' Address:
University Eye Clinic
Kantonsspital, Zürich, Switzerland
Present address:
Philellinon 9, GR. – Thessaloniki, Greece

ECHOGRAPHIC FINDINGS IN 34 PATIENTS WITH CHOROIDAL FOLDS

A.M. VERBEEK

(Nijmegen, The Netherlands)

INTRODUCTION

Choroidal folds are lines or grooves of the posterior fundus often arranged in a horizontal parallel fashion, seldom vertical or oblique, and seldom extending beyond the equator. For a long time they have been considered as a characteristic, although uncommon, sign of expanding orbital tumors (Vedel-Jensen 1959, Wolter 1974).

In 1969 Norton described the typical fluoresceinangiographic picture of this condition. A better detection of choroidal folds and differentiation from retinal folds was then achieved (Norton 1969, von Winning 1973). The concept that orbital tumors alone could give choroidal folding faded away in the period 1968–1979. In this period case histories of patients appeared with this symptom, showing only ocular disease or sometimes no proven pathologic condition (Hyvärinen 1970, Bird 1973, Newell 1973, Cappaert 1977, Gangemi 1977, Benson 1979). It also became evident that regression of the folding is possible (Kroll, Norton 1970) and that in case of orbital tumors the location of the folds is not of great value in localising the tumor (Newell 1973). The first purpose of this paper is to review all cases of choroidal folds and their etiology in literature and our own cases observed over the last three years. The second purpose is to show that diagnostic ultrasound can be very helpful in finding the cause.

When we review the etiology of the cases in the literature we can see that in only 26% an orbital cause was found; in 45% an ocular and in 15% C.N.S. disease was responsible for the folding. In 10% no reason could be found. (Table 1). In the *orbital cases* Graves disease, sinus disease and cavernous hemangioma are frequently found; in six cases no explanation for the exophthalmus and folding could be found. (Table 2). In the *ocular cases* hypermetropia, macular degeneration, hypotony and posterior scleritis have a high score. (Table 3). In central nervous system disease papilloedema of different etiology caused folding of the retinal pigment epithelium layer and Bruch's membrane in the surroundings of the optic disc (Bird 1973) (Table 4). In the last three years in our institute choroidal folds were seen in 34 patients, in 45 eyes, therefore 11 bilateral cases. (Table 5).

We excluded from this series patients with folds after buckle procedure

Table 1.

Etiology of choroidal folds	Literature
	No. of eyes
– Ocular	78
– Orbital	45
– C.N.S.	26
– e.c.i.	18
	167

Table 2.

Etiology of choroidal folds	Literature
Orbital cases	
	No. of eyes
– M. Graves	11
– Sinusitis	5
– Mucocele	2
– Haemangioma	6
– Pseudotumor	5
– Misc. tumors	8
– Exophth. e.c.i.	6

Table 3.

Etiology of choroidal folds	Literature
Ocular cases	
	No. of eyes
– Hypermetropia	17
– Macular degeneration	12
– Hypotony	12
– Posterior scleritis	9
– Post buckle procedure	9
– Trauma	6
– Tumor	3
– Miscellaneous	10
	78

and after cataract or fistulizing surgery. All patients had fluoresceinangiography and diagnostic ultrasound examination to start with. Our ultrasound equipment is a combination of a standardised A-scan Kretchtechniek 7200 MA and a Bronson-Turner real time B-scanner. Ultrasound diagnosis was made following the criteria of Ossoinig (Ossoinig 1974). At the ultrasound examination the following items were investigated. (Table 6). We found an ocular cause in nearly 45% of the cases. In this group we also frequently found hypermetropia (small axial length), normal posterior globe curvature, no signs of orbital sinus or ocular disease. (Fig. 1a, b). (Table 7). In only 20% an orbital cause was found. In the case of astrocythoma and neuroblastoma we were unable to differentiate the tissue. (Table 8).

In 16% CNS disease caused folding of the choroid. Three times we found a

Table 4.

Etiology of choroidal folds	Literature
C.N.S.	No. of eyes
12 patients with bilater papilloedema by raised intracranial pressure	24
2 patients with unilateral papillitis	2
	26

Table 5.

Etiology choroidal folds		Nijmegen
	No. of eyes	
Orbital	9	No. of patients: 34
Ocular	20	
C.N.S.	7	No. of bilateral
Spec. group	9	choroidal folds: 11
	45	

Table 6.

Choroidal folds

Ultrasound examination of both eyes:

A-scanning: Kretztechnik 7200 MA
 – axial length
 – periorbital bone ('sound permeability')
 – extraocular rectus muscle size
 – optic nerve size
 – paraocular/transocular examination for mass lesion

B-scanning: Bronson-Turner
 – curvature posterior part of the globe
 – thickening of the posterior coats
 – retrobulbar edema
 – topografic examination for mass lesion

Table 7.

Etiology of choroidal folds	Nijmegen
Ocular	No. of eyes
Hypermetropia bilateral	8
Hypermetropia unilateral	1
Harada/Chor. effusion	5
Choroidal metastasis	1
Post trauma	2
Subretinal haemorrhage	1
Senile mac. degen.	1
Prominent process e.c.i.	1
	20

369

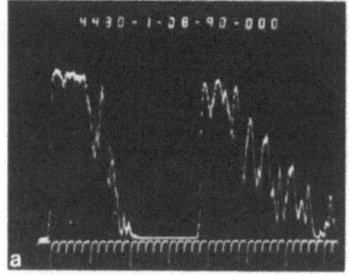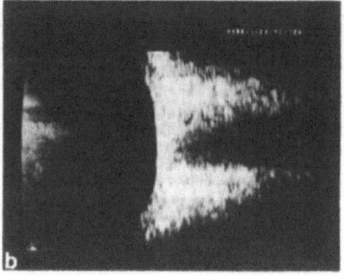

Fig. 1a. A-scan of 18.8 mm eye at central application of a patient with bilateral hypermetropia (+ 8 D) and choroidal folds.
   b. B-scan of the same eye with *normal* posterior pole curvature.

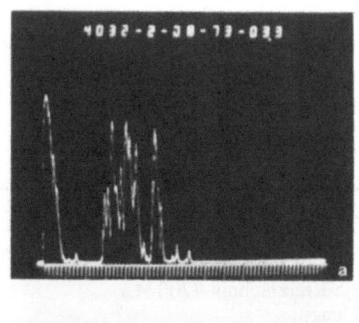

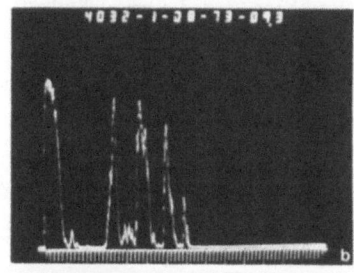

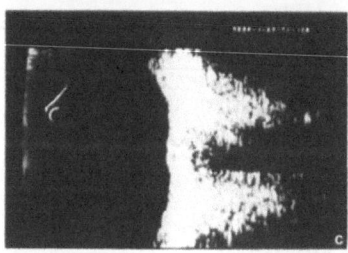

Fig. 2a. A-scan: normal optic nerve diameter
   b. A-scan: thickened optic nerve in a case of optic neuritis with choroidal folds.
   c. B-scan: papilloedema in case of optic neuritis with choroidal folds.

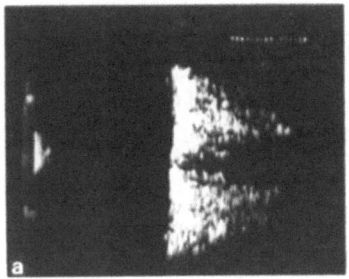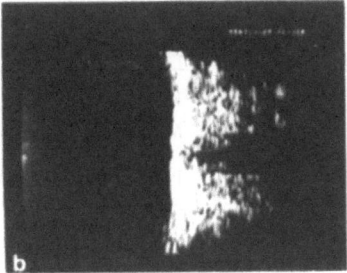

Fig. 3. Flattening of the posterior part of the globe.
  a. B-scan through the lens.
  b. B-scan by passing the lens (so flattening not an acoustic artefact of the lens).

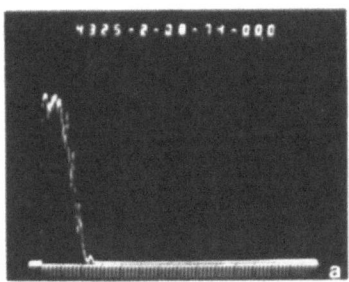

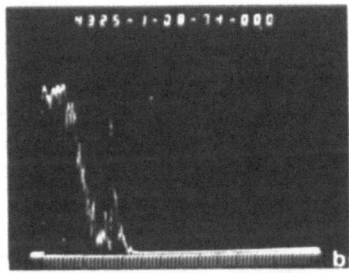

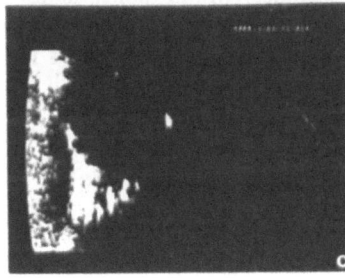

Fig. 4a. Normal A-scan pattern of sinus area. Sound probe perpendicular to maxillary bone
  b. Pathologic A-scan pattern of sinus area. Sound probe perpendicular to maxillary bone (sound permeability 'of the bone').
  c. B-scan pattern of pathologic sinus area.

371

Table 8.

Etiology of choroidal folds	Nijmegen
Orbital	No. of eyes
– M. Graves	2
– Mixed tumor	1
– Polyposis sinu-orbital	1
– Mucocele	2
– Muscle haematoma	1
– Neuroblastoma	1
– Astrocythoma IV	1
	9

Table 9.

Etiology of choroidal folds	Nijmegen
C.N.S.	No. of eyes
Benign intracranial hypertension	2
Intracranial tumor, papilloedema	2
Unilateral optic neuritis	3
	7

unilateral neuritis responsible. (Fig. 2a, b, c). (Table 9). Reviewing the files, the patient histories, the findings of routine ophthalmic examinations, having in mind the articles of Hyvärinen-Walsh and Cappaert-Purnell-Frank about benign choroidal folds we also found a special group covering 19% of our cases having many signs and symptoms in common. Clinically and echographic Table 10 and Table 11.

The flattening of the posterior part of the globe is shown in Fig. 3a, b and the 'sound permeability' of the bones in the sinus area in Fig. 4a, b. No signs of orbital mass lesion retrobulbar oedema, thickening of the posterior coats, and endocrinologically no signs for the existence of Graves disease were found.

CONCLUSIONS

As explanation for these findings, we think, like Hyvärinen and Cappaert, that chronic sinus disease, with and without symptoms, with and without roentgenological signs spreads in the orbit giving muscle and nerve swelling and scleral alterations (shrinkage) resulting in so called benign-choroidal folds. In our series of 34 patients in only three cases a real orbital tumor (or tumor expanding in the orbit) was responsible for choroidal folding.

Table 10.

Choroidal folds	Special group
Echographically:	
– Axial length	7/7
– Flattening posterior part of the globe	7/7
– Thickening posterior coats	0/7
– Sound permeability of the bones in the sinus area	4/7
– Thickened rectus muscle(s)	4/7
– Thickened optic nerve	6/7
– Retrobulbar oedema/mass lesion	0/7

Table 11.

Choroidal folds	Special group
Clinically:	
– Blurred vision	6/7
– Metamorphopsia	3/7
– Hypermetropia, hypermetropisation	7/7
– Horizontal folds pap. mac.	7/7
– Slight atypical visual field alterations	7/7
– Proptosis	0/7
– Motility disturbance	0/7
– History: sinus disease anterior scleritis	0/7

REFERENCES

Benson, W.E., Shields, J.A., Tasman, W. et al. Posterior scleritis, a cause of diagnostic confusion. Arch. Ophthalmol. 97: 1482 (1979).

Bird, A.C. & Sanders, M.A. Choroidal folds in association with papiloedema. Br. J. Ophthalmol. 57: 89 (1973).

Bullock, J.D. & Egbert, P.R. Experimental choroidal folds. Am. J. Ophthalmol. 78: 618 (1974).

Cappaert, W.E., Purnell, E.W. & Frank, K.E. Use of B-scan ultrasound in the diagnosis of benign choroidal folds. Am. J. Ophthalmol. 84: 375 (1977).

Dellaporta, A. Fundus changes in postoperative hypotony. Am. J. Ophthalmol. 40: 781 (1955).

Gangemi, F.E., Trempe, C.L. & Walsh, J.B. Choroidal folds. Am. J. Ophthalmol. 86: 380 (1978).

Hyvärinen, L. & Walsh, F.B. Benigne chorioretinal folds. Am. J. Ophthalmol. 70: 14 (1970).

Kroll, A.J. & Norton, E.W. Regression of choroidal folds. Trans. Am. Acad. Ophthalmol. & Otolaryng. 74: 515 (1970).

Newell, F.W. Choroidal folds. Am. J. Ophthalmol. 75: 930 (1973).

Norton, E.W. A characteristic fluorescein angiographie pattern in choroidal folds. Lang. Lecture. Proc. Roy. Soc. Med. 62: 119 (1969).

Ossoinig, K.C. & Blody, F.C. Pre-operative differential diagnosis of tumors with echography, part III. Intra-ocular tumor. Part IV Orbital tumors. (F.C. Blody, ed.) Current Concepts Ophthalmol Vol. 4 (17): 296 St. Louis: Mosbry (1974).

Vedel-Jensen, N. Retinal grooves caused by pressure of the globe. Acta Ophthalmologica (1959) p. 59.

Von Winning, C.H.O.M. Fluography of choroidal folds. 165th Neth. Soc. Meeting, The Hague, 167: 436 (1973).

Wolter, J.R. Parallel horizontal choroidal folds secondary of an orbital tumor. Am. J. Ophthalmol. 77: 669 (1974).

Author's Address:
Institute of Ophthalmology
University of Nijmegen
Philips van Leydenlaan 15
6500 HB Nijmegen
The Netherlands.

374

ULTRASONOGRAPHY AND PERCUTANEOUS ORBITAL ASPIRATION

H.W. SKALKA

(Birmingham, Alabama, U.S.A.)

Ultrasonically-guided percutaneous needle biopsy or aspiration is a well-established technique in abdominal and thoracic diagnosis (Elyaderani & Skolnick 1978, Wolf 1978, Reynes, *et al.* 1977, Goldberg 1978). Schyberg (1975), Westman-Naeser & Naeser (1978), Kennerdell, *et al.* (1979, 1980), and Spoor, *et al.* (1980), have described the technique of aspiration biopsy in orbital tumors, and Jakobiec & Chattock have used a similar technique for biopsy of tumors of the lid (Jakobiec & Chattock 1979), as well as for intra-ocular mass lesions (Jakobiec & Chattock 1978, Jakobiec, *et al.* 1979). The ophthalmic interest in this technique has centered exclusively on tissue diagnosis of mass lesions by the provision of biopsy material suitable for histologic examination.

The *therapeutic* possibilities of percutaneous ultrasonically-guided needle aspiration in selected cases of cystic orbital mass lesions have not heretofore been emphasized. While useful in terms of providing fluid biopsy material for confirmation (or alteration) of the diagnosis made on ultrasound (or other diagnostic) examination, the decompression of these cystic masses, which are often difficult to eradicate surgically without producing profound functional and cosmetic morbidity, provides temporary or permanent improvement or cure.

Four cases of cystic mass lesions of the orbit are herein briefly described. In each case, the original diagnosis was made (or substantiated) by pre-aspiration quantitative A-scan (Kretztechnik 7200 MA) and contact B-scan (Bronson-Turner) ultrasonography. After ultrasound localization, percutaneous needle aspiration was performed in each case, when appropriate under real-time contact B-scan guidance of the aspirating needle.

CASE 1

A two year old white female was referred with a six week history of slight ptosis and proptosis OS secondary to 'a mass in the orbit'. There was no history of trauma, and standard x-ray views of the orbits were reported as 'normal'. Ultrasonography revealed a firm, slightly compressible cystic mass lesion of low internal reflectivity in the superior orbit OS. Septae were present in one small part of the mass. A fluid-filled cyst, felt not to be a dermoid, was diagnosed, and percutaneous aspiration under B-scan guidance yielded 2 cc of slightly turbid brown fluid, with resolution of the patient's mild proptosis OS. Laboratory investigation revealed the fluid to contain hemolyzed red blood cells and some white blood cells. No tumor cells were identified. The patient's ptosis has since resolved.

CASE 2

A ten year old white female (Skalka & Callahan 1979a) was referred with a history of proptosis OD, stable for at least the preceding six months. Orbital x-rays, said to be 'normal', actually showed slight relative enlargement of the right orbit. The patient's birth had been difficult, and some facial bruising was apparently present at delivery; there was no other history of trauma; five mm of proptosis OD was present. Ultrasound examination OD revealed a firm cystic mass, located mainly in the nasal retrobulbar muscle cone (Fig. 1). The history, x-ray findings and ultrasound examination suggested a blood cyst, likely dating from birth trauma.

The patient underwent a modified (Wright 1976) lateral orbitotomy with drainage of approximately 6 cc of thick, chocolate-brown fluid and excision of as much of the cyst wall as could easily and atraumatically be performed.

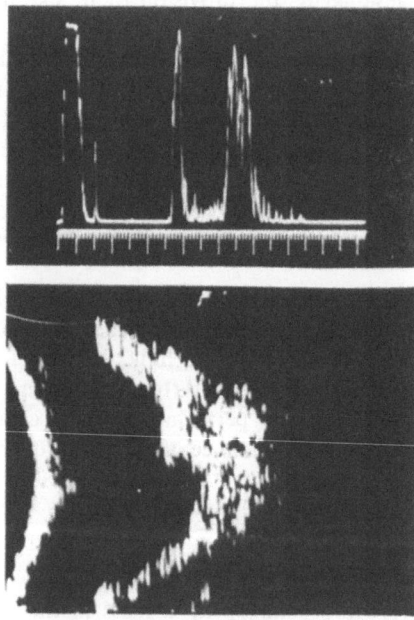

Fig. 1. Case 2: A-scan (tissue sensitivity) above, contact B-scan (80 db) below (probe oriented vertically) OD. Probes on temporal sclera, beams directed posteronasally. Large cystic mass may be seen in nasal muscle cone area.

376

The fluid which was drained stained strongly positive for iron, and sections of the cyst wall showed no evidence of an epithelial or endothelial lining. Over the next eight months, the patient's proptosis OD gradually returned, and repeat ultrasound examination showed a picture identical to that seen on the initial examination, except temporally and inferotemporally (the areas of the previous surgical excision). Percutaneous needle aspiration yielded approximately 5 cc of fluid, with marked resolution of proptosis. The proptosis OD again gradually recurred over the next several months, and a medial orbitotomy was performed with removal of more of the lesion wall and drainage of a copious amount of thick brown fluid (hemolyzed old blood). Immediately post-operatively no proptosis was present, but two months later the patient's right eye was again proptotic. Examination revealed significant proptosis OD, and ultrasound examination revealed large cystic spaces limited to the superior orbit and extending back to the apex (Fig. 2). Percutaneous aspiration yielded 4 cc of blood with decrease of proptosis. Visual acuity has remained at 20/20.

CASE 3

A 13 year old white male (Skalka & Callahan 1979b) had undergone exploratory orbital surgery OD elsewhere at age two for proptosis. An orbital lymphangioma was found, but could only be partially resected. The patient

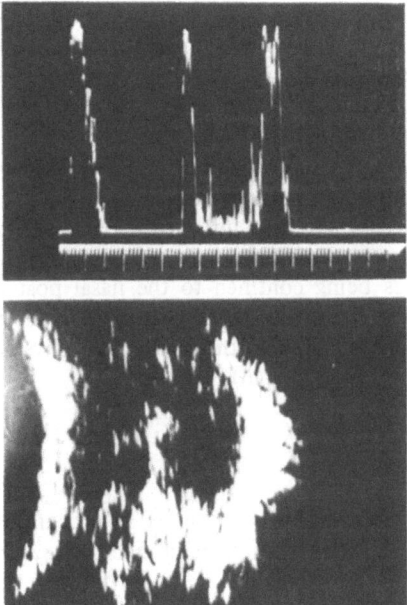

Fig. 2. Case 2: A-scan (tissue sensitivity) above, contact B-scan (80 db) below (probe oriented horizontally) OD. Probes on inferior sclera, beams directed superoposteriorly. Cystic spaces may be seen in superior orbit posteriorly.

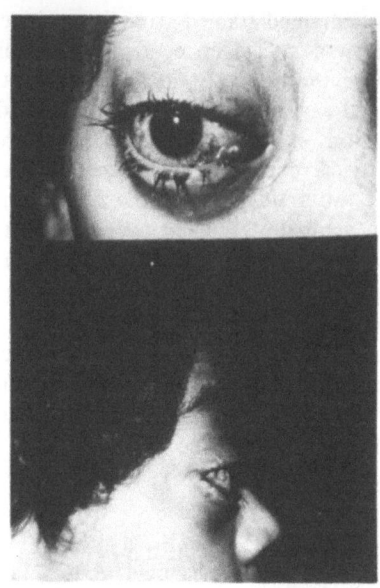

Fig. 3. Case 3: Appearance of proptotic OD before first aspiration.

was referred to us because of right orbital discomfort and increased proptosis (Fig. 3) following mild trauma. Ultrasonography OD revealed large cystic spaces filling the middle and posterior orbit. Our diagnosis was hemorrhage into the lymphangioma, and percutaneous needle aspiration of 15 cc of blood resulted in return of the patient's usual appearance (Fig. 4).

Six months later, the patient returned with severe proptosis and pain OD (Fig. 5). Two attempts at percutaneous aspiration were unsuccessful, and the patient was referred for repeat ultrasound examination. At this time, only diffuse hemorrhage was present in the anterior orbital tissues, with residual large cystic spaces being confined to the nasal posterior orbit. With these ultrasound findings, a long needle was directed to the nasal orbital apex and 20 cc of blood was aspirated, with resultant symptomatic relief and marked improvement of proptosis (Fig. 6).

CASE 4

A 39 year old Negro male (Skalka, *et al.* In preparation) was struck on the left brow, resulting in a subconjunctival hemorrhage and superficial lid skin abrasion OS. Two months later, marked proptosis developed OS (Fig. 7). X-rays were said to be 'negative', and the patient was referred for ultrasound examination. A massive cystic lesion of the posterior orbit was found OS (Fig. 8), and a cystic hematoma was diagnosed. Percutaneous aspiration of 10 cc of hemolyzed blood resulted in complete resolution of the patient's proptosis.

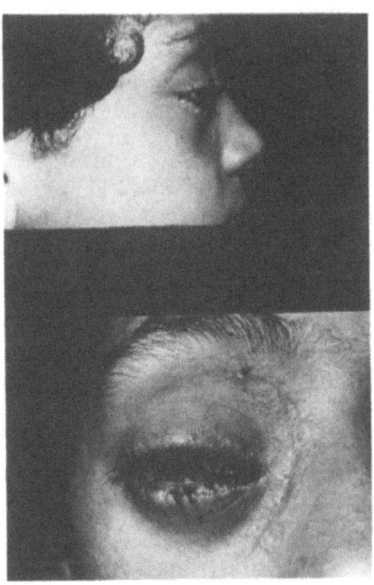

Fig. 4. Case 3: Patient's 'usual' appearance OD immediately after needle aspiration of 15 cc of non-clotting blood.

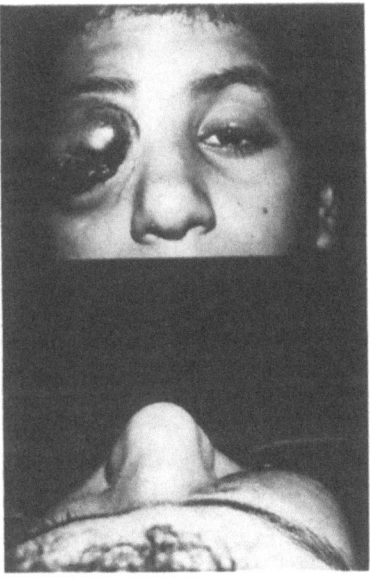

Fig. 5. Case 3: Patient's appearance before ultrasonically-guided needle aspiration.

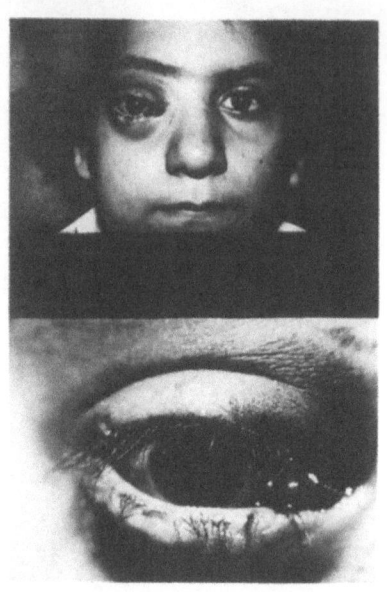

Fig. 6. Case 3: Appearance one week post-aspiration of 20 cc of blood.

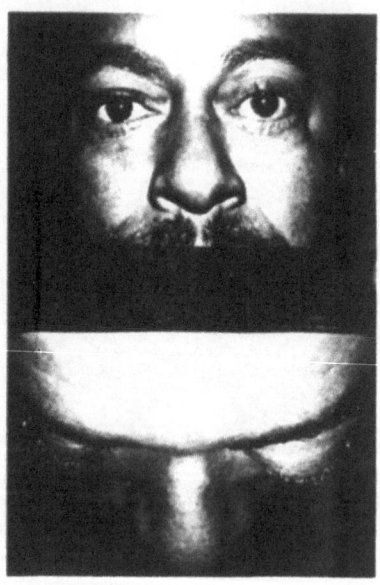

Fig. 7. Case 4: Patient's appearance, showing 10 mm of proptosis OS.

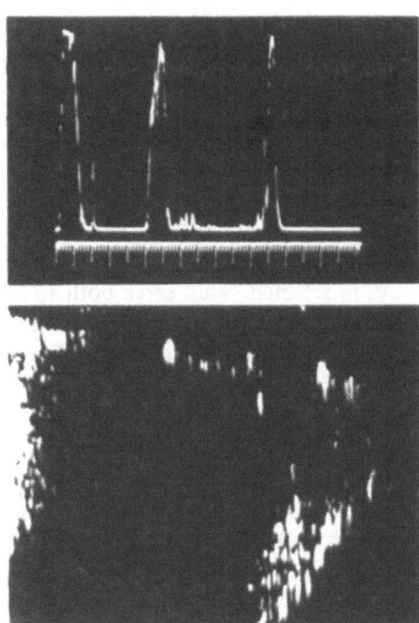

Fig. 8. Case 4: A-scan (tissue sensitivity) above, contact B-scan (80 db) below (probe oriented obliquely) OS. Probes placed on inferior sclera, beams directed superoposteriorly. Massive cystic lesion of superoposterior orbit may be seen.

Three months later, the patient again sustained trauma about his left eye, and his proptosis OS returned. Needle aspiration again relieved the proptosis, but repeat trauma ten days later produced epistaxis, and proptosis which was twice tapped and twice reformed. The patient was referred for repeat ultrasound examination.

The ultrasound examination was essentially unchanged, except for the finding of a bone defect in the superonasal orbit posteriorly. X-rays were obtained which showed 'indistinctness of the left sphenoid bone', and the patient was returned to his referring ophthalmologist for further work-up.

Neurosurgical evaluation (and subsequent surgery) disclosed an epidural hematoma communicating via a break in the left sphenoid bone with the cystic hematoma of the left orbit.

DISCUSSION

Ultrasonography, properly utilized and interpreted, is the most effective modality available for the detection, localization and diagnosis of orbital mass lesions. Together with computed tomography, it has made exploratory orbital surgery little more than a historical curiosity.

While quantitative A-scan can diagnose orbital mass lesions with a high degree of reliability (Ossoinig & Blodi 1974), some lesions do not lend themselves to precise ultrasonic differentiation (e.g. inflammatory pseudo-tumor vs. lymphoma), and a histologic diagnosis is always desirable, even in cases of benign lesions not generally considered surgical diseases. The adaptation of ultrasonically-guided percutaneous biopsy to ophthalmic mass lesions is commendable, and has already proven to be of value (Schyberg 1975, Westman-Naeser & Naeser 1978, Kennerdell, *et al.* 1979, Kennerdell, *et al.* 1980, Spoor, *et al.* 1980, Jakobiec & Chattock 1979, Jakobiec & Chattock 1978, Jakobiec, *et al.* 1979). Therapeutic aspiration of cystic orbital mass lesions utilizing ultrasound localization or under actual ultrasound guidance may, in selected cases, serve both to confirm a diagnosis and to decompress a mass lesion without recourse to the major operative procedure of orbital surgery, with its attendant morbidity.

Potentially toxic material, such as dermoid or hydatid cyst contents, should obviously not be aspirated, as liberation of these cyst contents into the orbital tissues via the cyst puncture wound or aspirating needle track may produce a marked inflammatory response. Careful pre-aspiration ultrasonography is therefore essential for the selection of cases amenable to this procedure. The presence of major arterial blood flow (e.g. A-V fistula) may be evaluated by A-scan or Doppler methods. The presence of a wall or capsule of demonstrable thickness (as opposed to a discrete surface only) may be determined, as well as the compressibility or rigidity of the lesion in question. Acoustic homogeneity or heterogeneity of the mass should be evaluated (e.g. septae as in an angiomatous lesion, or stronger reflectors as may be found within a dermoid or hydatid cyst). History, clinical findings, and radiologic or other studies will often provide additional information helpful in deciding whether percutaneous aspiration is appropriate in each individual case.

In our experience, sharp needles with short bevels have proven most useful (a large gauge needle would only be required for cases in which the fluid to be aspirated was very viscous). Longer-bevelled needles appear to be more prone to obstruction by cyst septae or walls, and require more rotatory movements for continued aspiration.

As demonstrated by the cases herein presented, percutaneous aspiration may be palliative rather than curative. However, many of these cystic orbital masses do not lend themselves to easy surgical extirpation short of orbital exenteration or craniotomy. If repeat aspirations become necessary, repeat ultrasonography should be performed to demonstrate the current configuration of the lesion to be aspirated.

In selected cases, ophthalmic ultrasonography can establish the presence, location, and probable nature of cystic orbital masses amenable to percutaneous needle aspiration; and can guide the aspiration procedure itself. This technique allows both diagnosis and therapy without the necessity of performing extensive and sometimes mutilating orbital surgery.

REFERENCES

Elyaderani, M.K. & Skolnick, L. Ultrasonic detection of abdominal abscesses and verification by percutaneous aspiration, Ultrasound in Medicine, Vol. 4, New York & London: Plenum Press, (1978) p. 167.

Goldberg, B.G. Ultrasonic aspiration biopsy techniques, Handbook of Clinical Ultrasound (de Vlieger, et al., eds.) New York: John Wiley & Sons (1978) p. 387.

Jakobiec, F.A. & Chattock, A. Aspiration cytodiagnosis of lid tumors. Arch. Ophthalmol. 97:1907 (1979).

Jakobiec, F.A. & Chattock, A. Ocular and adnexal tumors. (F.A. Jakobiec ed.) Birmingham: Aesculapius Publishing Co. (1978) p. 341.

Jakobiec, F.A., Coleman, D.J., Chattock, A., & Smith, M. Ultrasonically guided needle biopsy and cytologic diagnosis of solid intraocular tumors. Ophthalmology 86:1662 (1979).

Kennerdell, J.S., Dekker, A., Johnson, B.L., & Dubois, P.J. Fine-needle aspiration biopsy: Its use in orbital tumors. Arch. Ophthalmol. 97: 1315 (1979).

Kennerdell, J.S., Dubois, P.J., Dekker, A. & Johnson, B. CT-guided fine needle aspiration biopsy of orbital optic nerve tumors. Ophthalmology 87:491 (1980).

Ossoinig, K.C. & Blodi, F.C. Preoperative differential diagnosis of tumors with echography IV diagnosis of orbital tumors, Current Concepts in Ophthalmology, Vol. 4, (F.C. Blodi, ed.), St. Louis: C.V. Mosby Co., (1974) p.313.

Reynes, C.J., Chandresekhar, A., & Churchill, R.J. Ultrasound guided, percutaneous biopsy of peripheral lung masses, Ultrasound in Medicine, Vol. 3A, (D. White & E.A. Lyons, eds.) New York & London: Plenum Press, (1977) p. 1163.

Schyberg, E. Fine needle biopsy of orbital tumours, Acta Ophthalmol. Supp. 125:11 (1975).

Skalka, H.W. & Callahan, M.A. 'Congenital' hematic cyst of the orbit. Ann. Ophthalmol. 11:1103 (1979).

Skalka, H.W. & Callahan, M.A. Ultrasonically-aided percutaneous orbital aspiration. Ophthalmic Surgery 10:41 (1979).

Skalka, H.W. et al. In preparation.

Spoor, T.C., Kennerdell, J.S., Dekker, A., Johnson, B.L., & Rehkopf, P. Orbital fine needle aspiration biopsy with B-scan guidance. Am. J. Ophthalmol. 89:274 (1980).

Westman-Naeser, S. & Naeser, P. Tumours of the orbit diagnosed by fine needle biopsy. Acta Ophthalmol. 56:969 (1978).

Wolf, D.A. Ultrasonically guided amniocentesis in twin gestations, Ultrasound in Medicine, Vol. 4, (D. White & E.A. Lyons, eds.) New York & London: Plenum Press (1978) p. 633.

Wright, J.E. Surgery on the orbit. Operative Surgery (S. Miller, ed.) London: Butterworths & Co. (1976).

Author's Address:
Eye Foundation
University of Alabama in Birmingham
1720 Eighth Avenue South
Birmingham, Alabama 35233, U.S.A.

A COMPARISON OF ULTRASOUND AND C.T. SCANNING IN BLOW OUT FRACTURE OF THE ORBIT

R.A. ORD, M.M. LEMAY, J.G. DUNCAN & K.F. MOOS

(Glasgow, United Kingdom)

Orbital wall fractures are conveniently divided into two types; 'Impure' blow out fractures, in which the fracture is associated with violence transmitted through the bone, and 'pure' blow out fracture in which the fracture is produced by a hydraulic mechanism through the orbital soft tissues (Converse, *et al.* 1967, Cramer, *et al.* 1965). In practice, impure fracture is usually associated with other fractures of the facial skeleton and pure blow out fracture may be associated with concomitant ocular damage (Milauskas & Fueger 1966).

The experience of the authors is with a majority of impure blow out fractures, involving the malar complex. A majority of these patients suffered from diplopia and enophthalmos even after malar elevation and reconstruction of the orbital floor. Persistent diplopia can be explained by haemorrhage into the orbital fascia (Koorneef 1977, Putterman, *et al.* 1974), but it was the belief that enophthalmos might be due to undiagnosed orbital fracture.

The frequency of medial wall fracture has previously been noted (Jones & Evans 1967, Pearl & Vistnes 1978) and the current study has compared computed tomography (C.T.) and B-scan ultrasound examination of the medial wall.

METHOD

Twelve patients were selected for study. The patients were selected if they experienced diplopia, enophthalmos or had radiographic signs of extensive orbital fracture.

Ultrasound was performed on the Sonometrics 100 Ophthalmoscan (Coleman, *et al.* 1969) at Glasgow Western Infirmary (Fig. 1 & 2).

C.T. scanning was performed on the E.M.I. 5005 body scanner at Glasgow Royal Infirmary. The results were compared by a third party (Fig. 3).

RESULTS

The results of this survey have previously been reported (Ord, *et al.* 1980). Ultrasound and C.T. scanning are in agreement in ten out of twelve cases (Fig. 4).

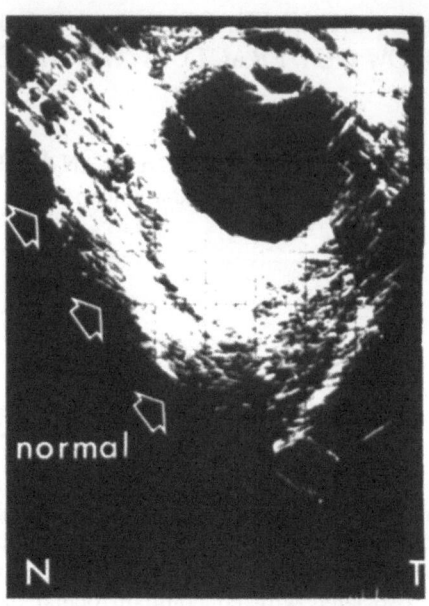

Fig. 1. B-scan echogram of the normal medial orbital wall (N = nasal, T = temporal).

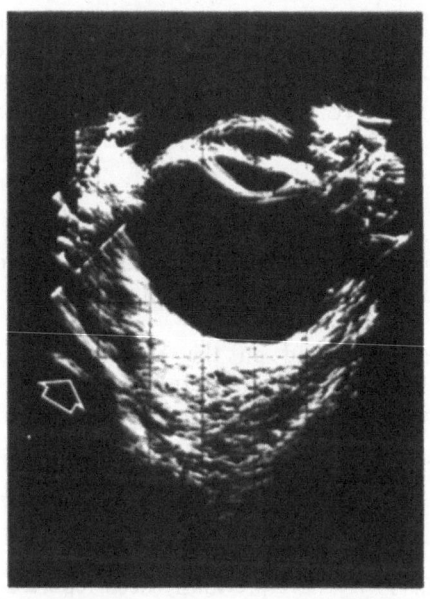

Fig. 2. A blow out fracture is visualised as a prolapse of orbital soft tissues with occasional bony fragments (arrow).

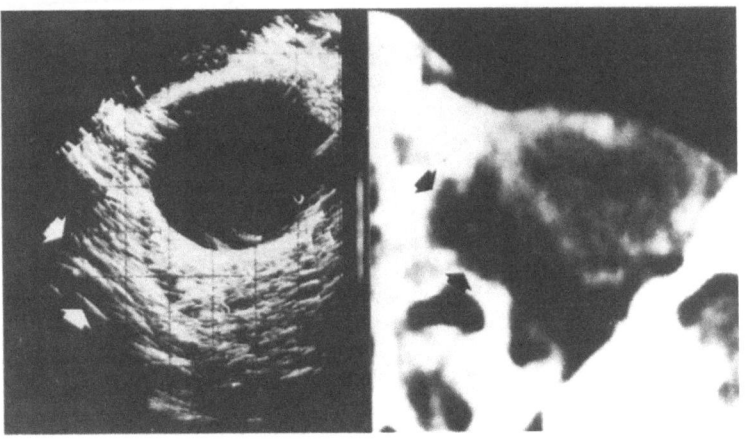

Fig. 3. Corresponding echogram and C.T. scan showing prolapse of orbital contents (arrows).

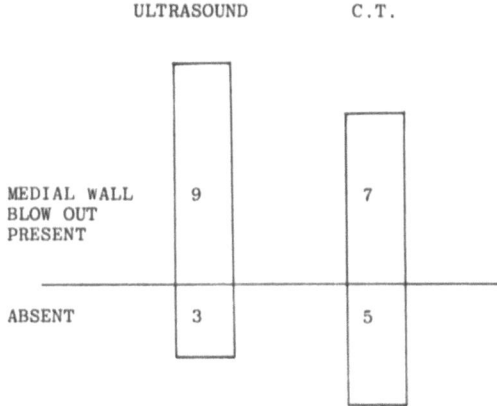

Fig. 4. Twelve cases of suspected medial wall blow out fracture. Comparison of ultrasonic and C.T. diagnosis.

There are five patients with X-ray signs, enophthalmos and diplopia and all of these had medial wall fractures with prolapse of orbital contents. Of the remaining two patients with definite medial blow out fractures one had X-ray signs alone and one had enophthalmos alone. Neither positive radiology nor the presence of enophthalmos alone was a reliable sign when considered alone (Ord, *et al.* 1980).

CONCLUSION

The results of the small series of patients with orbital fractures would suggest that medial wall fractures are common. The previous reports do not emphasise

387

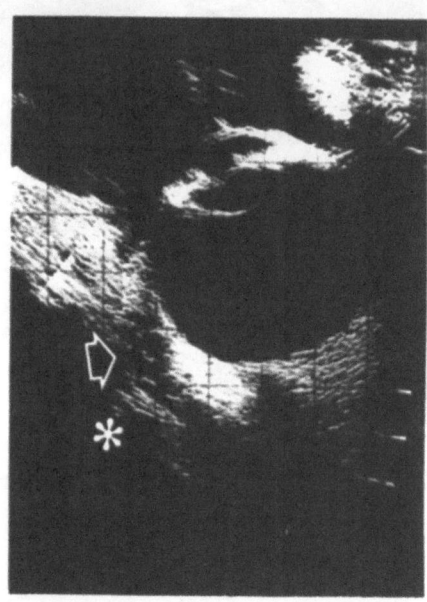

Fig. 5. A small anterior fracture. The soft tissue prolapse (asterisk) and the incarceration of the medial rectus (arrow) are demonstrated.

the frequency of trapping of the medial rectus muscle in the bony defect: this is most likely to happen if the fracture occurs anteriorly in the orbit (Fig. 5).

We believe that either investigation alone is a valuable adjunct to conventional clinical and radiological assessment.

ACKNOWLEDGEMENTS

The authors express their thanks to Mr. A. El-Attar, Mrs. A. Currie for the illustrations and to Miss O.M. Rankin who typed the manuscript.

REFERENCES

Coleman, D.J., Konig, W.F. & Katz, L. A hand operated ultrasound scan system for ophthalmic evaluation. Am. J. Ophthalmol. 68: 256 (1969).

Converse, J.M., Smith, B., Obear, M.F. & Wood-smith, D. Orbital blow-out fractures: A ten year survey. Plast. Reconstr. Surg. 39: 20 (1967).

Cramer, L.M., Tooze, F.M. & Lerman, S. Blow out fractures of the orbit. Brit. J. Plast. Surg. 18: 171 (1965).

Jones, D.E.P. & Evans, J.N.G. 'Blow-out' fractures of the orbit: An investigation into their anatomical basis. J. Laryng. 81: 1109 (1967).

Koornneef, L. New insights in the human orbital connective tissue. Arch. Ophthalmol. 95: 1269 (1977).

Milauskas, A.T. & Fueger, G.F. Serious ocular complications associated with blow out fractures of the orbit. Am. J. Ophthalmol. 62: 670 (1966).

Ord, R.A., Lemay, M.M., Duncan, J.G. & Moors, K.F. Computerised tomography and B-scan ultrasonography in the diagnosis of fractures of the medial orbital wall. Plast. Reconstr. Surg. (in Print) (1980).

Pearl, R.M. & Vistnes, L.M. Orbital blow-outs, an approach to management. Ann. of Plastic Surg. 1: 167 (1978).

Putterman, A.M., Stevens, T. & Urist, M.J. Non-surgical management of blow-out fractures of the orbital floor. Am. J. Ophthalmol. 77: 232 (1974).

Authors' Address:
Dept of Ophthalmology (Dr. Lemay)
Glasgow Western Infirmary
Glasgow, United Kingdom

A PROPOSED ORBITAL WALL ORIENT POINT FOR TOPOGRAPHIC AND QUANTITATIVE ECHOGRAPHY

V. DORN

(Zagreb, Yugoslavia)

Echographic orbita plane sections, depending on scanning type, have their characteristic acoustic appearance, as was demonstrated in skulls by Coleman (1977) and Kaneko, *et al.* (1977). Bidimensional B-scan display, in general, better documents shape, topography and topographic relations, than does the A-scan.

Based on anatomic elements, Buschmann (1971) & co-workers (Meier zu Eissen, *et al.* 1970, Staudt, *et al.* 1972) constructed the scheme for A-scan ultrasound orbital diagnostics. We tried, by means of A-scan echography, to get a 'three-dimensional' orbital walls picture and to construct an adequate scheme for clinical practice. We also tried to evaluate the ultrasound reflectivity of orbital walls.

MATERIAL AND METHODS

We made our measurements experimentally in 25 macerated human skulls (20 males and five females), i.e. 50 orbits. We performed echographic orbita examinations in four planes: horizontal $0-180°$, vertical $90°-(270°)$ and in both oblique planes $45°-(225°)$ and $135°-(315°)$ using TABO meridian determination. All measurements were performed by means of a standardized A-scan instrument 7200 MA, Nr 128, Kretztechnik FTZ-B-164/72 (Ossoinig 1973), with the probe NM 8/5 K, Nr 301. The 'tissue sensitivity', according to Ossoinig (1971), for our system combination instrument-probe was 65 dB. 10 mm echo amplitude, from 30 mm thick McGhan Silicone Gel Block reflector (Cat. Nr.25-10303), was obtained at $40 \mu s$ distance with 24.0 ± 0.7 dB. The ultrasonic orbital walls examination, on the macerated human skulls, were performed using the immersion technique (Fig. 1). Probeholder contrivance, provided with four joinaxle and two goniometers, enables the probe angling (in degrees) from medial position (the middle of orbital aperture) towards nasal, temporal, upwards and downwards in above mentioned four planes. Thus temporal probe angling explores nasal orbital wall, etc. Obtained results for orbital walls distances (in μs) and reflectivity in dB (measured echo amplitude was $1-2$ mm) in all four echographic plane sections of the orbits, with preliminary measurements of the anthropological data of the site of the orbits in the skull, made the construction of a three-dimensional scheme for clinical echographic practice possible (Dorn 1979).

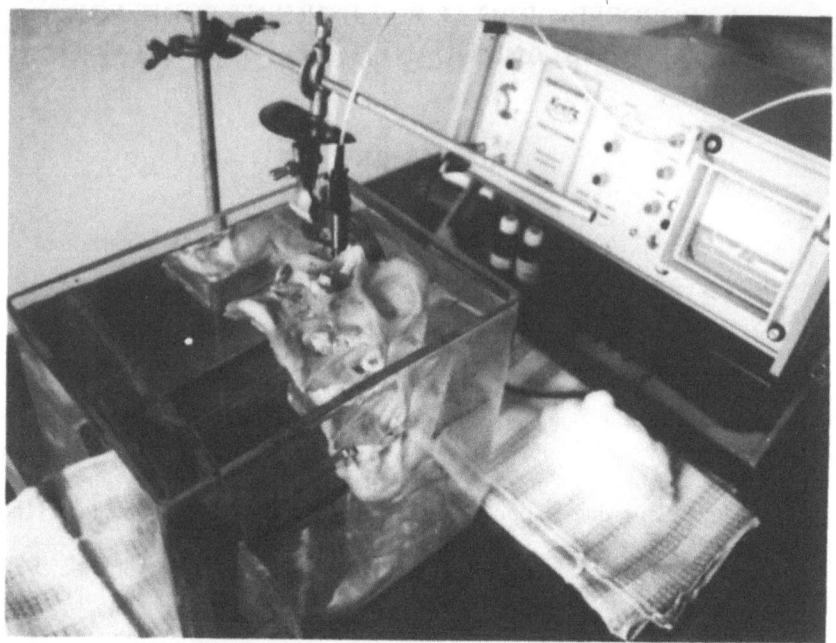

Fig. 1. The ultrasonic evaluation of orbital walls on the macerated human skulls using the immersion technique and Echo-Ophthalmograph 7200 MA Kretztechnik.

Although the orbital walls in sound reflection can be compared with large mirror-like surfaces (Ossoinig 1972), the exact measurements of these uneven and oblique bony surfaces showed the expected variability. Our results agree with the works of Baum (1963, 1965) and Buschmann (1968).

Evaluation of our results also revealed certain orbital areas with relatively little or constant variation, as well of location as of reflectivity, promising a good reliability, relative constant ultrasound reflectivity and, on the base of a suitable approach, easy location in echographic examination. So, we selected, on the medial orbital wall, the area of the orbital face of the lacrimal bone towards lacrimoethmoidal suture and lamina papyracea of ethmoidal bone — the reference point A. The lacrimal bone is built of compact substance, but the neighbouring lamina papyracea is very thin and often dehiscent (Whitnall 1921, Wolff 1948). The ultrasonic approach is from the lateral side and placing of the probe is suitable (Fig. 2).

Another area with a rather compact substratum and relative plane surface is point B on the medial part of upper orbital wall, more precisely the lateral face of the nasal part of frontal bone, above and behind the fovea or spina trochlearis. The approach from temporal and down is excellent (Fig. 3).

The third reference point C, is the area of the lateral orbital wall, the middle of orbital face of zygomatic bone, margo zygomaticus and anterior part of the orbital face of the great wing of sphenoid bone. The substratum is compact bone, the approach direction from the nasal side slanting from above, by suitable probe placing in the angle between the root of nose and the forehead (Fig. 4).

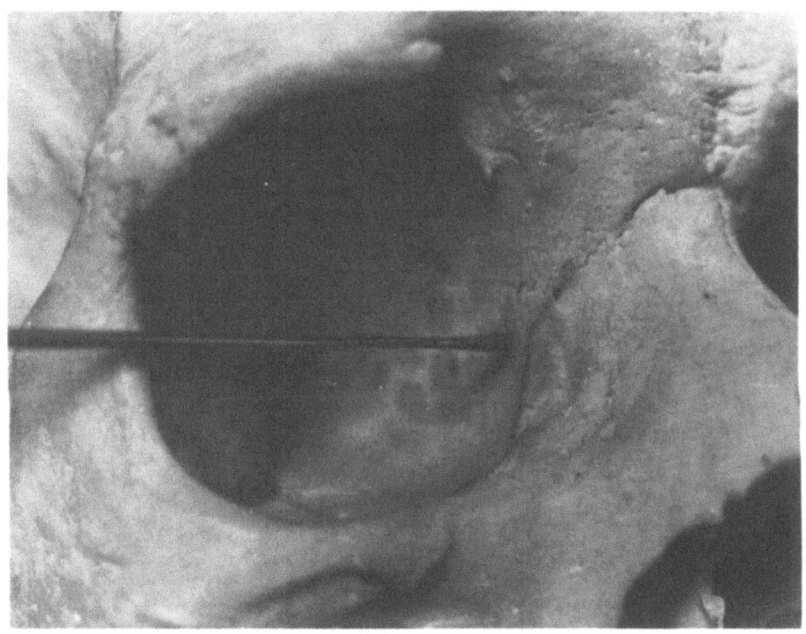

Fig. 2. The reference point A on the medial orbital wall. The probe indicates the ultra-sound beam direction.

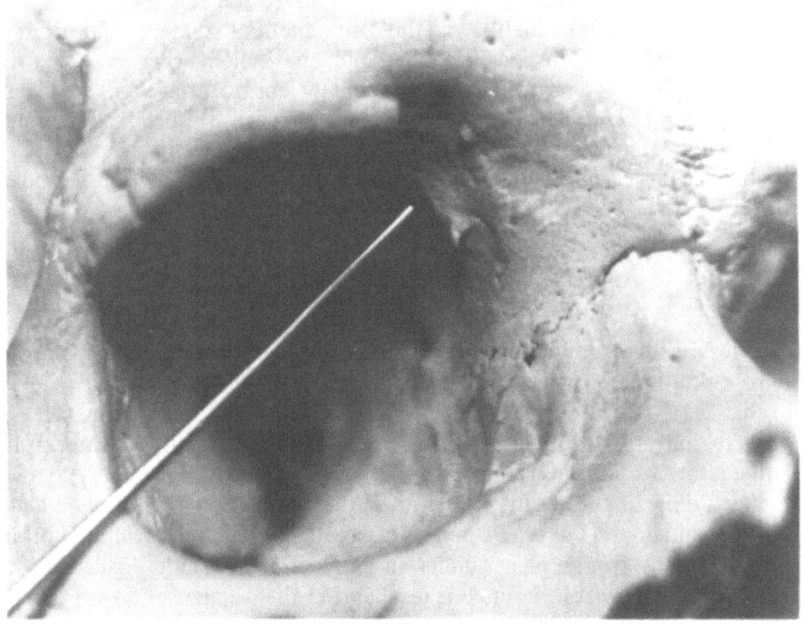

Fig. 3. Reference point B, above end behind fovea or spina trochlearis.

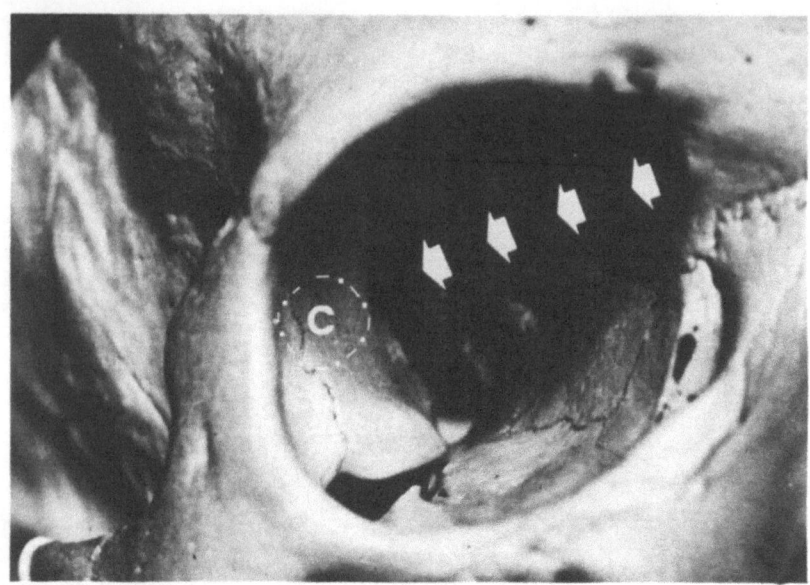

Fig. 4. The anatomical localisation of the reference point C on the lateral orbital wall. The arrows indicate ultrasound beam direction.

Additional experimental echographic examinations were performed to clarify whether or not these areas – the reference points A, B and C – give reliable and comparable values for location (distances, angles of probe position) and for reflectivity. On the same anatomic material (50 orbits of 20 males and five females macerated human skulls), using an immersion technique, we checked up (under goniometer control) the point A, placing the top of probe on the temporal orbital margin (Fig. 5). A similar procedure was conducted checking up the point B (Fig. 6). Checking up the point C, the probe was placed on medial orbital margin, in the angle between the root of the nose and glabella (Fig. 7).

RESULTS AND DISCUSSION

The results of examinations for all three points, separately for males and female skulls, are arranged in tables. Distances are given in μs (Table 1), mm (Table 2), angles in degrees (Table 3) and reflectivity (Table 4). The values in μs were converted in mm taking 1488 m/s for sound velocity in water. Water temperature was 22.5°C (Willard 1947, Poujol 1973).

According to the results it is shown that point A can be reached at the distance of about 51 μs (ca 38 mm), placing the probe on the temporal orbital margin, in the frontal plane, under an angle of 181° for the right orbit, i.e. 359° for the left orbit. Point B is reachable at the distance of 58 μs (43 mm), placing the probe on the temporal margin under an angle of 221° on the right, and 317° on the left orbit (frontal plane). Point C can be reached at the

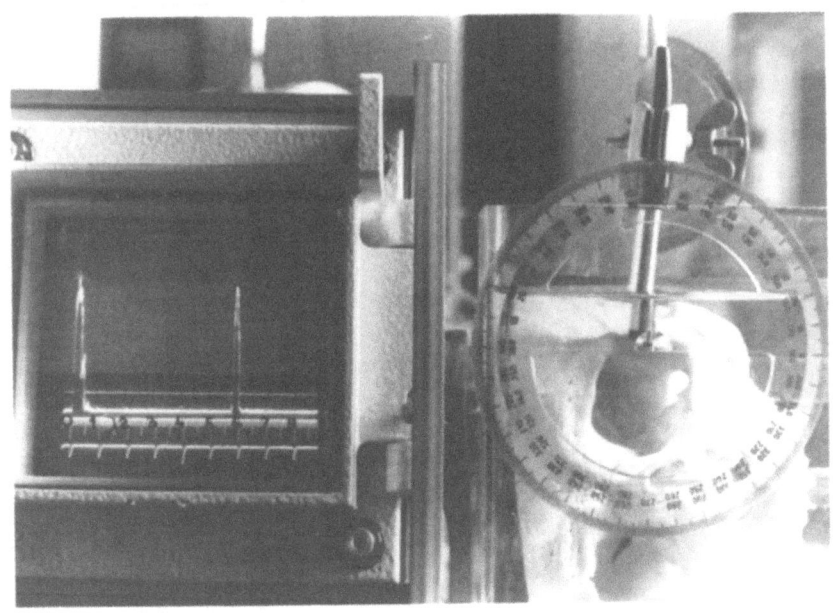

Fig. 5. The ultrasonic check up of the reference point A.

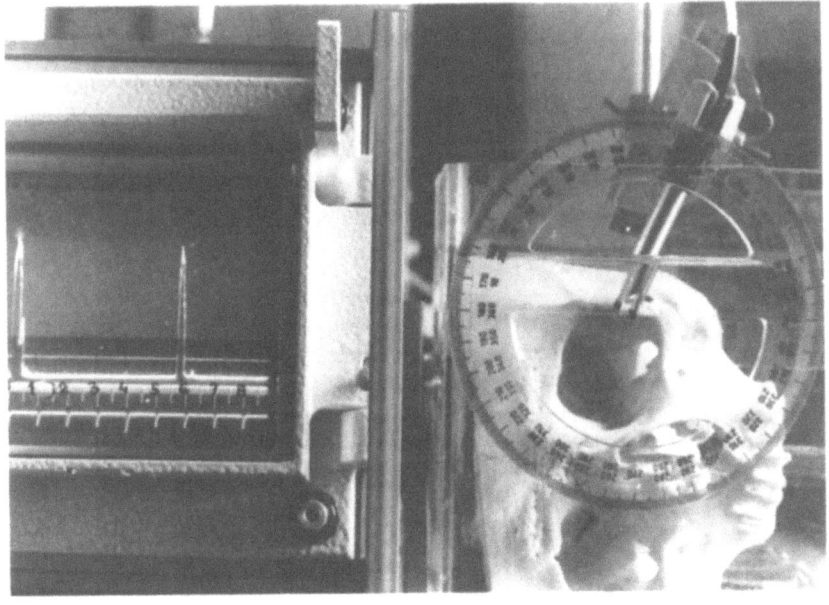

Fig. 6. The ultrasonic check up of the reference point B.

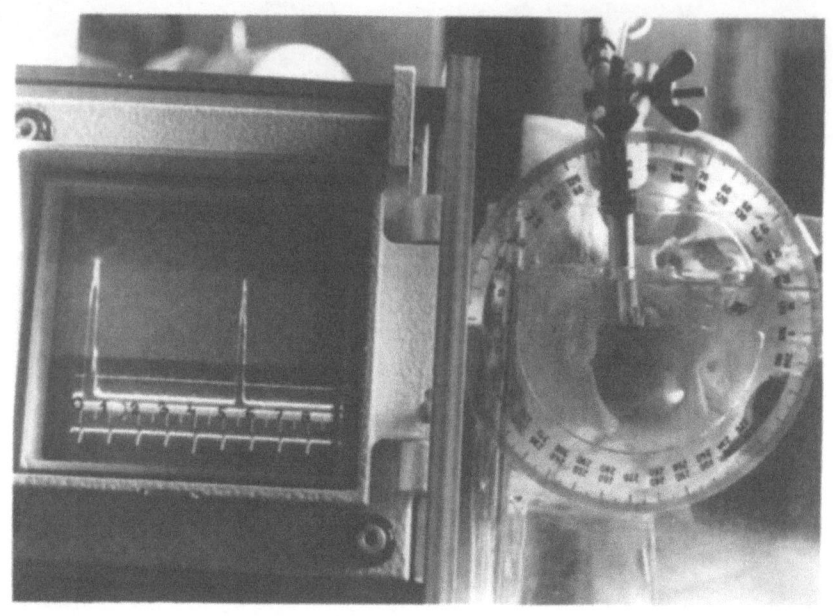

Fig. 7. The ultrasonic check up of the reference point C.

Table 1. Distances in microseconds of all three reference points (A, B, C) for right (R) and left (L) orbit. The results present mean values with standard deviation ($\bar{x} \pm s$). N = number of observations.

| | A | | B | | C | μs |
	R	L	R	L	R	L
Males (N = 20)	52.1 ± 1.9	51.6 ± 1.3	58.3 ± 2.1	58.3 ± 1.9	54.8 ± 1.5	54.3 ± 1.3
Females (N = 5)	47.8 ± 2.2	48.8 ± 1.1	56.4 ± 2.6	56.6 ± 2.3	54.0 ± 0.6	53.8 ± 1.6
Total	51.2 ± 2.7	51.1 ± 1.7	57.9 ± 2.3	57.9 ± 2.1	54.6 ± 1.5	54.3 ± 1.2

Table 2. Distances in millimeters for all three reference points. The μs values are converted in mm with 1488 m/s for sound velocity in watter at temperature of 22.5°C.

| | A | | B | | C | mm |
	R	L	R	L	R	L
Males (N = 20).	38.7 ± 1.5	38.4 ± 1.0	43.4 ± 1.6	43.3 ± 1.4	40.8 ± 1.1	40.4 ± 0.9
Females (N = 5)	35.6 ± 1.6	36.3 ± 0.8	42.0 ± 1.9	42.1 ± 1.7	40.2 ± 0.5	40.0 ± 1.2
Total	38.1 ± 1.9	38.0 ± 1.3	43.0 ± 1.7	43.1 ± 1.6	40.6 ± 1.1	40.4 ± 0.9

Table 3. Probe angling in degrees for reference points (A, B, C).

| | A | | B | | C | $\varkappa°$ |
	R	L	R	L	R	L
Males (N = 20)	181.8 ± 5.1	358.4 ± 1.9	221.6 ± 7.3	316.5 ± 7.3	16.7 ± 3.1	162.5 ± 3.9
Females (N = 5)	176.4 ± 4.2	361.0 ± 2.2	221.0 ± 4.2	320.0 ± 3.5	16.5 ± 2.9	163.2 ± 3.2
Total	180.7 ± 5.3	359.0 ± 4.6	221.4 ± 6.7	317.2 ± 6.8	16.6 ± 3.0	162.6 ± 3.5

Table 4. Relative dB values ($\bar{x} \pm s$) of reflectivity of all three reference points.

| | A | | B | | C | db |
	R	L	R	L	R	L
Males (N = 20)	14.9 ± 3.7	13.1 ± 3.8	16.0 ± 3.6	14.5 ± 3.8	10.6 ± 2.9	11.7 ± 3.0
Females (N = 5)	11.3 ± 3.1	11.7 ± 2.3	15.6 ± 2.9	15.1 ± 4.2	10.7 ± 1.5	9.3 ± 2.4
Total	14.2 ± 3.6	12.8 ± 3.5	15.9 ± 3.5	14.6 ± 3.9	10.6 ± 2.4	11.2 ± 2.9

distance of about $54\,\mu s$ (ca 40 mm), placing the probe on the medial orbital margin, under an angle (frontal plane) of $17°$ on the right, i.e. $163°$ on the left orbit and inclining the probe $50–70°$ nasal (in relation to the sagittal plane). Analysis of the variability of the data shows that point C is more reliable than points A and B. The reflectivity evaluation seems to indicate that point C is the most suitable place of the orbital walls as reference point.

CONCLUSION

The analysis of the orbital walls (location, reflectivity), by means of ultra-sonic A-scan technique in experiments on the macerated human skulls revealed a lateral orbital wall point with relatively constant reflectivity. This easy-to-find and approachable characteristic orbital wall point may be a convenient aid for quick orientation and comparative measurements in clinical echographic examination.

REFERENCES

Baum, G. Present status of orbital ultrasonography. Am. J. Ophthalmol. 56: 98 (1963).

Baum, G. A reappraisal of orbital ultrasonography: Series II. Trans. Am. Acad. Ophthalmol. Otolaryngol. 69: 943 (1965).

Buschmann, W. Probleme der Ultraschalldiagnostik in der Orbita. In: Diagnostica Ultrasonica in Ophthalmologia, SIDUO II. Acta fac. med. univ. brunensis, 35: 109 (1968).

Buschmann, W. & Staudt, J. Grundlagen der echographischen differential Diagnostik. In: Ultrasonographia medica, Vol. 1 (J. Böck & K. Ossoinig, eds) Wien: Verl. Wiener med. Akad. (1971) p. 395.

Coleman, J., Lizzi, F. & Jack, R. Ultrasonography of the Eye and Orbit. Philadelphia: Lea & Febiger (1977) p. 296.

Dorn, V. Elavucija kvantitativne ehografije kod eksperimentalnih imitacija intrabulbarnih lezija te ultrazvučnih presjeka orbite sa praktičnom primjenom u diferencijalnoj ehografskoj dijagnostici nalaza oka i orbite. Doktorska disertacija. Zagreb: Sveučilište u Zagrebu (1979).

Kaneko, A., Shigeyama, S. & Uchida, R. A new ultrasonic apparatus for the ophthalmological diagnosis using manual compound scanning. In: Ultrasound in Medicine 3A (D. White & R. Brown, eds.) New York: Plenum Press (1977) p. 917.

Meier zu Eissen, J., Staudt, J., Wilcke, G. & Buschmann, W. Topographisch anatomische Grundlagen für die Ultraschalldiagnostik im Orbitagebiet. Anat. Anz. 126: 21 (1970).

Ossoinig, K. Grundlagen der echographischen Gewebsdifferenzierung IV. Teil: Klinische Standardisation der Diagnostikanlage und Untersuchungstechnik. In: Ultrasonographia medica, Vol. 2 (J. Böck & K. Ossoinig, eds.) Wien: Verl. Wiener med. Akad. (1971) p. 83.

Ossoinig, K. Clinical echo-ophthalmography In: Current concepts in Ophthalmology Vol. 3 (F. Blodi, ed.) St. Louis: Mosby (1972) p. 101.

Ossoinig, K. Ein neues Gerät für die klinische Echo-Ophthalmographie. Vorschläge zur Standardisation wichtiger Geräte-Parameter. In: Diagnostica Ultrasonica in Ophthalmologia, SIDUO IV (M. Massin & J. Poujol, eds.) Paris: Centre National d'Ophtalmologie des Quinz-Vingts (1973) p. 131.

Poujol, J. Physique des Ultrasons. In: Echographie de l'oeil et de l'orbite. Bull. Soc. Ophthalmol. Fr. Numéro spécial (1973) p. 15.

Staudt, J., Kunz, G., Wilcke, G. & Buschmann, W. Topographisch-anatomische und statistische Untersuchungen im Orbitagebiet entsprechend dem ultraschalldiagnostischen Abtastvorgang bei Winkelabweichung um jeweils 30°. Anat. Anz. 131: 88 (1972).

Whitnall, S.E. Anatomy of the human orbit and accesory organs. London: Frowde (1921).

Willard, G. Temperature coefficients of ultrasonic velocity in solutions. J. Acoust. Soc. Am. 19: 235 (1947).

Wolff, E. The Anatomy of the Eye and Orbit, 3rd Ed, London: H.K. Lewis & Co. (1948).

Author's Address:
Dr. Vjekoslav Dorn, Department of
Ophthalmology, Faculty of Medicine,
University of Zagreb, Kišpatićeva 12.
YU-41000 Zagreb, Yugoslavia

SOME LESS IMPORTANT USE OF ULTRASOUND IN OPHTHALMOLOGY

V. MAZZEO

(Ferrara, Italy)

In 1966 at the Münster Symposium Prof. Arvo Oksala a pioneer in ultrasound diagnostics mentioned all the fields in which ultrasound could be used in his review based on the 173 papers already published at that time: '. . . intraocular tumors, vitreous opacities, intraocular foreign body, detachment of the Retina and the Choroid and between other pathological conditions: diseases of the orbit, exophthalmos, lids, lens. . . '. This Congress has shown the advances made in the past 14 years. If one examines the enormous amount of existing ultrasound literature it is evident that pathology of the lids and lacrimal sac is the least considered. In fact one must go back to 1959 and 1960 to find two papers by Oksala about the use of ultrasound in a case of chalazion and in an acute dacryocystitis. The author himself mentions them as curiosities but points out how, even in that case, ultrasound examination could give some comprehensible and meaningful answer.

It is possible to utilize ultrasound, using an A-scan Kretztechnik 7200 MA with an 8 Mhz unfocused probe, both in lids and skin pathology, even outside the ocular region.

In this last field clinical inspection and palpation cannot be substituted and the biopsy gives the most useful diagnostic information. But sometimes ultrasound examination can be tried since it is non-invasive and, the pattern of the response in this area may be similar to echographic patterns found in pathological situations which are usually well studied by this diagnostic tool, i.e. ocular and orbital tumors. Summarising it is possible to find echographic patterns characteristic of an already unknown pathology.

In a 14-day-old female baby with an evident palpebral haemangioma, the u.s. examination performed by putting the probe on the mass (Fig. 1) revealed an echotrace similar to the pattern of a cavernous haemangioma of the orbit (Ossoinig, *et al.* 1975). A large inferior lid haematoma had the same echopattern as the citrated blood phantom (Ossoinig 1971) or Till's tissue model (Till 1978).

A clinically diagnosed subcataneous cyst at the superior-internal angle of the orbital arcade at u.s. revealed a high internal reflectivity with a slight 'kappa' angle; the hystopathologic answer was a benign haemangio-endothelioma.

Cysts do not occur strictly in the lids, they are mainly found at the

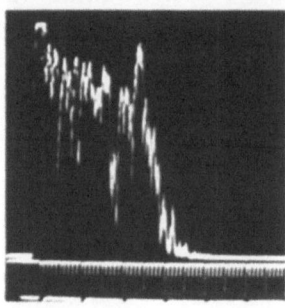

Fig. 1. Cutaneous haemangioma. Characteristic 'Kappa' angle.

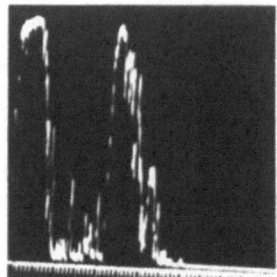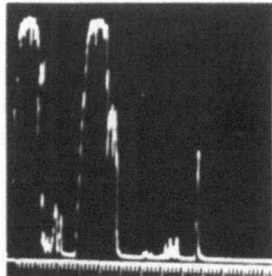

Fig. 2. Serous-mucous cyst near the lacrimal sac, which had been operated some years before. 2a: parabulbar projection. 2b: toward the lacrimal bone.

external contour of the orbit or within the orbit. Internal reflectivity changes with the cystic content; a serous-mucous cyst will show very low reflectivity or none at all (Fig. 2), while an epidermoidal cyst will show a variable internal reflectivity due to its inhomogeneous content.

A case that should be considered in the chapter of the cysts is one of a young man who had been operated on for a left maxillary sinus cyst, via an external skin incision, at the age of 17. At the age of 37 years, a slight exophthalmus and hypertropia of the left eye was noticed with the duration of a month. U.s. examination revealed a serous cyst behind the inferior orbital arcade (Fig. 3a) and when the probe was placed on the scar, where the bony wall had been removed, the echotrace was characteristic for an enormous acoustically silent serous cyst (Fig. 3b). The diagnosis of a relapse of the cyst in the sinus with orbital extension was made. In fact even in the absence of bone the sound could never have been transmitted through air. Surgery via the superior gingival fornix confirmed the diagnosis.

Cutaneous pathology cannot always be examined by our contact A-scan, especially when it is very superficial. But when it reaches dimensions bigger than the so-called 'dead zone' of the transducer, it is sometime easy to find a characteristic echo pattern.

The echotrace of a soft scalp lump in a man operated for a sarcoma of the forehead bone was similar to the pattern of the lymphoma-sarcoma-pseudotumor group (Fig. 4).

400

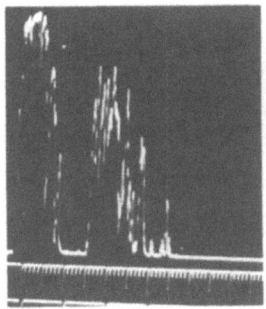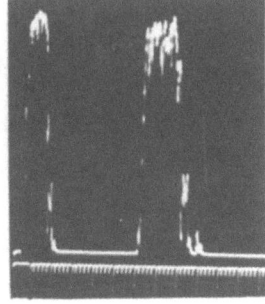

Fig. 3. Serous cyst. 3a: parabulbar projection. 3b: left maxillary sinus (see text).

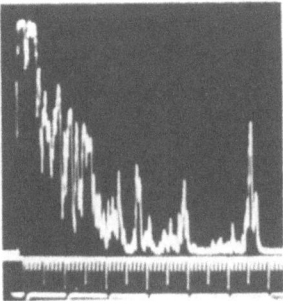

Fig. 4. Soft scalp lump in a sarcoma of the forehead bone. Low internal reflectivity.

The ultrasound answer based on tissue texture (Gallenga, *et al.* 1971, Hodes 1976, Freyler 1976) does not change with the body site. This similarity exists even in the group of orbital or bulbar carcinomas, whose pathognomical echo-pattern is the so-called 'V' shape (Ossoinig, *et al.* 1975, Mazzeo, *et al.* 1979). All the cases dealt with more or less large lid epitheliomas. In some cases, the 'V' shape was clear, while in others there was an internal acoustic discontinuity and a medium to high reflectivity (Fig. 5). In a case of metastatic cutaneous infiltration to both lower lids from a mamma carcinoma, traces with an increased reflectivity (Fig. 6, left) and a 'V' shape were found (Fig. 6, right). In this case the extremely high reflectivity of the carcinomatous tissue overlaps the attenuation that occurs in normal tissues.

Finally, ultrasound may be used in assessing bone defects especially in periorbital malignancies. At 8 MHz bone strongly reflects sound. Dispute still occurs on whether transmission through *healthy* extremely thin bone, like the one dividing the orbit from the ethmoid sinus, occurs when air is excluded from the sinus. Some authors state that transmission occurs only when bone lesions are present (Till 1975, Hauff & Till 1979). Others state that the only unsurpassable barrier is the bone to air interface and not intact bone (Ossoinig 1977).

In dacryocystorhinostomy the bone defect is due to the surgical procedure. It is therefore possible by putting the probe on the skin to find the surgical break and to measure it, going step by step along the surgical

401

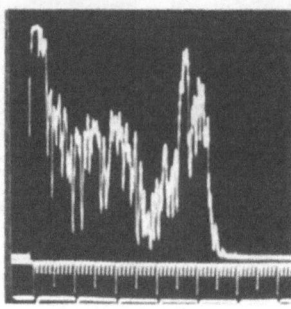

Fig. 5. Epithelioma of the upper lid. Transverse projection through the mass. Internal acoustic discontinuity.

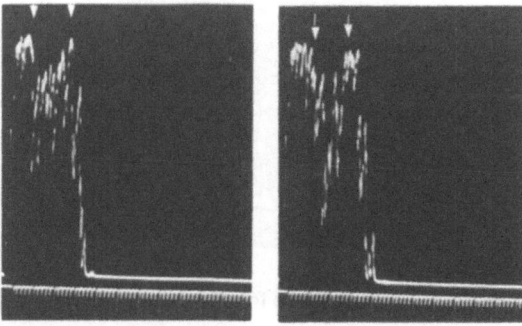

Fig. 6. Metastasis from a mamma carcinoma to both lower lids (arrows). 6a: Increasing internal reflectivity; 6b: 'V' shape.

scar. Of course tearing absence and irrigation through the lacrimal point give the best information about the functioning of the opening.

In conclusion ultrasound examination plays only an accessory role in all the above mentioned pathological situations and at least the chapter of 'curiosities' may have been increased.

REFERENCES

Freyler, H., Egerer, I. Echography and Histological studies in various eye conditions. Arch. Ophthalmol. 95: 1385 (1977).

Gallenga, R., Bellone, G., Gallenga P.E. & Pasquarelli A. Ultrasonografia clinica dell'occhio e dell'orbita in Recenti acquisizioni di semeiotica oculare. Firenze: Edizioni S.O.I. (1971).

Hodes, B.L. Tissue Texture: The histologic basis for standardized A-scan diagnosis in Ophthalmology in Ultrasound in Medicine 3B (D.N. White & R. Brown, eds.). New York Plenum Press. (1977) p. 1895.

Mazzeo, V., Scorrano, R., Gallenga, P.E., Rossi A. Echography in choroidal metastatic tumors. Second WFMB Miyazaki (1979) Abstract book, p. 159.

Hauff, W., Till P. Echographic findings in orbital mucoceles In: Diagnostica Ultrasonica in Ophthalmology (H. Gernet, ed.). Münster: Remy Verlag (1979) p. 151.

Oksala A. Diagnosis by ultrasound in acute dacryocistitis. Acta Ophthalmol. Kbn 38: 100 (1960).

Ossoinig K. Grundlaghen der Klinische standardisation der diagnostikanlage und der untursuchungstechnik. In: Ultrasonographya Medica III (Böck & K. Ossoinig, eds.) Wein: Wiener Med Akad (1972) p. 83.

Ossoinig K. A-scan echography and orbit disease. Mod. Probl. Ophthalmol. 14: 203 (1975).

Ossoinig K. Echography of the Eye, Orbit and Periorbital Region in Orbit Roentgenology (P.H. Arger, ed.) New York: Wiley & sons (1977) p. 224.

Ossoinig K., Till P. A ten years study of Clinical Echography in orbital diseases. Bibl. Ophthalmol. 83: 200 (1975).

Till P. Echography in Rhinogenic Orbital conditions Mod. Probl. Ophthalmol. 14: 273 (1975).

Till P. Solid tissue model for the standardization of the Echo-Ophthalmograph 7200 MA Kretztechnik. Documenta Ophthalmologica 41: 205 (1976).

Author's Address:
Clinica Oculistica
Università di Ferrara
Corso Giovecca, 203
44100 Ferrara, Italy

DIGITAL PROCESSING AND IMAGING MODES FOR CLINICAL ULTRASOUND

F.L. LIZZI, D.J. COLEMAN, E. FELEPPA, J. HERBST & N. JAREMKO

(New York, U.S.A.)

A computer-based ultrasound system has been designed and constructed to provide new approaches to processing, analyzing, and displaying clinical ultrasonograms. (c.f. Lizzi, et al. 1979, 1980). Over the past year, the system has been applied in ophthalmic examinations, and it has been continually refined and expanded as clinical trials proceed.

During a patient examination, the system digitizes and stores RF echo signals from a complete set of adjacent scan lines and immediately generates B-scan images for inspection from the digitized signals; the system also provides a comprehensive series of time- and frequency-domain processing capabilities for characterizing scanned tissue structures. Data storage and retrieval facilities permit interactive processing, and provide a large clinical data base to support retrospective studies. The salient features of the system are outlined in the following sections.

SYSTEM CONFIGURATION AND DATA ACQUISITION

The configuration of the system is shown in Fig. 1. The central unit is a DEC PDP 11/60 minicomputer with 128 KBytes of semiconductor memory. A pair of RK06 disk drives provides 28 MBytes of removable storage for data and computational results. A tape drive provides long term archival storage on magnetic tape. An imaging system with a microprocessor-controlled digital scan converter is interfaced with the Unibus structure of the mini-computer, and an ancilliary 'joy-stick' module provides operator interaction with displayed images and graphs.

In clinical operation, RF data are acquired from the focal region of a broad-band transducer, usually employing a 10-MHz center-frequency. A conventional ultrasonic system is used to survey the eye and to assure that the lens is avoided in all quantitative scans. An optical encoder provides signals to trigger data acquisition from 100 equally spaced sector-scan lines; the angular increment between lines usually is set at 0.35 degrees.

Along each scan line, RF signals from a preset range increment are automatically sampled, digitized, and stored in a line buffer. Typically, 1024, 6-bit samples are acquired at a sampling frequency of 100 MHz. (This

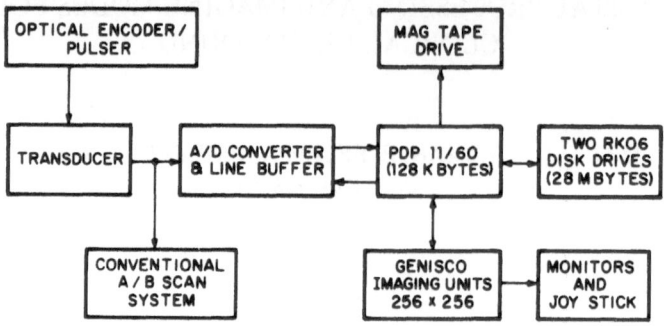

Fig. 1. Block diagram of the clinical computer system.

high sampling rate is well above the Nyquist limit, and permits post-processing improvement in signal resolution.) The buffered series of samples from each line is transferred to the PDP 11/60, whose memory is used to store the 100 KByte block of data obtained from an entire 100-line scan. The actual scan operation and concurrent DMA data transfer require only 0.2 s; a subsequent quiescent period of 0.6 s is required for transferring scan data to a disk. Thus, data from a 100-line scan can currently be acquired at 1.2 frames/s, which is more than adequate for most clinical situations. Alternatively, M-mode data can be acquired in a similar manner, but under the control of an external pulse generator which triggers transducer excitation and data acquisition.

Acquired data can be processed in a variety of ways using a basic 'Sig-Pro' software package specially developed for the ultrasound system. This package provides versatility and modular programming techniques that greatly facilitate the testing and refinement of processing approaches. When specific processing techniques prove particularly useful, special-purpose software, tuned for speed and efficiency, is developed to expedite routine application.

The first step in examining clinical data is the generation of a B-scan presentation of the stored RF echo signals. These signals are digitally rectified and smoothed, and are displayed in a gray-scale format on a video monitor, as shown in Fig. 2. Inter-line interpolation is used to derive a 200-line display from the original 100-line scan. These operations are performed within 6 s so that each scan can be viewed during patient examination. (Spatial image reformatting to account for the scan line pattern is available, but is not needed for most studies.)

The speed of data acquisition and B-scan display easily accommodates digitizing and viewing up to 20 scans per patient. The data from 20 scans represents 2 MBytes, so that at least ten patients can be examined before requiring a new disk or the transfer of scan data to magnetic tape.

DATA PROCESSING

A variety of processing techniques can be applied to stored scan data. These techniques can be described conveniently in terms of three categories: image processing, RF analysis, and image synthesis.

406

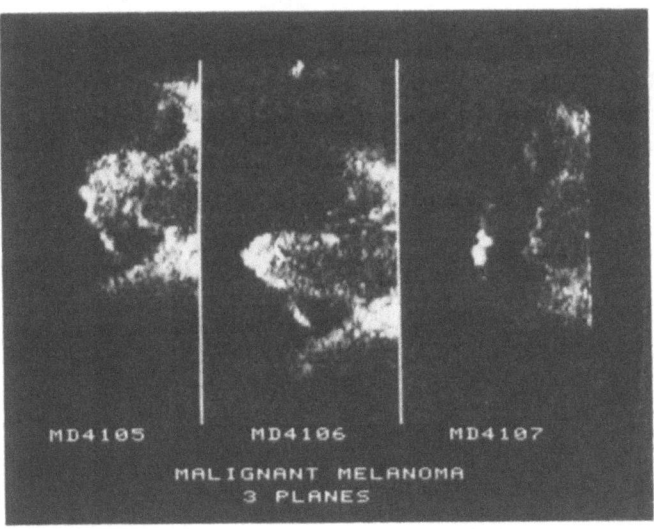

Fig. 2. Computer-generated B-scan images of three, adjacent planes through a choroidal melanoma.

The first category, image processing, manipulates video B-scan signals as shown in Fig. 2. Image processing includes gray-scale manipulations (e.g., logarithmic and squared gray scales), color and isometric modes, and feature-enhancement techniques (e.g., differential and gradient imaging).

The second data processing category is graphically presented RF data analysis. The tissue area to be examined is selected by using the joy-stick module to superimpose a box over the region of interest as shown in Fig. 3. After a simple statement is entered at the operator console, RF signals from within the demarcated area are analyzed in the prescribed manner, and the results are displayed in an annotated, graphical format adjacent to the B-scan image.

In the example shown in Fig. 3, a normalized power spectrum has been computed from the RF signals within the demarcated 2 × 2 mm region. Spectral analysis involves the following operations. RF data for each line are retrieved from storage, and multiplied by a Hamming (window) function; then, a Fast Fourier Transform (FFT) subroutine is applied to each line. The squared amplitudes of the FFT computations are averaged and then normalized with respect to the spectrum obtained for a glass-plate reference echo. Finally, the normalized spectrum is converted to dB units (dBr) relative to the glass-plate spectrum, and displayed in annotated graphical format as shown. The programmed sequence of operations is executed in less than 30 s.

The size of the demarcated area is adjustable; most often, it encloses either a 1 × 1 mm or a 2 × 2 mm square. The number of distinct, analyzed areas is also adjustable so that larger tissue elements can be examined in their entirety as an ensemble. This is particularly valuable in tracking detached retinas, vitreous membranes and superficial layers in tumors (Lizzi, *et al.* 1978, 1979b).

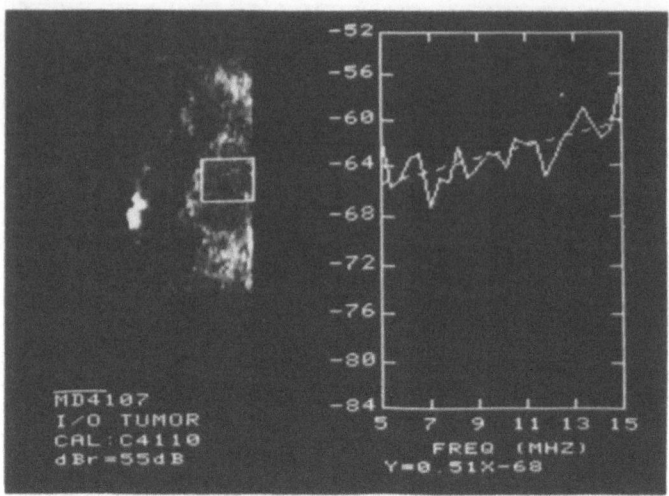

Fig. 3. Computer-generated B-scan with a superimposed rectangular analysis region (positioned by a joy-stick), and resultant graphical display showing the normalized power spectrum of RF data from the scan-line segments defined by the analysis rectangle.

Other analyses can be applied to demarcated areas. These include multiple- or single-line A-scan displays (video and RF signals), coherently integrated and deconvolved A-scan displays (M-mode scans), deconvolution (for axial resolution improvement), cepstral analysis (for biometry) and histogram computations. The analysis is specified by a simple statement entered at a computer terminal prior to joy-stick operation.

The third category of digital techniques synthesizes special images after specific RF data processing has been applied. Usually, these procedures involve digital filtering applied to the entire block of RF data. An example of such filtering is shown in Fig. 4. Here, digital band-pass filters have operated on stored RF data to isolate signal components in three contiguous frequency bands. An image is then generated from the filtered data in each band. The three images depict the low-, middle-, and high-frequency ranges, and are useful in assessing reflectivity as a function of frequency prior to more detailed, quantitative analysis. Signals in each band are normalized with respect to the glass plate reference echo so that gray scale can be compared, quantitatively, in the three band-pass images. In addition, band-pass images can be color coded and superimposed to present spectral data in a format that is visually striking and easy to interpret.

Other processing can be applied in a similar fashion. For example, deconvolution is often used to produce images of detached retinas; surfaces separated (in range) by about $120\,\mu m$ can be distinctly imaged.

SUMMARY

A flexible computer system is now being used in a variety of clinical ultrasonic research projects. The system operates conveniently in clinical data

408

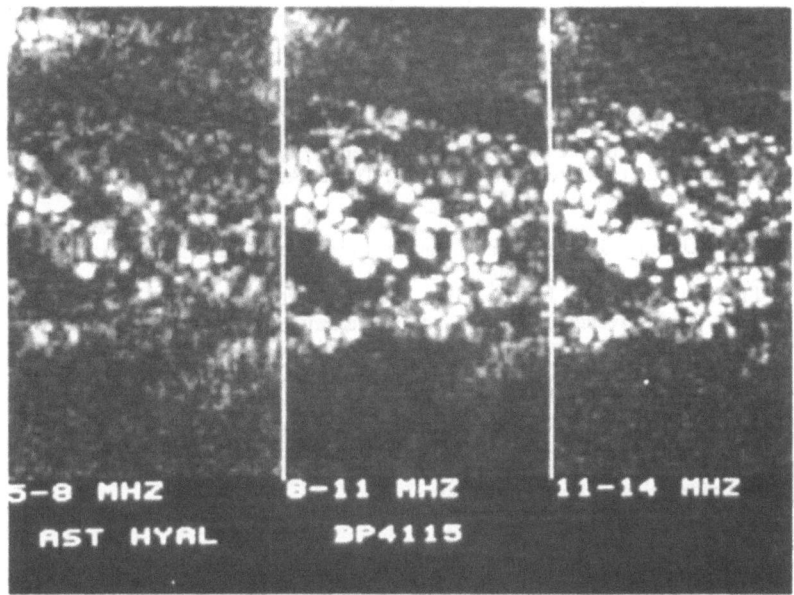

Fig. 4. Band-pass images of asteroid hyalosis (consisting of a dispersion of small particles in the vitreous humor) showing higher reflectivity in the high-frequency band, consistent with Rayleigh scattering.

acquisition, and provides gray-scale images during patient examination. A variety of processing and analysis techniques support complete evaluation of B-scan data and provide new types of frequency-domain data for tissue characterization. Additional processing methods generate band-pass-filtered and deconvolved images to enhance assessment of tissue properties.

Data from any particular scan can be examined by all techniques so that a complete evaluation can be made. Since an archival data library is maintained, cases can be analyzed in retrospective studies to evaluate newer processing concepts as they are made available.

ACKNOWLEDGEMENTS

The authors thank Dr. David Hom for his contributions to the design and implementation of computer software; Ms. Mary Smith, Mr. Mark Rondeau, Ms. Maureen Vogt, and Ms. Cindy Tynik for their utilization of the system in the clinical setting; and Ms. Ilene Rocklin for her assistance in documenting the work.

SUPPORT

This work is supported by U.S. Public Health Service Grants EY-01212 and EY-03183 administered by the Eye Institute of the National Institutes of Health.

409

REFERENCES

Lizzi, F.L., Coleman, D.J., Franzen, L., & Feleppa, E.J., 'Use of a Spectrum Analysis System for Characterization of Malignant Melanoma,' Ultrasound in Medicine, Vol. 4, (D. White & E.A. Lyons, eds.) New York: Plenum Press (1978).

Lizzi, F.L., Feleppa, E.J., Herbst, J., Jaremko, N., & Coleman, D.J., 'Computerized Ultrasonic Characterization of Ocular Tissue,' Annual Meeting, Acoustical Society of America, Boston, MA (1979a).

Lizzi, F.L., Feleppa, E.J., Herbst, J., Rosenberg, S., and Hom, D., 'Digital Tissue Analysis in Ophthalmic Ultrasound', Fourth Ultrasonic Tissue Characterization Seminar, National Bureau of Standards, Gaithersburg, MD (1979b).

Lizzi, F.L., Feleppa, E.J., Herbst, J. & Jaremko, B., 'Digital Spectral, Cepstral, and Image-Processing Techniques for Tissue Characterization,' Fifth Ultrasonic Tissue Characterization Seminar, National Bureau of Standards, Gaithersburg, MD (1980).

Lizzi, F.L., Herbst, J., Feleppa, E.J., Rosenberg, S., Jaremko, N., Hom, D., & Coleman, D.J., 'Digital Signal and Image Processing in Clinical Ophthalmic Ultrasonography,' AIUM Conference, Montreal, Canada (1979c).

Authors' Addresses:
Riverside Research Institute (Dr. Lizzi)
80 West End Avenue
New York, U.S.A.
Cornell University Medical College (Dr. Coleman)
New York, U.S.A.

IN VIVO CHARACTERIZATION OF
INTRAOCULAR MEMBRANES

A.L. BAYER & J.M. THIJSSEN

(Nijmegen, The Netherlands)

INTRODUCTION

Up till now echografic signals have been mainly used for visual evaluation by a clinician. For this purpose the signal is rectified, filtered, and often compressed, rendering a one sided peak pattern, known as the video-signal. In this processing the received signal is irreversibly distorted, causing a loss of information. It is this information that may yield valuable parameters of the acoustic properties of the considered tissue. Though some results have been reported on tissue characterization by analysis of A-scan video signals (Mountford & Wells 1972, Thijssen, *et al.* 1980), the undistorted RF-signal is much more appropriate for quantitative analysis.

A method to extract the actual physical tissue information from the RF-signal is a signal processing procedure called inverse filtering or deconvolution. The aim of such filtering is to remove, to a certain extent and with particular restrictions, the characteristics of the equipment in order to obtain the pure acoustic characteristics of the tissue.

Deconvolution has been proposed by several authors (Beretzky 1977, Herment 1980, Jones & Cole-Beuglet 1979, Kruizinga & Thijssen 1978, Martens, *et al.* 1980, Papoulis & Chamzas 1979), mostly as part of a mapping procedure of the acoustic tissue impedance, so called impediography (raylography). Until now much emphasis has been laid on mathematical procedures rather than practical applicability. Many workers implicitly assume an invariant sound pulse, neglecting the inhomogeneous character of the sound field of the transducer. Jones (1979) announced the study of these effects, but no practical results have been reported so far.

In this study, meant to evaluate the applicability of deconvolution to echographic signals obtained from the eye, in particular membrane echoes, the emphasis has been on such effects, and attempts have been made to define the limits of applicability and the optimization of the signal to noise ratio.

PRINCIPLE OF INVERSE FILTERING

In a simple approach to echo formation, a transmitted pulse interacts with the tissue, and the backscattered sound is picked up by a receiver system. The

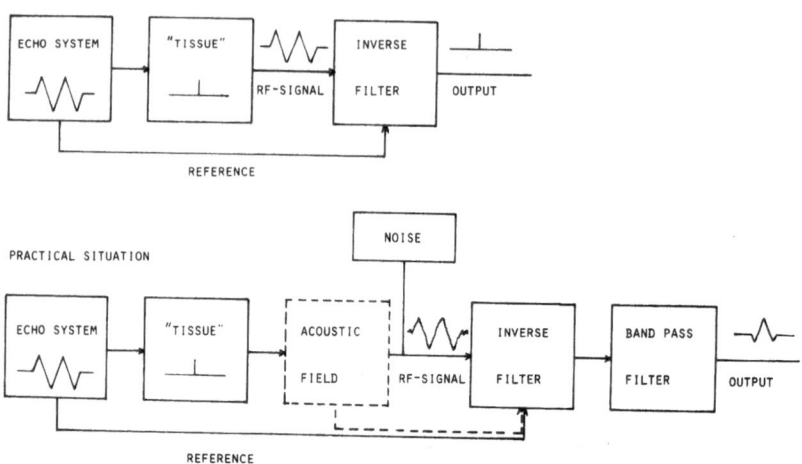

Fig. 1. Schematic model of echo formation.

resulting RF-signal then merely depends on the characteristics of the echo-system, consisting of pulser, transducer and receiver, and those of the tissue. If these components may be considered as linear systems, the components are interchangeable and the overall system can then be described mathematically as a convolution of the impulse responses of the echosystem and the tissue. Fig. 1 shows this process schematically. The tissue response is depicted as a single (Dirac) pulse, as if the tissue only consisted of one interface.

In principle it should be possible to compensate for the convolution with the echosystems response, provided it is known. This compensation is accomplished in an inverse operation, called inverse filtering or deconvolution. Under ideal circumstances this operation yields the exact tissue impulse response. In the case of a flat multilayered tissue structure, this would mean a series of Dirac pulses with well defined sign, amplitude and time of flight.

In practice, the echoformation model has to be extended by two substantial components. Firstly noise, electronic as well as digitization noise, is present in the signal. The inverse filter emphasizes noise beyond proportion, thus necessitating the use of additional bandfiltering. This results in an output signal with diminished resolution and of an oscillating character.

Secondly the path to the tissue and back to the transducer may be of considerable influence. Besides dispersive attenuation in the traversed tissue, which is considered small in a superficial and liquid filled organ like the eye, the inhomogeneous sound field is a cause of alterations of the received pulses. This influence, that has linear system characteristics (Robinson 1974), should also be compensated for, but this can not always be performed exactly because of the uncertainty about the exact tissue location in an *in vivo* situation.

412

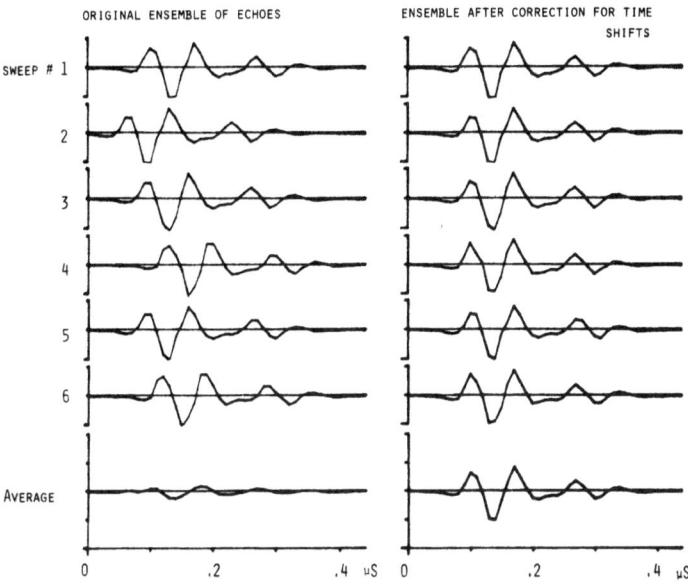

ORIGINAL ENSEMBLE OF ECHOES   ENSEMBLE AFTER CORRECTION FOR TIME SHIFTS

SWEEP # 1

2

3

4

5

6

AVERAGE

0   .2   .4 µS 0   .2   .4 µS

Fig. 2. The effect of aligning on the averaging procedure.

REDUCTION OF NOISE

As stated above, the presence of noise obligates the use of additional band-filtering. The stronger the noise power is, the narrower the passband must be, and the worse the output resolution is. Reduction of the noise may therefore enhance the ultimate resolution. This reduction may be achieved by averaging consecutive sweeps, provided the signal waveform does not vary too much. Fig. 2 shows how an ensemble of sweeps may be disaligned for instance due to hand and eye movements. Considerable loss of signal power or even severe distortion of the average signal, due to non-coherent superposition may result. After application of an aligning procedure, which uses the signals phase spectrum, no loss of signal power occurs. The procedure we have developed for this purpose may be called coherent averaging. Fig. 3 shows the consequences of the procedure in the signal spectrum. Straightforward averaging yields a considerable reduction of the noise level, visible outside the signal band, but there may also be a loss of signal power (See band around 7 MHz). After aligning, the signal power is not affected but the noise is diminished, resulting in a considerable improvement of signal to noise ratio (SNR). After such an optimization of this SNR, a better output resolution can be achieved.

INFLUENCE OF THE ACOUSTIC FIELD

The returning signal is effected not only by the acoustic tissue characteristics, but also in a considerable way by the shape, orientation and position of the

413

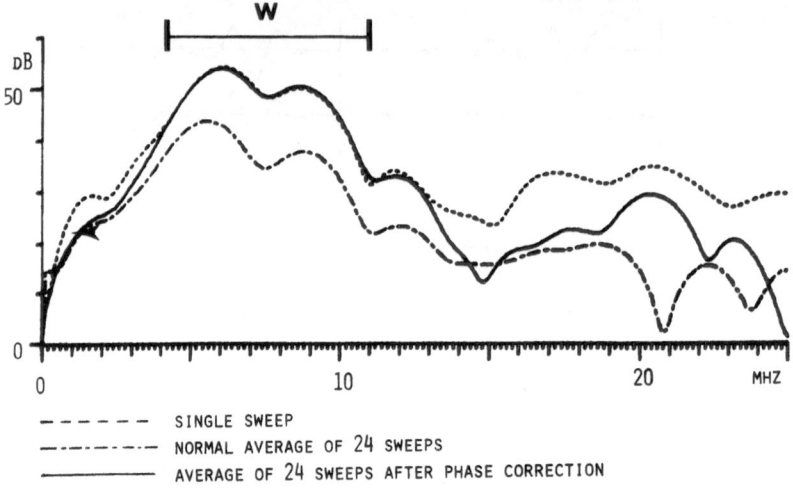

Fig. 3. Effect of aligning on the spectrum of the average; the interval W indicates the relevant signal band.

tissue (membrane) with respect to the non-homogeneous sound field. *In vivo* these circumstances cannot be controlled or determined very well. The position may be estimated in one coordinate, along the beam axis, from the time of flight. We consider intraocular membranes to be flat, so the only undefined factor that remains *in vivo* for such structures is their orientation. If variations in orientation are of little influence on the echo waveform, reliable results may be obtained *in vivo*.

The influence of the incidence angle on reflections from a flat plate has been studied for both flat and medium focused transducers. Fig. 4 shows the logarithmic spectra as a function of angle of incidence of the sound on a brass plate reflector, both for a flat transducer ($\emptyset$ 5 mm) at an axial distance of 20 mm and for a focused transducer (focal length 60 mm) in focus. The spectra clearly display the enormous sensitivity, in both magnitude and spectral content, to slanting of the plate if a flat transducer is used. The spectra of the focused transducer are much more constant. As a result the echo waveform varies much less. For our purposes, the echo waveform of the focused transducer showed a sufficient constancy in an area of 8 mm depth around focus and angles of incidence up to 3 to 4 degrees. For this transducer, these applicability limits about coincide with a reduction of echo amplitude with respect to normal incidence by a factor of two.

RESULTS

In vitro

Deconvolution was applied to a thin polyethylene membrane (170 μm). Fig. 5 in the middle shows the reflection from this membrane, that was placed in

414

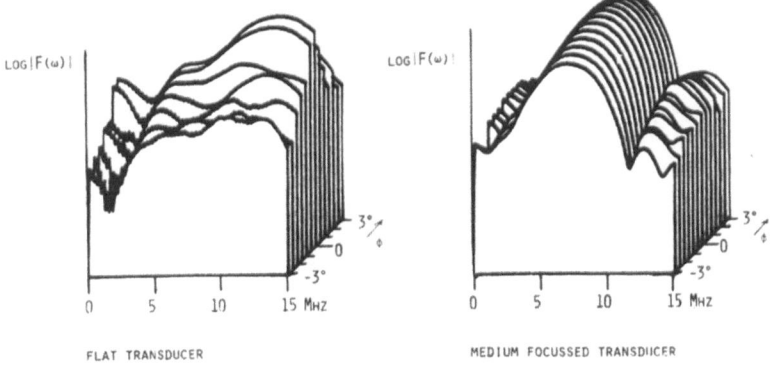

LOG |F(ω)|

3°
0
-3°

0   5   10   15 MHZ

FLAT TRANSDUCER

LOG |F(ω)|

3°
0
-3°

0   5   10   15 MHZ

MEDIUM FOCUSSED TRANSDUCER

Fig. 4. Dependence of logaritmic spectra of a plate echo on the angle of incidence.

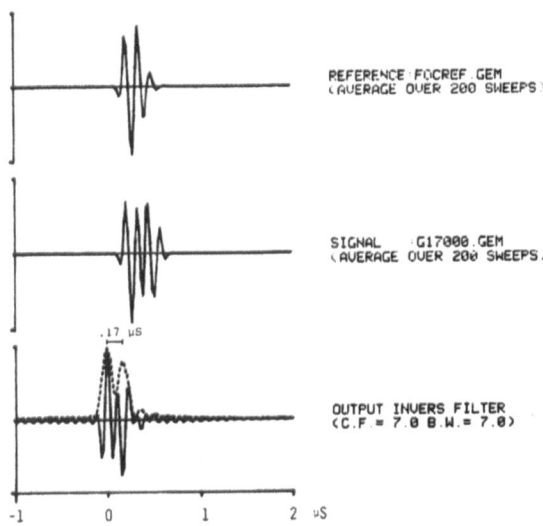

REFERENCE FOCREF.GEM
(AVERAGE OVER 200 SWEEPS)

SIGNAL   G17000.GEM
(AVERAGE OVER 200 SWEEPS)

.17 µS

OUTPUT INVERS FILTER
(C.F.= 7.0 B.W.= 7.0)

-1   0   1   2 µS

Fig. 5. Inverse filter output for membrane of polyethylene.

focus. On top is the reference echo, obtained from a brass plate in the same configuration. On the bottom, the result of the inverse filtering (and additional application of a 7 MHz wide bandfilter) clearly resolves the front and rear interface of the membrane. The ripple is an 11 MHz artifact, due to a peculiarity of the transducer used. The difference in time of arrival, equivalent to a tissue thickness of 120 micrometers, as well as the signs and magnitudes of the individual echoes can be extracted easily. Strong damping within the layer is the cause of the rear echo being much lower than the front one.

415

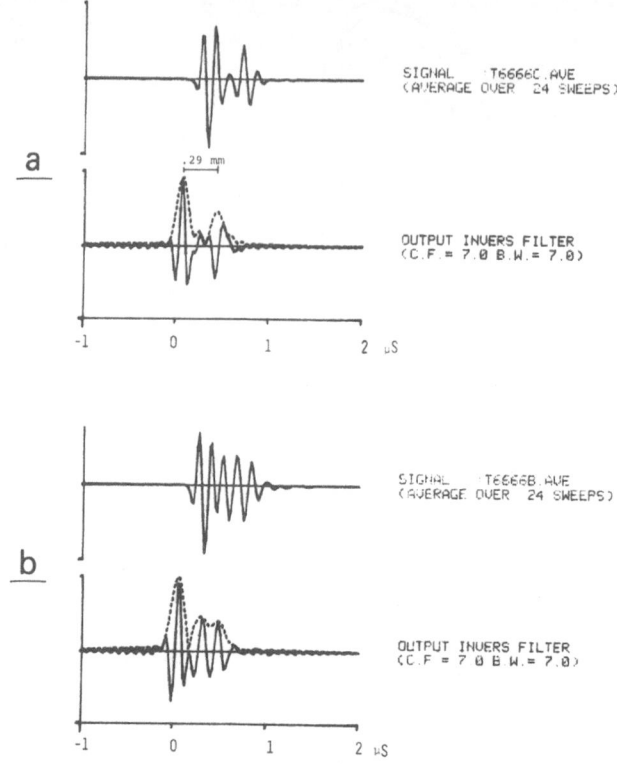

Fig. 6. Result of deconvolution on registrations of a detached retina.

In vivo

Figs. 6 & 7 show the preliminary *in vivo* results. Not all echoes can be processed in this way because of effects of the acoustic field. The traces shown here however, were obtained within the usable part of the field of the transducer. Fig. 6 concerns registrations of a detached retina. After inverse filtering the front echo is clearly displayed, with well defined sign and magnitude. In the first recording the same holds true for the rear echo, indicating a local retinal thickness of 290 μm. The low amplitude of the rear echo and it's ambiguity in the other registration suggest a less specular character of the reflection from the interface between retina and subretinal fluid. Fig. 7 shows the output in case of choroidal detachment. After processing three echoes can be distinguished, presumably corresponding to vitreous-retina, retina-choroid and choroid-fluid interfaces.

DISCUSSION

Inverse filtering techniques have shown their potential to improve the resolution of echographic signals from thin layers, provided they are obtained

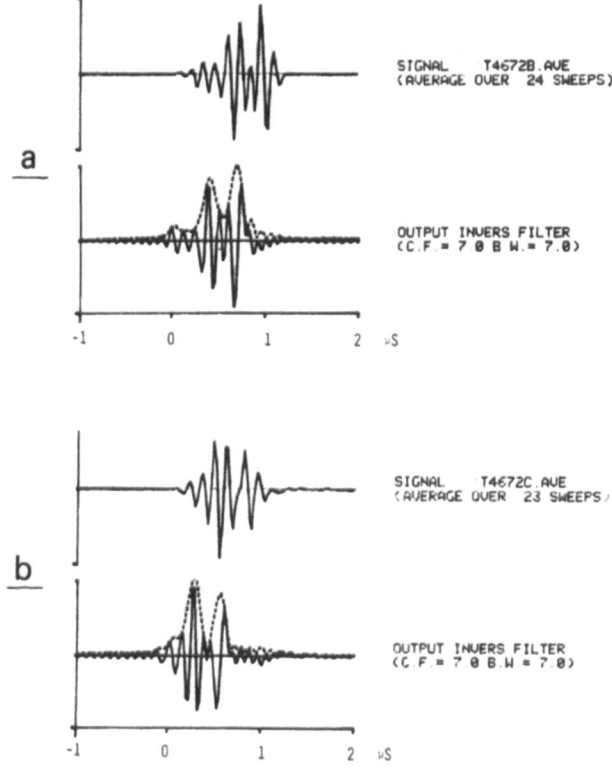

Fig. 7. Deconvolution results for a choroidal detachment.

with a focused transducer and lie within a restricted area around focus and limited angle of incidence. Our *in vivo* results indicate that an improvement of axial resolution by a factor of two can be achieved. Simultaneously the signs of individual echoes are produced, as well as the received amplitudes. The latter though is less reliable, because of the strong influence of the angle of incidence on it. Therefore, reliable quantitative conclusions about the relations of acoustic impedances of adjacent layers cannot yet be drawn. Processing of *in vivo* obtained intraocular membranes yields different patterns for retinal and choroidal detachment. Not enough cases have been evaluated yet to draw conclusions about the possibilities in characterizing the tissues adequately.

REFERENCES

Beretzky, I. Detection and characterization of arterosclerosis in a human arterial wall by raylographic techniques, an in vivo study. In: Ultrasound in Medicine Vol. 3B (D.N. White & R.E. Brown, Eds.) New York: Plenum Press (1977) p. 1597.
Herment, A. 'Impediography': Principle, applicability, results. In: Ultrasonic Tissue Characterization (J.M. Thijssen, Ed.) Alphen aan de Rijn: Stafleu (1980) p. 186.

Jones, J.P. & Cole-Beuglet, C. In vivo characterization of several lesions in the eye using ultrasonic impediography. In: Acoustic imaging, Vol. 8 (A.F. Metherhell, Ed.) New York: Plenum Press (1980) p. 539.

Kruizinga, R. & Thijssen, J.M. Determination of the times of arrival and the amplitude of echoes by inverse filtering of the power spectrum. In: Proc. 3rd Europ. Cong. Ultrasonics in Medicine, Bologna (1978) p. 161.

Martens, W.L.J., Somer, J.C., Hoeks, A.P.G. & Smeets, F.A.M. 'Optimal' inverse filtering and matched filtering, and their relations to in vivo echographic tissue characterization. In: Ultrasonic Tissue Characterization, (J.M. Thijssen, Ed.) Alphen aan de Rijn: Stafleu (1980) p. 245.

Mountford, R.A. & Wells, P.N.T. Ultrasonic liver scanning: the A-scan in the normal & liver cirrhosis. Phys. Med. Biol. 17: 261 (1972).

Papoulis, A. & Chamzas, C. Improvement of range resolution by spectral extrapolation. In: Untrasonic Imaging, 1: 121 (1979).

Robinson, D.E. Nearfield transient radiation patterns for circular pistons. IEEE Trans. ASSP 22: 395 (1974).

Thijssen, J.M., Bayer, A.L. & Cloostermans, M. Computer assisted echography: Statistical analysis of A-mode video echograms obtained by tissue sampling. In press: Med. Biol. Engng. & Comp.

Authors' Address:
Biophysics Laboratory of the Institute of Ophthalmology
University of Nijmegen, The Netherlands

THE RECOGNITION OF DETACHED RETINA AND VITREOUS MEMBRANES BY MEANS OF RADIO FREQUENCY SIGNAL ANALYSIS

H.G. TRIER, D. DECKER, R. MÜLLER-BREITENKAMP,
K. IRION & K.J. OTTO

(Bonn/Stuttgart, F.R.G.)

INTRODUCTION

A doctor who becomes aware of the fact that he is not able to evaluate tissue echograms fully himself, may become interested in being aided by a computer. For almost ten years now (SIDUO IV) the Bonn/Stuttgart group has been continuously engaged in computer analysis of A-mode and RF-signals for improved tissue differentiation in the eye. Since 1973 we have specialised on the radio frequency (RF)-signal. This signal carries maximum information on tissue structure and is clearly superior to the A-mode or the lines forming the B-mode image (Trier & Reuter 1973a, b, Decker, *et al.* 1973, Trier 1974). Since 1977 the developed technique has been granted for clinical evaluation *in vivo* in the University Eye Clinic, Bonn, to collect statistical data.

In the meantime, other groups (Coleman & Lizzi, New York, Thijssen, Nijmegen) have followed in the same direction. The methodical approach, however, shows some differences, dependent upon the equipment and strategy used. Fundamentally, the original RF-signal can be analysed either in the time domain, or in the frequency (spectral) domain.

METHOD

Our group's approach is especially characterized by:
- use of reference signals (Trier, *et al.* 1977a)
- signal analysis both in the time and frequency domain (Reuter & Trier 1972, Trier & Reuter 1975)
- time averaging technique in time domain analysis
- combination of extracted features in feature sets (Decker, *et al.* 1973, 1977a).

Signal acquisition

The region of interest is identified in the eye and then examined using a broadband system with the following characteristics:
- hand held transducer, ∅ 1/2 in., focused at 50 mm, with water stand off, nominal frequency 15 MHz

- pulse length ca 200 ns (- 10 dB)
- receiver band width 5–30 MHz (- 3 dB)
- time window 2 μs
- A/D-conversion with 9 bit (y), sampling rate 256 MHz (equiv.)
- data intermediate storage and transfer on tape/disc via minicomputer.

Details of signal acquisition are described elsewhere (Trier & Reuter 1973b, Reuter, *et al.* 1975, Trier 1977b, Lepper, *et al.* 1978).

Signal processing

Signal processing of RF-signals is done on a small real-time computer (PDP 11/40) and proceeds in a semi-automated way. The software shows a modular structure and allows interactive corrections under display control. A bandwidth of 5–22 MHz was evaluated. (Decker 1977, Decker, *et al.* 1980).

THIN LAYER EXAMINATION

One of the main applications of the system is the examination of thin layers. Conventional A- and B-mode techniques do not give any information on tissue layers smaller than 1 mm approximately, besides integrated amplitude information. By means of sophisticated computer aided techniques, however, the thin layer structure of the tissue can be characterized in a double way:

(1) by accurate measurement of the layer thickness (down to 60 μ at a sound velocity of 1500/s) and

(2) by description of the boundaries, that means of the anterior and posterior surfaces of the thin layer (Trier, *et al.* 1979).

For this potential the following clinical applications are promising:

- Vitreoretinal diseases, especially detection and differentiation of retinal detachment vs vitreous membranes before vitreous surgery.
- Differentiation of tumours by means of proximity layer characterization (Nachbarschichtanalyse, Trier 1980).

VITREORETINAL DISEASES

The following part deals with vitreoretinal diseases. The question whether an unknown intraocular membrane really can be considered to be a detached retina or a type of a vitreous membrane can be solved by two different strategies (Fig. 1)

Direct approach: Direct signal analysis of the membrane signal. The features of the unknown membrane have then to be compared with the appropriate features of detached retina and vitreous membrane.

Indirect approach: For this purpose the eye's back wall lying under the unknown membrane is examined with the system to find out, whether a normally attached retina can be found. The corresponding steps are: comparison of the prescleral layers of the unknown back wall echogram with the feature sets of: (1) normal back wall and (2) back wall without retina.

420

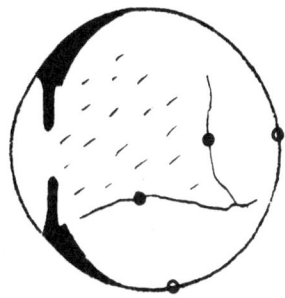

Detached Retina   vs   Vitreous Membrane
●   DIRECT   Diagnostic Approach
○   INDIRECT Diagnostic Approach

Fig. 1. Diagnostic strategies for the detection of retinal detachment, schematically.

The results of both approaches together lead to the final diagnostic decision. This double strategy is not new; however, new are the chances to solve this old problem by computerized techniques. For this application the following signal processing steps are made:

Automated quality assurance

By means of various plausibility criteria disturbed signals are recognized, and according to the degree of disturbance restored or rejected. Disturbances may arise e.g. from faults in the recording system, insufficient angle of incidence and lacking cooperation ability of the patient. The number of restored and rejected echograms is registered.

The formation of file-specific representative echograms

By means of controlled averaging (after time alignment) in the time domain of echograms, which are recorded from one location of the examined tissue, one or more representative echograms are constructed. To characterize tissues the number of representative echograms and the dispersion between single echograms and average echograms are used (Fig. 2).

Determination of layer thickness

The distance of boundaries can be determined by various methods: visually; inverse filtering, interference spectrum; autocorrelation; cross correlation. A comparison of these methods for retinal thickness measurement was given at SIDUO VII (Decker & Trier 1979). The visual method is especially limited in applicability and resolution, even after preprocessing. The relevant techniques are:

Interference spectrum. Transformation of the echogram produced by two surfaces into the frequency domain yields an interference spectrum, which shows equidistant maxima and minima (Δf). From Δf the correspondent

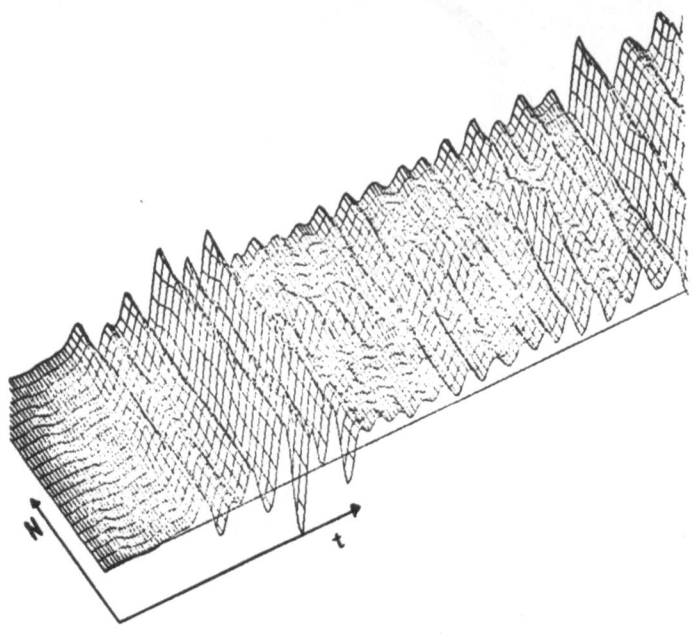

Fig. 2a. Isometric view of an echo signal series, as a means for qualitative evaluation of homogeneity.

distance Δs of the boundaries can be calculated for a given sound velocity (Fig. 3). Under the premises of a 5...22 MHz analysed frequency range and of the presence of at least four minima for a reliable thickness measurement the resolution is Δs min = 125 μm; the accuracy ± 10%. In clinical routine these values cannot be reached, because the transducers mostly do not provide the necessary regular spectral characteristics. This technique is, therefore, restricted on tissue layers of ⩾ 180 μm.

Cross correlation. Correlation of a reference echogram from a flat target with the tissue echogram leads to the cross correlation function (Fig. 4). By its evaluation layer thickness down to Δs min = 60 μm can be measured; the accuracy being ± 3% of the layer thickness. Compared with the spectral technique above, cross correlation is not only more powerful in resolution, but also applicable in case of more than two boundaries, which is the clinical situation of the eye wall.

In vivo results for thickness of retina, choroid, detached retina and retina overlying a choroidal tumour were presented at SIDUO VII (Decker & Trier 1979). Registration of retinal and choroidal thickness in dependence on time, provides information on circulation dependent pulsation of these layers; such measurements in humans without anesthesia were reported by Lepper 1978.

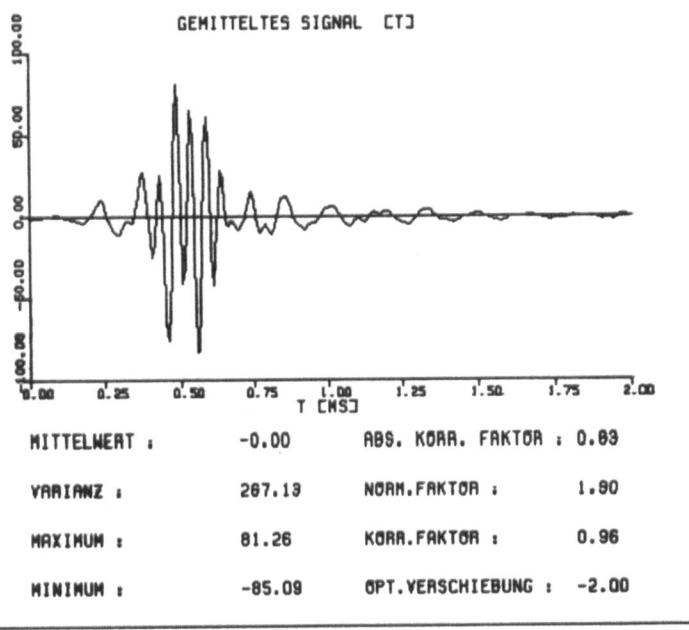

GEMITTELTES SIGNAL [T]

MITTELWERT :	-0.00	ABS. KORR. FAKTOR :	0.83
VARIANZ :	267.13	NORM.FAKTOR :	1.80
MAXIMUM :	81.26	KORR.FAKTOR :	0.96
MINIMUM :	-85.09	OPT.VERSCHIEBUNG :	-2.00

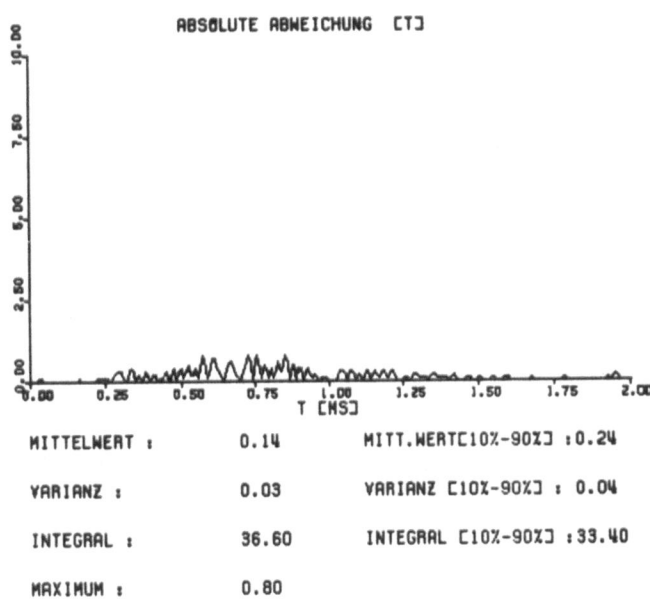

ABSOLUTE ABWEICHUNG [T]

MITTELWERT :	0.14	MITT.WERT[10%-90%] :	0.24
VARIANZ :	0.03	VARIANZ [10%-90%] :	0.04
INTEGRAL :	36.60	INTEGRAL [10%-90%] :	33.40
MAXIMUM :	0.80		

Fig. 2b. The lower curve demonstrates the absolute maximal deviation between a representative, averaged signal (upper part) and all the signals of one file, in the case of detached retina (old peripheral detachment, case Nr. MAR 633).

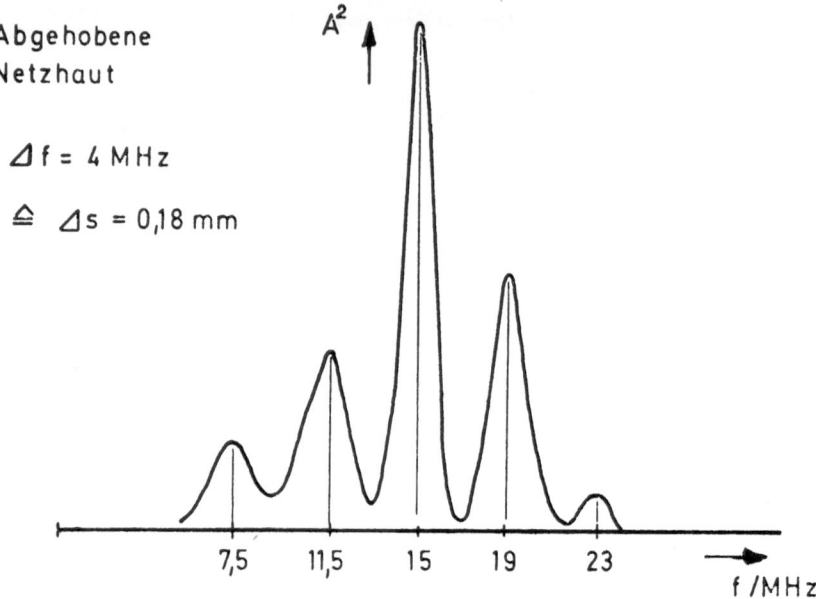

Abgehobene
Netzhaut

$\Delta f = 4\,MHz$

$\triangleq \Delta s = 0{,}18\,mm$

A^2

7,5   11,5   15   19   23

f /MHz

Fig. 3. Thickness determination of detached retina using the spectral distribution, schematically.

The analysis of the boundary surface in the frequency domain

According to the roughness r of a surface in relation to the wave length λ a distinction is made between: (Fig. 5)

    (a) specular surfaces with $r \ll \lambda$

    (b) scattering surfaces with $r \leqslant \lambda$ and with a homogeneous distribution of scattering elements

    (c) structured surfaces with $r \geqslant \lambda$ and an inhomogeneous distribution of scattering elements.

The corresponding spectral distributions (amplitude spectrum) are distinguished as follows:

    ad (a) Single peak distribution (similar to a Gaussian distribution with $f_c \approx f_N$.

          (f_c = centre frequency of the distribution,

           f_N = nominal frequency of the transducer).

    ad (b) Single peak distribution with $f_c > f_N$.

    ad (c) Multi peak or asymmetrical distribution, respectively.

Echo amplitude (reflectivity) of the boundaries or echo ensembles

Compared to a reference signal, this evaluation is performed with the RF-signal and the derived computer-made A-mode signal.

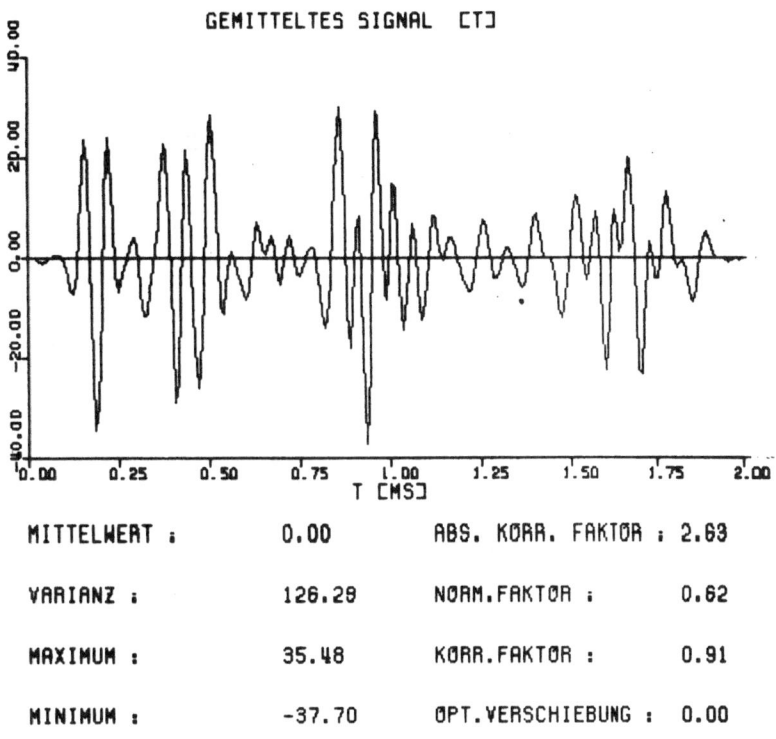

GEMITTELTES SIGNAL [T]

MITTELWERT :	0.00	ABS. KORR. FAKTOR : 2.63
VARIANZ :	126.29	NORM.FAKTOR : 0.62
MAXIMUM :	35.48	KORR.FAKTOR : 0.91
MINIMUM :	-37.70	OPT.VERSCHIEBUNG : 0.00

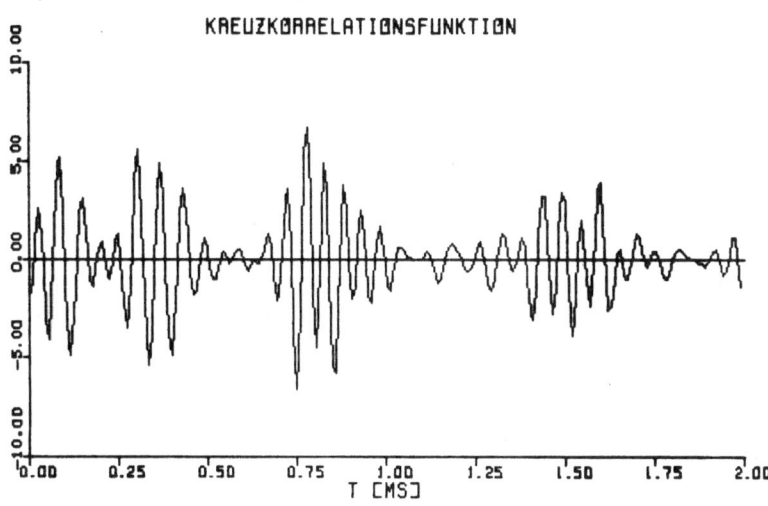

KREUZKORRELATIONSFUNKTION

Fig. 4. Representative, averaged echogram (upper part) and correspondent cross correlation function (lower part) in a case of normal retinochoroidal layer (case Nr. MAR 913).

425

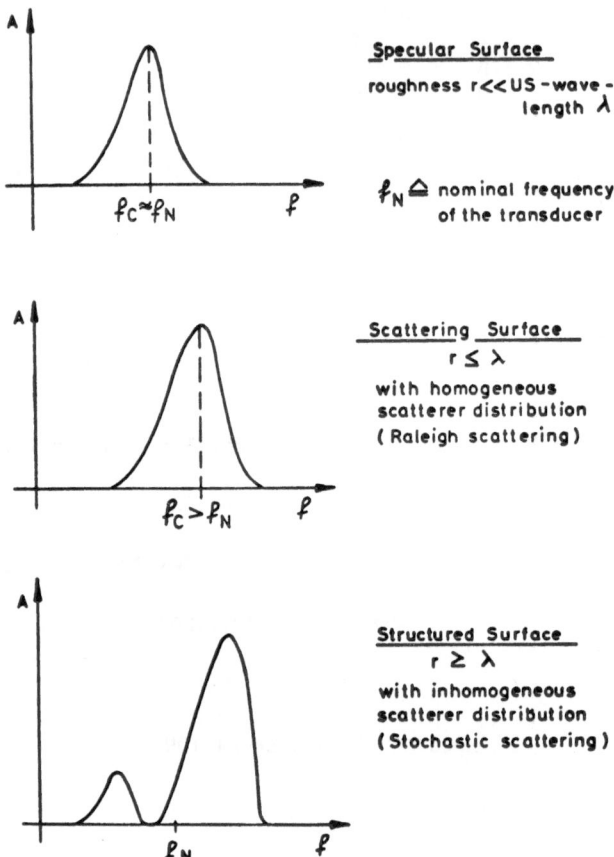

Specular Surface

roughness r<<US–wave–
length λ

$f_N \triangleq$ nominal frequency
of the transducer

Scattering Surface
$r \leq \lambda$

with homogeneous
scatterer distribution
(Raleigh scattering)

Structured Surface
$r \geq \lambda$

with inhomogeneous
scatterer distribution
(Stochastic scattering)

Fig. 5. Spectral classification of boundaries (surfaces), schematically.

EXAMPLES OF TISSUE DIFFERENTIATION

From a parameter printout (Fig. 6), we try to extract features in data sheets. The full printout contains for every patient's file the significant properties for the characterization of the examined tissue layers like distance and structure of the boundary surfaces as well as data on the spatial inhomogeneity (Decker & Irion 1980). From such data sheets, Table 1 has been composed.

(a) *Direct diagnostic approach:*

The characterization of boundaries in a case of detached retina is shown in the upper left part of Table 1. Please note that in part (25%) of the echograms the retina was thickened and an interior echo structure was found in the retinal layer, indicated here as 'additional layer'. The second thing to note is, that the centre frequency of the posterior retinal surface is higher than that of the anterior retinal surface.

426

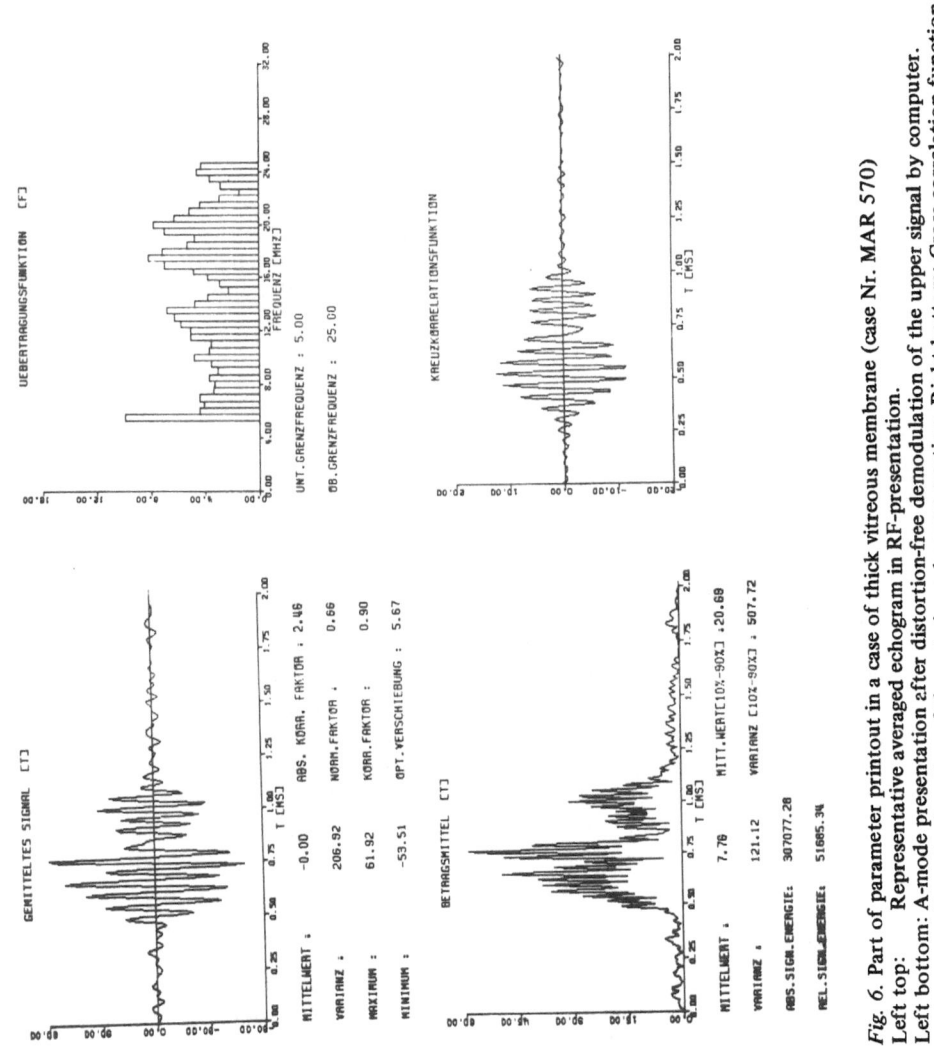

Fig. 6. Part of parameter printout in a case of thick vitreous membrane (case Nr. MAR 570)
Left top: Representative averaged echogram in RF-presentation.
Left bottom: A-mode presentation after distortion-free demodulation of the upper signal by computer.
Right top: Transfer function of the anterior echogram portion. Right bottom: Cross correlation function.

427

Table 1. Preliminary results in detached retina.

Features	Detached retina		Vitreous membrane	
boundary surfaces	I	II	I	II
layer thickness/μm	128 const		120...700 var	
centre frequency/MHz	10.5	14.5	15.5...17.5	17.5
spectral type	SP	SP	ST	ST, FS
additional layer Δ s/μm	–	95 var	120...200 var	–
reflectivity/dB	– 28		– 32	

	Back wall without retina			Normal back wall (retina and choroid)		
boundary surfaces	I	II	III	I	II	III
layer thickness/μm	150..240	240..440 const		133 const	540 const	
additional layer Δs/μm	–	90..220 var	–	–	100 const	–
centre frequency/MHz	–	80..13.5	8.5..16.0	12.6	14.5	14.0
spectral type	FS	SP	SP	SP	SP	SP
reflectivity/dB	– 30			– 20		

Spectral type of surfaces	Layer thickness	Reflectivity
SP: specular surface	const = constant per file and per patient (n files)	dB-level referenced to a flat target reflectivity
ST: scattering surface		
FS: structured surface	var = constant per file; variable per patient (n files)	$(15\,\text{mV} \stackrel{\wedge}{=} 0\,\text{dB})$

The right upper part of Table 1 shows a vitreous membrane. Typically layer thickness is variable in one membrane, in contrast to detached retina. Thickness ranges between 120–700 μm or more. Dominating frequencies of front and back surface are higher than in detached retina. Reflected energy is markedly lower than in detachment, which seems to fit the clinical experience in A- and B-mode. However, here the reflectivity of the surface echo alone can be utilized for differentiation, without electronical summation effects over the whole layer, which are involved in normal A-mode reflectivity.

(b) *Indirect diagnostic approach:*

In the right lower part of Table 1 the normal rear wall outside the macular region is characterized by a first layer of about 133 μs. The choroid – that is the distance between the presumable back surface of the retina and the sclera – is about 540 μs. In part of the patients an additional echo can be seen. This might be an interior choroidal structure. The layers have a constant thickness in one patient. The dominating spectral frequency increases only slightly from retina towards choroid. A case of back wall without retina is shown in the lower left part of Table 1. The typical first layer with the thickness of retina is absent here. In contrast to retina, the first layer (pigment epithelium and choroid) varies in thickness in one patient. Spectral behaviour has a broader variability; reflectivity may be less than for the retinal surface. In conclusion, Table 2 demonstrates some additional findings in detached retina. We feel that for the present the echographic findings regarding the

Table 2. Tissue features for the recognition of detached retina and vitreous membrane; examples of 4 clinical cases:

Upper part: Direct diagnostic approach. Left: detached retina. right: vitreous membrane.

Lower part: Indirect diagnostic approach. Left: back wall without retina. right: normal back wall (without scleral features).

Statistical results in cases of detached retina	
(A)	A dependence of the features of detached retina on age and sex of the patients can not be proved statistically.
(B)	Retinal thickness D of old and recent detachment: Collective without consideration of the patients age (61 patients): Old detachment (> 1 month) $D = 123\,\mu m$ Recent detachment (< 1 month) $D = 133\,\mu m$ Patient group of 50–60 years (18 patients). Old detachment $D = 124\,\mu m$ Recent detachment $D = 137\,\mu m$ (coefficient of variation: 30%)
(C)	Structure of the retinal boundaries Scattering or fine-structured boundaries are obtained with Old detachment 60% Recent detachment 12.5%

interior structure of retina and choroid have not yet been fully correlated with histology. However, we suppose that vitreoretinal applications will, in the near future, profit first in clinical use from the ten years research history in computer-aided signal analysis of the eye.

ACKNOWLEDGEMENT

This study was supported by grants: DFVLR-BPT 01 VI 047 and 057 from the Bundesminister für Forschung and Technologie.

REFERENCES

Decker, D., Epple, E., Leiss, W. & Nagel, M. Digital computer analysis of time-amplitude ultrasonograms from the human eye. II. Data processing. J. Clin. Ultrasound 1: 156 (1973).

Decker, D., Trier, H.G., Nagel, M., Reuter, R., Epple, E. & Lepper, R.-D. Rechnergestützte Ultraschall-Diagnostik in der Ophthalmologie. In: Medizinische Physik (W.J. Lorenz, ed. Proc. 7. Wiss. Tag. Dtsch. Ges. Med. Physik, Heidelberg 1976, Bd. 2, Heidelberg: Hüthig-Verlag (1977) p. 195.

Decker, D. Entwicklung rechnergestützter Auswertungsverfahren zur Gewebsdifferenzierung mit Ultraschall. In: Proc. Symp. Ultraschall in der medizinischen Diagnostik und Therapie, DFVLR Köln, Feb. 1977, Wissenschaftliche Berichte der DFVLR (1977) p. 97.

Decker, D. & Trier, H.G. Das Projekt 'rechnergestützte Gewebsdifferenzierung' der Arbeitsgemeinschaft Bonn/Stuttgart. II. Ergebnisse der Anwendung an dünnen Gewebsschichten im Auge. Proc. SIDUO VII, Münster 1978. In: Diagnostica Ultrasonica in Ophthalmologia (H. Gernet, ed) Münster: Remy (1979) p. 40.

Decker, D., Trier, H.G., Epple, E., Reuter, R., Nagel, M. & Lepper, R.-D. Computer-aided tissue differentiation in ophthalmology. Workshop: Engineering: 'Automatic

429

and computer-aided sonography' 3. Europ. Congr. Ultrasonics in Medicine, Bologna 1978. In: Investigative Ultrasonology 1. Technical Advances (C.R. Hill & C. Alvisi, eds.) London: Pitman Medical (1980) p. 29.

Decker, D. & Irion, K. Examination of thin tissue layers. 5. Int. Symp. Ultrasonic Imaging and Tissue Characterization, Gaithersburg, USA, 1980 (in press).

Lepper, R.-D. Ultraschallmessungen an der Rückwand des lebenden menschlichen Auges. Diss. Math.-nat. Fakultät Bonn 1978.

Lepper, R.-D., Reuter, R. & Trier, H.G. Digitization of high-frequency ultrasonic signals for tissue differentiation in ophthalmology. Biomed. Techn. 23: 75 (1978).

Reuter, R. & Trier, H.G. Beitrag zur Informationserfassung an Echogrammen in der Ophthalmologie. In: Proc. Medizin-Technik, Stuttgart 1972.

Reuter, R., Lepper, R.-D., Trier, H.G., Decker, D. & Nagel, M. Fortschritte bei der Erfassung schneller Ultraschallsignale und ihr Wert für die maschinelle Signalverarbeitung in der Ultraschalldiagnostik. Biomed. Techn. 20 (Ergänzungsband): 343 (1975).

Trier, H.G. & Reuter, R. Eine Anlage zur halbautomatischen Klassierung verschiedener Formen von Gewebsechogrammen in Zeit-Amplituden-Darstellung. In: Proc. SIDUO IV, Paris 1971 (Massin, M. & J. Poujol, eds.) Paris: Centre National d'ophtalmologie des Quinze-Vingts (1973) p. 87.

Trier, H.G. & Reuter, R. Digital computer analysis of time-amplitude ultrasonograms from the human eye. I. Signal acquisition. J. Clin. Ultrasound 1: 150–154 (1973).

Trier, H.G. Gewebsdifferenzierung mit Ultraschall. Habil. schrift Bonn 1974; Bibl. Ophthalmol. No. 86 Basel: Karger (1977).

Trier, H.G. & Reuter, R. Der Einfluß von Impulseigenschaften auf die Echo-Umhüllende. Proc. SIDUO V, Gent 1973. In: Ultrasonography in ophthalmology. Bibl. Ophthalmol. No. 83, Basel: Karger (1975) p. 2.

Trier, H.G., Decker, D., Lepper, R.-D. & Reuter, R. Reference signals in the field of ultrasonogram analysis. Engineering aspects. In: Ultrasound in Medicine, Vol. 3B. (D. White & R.E. Brown, eds.) New York & London: Plenum Press (1977) p. 1965.

Trier, H.G. Entwicklung von objektiven Verfahren der Gewebsdifferenzierung aus dem A-Bild und HF-Echogramm sowie ihre Anwendung in der Ophthalmologie. Proc. Symp. Ultraschall in der medizinischen Diagnostik und Therapie, DFVLR Köln, Feb. 1977. Köln: Wissenschaftliche Berichte der DFVLR (1977) p. 65.

Trier, H.G., Lepper, R.-D. & Reuter, R. Das Projekt 'rechnergestützte Gewebsdifferenzierung' der Arbeitsgemeinschaft Bonn/Stuttgart. I. Stand der Methodik in vivo. Proc. SIDUO VII, Münster 1978. In: Diagnostica Ultrasonica in Ophthalmologia, (H. Gernet, ed) Münster: Remy (1979) p. 35.

Trier, H.G. Ultrasonic tissue characterization in the eye and orbit. In: Ultrasonic Tissue Characterization (J.M. Thijssen, ed.) Alphen aan den Rijn: Stafleu (1980) p. 45.

Authors' Addresses:
Klinisches Institut für experimentelle
Ophthalmologie der Universität Bonn
(Dr. Trier, Dr. Müller-Breitenkamp & Dr. Otto)
Bonn, F.R.G.

Institut für Biomedizinische Technik der
Universität Stuttgart (Dr. Decker & Dr. Irion)
Stuttgart, F.R.G.

430

MEASUREMENT OF ULTRASOUND ATTENUATION IN TISSUES FROM SCATTERED REFLECTIONS: IN-VITRO ASSESSMENT OF APPLICABILITY

J.M. THIJSSEN, M. CLOOSTERMANS & A.L. BAYER

The attenuation of ultrasound may become a useful parameter in *in-vivo* tissue characterization. A simple approach using the video signal of A-mode equipment and decompressing the amplitude levels has proven to yield significant information (c.f. Thijssen *et al.* 1980, 1981). Since the A-mode signal contains only disturbed frequency information a better signal for studying the frequency dependence of tissue interaction is of course the radio frequency (RF) echogram. Two parameters may be derived then, i.e. the attenuation per centimeter tissue at a particular frequency (e.g. the center frequency of the transducer), and the frequency dependence of the interaction of ultrasound with tissue expressed by the spectral slope, i.e. the spectral power relative to some internal (i.e. another tissue sample) or external reference power spectrum. The attenuation and the frequency dependence can by summarized by the so-called tissue transfer function, or tissue impulse response (Kak & Dines 1978, Dines & Kak 1979).

In this kind of approach the transmission of ultrasound is measured, or alternatively, the reflections from tissue boundaries are used (Lizzi *et al.* 1976). Another approach is to analyse the scattered echoes from a tissue region and take a reference from another region of the same tissue. This latter method has been discussed by Kuc & Schwarz, 1979, who with particular assumptions derived an optimal strategy for taking samples along the ultrasound beam (i.e. in depth from a single RF-echogram). Coleman & Lizzi (1979) published results on intra-ocular tumours and further data are given in this volume (Coleman & Lizzi 1981). A survey of the described techniques is given by Berger & Perrin (1980).

The aim of the present study is to investigate the limitations of the RF analysis. The first limitation is caused by the sound field of the transducer. The lateral inhomogeneities may be reduced by focusing (cf. Filipczynski 1976, Kossoff 1979), but with broadband transducers they still may have to be considered and any asymmetry in depth around the focus may also be important. The second limitation may be the inhomogeneity of the tissue itself. We are attempting to answer the question as to whether axial tissue sampling and subsequent averaging of the results is sufficient to obtain reliable estimates of the attenuation and the spectral slope.

© *1981. Dr W. Junk Publishers, The Hague*

METHODS

The equipment

The A-mode apparatus is home made and it has a bandwidth of 20 MHz. The output impedance of the transmitter is adapted to the 50 Ω load of the cable. The transducer is tuned by means of a built-in transformer and it has been manufactured by Oldelft Inc. The transmission pulse and the spectrum of it can be found in Thijssen (1981) in this volume, (i.e. a 7.5 MHz center frequency and a 4 MHz bandwidth ($Q \simeq 2$)).

The transducer has a diameter of 15 mm and is focused at 60 mm. The RF signal is lineary amplified and fed into a transient digitizer (Biomation 8100). This transient recorder is linked with a digital computer system (Digital Equipment Corp. PDP 11/34, 128 K memory) and all controls are software manipulated. The data are stored on magnetic disk prior to further frequency analysis. The digitization is performed in a 50 MHz sampling rate and a time window of 15 mm is obtained by collecting 1024 samples. In order to decrease the electronic and digitization noise 200 identical echograms are collected in rapid succession and are continuously averaged. This average is then stored for further analysis. Since we have performed *in-vitro* measurements the transducer has been fixed in a apparatus that enables accurate lateral and axial displacement of the transducer with respect to the tissue volume. The set-up of the measuring and analysis system is schematically shown in Fig. 1. We have used 35 different lateral positions in a single measurement in our attempt to obtain an estimate of the tissue parameters and their accuracy.

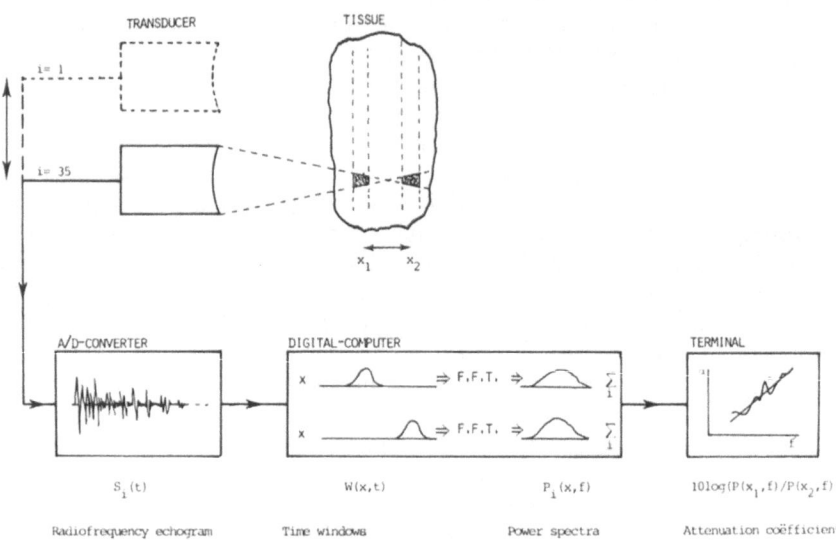

Fig. 1. Scheme of measuring and analysis system. Echograms are collected from 35 lateral positions. Echograms are segmented by Hanning windows w(t). Power spectra of segments are averaged over lateral positions. Slope of the attenuation coefficient from the plot of log difference spectra (averaged over depth) v.s. frequency.

The measurements were performed with a tissue model (Till 1976) and with a preserved liver. The animal (goat) was anaesthetized with Nembutal (30 mg/kg) and blood clotting was prevented by an intravenous injection of Heparine (10^4 I.E.). The animal was sacrificed immediately before the preparation of the liver. The liver was perfused in-situ with ringer solution and thereafter with formalin (4%) via the vena porta.

After four days storage of the liver in formalin small cubes of $10-15$ cm^3 were excised. Care was taken to avoid large vessels running through the tissue samples. According to Bamber *et al.* (1979) the preserved liver is acoustically almost identical to fresh liver.

Data analysis

The time averaged RF echograms are segmented in time windows of a duration Δt (see Fig. 1). In order to prevent side lobes occurring in the spectrum a Hanning window shape ($w(t)$) is used for the segmentation. The time window corresponds to a tissue sample in depth Δx, hence

$$\{(t + \Delta t), t\} \leftrightarrow \{(x + \Delta x), x\} \tag{1}$$

The RF segment $s_{\Delta t}(t)$ yields a power spectrum P:

$$s_{\Delta t}(t) \overset{\text{FFT}}{\Longrightarrow} P_i(x, f) \tag{2}$$

Where i stands for the number of lateral position code of the transducer. The power spectra from a particular depth are averaged over the lateral positions yielding:

$$P(x, f) = \frac{1}{N} \sum_{i=1}^{N} P_i(x, f) \qquad (N = 35) \tag{3}$$

Next a similar power spectrum is introduced to serve as a reference. We have taken the spectrum obtained from the focal region of the transducer, so:

$$P(o, f) = P(x_{foc}, f) \tag{4}$$

The tissue spectra are then divided by this reference spectrum, or if the logarithmic spectrum is taken, the log-difference spectrum is obtained:

$$\Delta P_x(f) = \log P(x, f) - \log P(o, f) \tag{5}$$

generally it is more convenient to calculate the power in decibels:

$$\Delta B_x(f) = 10 \{\log P(x, f) - \log P(o, f)\} \tag{6}$$

The attenuation coefficient from a tissue sample of thickness l can be calculated from the average difference spectrum that is obtained by grouping the log-spectra with a depth distance of $2l/3$ (c.f. Kuc & Schwartz 1979).

$$\Delta B(f) = E\{B_x(f)\} = \frac{1}{n}\sum_{i=1}^{n}[\Delta B_{x_i}(f) - \Delta B_{x_i + 2l/3}(f)$$

$$\text{with } x_n \leqslant l/3 \tag{7}$$

With this procedure the reference spectrum is removed from the calculations. With the assumption that the attenutation coefficient is proportional to the frequency it follows:

$$\Delta B(f) = -10\log(e)\mu_0|f|\frac{1}{n}\sum_{i=1}^{n}(x_i - (x_i + 2l/3))$$

$$= 4.35\,\mu_0\,|f|\,2l/3 \tag{8}$$

and:

$$\Delta B(f)/(2l/3) = \alpha = \alpha_0|f|, \text{with } \alpha_0 = 4.35\,\mu_0 \tag{9}$$

Field effects

In these measurements the transducer was axially displaced in order to obtain spectra from the same piece of tissue but at different axial positions within the sound field (making x only an axial field coordinate). The result of the spectra obtained from a piece of preserved liver are shown in Fig. 2. The center of the x-axis corresponds to the site of the focus, and therefore, the

INFLUENCE OF THE BEAMWIDTH AND FIELDEFFECTS ON THE POWERSPECTRA AS A FUNCTION OF DISTANCE TO FOCUS AND FREQUENCY.

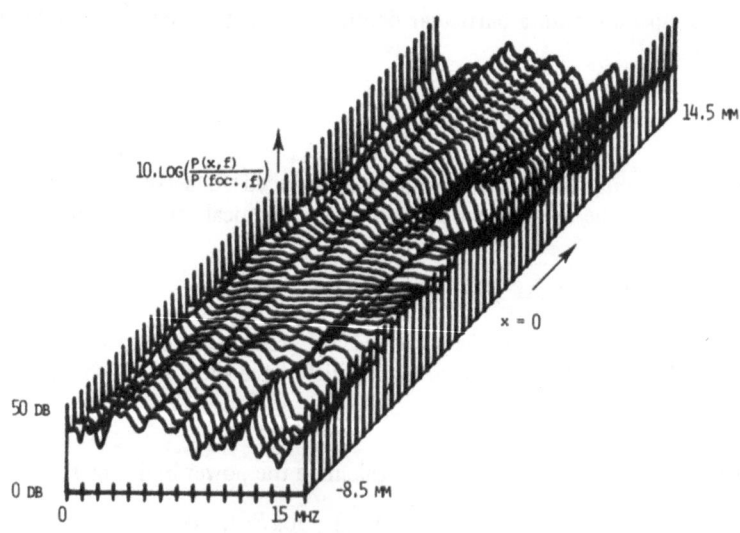

Fig. 2. Relative power spectra (log difference spectra) for preserved tissue as a function of depth. By axial movement of the transducer all spectra are obtained from the same tissue volume. Clear demonstration of field effects. $x = 0$ corresponds to focus.

log-difference spectrum is a horizontal straight line. In front of and behind the focus considerable deviations from a horizontal line are evident and the riples on the spectra (scalloping) are caused by the fact that interference effects (due to interaction of ultrasound with tissue) are frequency dependent as is the sound field itself. Moreover, the change of the diameter of the sound field around the focus results in a gradual increase of the scalloping riples. It may be concluded that if the slope of the relevant part of the log-difference spectrum is considered, the depth of the position from which the spectra are obtained is greatly influencing the result. So even with a focused transducer one has to be very cautious in the interpretation of results.

RESULTS

In vitro attenuation measurements

The logarithmic spectra as a function of depth in the medium (i.e. fixed axial distance of transducer to tissue) are shown in Fig. 3, again for the tissue model (left) and preserved liver (right). It is difficult to appreciate details about the interaction of ultrasound with the media in this kind of picture. The spectra have been averaged over the lateral positions as described in 'Methods'.

The log-difference spectra (dB-scale) are displayed in Fig. 4. The x-coordinate is set to zero in the focus and the reference spectrum is taken from this point. The gradual decline of the high frequency part of the spectra with increasing penetration depth becomes clearly visible. The expected and demonstrated symmetry of field effects around the focus enables in this case further evaluation of the attenuation coefficient with the data in Fig. 4.

The attenuation slope is obtained from the log-difference spectra according to Form. 9 in 'Methods' as shown in Fig. 5. The straight line is the linear regression line through the measured curve. The data yield almost identical values of the order of $1 \, dBcm^{-1} \, MHz^{-1}$ for the tissue model and the liver. It should be noted that the frequency scale has been limited from 3 to 10 MHz because of noise interference.

DISCUSSION

The effect of the ultrasonic field on the estimation of the attenuation coefficient has been minimized by positioning the focus exactly in the centre of the tissue volume. Our measurements indicated that this simplification no longer holds in assymmetrical conditions. Further research to account for this problem will be reported elsewhere. The high degree of averaging we have applied to our data has to be reduced in *in-vivo* measurements. A reduction of the temporal averaging with a factor of 8 to 25 sweeps (0.5 s acquisition time) seems a reasonable first step. The next step has to be the reduction of the lateral measurements. We have found a variability (standard deviation/mean) in the estimates of the attenuation coefficient for liver tissue of 10%.

435

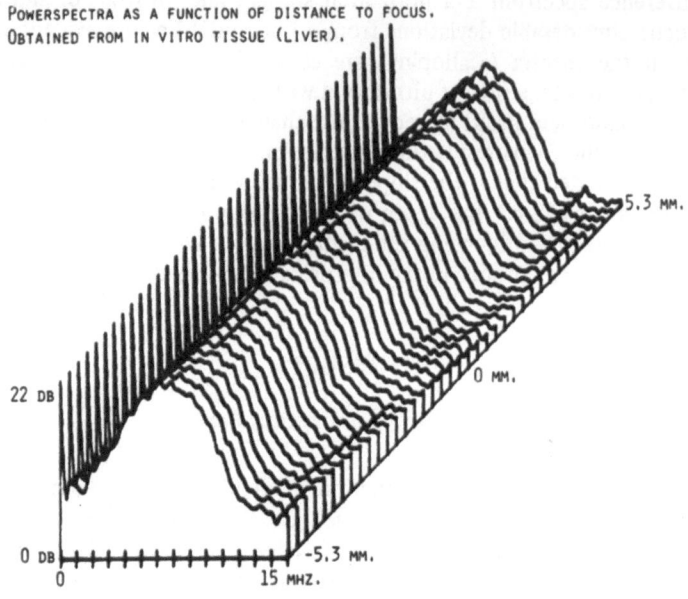

POWERSPECTRA AS A FUNCTION OF DISTANCE TO FOCUS.
OBTAINED FROM IN VITRO TISSUE (LIVER).

5.3 MM.

0 MM.

22 DB

0 DB   -5.3 MM.
  0   15 MHZ.

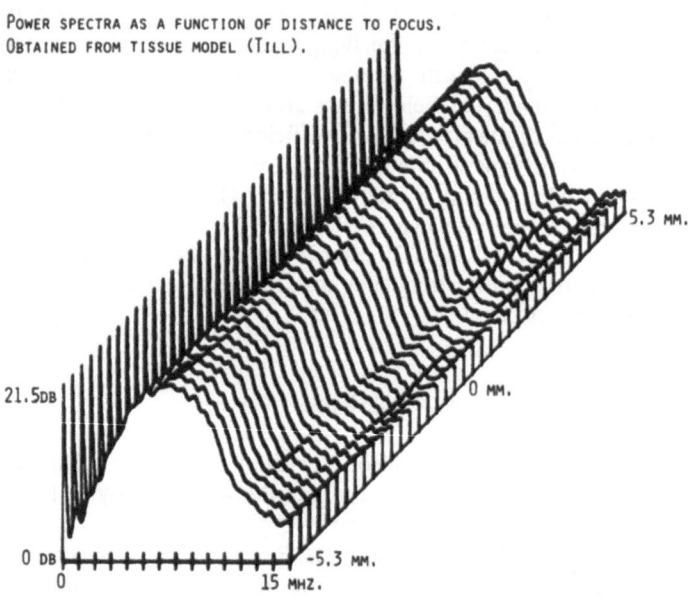

POWER SPECTRA AS A FUNCTION OF DISTANCE TO FOCUS.
OBTAINED FROM TISSUE MODEL (TILL).

5.3 MM.

0 MM.

21.5DB

0 DB   -5.3 MM.
  0   15 MHZ.

Fig. 3. Logarithmic power spectra with fixed distance of transducer to tissue (see Fig. 1).
Bottom: tissue model (Till 1976). Top: preserved liver.

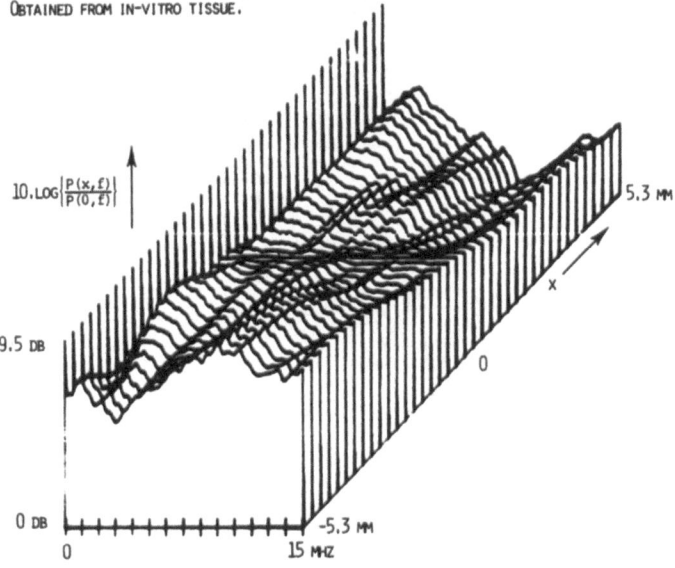

RELATIVE POWERSPECTRA AS FUNCTION OF DISTANCE TO FOCUS AND FREQUENCY.
OBTAINED FROM IN-VITRO TISSUE.

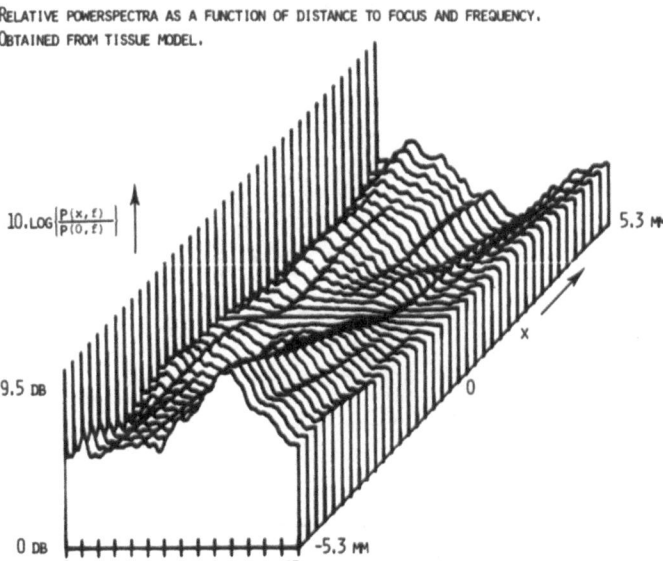

RELATIVE POWERSPECTRA AS A FUNCTION OF DISTANCE TO FOCUS AND FREQUENCY.
OBTAINED FROM TISSUE MODEL.

Fig. 4. Log difference power spectra from data in Fig. 3.

437

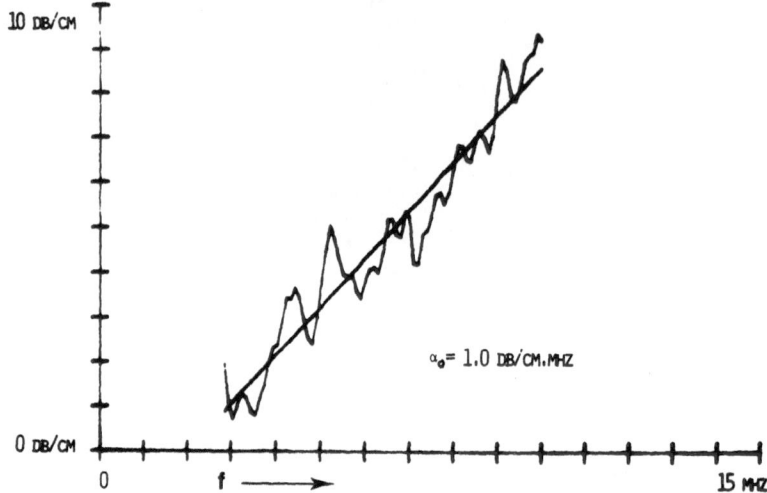

ATTENUATION AS FUNCTION OF FREQUENCY, OBTAINED FROM IN-VITRO TISSUE

$\alpha_o = 1.0$ DB/CM.MHZ

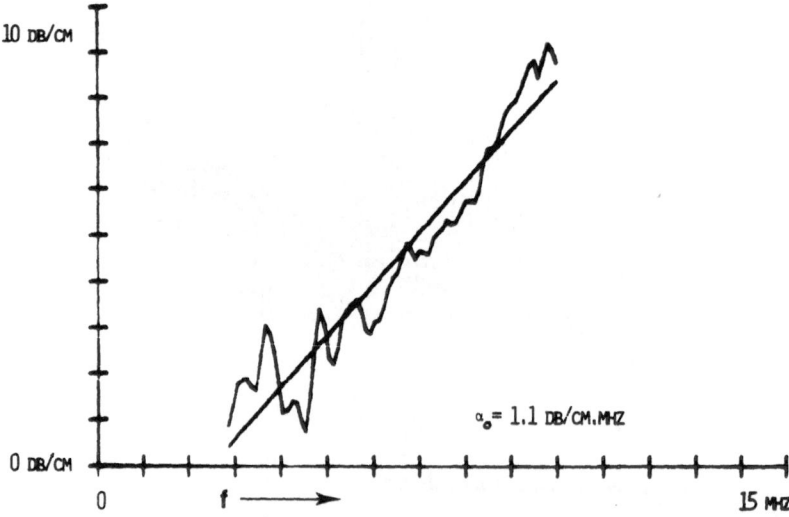

ATTENUATION AS FUNCTION OF FREQUENCY, OBTAINED FROM TISSUE MODEL

$\alpha_o = 1.1$ DB/CM.MHZ

Fig. 5. Slope of attenuation coefficient, α_0, obtained from slope of linear regression line through attenuation data from Fig. 4.

438

Reduction again by a factor of four yields an increase in the variability by another factor of two. The reduction of the accuracy may be partly reversed by increasing the bandwidth of the transducer.

REFERENCES

Bamber, J.C., Hill, C.R., King, J.A., & Dunn, F. Ultrasonic propagation through fixed and unfixed tissues. Ultrasound in Med. & Biol. 5: 159 (1979).

Berger, G., & Perrin, J. Attenuation principles and measurements for tissue characterization. In: Ultrasonic Tissue Characterization: Clinical Achievements and Technology Potentials (J.M. Thijssen, ed.) Alphen a/d Rijn: Stafleu, (1980). p. 117.

Coleman, D.J., & Lizzi, F.L. Computer processed acoustic spectral analysis of ophthalmic tissues. Trans. Am. Acad. Ophthalmol. Otolaryngol. 68: 256 (1979).

Coleman, D.J., & Lizzi, F.L. Absolute absorption and reflectance constants of ocular tissue. pp. 96 in this volume.

Dines, K.A., & Kak, A.C. Ultrasonic attenuation tomography of soft tissues. Ultrason. Imag. 1: 16 (1979).

Filipczynski, L., Lypacewicz, G. & Salkowski, J. Intensity determination of focused ultrasonic beams by means of electrodynamic and capacitance methods. Proceedings of Vibration Problems 15: 4 (1974).

Foster, F.S. & Hunt, J.W. Transmission of ultrasound beams through human tissue-focussing and attenuation studies. Ultrasound in Med. & Biol. 5: 257 (1979).

Gammel, P.M., Le Croisette, D.H. & Heyser, R.C. Temperature and frequency dependence of ultrasonic attenuation in selected tissues. Ultrasound in Med. & Biol. 5: 269 (1979).

Kak, A.C., & Dines, K.A. Signal processing of pulsed ultrasound. IEEE Trans. Biomed. Engng. 4: 321 (1978).

Kossoff, G. Analysis of focussing action of spherically curved transducers. Ultrasound in Med. & Biol. 5: 359 (1979).

Kuc, R. & Schwartz, M. Estimating the acoustic attenuation coefficient slope for liver from reflected ultrasound signals. IEEE Trans. Sonics Ultrason. SU 26: 363 (1979).

Lizzi, F.L., Katz, L., St. Louis, L., & Coleman, D.J. Applications of spectral analysis in medical ultrasonography. Ultrasonics 14: 77 (1976).

Thijssen, J.M., Bayer, A.L., & Cloostermans, M. Computer assisted echography: statistical analysis of A-mode video echograms obtained by tissue sampling. Med. & Biol. Engng & Comp. In press (1981).

Thijssen, J.M. & Verbeek, A.M. Computer analysis of A-mode echograms from choroidal melanoma. pp. 123 in this volume.

Authors' Address:
Biophysics Laboratory of the Institute of Ophthalmology
Univ. of Nijmegen
6500 HB Nijmegen, The Netherlands

ACOUSTIC MEASUREMENTS OF VITREOUS MEMBRANE AND RETINA THICKNESS REFLECTIVES

S. CHANG, D.J. COLEMAN & F.L. LIZZI

(New York, U.S.A.)

ABSTRACT

Ultrasonic evaluation of vitreous membranes and retinal detachment generally has been accomplished by analysis of amplitude variation and two-dimensional B-scan patterning to differentiate between these two echo complexes. Specific acoustic reflectance differences are augmented by the use of computers, allowing thickness measurements of retina (normally 170 to 210 microns) and membrane thickness (normally 250 microns and greater) in order to further distinguish between these two patterns.

Specific reflectances are measured by spectrum or frequency domain analysis. Discrimination of retinal thickness variations produced by peri-retinal membranes is also enhanced by use of thickness measurements.

The application of these measurements to selection of patients for vitreo-retinal surgical procedures will be discussed elsewhere.

Authors' Addresses

The New York Hospital-Cornell Medical Center (Dr. Chang, Dr. Coleman)
New York, U.S.A.

Riverside Research Institute (Dr. Lizzi)
New York, U.S.A.

THE SIGNIFICANCE OF THE S-SHAPED AMPLIFIER
CHARACTERISTICS IN ECHOGRAPHIC TISSUE DIAGNOSIS

K.C. OSSOINIG

(Iowa City, Iowa, U.S.A.)

The importance of S-shaped amplification characteristics for echographic tissue diagnosis has been recognized for many years. The significance of the S-shaped amplification curve has been discussed extensively and has been generally accepted in the field of ophthalmic ultrasound. But little consideration has been given so far to the clinical significance of details of the S-shaped curve. As a consequence, instrument designs with varying shapes of S-curves and varying totals and distributions of dynamic ranges have been introduced without repeating the success in tissue diagnosis obtained with the standardized 7200 MA Kretztechnik.

All portions of the S-shaped amplifier characteristic curve have their specific function and must contain the appropriate amounts of dynamic range. The upper portion of the curve, for instance, determines whether it is easy (or even possible) to detect and differentiate highly reflective lesions, and to display normal extraocular muscles. The central portion of the curve is crucial for measurements (e.g., of the size of the optic nerve and extraocular muscles). The lower portion of the curve is important for the detection and differentiation of low-reflective lesions. A prominent example is the detection of diffuse homogeneous opaqueness of the vitreous as is seen in long-standing vitreous hemorrhages that have not formed membranes or pseudomembranes. At tissue sensitivity, such a homogeneous opaqueness produces a few little blips along the base line only. At 6 dB higher system sensitivity $(T + 6)$, such a condition, however, causes a continuous chain of low spikes (Fig. 1), which clearly indicate that this vitreous is opaque. This diffuse opaqueness of the vitreous can not be demonstrated echographically if the lower portion of the S-shaped amplifier characteristic curve does not have a sufficient amount of dynamic range, which should be 16 dB (between a 1 mm and a 30 mm high signal). An example from our past experience in standardizing 7200 MA's (at the Standardization Center in Iowa City, Iowa U.S.A.) will help to explain and emphasize the importance of this lower portion of the curve.

While working at the Bascom Palmer Eye Institute in Miami, Dwain Fuller, using the 7200 MA #168 (since 1975), successfully detected diffuse opaqueness of the vitreous as described above. When he moved to Dallas in 1977 and began using the 7200 MA #167, Fuller failed to detect diffuse

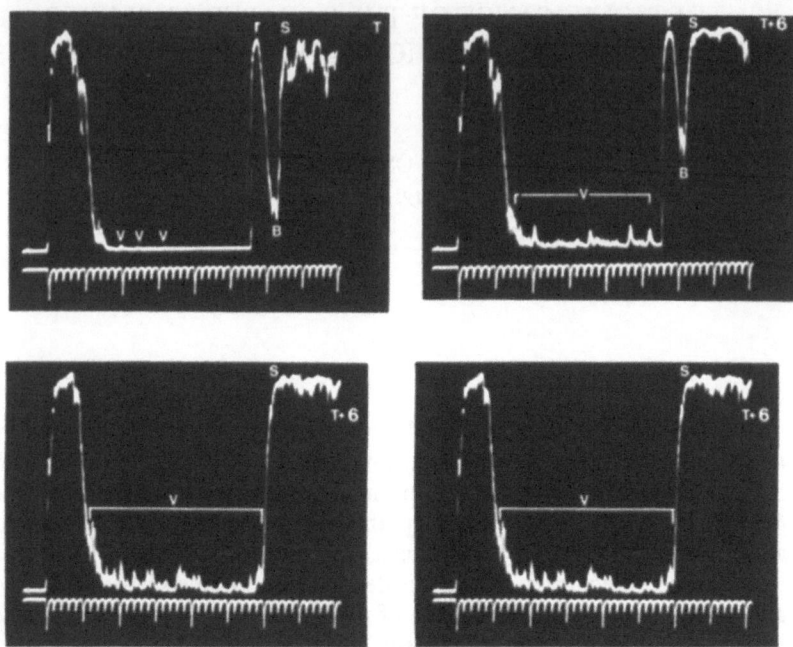

Fig. 1. A-scan echograms (standardized 7200 MA) of eye with diffuse vitreous opaqueness (old non-organized hemorrhage) and hemorrhagic retinal detachment. At tissue sensitivity (T), only a few blips are recorded from the vitreous (top echograms), which fail to indicate the great density of the vitreous opaqueness. The bottom echograms that were obtained with a 6 dB higher sensitivity (T + 6), however, show a continuous chain of low spikes clearly indicating that the vitreous is totally opaque. v vitreous opacities; r retinal detachment, B subretinal blood; S choroid and sclera.

opaqueness of the vitreous in a case. He contacted us immediately and we arranged to compare both machines (#167 and #168) with our standard in Iowa City. It was immediately apparent that there was a minor but significant difference in the course and dynamic range of the lower portion of the S-shaped curve in machine #167 (Fig. 2). It should be emphasized that the overall dynamic range in both amplifiers (#167 and #168) was 33 dB (as is standard); in unit #167, however, the distribution of the dynamic range was different in that the dynamic range was shifted toward the central and upper portions of the curve. The lower portion of the curve (1–30 mm signal height) had only 13 dB (= − 3 dB). We corrected the shape of the S-curve in this machine (Fig. 3), and Fuller has had no problem in detecting and quantitating diffuse opaqueness of the vitreous since that time.

This experience demonstrates how important the exact standardization of the S-curve is, and that even a 'minor' deviation from the standard can cause diagnostic problems. Since this experience in 1977, we have been very careful

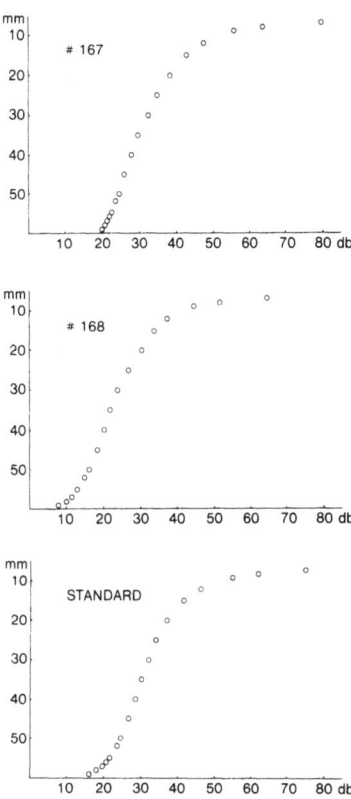

Fig. 2. Plotted amplifier characteristic curves of machine #167 prior to corrective calibration (top), of correctly calibrated machine #168 (center) and standard curve (bottom).

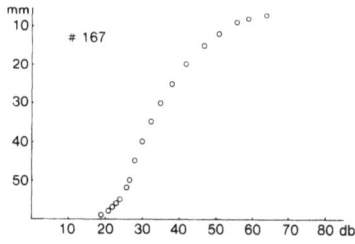

Fig. 3. Plotted amplifier characteristic curve of machine 7200 MA #167 after recalibration.

to maintain the specifically high dynamic range in the lowest portion of the S-shaped curve in all machines calibrated in Iowa City (and in Vienna, Austria).

Author's Address:
Dept. of Ophthalmology
The University of Iowa
Iowa City, IA 52242, U.S.A.

443

COMPARATIVE MEASUREMENTS ON DIFFERENT PULSE-ECHO SYSTEMS USING TEST REFLECTORS

W. HAIGIS, R. REUTER & R.D. LEPPER

(Würzburg, F.R.G.)

INTRODUCTION

Quantitative evaluation of echographic signals has become more and more important in the last years and is now a widely employed tool for differential diagnosis. The implementation of this method, however, is largely influenced by the technical performance of the ultrasonic system being used.

Principally, there are no basic technical difficulties involved in measuring and checking the main system features. Such measurements, however, require the employment of highly sophisticated equipment by trained personnel. Therefore, different working groups have developed a number of relatively simple methods allowing the most important functional characteristics to be checked clinically (Buschmann, et al. 1977, Ossoinig & Patel 1977, Till & Ossoinig 1977, Haigis & Buschmann 1979, Reuter 1979, Haigis & Buschmann 1980, Reuter, et al. 1980). One of these methods, the application of test reflectors for calibration and performance control, will be presented in this paper.

TEST REFLECTORS

The test reflectors we are using (Trier 1969, Buschmann, et al. 1977, Haigis & Buschmann 1979, Haigis & Buschmann 1980) are working standard plane echo interfaces according to the definition given in the IEC draft 29D (International Electrotechnical Commission 1979). They consist of discs, some 30 mm in diameter, 5 mm thick, made out of HEMA material, from which soft corneal contact lenses are manufactured. This material is available in constant quality and good long term stability with water contents of 38, 72, and 88%. There are three different types of reflectors, labeled W38, W72 and W88 respectively. Some of the physical properties of test reflector W38 are listed in Table 1. The surface finish of this type of reflector lies well within 1 μm.

From these data the reflectivity R expressed in decibels below a perfect reflector can be calculated according to

$$R = 20\,\text{dB} \cdot \log \frac{Z_2 - Z_1}{Z_2 + Z_1}$$

where $Z_1 = 1.48 \cdot 10^5$ g/(cm^2 sec) is the characteristic impedance of water (Wells 1977).

Table 1. Working standard plane echo interfaces: Physical properties of test reflector W38, made out of Polyhydroxyethylmetacrylat (HEMA) with 38% water contents. Measured at room temperature $T = 300\,\text{K}$, for frequencies $5-15\,\text{MHz}$. (ρ = density, c = velocity of sound, Z = acoustic impedance, r = reflectivity).

$\rho \left[\text{g/cm}^3 \right]$	$c \left[\text{m/sec} \right]$	$Z \left[10^5 \dfrac{\text{g}}{\text{cm}^2 \text{sec}} \right]$	$r \left[\% \right]$
1.149 ± 0.025	1689 ± 51	1.94 ± 0.07	13.4

The results are shown in Table 2. The value of $-17.4 \pm 4.2\,\text{dB}$ for the W38 reflector was calculated from the data in Table 1, whereas the other figures were experimentally deduced relating the respective reflectivities to the W38 reflector.

Table 2. Reflectivities in dB below perfect reflector of working standard plane echo interfaces W38, W72 and W88.

W38	W72	W88
− 17.4 ± 4.2	− 24.9 ± 4.5	− 34.7 ± 5.1

These test reflectors can be used

(1) as a reference to compare different ultrasonographic systems
(2) to measure some characteristic features of a specific system and thus get important data on its performance
(3) to establish a reference to which the reflectivities of pathologic structures can be related, thus allowing comparison of clinical experience gained with different instruments.

COMPARISON OF THE SENSITIVITY OF DIFFERENT INSTRUMENTS OF THE SAME MAKE

To compare the sensitivities of nine units of the Kretztechnik 7200 MA we have measured the amplification settings necessary to produce a 10 mm echo of a W38 reflector, situated in saline at a distance based on 30 μs time of flight. The results are shown in Fig. 1. Each measurement was performed with the original 8 MHz standard probe delivered with the main unit. Some additional results were also gained with two 8 MHz flat stalked transducers (NM 8/5 AG, 8 MHZ/3.5 Fl). It can be seen from Fig. 1 that even in standard-ized equipment sensitivity differences of up to 21 dB can be found. These differences do not stem from possible inaccuracies in the dB-scalings. These have been checked and found satisfactory in practically all units.

446

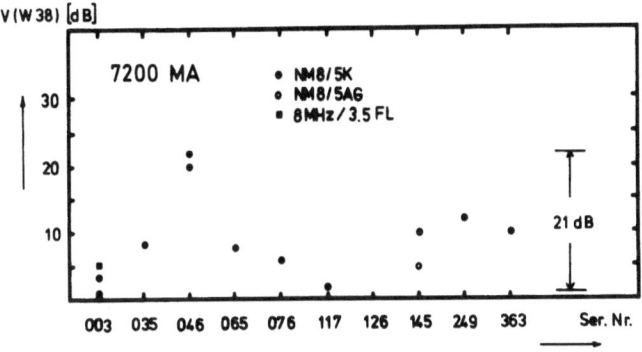

Fig. 1. Comparison of the sensitivities of different Kretz 7200 MA instruments. The horizontal axis is given by the serial numbers of the respective units.

In principle, these measurements can also be performed with a tissue model as designed by Till (Till & Ossoinig 1977) although in some instruments the available sensitivity range might not be high enough to allow the tissue sensitivity setting to be measured. Of course, the Echosimulator (Reuter 1979, Reuter, Trier & Lepper 1980) of the Bonn group can also be applied, but only to check the sensitivity of the electronics. To compare reproducibility of the W38 standard setting and the tissue sensitivity we performed double blind experiments with both phantom and reflector. The results of 15 measurements are displayed in Fig. 2. It turns out that the reproducibility of both procedures lies well beyond 1 dB, with a somewhat smaller standard deviation with our test reflector.

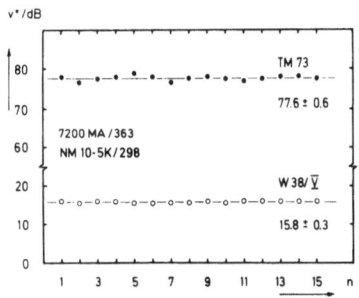

Fig. 2. Comparison of reproducibility of tissue sensitivity setting (tissue model TM73 (Till)) and W38 standard setting (test reflector W38/V).

USING TEST REFLECTORS TO CHECK EQUIPMENT PARAMETERS

Fig. 3 shows the results of a simple measurement, the so-called preset gain-distance variation of the Ocuscan 400, performed for constant 1 div- and 2 div-amplitudes with three types of test reflectors. We know from their respective reflectivities – as listed in Table 2 – that this measurement should yield two families of curves, where the spacing of the traces is given by the differences in reflectivities.

447

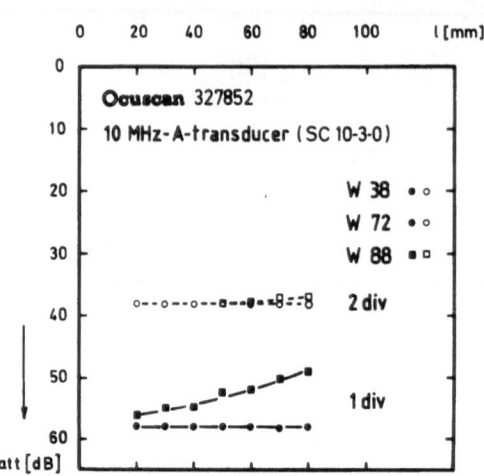

Fig. 3. Preset gain – distance variation (in destilled water) for the Ocuscan 400, taken with a 10 MHz A-transducer.

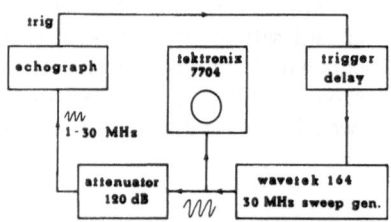

Fig. 4. Block diagram for some electronic measurements on echographic systems.

It can be seen from Fig. 3 that the maximum attenuation of this particular unit is obviously not high enough to display these differences properly. Also the indicated attenuation value could be incorrect. To verify this suspicion we were using the experimental set-up shown in Fig. 4. The Echosimulator, too, could have done the same job. Fig. 5 reveals that in fact there is a difference between indicated and true attenuation. This check on the dB scaling was done at 10 MHz; using other frequencies we found similar deviations, yet with differing numerical values. With the aid of such a correction curve we are eventually able to determine the gain characteristic of the instrument, again utilizing a test reflector. Fig. 6. shows the resultant A-mode display characteristic of the Ocusan unit.

The full-dotted curve would lead us to think that there is an S-shaped gain function. The open circles, however, represent the true gain characteristic, calculated from the graph labeled 'ind' and making allowance for the incorrect dB-scaling. The characteristic is essentially linear as can easily be derived. It should be pointed out that again different frequencies yielded different display characteristics.

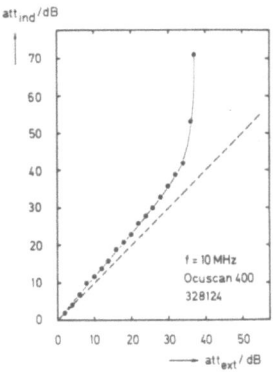

Fig. 5. Relation between indicated attenuation (att$_{ind}$) and true attenuation (att$_{ext}$) for one Ocuscan 400, at 10 MHz.

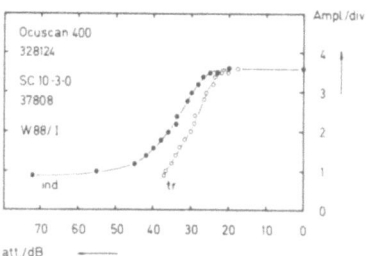

Fig. 6. A-mode display characteristic of one Ocuscan 400.

COMPARING THE ECHO DETECTION RANGES OF DIFFERENT INSTRUMENTS

The above mentioned measurements are necessary not only to provide a safe basis for quantitative echography but also in order to answer a question the clinician is really interested in, namely: which lesion can be detected with a particular instrument.

Fig. 7 depicts the reflectivities of some artificial reflectors and of some structures met in the human eye, expressed – in accordance with the IEC recommendations (International Electrotechnical Commission 1979) – in decibels below a perfect reflector (Haigis & Buschmann 1980). The data have been obtained with the 7200 MA and an 8 MHz flat stalked transducer. This figure has to be compared with the echo detection ranges of different instruments as shown in Fig. 8. Four Ocuscans 400 are compared with one 7200 MA.

The shaded areas on the high reflectivity side of the vertical scale correspond to the region, where echoes are too strong to be displayed as 10 mm

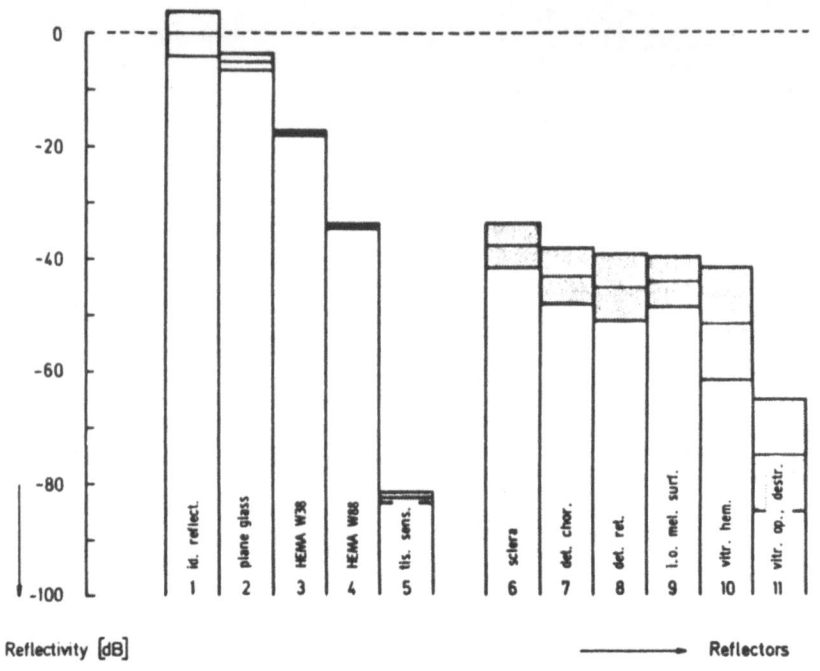

Fig. 7. Reflectivities of some artificial reflectors and of some tissue structures, taken with a 7200 MA and an 8 MHz flat stalked transducer (8 MHz/3.5 Fl).

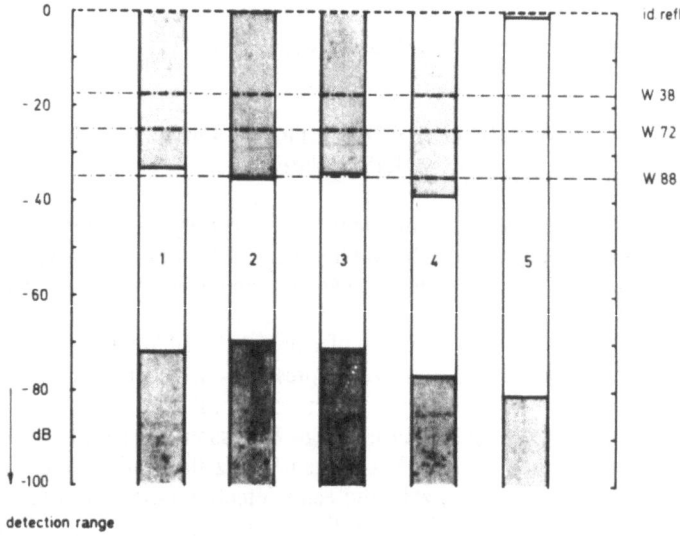

Fig. 8. Echo detection ranges of 4 Ocuscan 400 (Nrs. 1, 2, 3, 4) and one 7200 MA (Nr. 5)

450

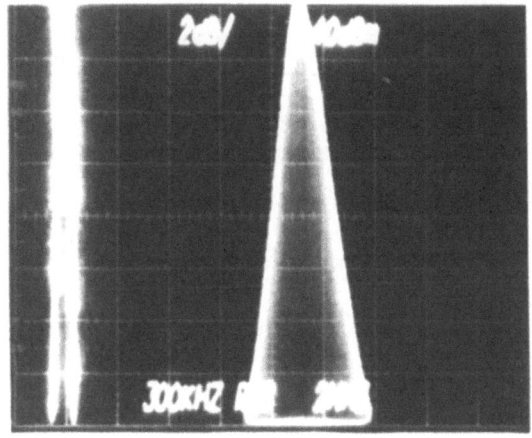

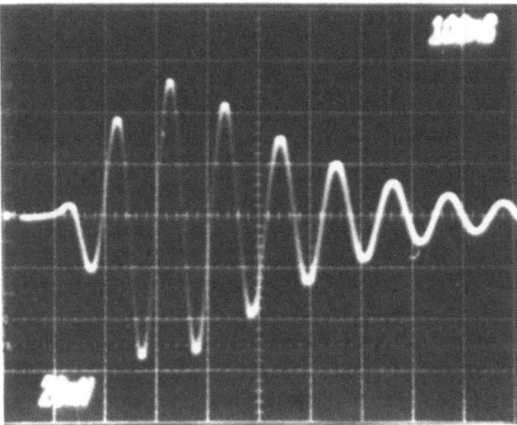

Fig. 9. Frequency and time domain signals of the echo from a W38 reflector, using a 10 MHz flat stalked transducer.

standard amplitudes. In this detection range three broken lines standing for the reflectivities of test reflectors W38, W72 and W88 provide a reference scale.

The upper limits of the shaded areas on the low reflectivity side are given by the maximum sensitivity available with a specific instrument. These values were calculated for 10 MHz as described in the foregoing.

The echo detection range of the 7200 MA is a bit higher than that of the Ocuscans with the least sensitive Ocuscan covering a range some 11 dB smaller than the 7200 MA range. Strong echoes, of course, can be seen with the Ocuscan. They only cannot be attenuated down to be displayed as 10 mm standard amplitudes.

451

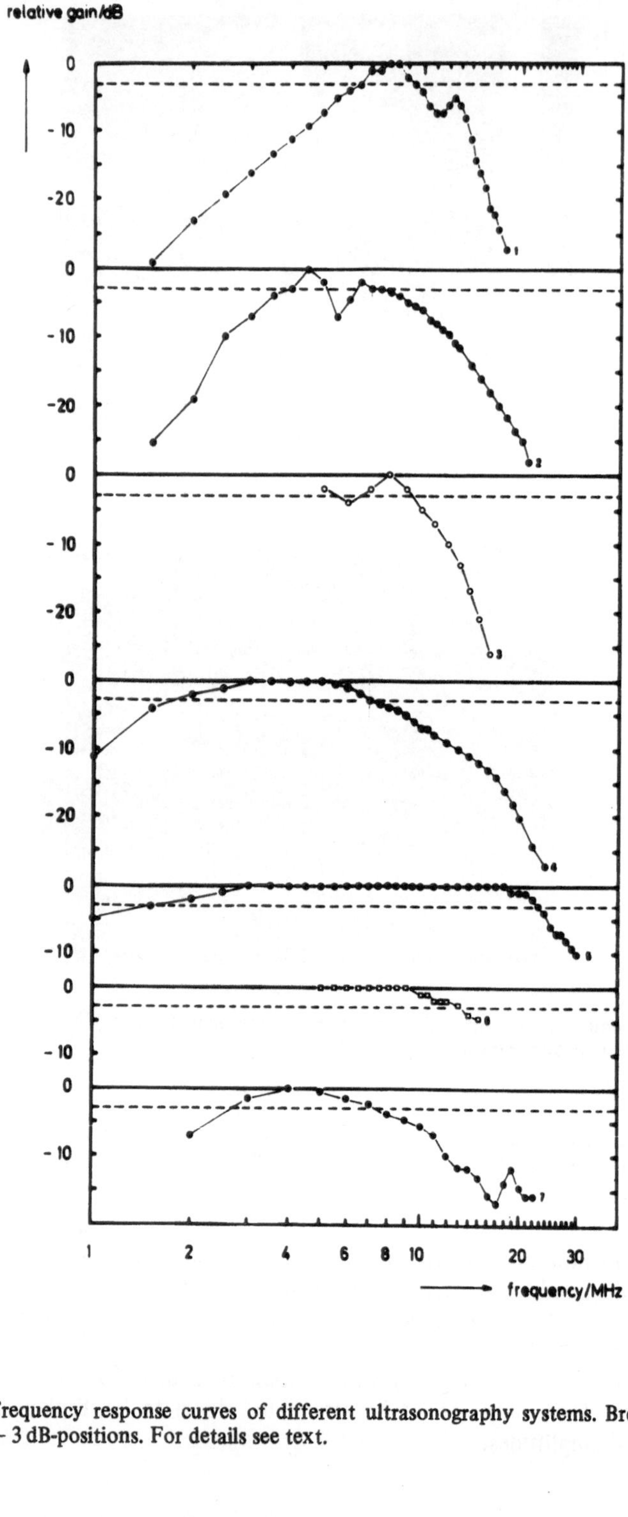

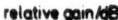

Fig. 10. Frequency response curves of different ultrasonography systems. Broken lines indicate — 3 dB-positions. For details see text.

452

FREQUENCY RELATED CHARACTERISTICS OF ULTRASONIC SYSTEMS

The interaction of ultrasound with biological tissue leads to an amplitude, phase and frequency modulation of the transmitted signal and it is this modulation which essentially carries the information about a specific tissue. We therefore need to know about the frequencies actually emitted as well as the frequency-dependent signal processing in an ultrasound system.

Applying electronic spectrum analysis (Tektronix 7L12) to an echo from a W38 reflector we get the spectrum of a 10 MHz flat stalked transducer as shown in the upper half of Fig. 9. It can be seen that this transducer is of the narrow-band type with a center frequency of some 9.3 MHz. An evaluation of the time domain signal from the lower part of Fig. 9 — according to the IEC recommendations — yields the same result of 9.3 MHz for the working frequency, which in this case is a well defined quantity. Apart from the apparent difference between working and nominal frequency it can be noted that for a narrow-band transducer like this one there is good agreement between working frequency and spectral center frequency. To find out about the frequency dependent signal processing we have measured the frequency response functions of various commercially available echography systems making use of the experimental set-up of Fig. 4. The resulting curves are shown in Fig. 10. They belong to three different Kretz 7200 MA units (Nrs. 1, 2, 3), one Kretz 7100 MA (Nr. 4), one Sonometrics Ophthalmoscan (Nr. 5), one Sonometrics Ocuscan 400 (Nr. 6), and one Xenotec Model 500 (Nr. 7). From the upper three graphs it follows again that there are still differences in the frequency responses of the standardized Kretz 7200 MA units. Also, there are relative minima more than 3 dB below maximum gain.

Contrary to these narrow-band units the Sonometrics Ophthalmoscan presents a very smooth response function over a wide range of frequencies with a 3 dB-bandwidth of some 23 MHz. Also, the Ocuscan is rather of the broad-band type, which does not hold for the Kretz 7100 MA and the Xenotec Model 500, the latter instrument revealing an additional response maximum at some 20 MHz, which is 10 dB down from the main maximum at frequencies of 4 to 5 MHz. I would like to remark that just recently we received an improved version of the Xenotec Model 500 which apparently has a much broader response function than the one presented here. However, we had not yet had a chance to perform exact measurements on this new machine.

USING THE EFFECT OF ABSORPTION ON THE FREQUENCY SPECTRUM TO DETERMINE LOW FREQUENCY SPECTRAL SIDE LOBES

Looking for a simple measurement technique to get an impression of the bandwidth or of possible low frequency components in the spectrum of a

453

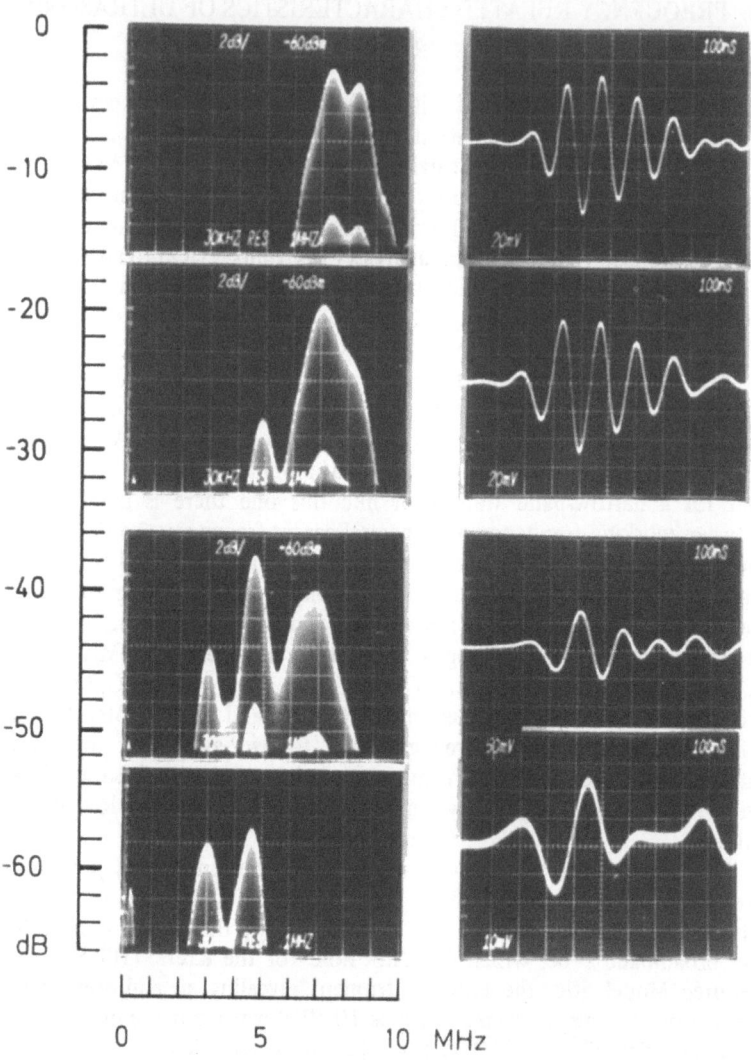

Fig. 11. Effect of absorption of ultrasound by silicone oil on frequency spectrum and R.F. signal. Transducer: 8 MHz focused Kretz standard transducer. Distances between transducer and plane steel reflector in silicone oil (AP 500) from top to bottom: 3 mm, 6 mm, 18 mm, 33 mm.

transducer we examined an 8 MHz standard Kretz transducer immersed in highly absorbing silicone oil (AP 500). Increasing the distance between transducer and a plane steel reflector we got the spectra shown on the left side of Fig. 11, together with the corresponding R.F. signals on the right. Two effects can clearly be seen:

    (1) Increasing the distance causes all of the spectral amplitudes to decrease.

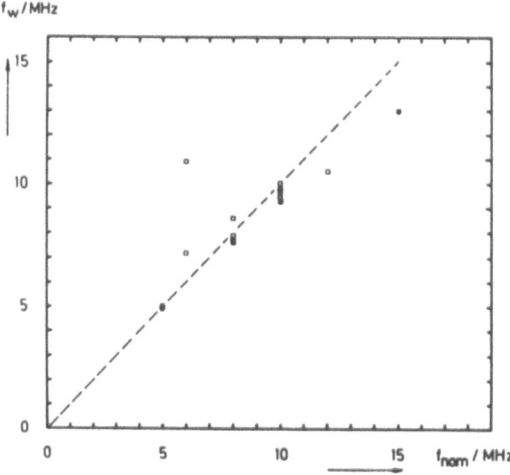

Fig. 12. Comparison between working frequency f_w and nominal frequency f_{nom} for several transducers.

(2) Higher frequency components decrease faster than lower frequencies, as is to be expected from the frequency dependance of absorption.

The overall effect results in an effective shift to lower frequencies. With the transducer used there are even two main low frequency components at 3 MHz and 4.7 MHz. The important feature of Fig. 11 is that this shift in the effective frequency is also clearly visible in the time domain signals. Therefore, in a clinical situation, the determination of the R.F. waveform after penetration of highly absorbing silicone oil provides a simple check to detect strong low frequency components.

Spectrum analysis yields the most complete data on transducer frequencies, but is generally not available in a clinic laboratory. Thus we measured the working frequencies of different transducers according to the IEC draft and compared these values with the figures specified by the manufacturers. The results are shown in Fig. 12, where different symbols correspond to transducers of different manufacturers. It can be seen that although there is often good agreement between working and nominal frequency, severe deviations can also be found.

SUMMARY

Comparative measurements on various ultrasonic systems for ophthalmic use illustrated the problems existing in the field of standardization of such equipment.

Test reflectors and synthetic electronic echoes enable one to measure some important system parameters and provide a basis for comparing both

455

the performance of different instruments and the clinical results gained with these machines. Checking the R.F. waveform of a pulse having traveled through silicone oil allows for clinical determination of strong side lobes, especially on the low frequency side of the spectrum of a transducer.

REFERENCES

Buschmann, W., Linnert, D. & Eysholdt, E. Measurement of Equipment Sensitivity in Diagnostic Ultrasonography. In: Ultrasound in medicine, Vol. 3B. (D. White & R. Brown eds.) New York: Plenum Publishing Corp. (1977) p. 1925.

Haigis, W. & Buschmann, W. Sicherung gleichbleibender echographischer Untersuchungsbedingungen über längere Zeiträume. In: Verhandlungsbericht SIDUO VII (H. Gernet, ed.) Münster: R.A. Remy-Verlag (1979) p. 59.

Haigis, W. & Buschmann, W. Die Benutzung von Testreflektoren zur schnellen klinischen Uberprüfung von Geräten für die ophthalmologische Ultraschalldiagnostik. In: Biomed. Technik, Bd. 25, Ergänzungsband, Berlin: Verlag Schiele & Schön (1980) p. 53.

International Electrotechnical Commission, Tech. Comm. 29: Electroacoustics, Sub-Comm. 29D: Ultrasonics. Draft: Methods of measuring the performance of ultrasonic pulse-echo diagnostic equipment (1979).

Ossoinig, K.C. & Patel, J.H. A-Scan Instrumentation for Acoustic Tissue Differentation. In: Ultrasound in medicine, Vol. 3B. (D. White & R. Brown, eds.) New York: Plenum Publishing Corp. (1977) p. 1955.

Reuter, R. Der Zusammenhang klinisch relevanter Gerätefunktionen im A- und B-Bild und ihre Überprüfung durch ein differenzierungsfähiges Testprogramm. In: Verhandlungsbericht SIDUO VII (H. Gernet, ed.) Münster: R.A. Remy-Verlag (1979) p. 44.

Reuter, R., Trier, H.G. & Lepper, R.-D. Der 'ECHOSIMULATOR', ein Funktionsgenerator zur Messung relevanter Eigenschaften von Ultraschalldiagnostik-Geräten. Biomed. Technik, 25: 163 (1980).

Till, P. & Ossoinig, K.C. First Experiences with a Solid Tissue Model for the Standardization of A- and B-Scan Instruments in Tissue Diagnosis. In: Ultrasound in medicine, Vol. 3B. (D. White & R. Brown, eds.) New York: Plenum Publishing Corp. (1977) p. 2167.

Trier, H.G. Lichtdurchlässige, feststoffähnlich bearbeitbare Kunststoffe mit Schallgeschwindigkeiten unter 2000 m/sec. In: Proc. I. Weltkongress Ultraschalldiagnostik Med. und SIDUO III Vol. 2 (1969) p. 199.

Wells, P.N.T. Biomedical Ultrasonics, London: Acad. Press (1977).

Authors' Addresses:
University Eye Clinic (Dr. Haigis)
Würzburg
F.R.G.
Institut für experimentelle Ophthalmologie der Univesität (Dr. R. Reuter, Dr. Lepper)
Bonn
F.R.G.

RELIABILITY AND ACCURACY OF TM (TISSUE MODEL) FOR CALIBRATION OF STANDARDIZED A-SCAN INSTRUMENTATION

P. TILL & V. SCHEIBER

(*Vienna, Austria*)

Acoustic differentiation is largely based on quantitative A-scan echography (Ossoinig 1974). In order to obtain useful, reliable and comparable results, standardized A-scan instrumentation is set at a defined, reproducible, rather high system sensitivity ('tissue sensitivity'). Citrated blood models have been used since 1966 as the only standard for setting an A-scan instrument at tissue sensitivity. The use of these biological tissue models, at preparation of the cell suspensions and the procedure of finding tissue sensitivity have been described in detail (Ossoinig 1974). The time-consuming preparation of such tissue models, their lack of durability and the limited accuracy inherent in any biological system such as this were considerable disadvantages. For these reasons calibration of standardized A-scan instrumentation remained difficult and restricted to some major centers.

During 1975 P. Till succeeded in finding a suitable material and developed a solid tissue model (TM) to replace the blood model. This tissue model consists of a silicone resin (Wacker Sil Gel 604) containing a specified number of glass micro-beads (S 100) in equal distribution. The TM permits a quick, simple and accurate tissue sensitivity adjustment. With the help of this technical standard, every examiner may set his instrument at tissue sensitivity himself. Most diagnostic techniques (i.e. basic examination, topographic, quantitative and kinetic echography) are performed or at least initiated at tissue sensitivity.

METHODS

Fig. 1 illustrates the TM and the application of the probe to the TM surface to obtain a regular echogram of medium spike height (the signal-free triangles above and below the TM spikes are of equal size). The system sensitivity required to display the medium-high spikes is the tissue sensitivity of the instrument/probe combination used (Kretztechnik-Unit 7200 MA and 8 MHz probe).

Blind studies have been undertaken to examine the accuracy and reliability of three charges each consisting of ten TMs and 15 replications for each TM. One examiner adjusted the sensitivity of the instrument by using the

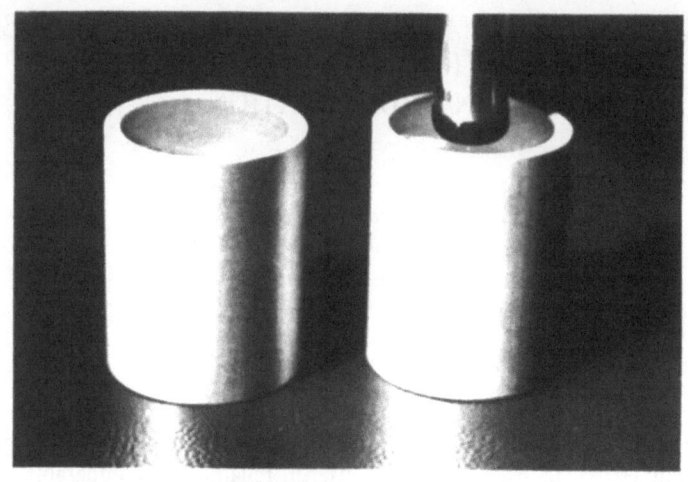

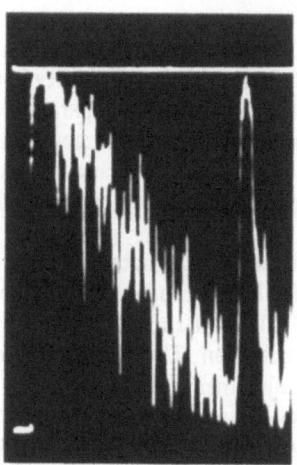
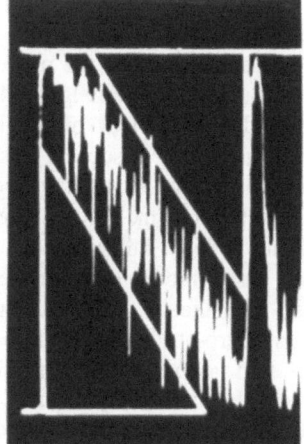

Fig. 1. Top: TM surface is wetted with water and the probe is placed on the surface. Now the probe is angled and shifted slightly to obtain a regular echogram.

Bottom: TM echogram of medium spike height displayed with tissue sensitivity. The echo-free triangles above and below the TM spikes have equal size.

dB-control dial without observing the dB gradation. Another examiner who had nothing to do with the adjustment itself, read resultant dB values without communicating them to the first examiner. This procedure was repeated 15 times using the same TM. Each time the probe was completely removed from the TM, water was reapplied to the TM surface, and the dB-control dial was set to zero before the next adjustment was performed.

Table 1. Components of variance of the three charges.

| Charge | 1 | | 2 | | 3 | |
Cause	v.c.	%	v.c.	%	v.c.	%
TM	0.156	43	0.114	38	0.214	38
repl.	0.203	57	0.189	62	0.350	62

RESULTS

(1) For each of the three charges a hierarchical analysis of variance was done with ten tissue models and 15 replications (repl.) per TM. Then components of variance (v.c.) attributable to TMs were determined (Table 1). In each charge the distribution of the percentages are very similar (40% due to TM, 60% due to repl.). In charge 3 the values of variance components are almost twice the values of the other charges. In Table 2. the minimum and maximum values and the range of the ten means within each charge are demonstrated.

Table 2. Regions of the mean values of the three charges.

Charge	1	2	3
$\bar{x}_{min.}$	69.87	70.25	70.22
$\bar{x}_{max.}$	71.11	71.35	71.68
Range	1.24	1.10	1.46

(2) An overall hierarchical analysis of variance with the factors 'charges', 'TMS' and 'replications' (nested within each TM) gives the following components of variance (Table 3). The component of variance due to charges is very small and statistically not different from zero.

Table 3. Components of variance.

Cause	v.c.	%
Charges	0.030	7
TMs	0.161	37
Repl.	0.248	56

(3) The Bartlett-test was applied to test a significant difference between the ten standard deviations based on 15 replicated measurements in each charge. Only in charge 1 a difference was found with error-probability $p < 0.01$, but this difference seems not relevant because the values do not vary much in relation to the high mean values (Table 4). The coefficient of variation was in the order of $0.1 - 1.0\%$. The standard deviations of charge 3 are seen to be higher than in the other charges.

(4) A comparison of the standard deviations between the three charges results in a statistically significant difference between charge 3 and the other

459

Table 4. Standard deviations of the three charges.

Charge	1	2	3
$s_{min.}$	0.25	0.29	0.45
$s_{max.}$	0.63	0.57	0.72
χ^2_9	24.70	9.46	3.82
p	< 0.01	n.s.	n.s.

χ^2_9 = Bartlett's test-statistic (chi-square with 9 degrees of freedom).
p = error probability in Bartlett-test.
n.s. = not significant.

charges ($p < 0.01$). The precision of the measurements of charge 3 is less than those of the other charges. The test was done by means of Scheffe's multiple comparisons (Scheffe 1964).

(5) Eighteen unexperienced examiners adjusted tissue sensitivity with the same TM three times (18 persons, three repl. per person). An analogous computation which led to Table 1 gives the following components of variance:

due to persons = 0.182 (46%)
due to repl.   = 0.215 (54%).

There is a higher proportion of the variance components due to persons than to TMs as in Table 1. The precision of the replications is in good agreement with those in Table 1.

DISCUSSION

Comparison of standard deviations between the three charges results in a statistically significant difference between charge 3 and the other charges (1 & 2). This is explained by the fact that charges produced more recently (charge 1 & 2) had a more homogeneous distribution of the glass micro-beads in the resin that TMs manufactured previously (charge 3). Accuracy of measurements of charge 3 is less than in charge 1 & 2, but deviations less than 0.9 dB for tissue sensitivity do not have a serious influence on tissue diagnosis. The accuracy of all three charges can be considered as sufficient. Reliability and accuracy of TM is also demonstrated by means of replicated measurements performed by unexperienced examiners; the precision of the replications is in good agreement with that of skilled examiners. Since 1975 annual comparison of TM with citrated blood model was done; acoustic parameters of 'standard TM 001' remained unchanged until now.

REFERENCES

Ossoinig, K.C. Quantitative Echography – The Basis of Tissue Differentiation. J. Clin. Ultrasound, 2: 33 (1974).
Ossoinig, K.C. Preoperative Differential Diagnosis of Tumors with Echography: I. Physical Principles and Morphological Background of Tissue Echograms. In: Current Concepts in Ophthalmology, Vol. 4 (F.C. Blodi, ed.) St. Louis: Mosby (1974) p. 264.

Scheffe, H. The Analysis of Variance. New York: Wiley & Sons (1964)

Till, P. Solid Tissue Model for the Standardization of the Echo-Ophthalmograph 7200 MA (Kretztechnik). Docum. Ophthalmol. 41: 205 (1976).

Till, P. & Ossoinig, K.C. First Experience with a New Solid Tissue Model for the Standardization of A- and B-scan Instruments used in Tissue Diagnosis. In: Ultrasound in Medicine, Vol. 3B: Engineering Aspects. (D. White & R.E. Brown, eds.) New York: Plenum (1977) p. 2167.

Authors' Addresses:
Univ. – Doz. Dr. P. Till
II. Univ. – Augenklinik
Alserstrasse 4
A-1090 Vienna, Austria

Dr. V. Scheiber
Institute for Statistics and Documentation in Medicine
University of Vienna
A-1090 Vienna, Austria

COMPARATIVE MEASUREMENTS ON ULTRASONIC PULSE-ECHO EQUIPMENT WITH THE ECHOSIMULATOR

R. REUTER, R.-D. LEPPER & W. HAIGIS*

(Bonn/*Würzburg, F.R.G.)

Conditioned by the historical development, today's ophthalmological diagnostic ultrasonic instruments differ considerably in their properties. Buschmann (this book) deals in more detail with this subject. Within the scope of standardization, quality control, and further development, enlarged 'diagnostics' of diagnostic equipment are nowadays required. Haigis & Till (this book) report about comparative measurements by means of test reflectors. I want to demonstrate in addition some measurement results gained with the ECHOSIMULATOR, which we reported about during SIDUO VII.

The tests served not only for localizing possible defects, but also for characterizing the instruments. Fig. 1 gives a number of relevant electrical parameters of ultrasonic impulse instruments. The measurement of the frequency response stands first. This is most important also for B- and C-mode display, although it might be pretended that by these modes only the amplitude modulation of the echoes is used.

Fig. 2a shows frequency responses of eight instruments, model 7200 MA (Kretz). The equipment concept is relatively narrow-banded and designed for 8 MHz medium frequency. At this frequency the variation of amplitude values is about 10 dB. The deviations increase with higher frequencies and reach 20 dB at 16 MHz. Fig. 2b indicates frequency responses of seven instruments, model Ocuscan 400 (Sonometrics). Ten MHz is indicated as the operating frequency. Here the variation is about 3 dB and reaches 14 dB at 15 MHz. Generally, the run of the frequency responses is flatter, compared with type 7200 MA. Thus, a greater bandwidth of the receiver is available. In Fig. 2c the frequency responses of some other ophthalmological ultrasonic equipment are plotted. If active components are used for varying the amplification, there is often a risk of affecting the frequency response additionally. As the Ocuscan 400 has such an electronic attenuator, its effect was tested. Fig. 3 shows above the frequency responses at the adjustment '0 dB', below at a 30 dB lower amplification. It is clearly observable that different amplification factors change the frequency response.

Why should one measure the frequency response?
It might be remembered that the extent of reflexion and scattering in tissue and, thus, tissue display depend on the frequency used. Frequency characteristics are of great importance especially for tissue differentiation:

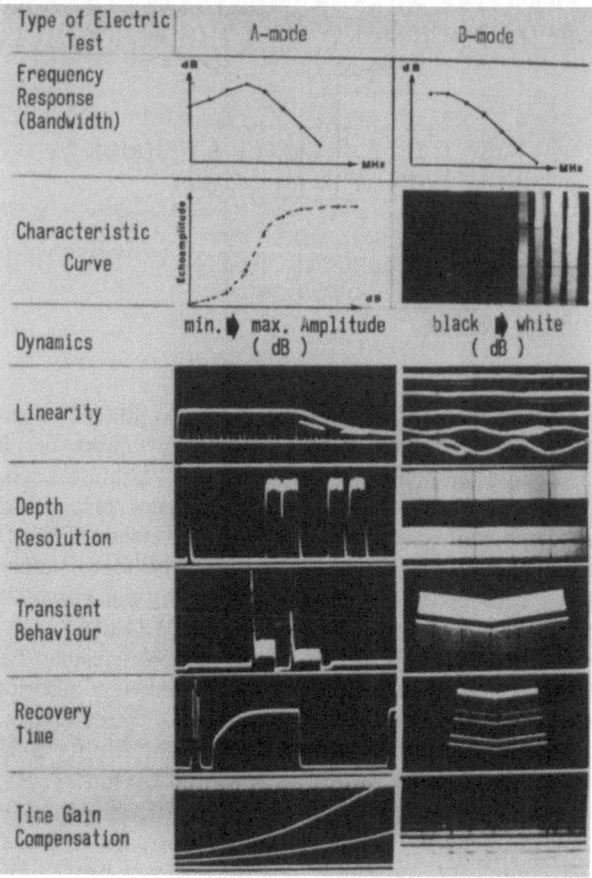

Type of Electric Test	A—mode	B—mode
Frequency Response (Bandwidth)		
Characteristic Curve		
Dynamics	min. ◆ max. Amplitude (dB)	black ◆ white (dB)
Linearity		
Depth Resolution		
Transient Behaviour		
Recovery Time		
Time Gain Compensation		

Fig. 1. System performance characteristics of pulse-echo equipment.

    (a) for the usual visual diagnostics on the screen. It should be mentioned that Ossoinig based his concepts on a defined frequency response of the Kretz 7200 equipment;

    (b) for computer-aided analysis of the echograms.

The bandwidth of the echoes is practically always larger than that of the transmitted pulse train. The reasons are: phase shifting, interferences, and scattering of small object structures. Because the transducer 'hears' only a small topographic area from the sound field that was generated by the transducer itself, complex broad-band oscillations result.

By means of computer-aided signal processing, i.e. Fourier transformation, additional information can be gained from such pulse trains, which would not be possible by visual evaluation of the echogram only. Trier & Decker during SIDUO VII and Lepper (1978) described a clinically used method for differentiating thin layers of the ocular back-wall. Coleman & Lizzi confirmed in September 1979 the usefulness of this method. But frequency analyses are

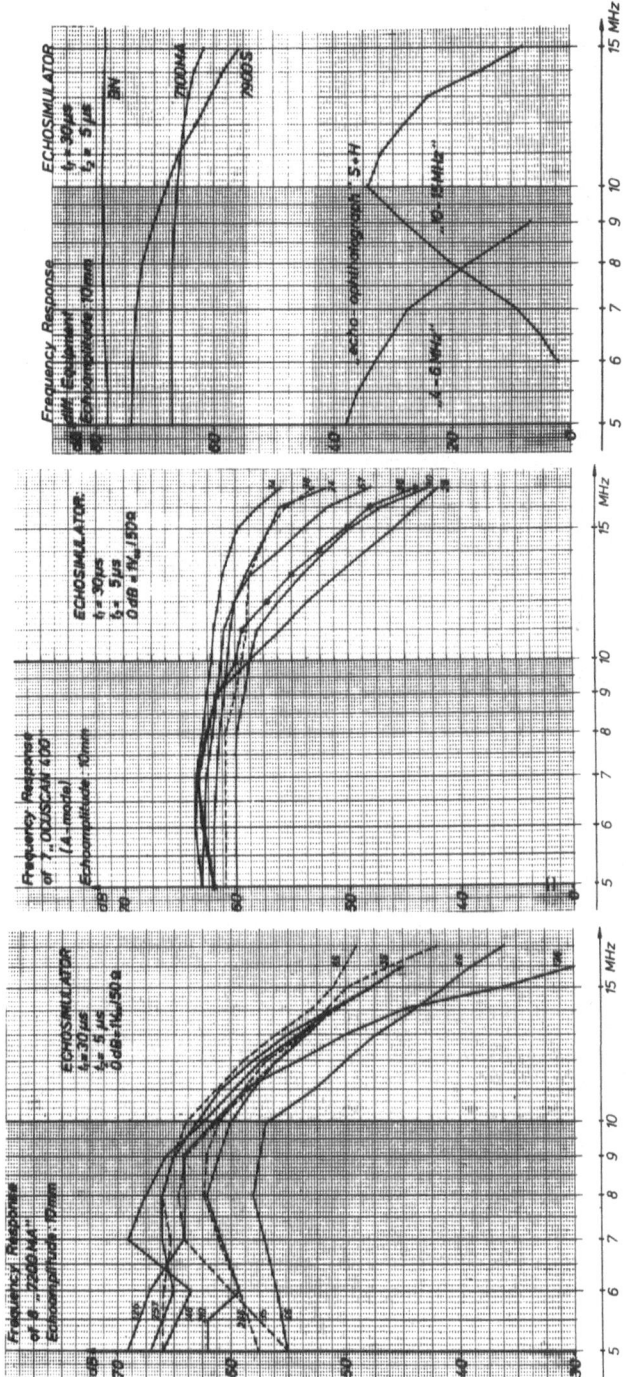

Fig. 2a. Frequency response characteristics of eight instruments of the type 7200 MA (Kretztechnik). (b) Frequency response characteristics of seven instruments of the type Ocuscan 400 (Sonometrics). (c) Frequency response characteristics of some other types.

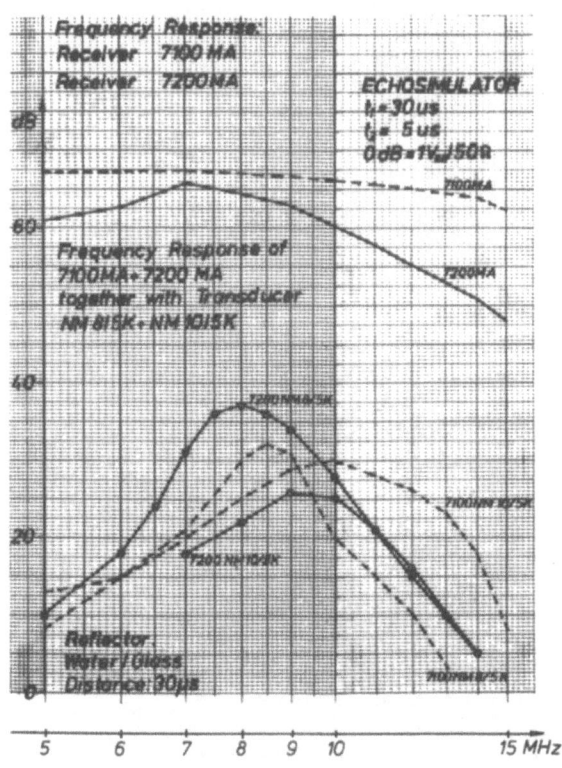

Fig. 3. Influence of amplification on frequency response characteristics of the Ocuscan 400. Upper curves 0 dB, lower curves − 30 dB.

useful only, if a minimum bandwidth is available. This bandwidth, decisive for every tissue differentiation, is determined as well by the receiver, as by the characteristics of the transducer.

In Fig. 4 the receiver's frequency response of a 7100 MA-equipment, below that of a 7200 MA are shown. In the lower part of the picture, the dependence of the frequency response on the transducer types NM 8/5 K and NM 10/5 K can be seen. For these measurements the transmitter of the ultrasonic instruments was substituted by the ECHOSIMULATOR (Fig. 5). A plane silicate glass plate served as reflector. The water/glass interface gives sufficiently high echo amplitudes, even with a low transmitter voltage. The following measurements, referred to the amplitudes, were always performed with medium frequencies, deduced from the maximum of the frequency responses. For a pre-set input voltage the characteristic curve of a receiver defines the echo height of A- and M-mode display (Fig. 6a), or the brightness value of B- and C-mode respectively (Fig. 6b). From the characteristic curves

466

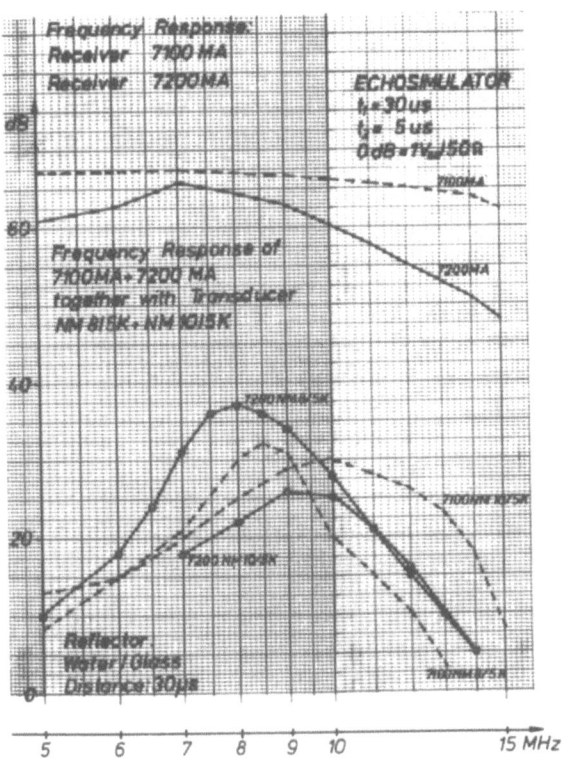

Fig. 4. Comparison of frequency response characteristic of the receiver to the frequency response characteristic curve of the receiver plus a transducer (8 MHz, or 10 MHz).

in Fig. 6a, besides their shapes (linear parts, logarithmic or S-shaped), also the displayable dynamics can be seen, as can the amplitude relation of the echoes, which can be displayed without changing the amplification. If this factor is added to the possible amplification variation, the total dynamics of each individual equipment may be determined.

Fig. 7a demonstrates the operating range and the echo-detection capability of nine instruments, model 7200 MA. In Fig. 7b the same parameters for other echo impulse instruments are given. The hatched bars on the left give the amplification factor necessary to get a 10 mm echo height on the screen from a test reflector W38. The dotted bars on the right indicate the input voltages of the ECHOSIMULATOR, needed to get the same echo height. The white bars correspond to the reserve amplification available. It could have been expected that a certain proportionality between the 'natural' echo amplitude of the W38, and the electrical 'artificial' echo amplitude would be found. But, obviously, this was not true. Low hatched bars point to a higher efficiency of the transducer. In this case the transducer was mostly more narrow-banded, and/or a lower amplification was necessary because of a more favourable

467

transmitter spectrum. The height of the dotted bars gives a measure for the sensitivity of the receiver. It cannot be excluded that this feature is primarily more constant in the 7200 MA-series. The basic adjustment of the amplification factor by means of reference reflectors may lead to the measured differences. It remains an open question whether or not it is really irrelevant for the transmission of an in vivo-echo how the relation between reflection factor of the object is examined, and how the resulting echo height on the display is standardized. After all, the 7200 MA instruments show differences in the range of 25 dB. This corresponds to the voltage ratio 1:20 at the amplifier input, or to the power ratio 1:400, referred to transmitter and transducer. If 'outsiders', as i.e. the 'echo-ophthalograph', or a 7900 S are included, these values increase to 1:50 (referred to the voltage), or to 1:2500 (referred to power ratio).

Further measurements dealt with linearity, electrical depth resolution, transient response, and recovery time after the transmitted impulse of the instruments. We will deal with this in another paper.

These results demonstrate that when comparing a single type of today's ultrasonic equipment, considerable differences with regard to important

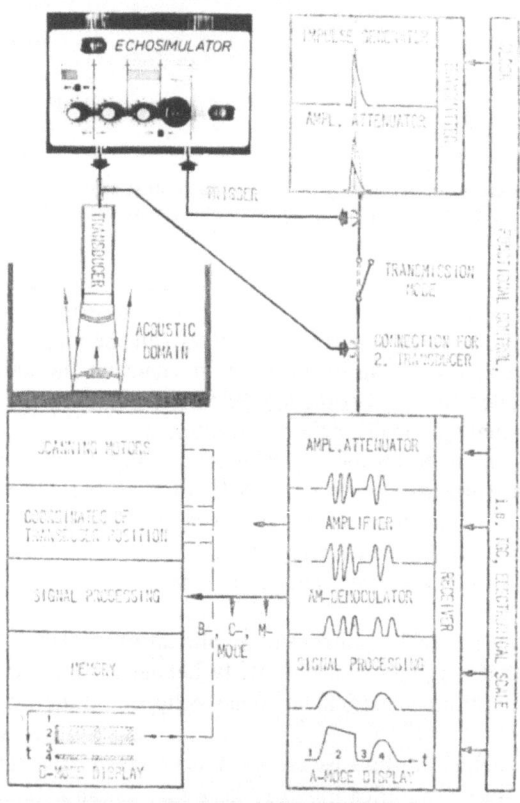

Fig. 5. Scheme of measurements by using the Echosimulator.

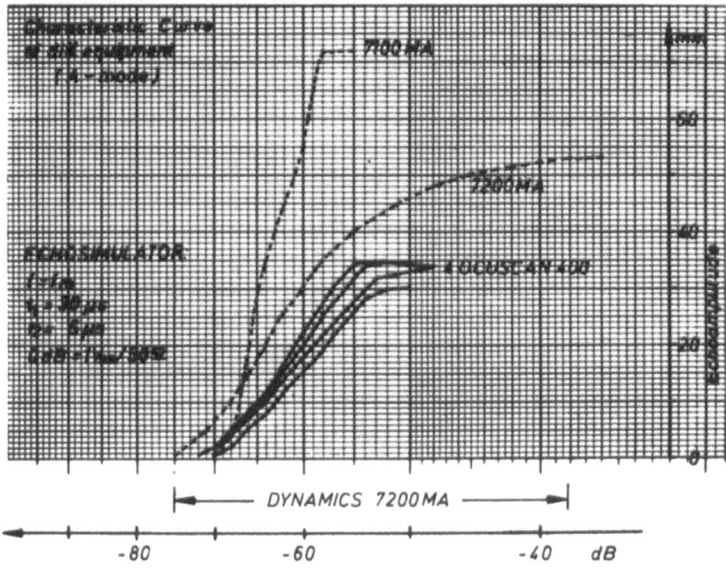

Fig. 6a. Dynamic range (input range in dB) of A-mode display of various types of equipment.

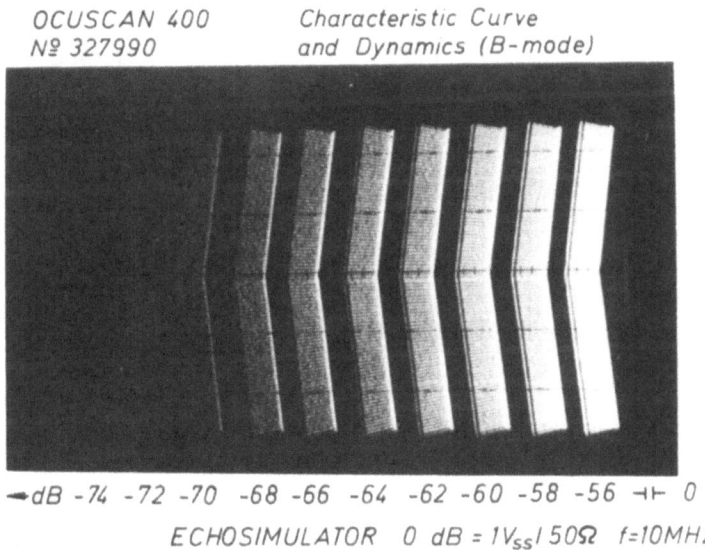

Fig. 6b. Dynamic range of B-mode display shown by attainable grey range.

469

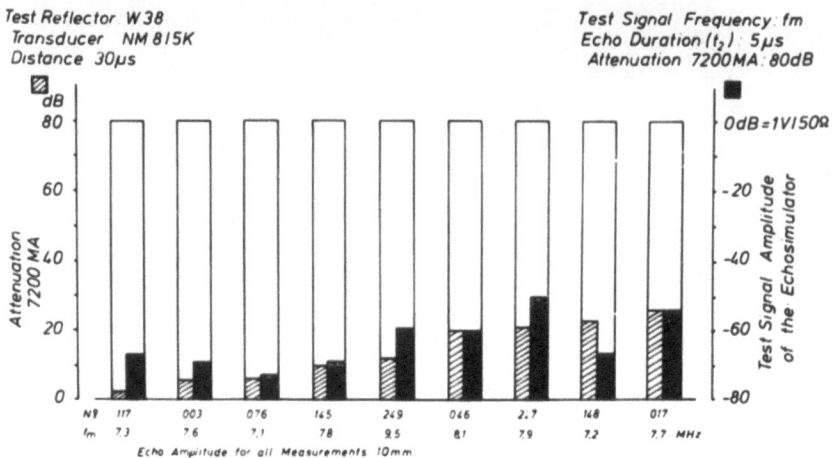

Fig. 7a. Investigation of sensitivity of nine instruments 7200 MA (Kretztechnik). Hatched bars: attenuator position yielding a 10 mm echo from a W38 reflector. Dotted bars: voltage from echosimulator producing 10 mm display height.

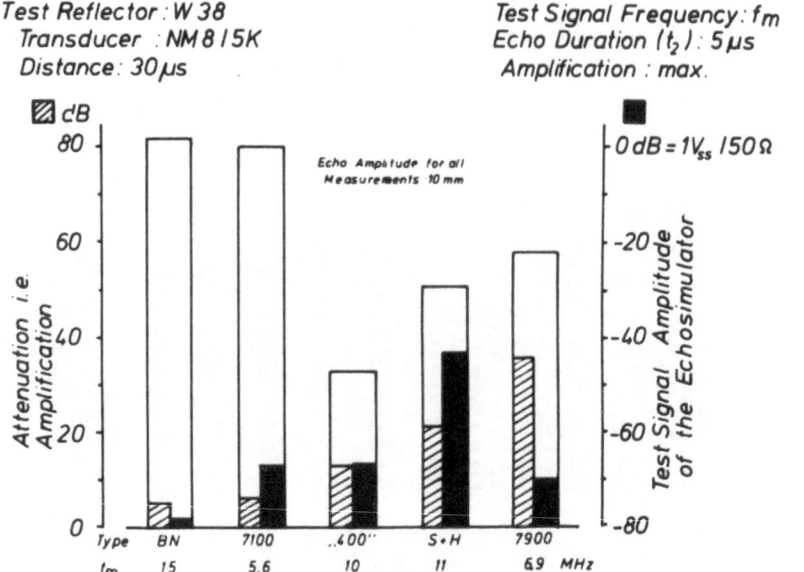

Fig. 7b. Same measurements for different types of instruments.

properties may still appear, in spite of final control, or calibration, respectively. The comparability of their examination results is thus restricted. On the other hand, the application of the electrical test signal by means of the ECHOSIMULATOR has proved suitable in discovering and compensating for such differences (quality assurance).

470

REFERENCES

Carson, P.L. Rapid evaluation of many pulse echo system characteristics by use of a triggered pulse burst generator with exponential decay. J. Clin. Ultrasound 4: 259 (1976).

Coleman, D.J. & Lizzi, F.L. In vivo choroidal thickness measurement. Am. J. Ophthalmol. 88: 369 (1979).

International Electrotechnical Commission, Technical Committee No. 29 Electroacoustics, Sub-Committee 29 D: Ultrasonics. Draft: Methods of measuring the performance of ultrasonic pulse echo diagnostic equipment. 29 D (secretariat) June 13, 1978, Suppl. May 1979.

Lepper, R.-D. Ultraschallmessungen der Rückwand des lebenden menschlichen Auges Diss. Bonn (1978).

Lepper, R.-D. Trier, H.G. & Reuter R. Beispiele für die Anwendung des Testprogramms mit Echosimulator an Geräten der Serie 7200 MA Kretztechnik In: Ophthalmologia Diagnostica Ultrasonica (H. Gernet, ed.), Münster: Remy Verl. (1979).

Reuter, R. Der Zusammenhang klinisch relevanter Gerätefunktionen im A- und B-Bild un ihre Überprüfung durch ein differenzierungsfähiges Testprogramm In: Ophthalmologia Diagnostica Ultrasonica (H. Gernet, ed.) Münster: Remy Verl. (1979).

Reuter, R. Klinisch einsetzbares Verfahren zur ergänzenden Prüfung von Ultraschall-Diagnostikgeräten Proc. Ultraschalldiagnostik in der Medizin; Dreiländertreffen Davos, Februar 1979, Stuttgart: Thieme-Verl. (1980).

Reuter, R., Trier, H.G. & Lepper, R.-D. Ein elektrisches Prüfverfahren und Prüfgerät für Ultraschalldiagnostik-Anlagen. Acta Medicotechnica 28, 58 (1980).

Reuter, R., Trier, H.G. & Lepper, R.-D. Der Echosimulator, ein Funktions generator zur Messung relevanter Eigenschaften von Ultraschalldiagnostik-Geräten Biomed. Techn. 25, 163 (1980).

Till, P. Solid tissue model for the standardization of the echo-ophthalmograph 7200 MA (Kretztechnik). Docum. Ophthalmol. 41, 205 (1976).

Trier, H.G. Lichtdurchlässige, feststoffähnlich bearbeitbare Kunststoffe mit Schallgeschwindigkeit unter 2000 m/s. Proc. I. Weltkongr. Ultraschalldiagnostik Med. and SIDUO III, Vol. 2, 199 (1969).

Williams, C. & Holmes, J.H. Pulse generator for verification of ultrasound equipment performance. In: Diagnostic Ultrasound, Vol. 3: 308 (1974).

Authors' Addresses:
R. Reuter, R.-D. Lepper
Klinisches Institut für experimentelle
Bonn (Venus berg)
F.R.G.

W. Haigis
Univeristy Eye Clinic
Würzburg
F.R.G.

REFERENCES

A NEW DEVICE FOR OCULAR BIOMETRY

R.-D. LEPPER & H.G. TRIER

(Bonn, F.R.G.)

Measuring the eye length and its different parts is of interest for several ophthalmological questions. Nowadays the ultrasonic biometry is very often used, as it is the only simple method to get information about the different axial distances of the eye.

For this purpose the transit times of the reflected sound waves are measured. These times have to be multiplied with the individual sound velocities to get the 'mm'-values. The transit times are very often deduced from A-mode-photographs. This technique, however, is quite time consuming and has limited resolution only.

To improve resolution and minimize time consumption, electronic clocks have been used since 1966 (Coleman & Carlin 1967). Typically, these measuring systems define two sensitive time gates of variable position and length during the echo transit time. Whenever a signal reaches a trigger level during the first gate an electronic clock is started. It is stopped if during the second gate another echo signal reaches the trigger level. The systems display the results in μs or in mm. Several instruments allow one to switch sound velocity for the calculation of mm. To measure the three different ocular distances (anterior chamber depth, lens thickness, and vitreous body length) with the instruments commercially available, the two gates have to be sequently positioned onto the corresponding echoes of the eye. In the mean time, however, the measuring axis has probably changed.

To overcome this, we developed a system capable of measuring the three distances simultaneously (Trier, *et al.* 1973, Lepper, *et al.* 1980) (Fig. 1). Four clocks (10 MHz counting frequency) are started simultaneously with the transmitting pulse, and stopped one by one by corresponding echo signals. The four values describing the transit times are read out to a computer to form a measurement protocol. The system evaluates each sound path through the eye, i.e. the measuring rate is 1000/s.

On the basis of this hardware several measuring techniques can be performed, statical and dynamical measurements. The statical measurements give information about the axial length of the eye and its three parts. For this purpose a user-selectible number of measurements for the different ocular parts is averaged to form one data printout. Before being averaged the set of data is checked by means of a plausibility criterion. By this, apparent

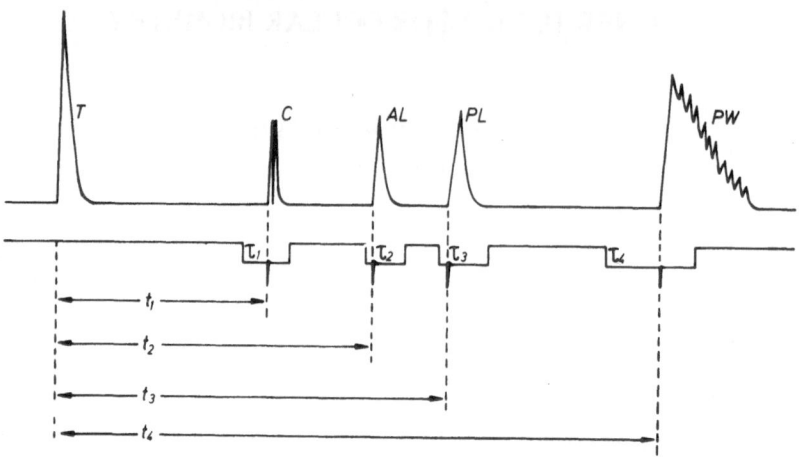

Fig. 1. Measurement scheme of the biometric device.
Four gates with alterable lengths $\tau_1 - \tau_4$ are positioned to four corresponding echoes.
Four clocks $t_1 - t_4$ are started by the transmitting pulse.
Four 'needles' pointing downwards the gate notches indicate a stop of the corresponding clock.

  T = transmitter pulse
  C = corneal echo
 AL = anterior lens surface
 PL = posterior lens surface
PW = posterior wall of the eye

measurement errors are excluded. In addition to the evaluation of the different axial lengths all accepted individual values are collected to form one histogram. By means of this histogram the selection of one single data set out of all is markedly improved. Fig. 2 gives an example. The data thus found are input data, for instance for lens implantation calculations (Gernet 1978). Up to now, we had approximately 120 patients being measured. Fig. 3a gives a histogram of the so far measured ocular lengths. Fig. 3b demonstrates the corresponding variation of the depth of the anterior chamber. The great variability of the displayed measures clearly demonstrates that implanting a standard lens of e.g. 19 D is not adequate for a true patient's care. We have to keep in mind that 1 D variation of the implant lens leads to approximately 1.5% variation of aniseiconia. A change of the calculated power of the lens to be implanted of 1 D may be caused by approximately 0.3 mm variation of the ocular length or by 0.5—1 mm variation of the anterior chamber depth.

Another way of treating the values derived from the electronic clocks is their display in an M-mode fashion. Fig. 4a & 4b give examples. During these experiments the patient (an 18-year-old girl) had to accommodate from 2 m to 0.15 m. The total ocular length remains nearly constant. The front surface of the ocular lens moves towards the cornea thus reducing the depth of the anterior chamber. The rear wall of the lens remains almost in place. Due to accommodation the lens thickness changes by approximately 8%.

So far, the measuring errors involved have not been discussed. The accuracy is affected by several factors. Among these the interaction of the sound

474

DATUM 08-SEP-80, ZEIT 15:59:04, PATIENT K█████,K██ 3.11.18 (OP.LA.VORG) RA
    32 MESSUNGEN, DAVON   32 AUSGEWERTET, HIERBEI ERGABEN SICH FOLGENDE WERTE:
HORNHAUT+VORDERKAMMER (C=1531.0 M/SEC)   4.38 +/-   0.07 USEC BZW.   3.36 +/-   0.06 MM
LINSE (C=1641.0 M/SEC)   5.19 +/-   0.15 USEC BZW.   4.26 +/-   0.12 MM
GLASKOERPER (C=1531.0 M/SEC)   20.40 +/-   0.19 USEC BZW.   15.62 +/-   0.14 MM
            AUGENLAENGE ALSO   29.97 +/-   0.12 USEC ODER   23.23 MM

DATUM 08-SEP-80, ZEIT 15:59:06, PATIENT K█████,K██ 3.11.18 (OP.LA.VORG) RA
    32 MESSUNGEN, DAVON   32 AUSGEWERTET, HIERBEI ERGABEN SICH FOLGENDE WERTE:
HORNHAUT+VORDERKAMMER (C=1531.0 M/SEC)   4.38 +/-   0.07 USEC BZW.   3.36 +/-   0.06 MM
LINSE (C=1641.0 M/SEC)   5.21 +/-   0.10 USEC BZW.   4.27 +/-   0.09 MM
GLASKOERPER (C=1531.0 M/SEC)   20.32 +/-   0.14 USEC BZW.   15.55 +/-   0.11 MM
            AUGENLAENGE ALSO   29.91 +/-   0.10 USEC ODER   23.18 MM

DATUM 08-SEP-80, ZEIT 15:59:07, PATIENT K█████,K██ 3.11.18 (OP.LA.VORG) RA
    32 MESSUNGEN, DAVON   32 AUSGEWERTET, HIERBEI ERGABEN SICH FOLGENDE WERTE:
HORNHAUT+VORDERKAMMER (C=1531.0 M/SEC)   4.39 +/-   0.06 USEC BZW.   3.36 +/-   0.04 MM
LINSE (C=1641.0 M/SEC)   5.18 +/-   0.15 USEC BZW.   4.25 +/-   0.12 MM
GLASKOERPER (C=1531.0 M/SEC)   20.33 +/-   0.12 USEC BZW.   15.54 +/-   0.10 MM
            AUGENLAENGE ALSO   29.90 +/-   0.05 USEC ODER   23.17 MM

DATUM 08-SEP-80, ZEIT 15:59:09, PATIENT K█████,K██ 3.11.18 (OP.LA.VORG) RA
    32 MESSUNGEN, DAVON   32 AUSGEWERTET, HIERBEI ERGABEN SICH FOLGENDE WERTE:
HORNHAUT+VORDERKAMMER (C=1531.0 M/SEC)   4.38 +/-   0.07 USEC BZW.   3.36 +/-   0.06 MM
LINSE (C=1641.0 M/SEC)   5.20 +/-   0.13 USEC BZW.   4.27 +/-   0.10 MM
GLASKOERPER (C=1531.0 M/SEC)   20.31 +/-   0.11 USEC BZW.   15.54 +/-   0.09 MM
            AUGENLAENGE ALSO   29.89 +/-   0.05 USEC ODER   23.17 MM

DATUM 08-SEP-80, ZEIT 15:59:10, PATIENT K█████,K██ 3.11.18 (OP.LA.VORG) RA
    32 MESSUNGEN, DAVON   32 AUSGEWERTET, HIERBEI ERGABEN SICH FOLGENDE WERTE:
HORNHAUT+VORDERKAMMER (C=1531.0 M/SEC)   4.38 +/-   0.07 USEC BZW.   3.36 +/-   0.06 MM
LINSE (C=1641.0 M/SEC)   5.20 +/-   0.13 USEC BZW.   4.27 +/-   0.10 MM
GLASKOERPER (C=1531.0 M/SEC)   20.36 +/-   0.14 USEC BZW.   15.59 +/-   0.11 MM
            AUGENLAENGE ALSO   29.95 +/-   0.10 USEC ODER   23.21 MM

HAEUFIGKEITSVERTEILUNG ALLER AUSGEWERTETEN MESSWERTE

VORDERKAMMERTIEFE

0   1   2   3   4   5   6   7   8   9   10 MM

LINSENDICKE

0   1   2   3   4   5   6   7   8   9   10 MM

GLASKOERPERLAENGE

13   14   15   16   17   18   19   20   21   22   23 MM

Fig. 2. Printout of a biometric measurement. The date and time of measurement are documented, likewise the patient's name. The printout shows the number of measurements and the number of accepted values. The depth of the anterior chamber, the lens thickness, and the vitreous body length are given in [μs] transit time on the left, and [mm] calculated with adequate speed of sound on the right. The twofold standard deviation of each value is given. The histograms present all accepted values in one.

475

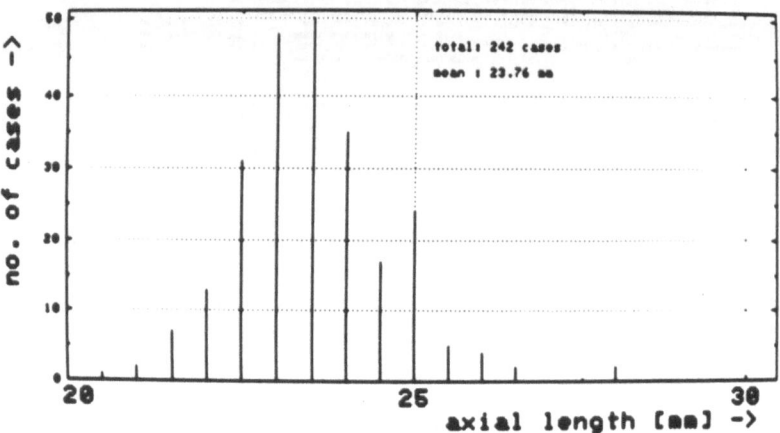

Fig. 3a. Histogram of the axial length of patients coming for lens implantation.

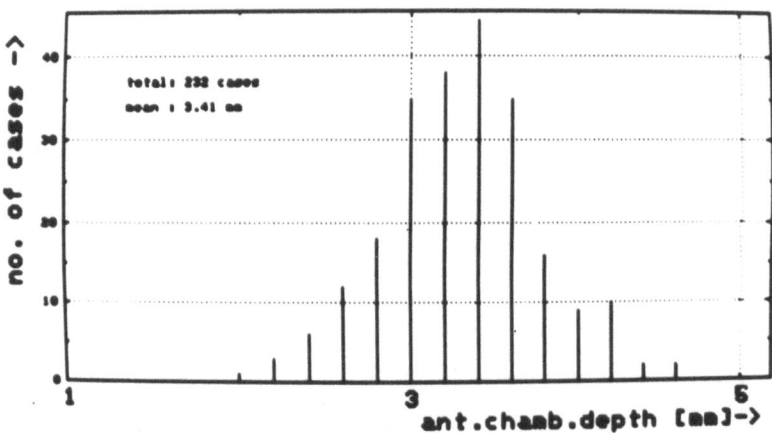

Fig. 3b. Histogram of the depth of the anterior chamber of our patients.

field and the shape of the reflecting target is of interest. To simulate the interaction of the transducer's sound field and the posterior ocular wall a hollow semisphere was scanned rectangularly by a transducer. The measured distances roughly correspond to the theoretical values calculated according to the curvature of the test object. However, there are several values situated on a circle which show differences up to nearly 1 mm to the theoretical values. These effects are probably due to an interaction between side lobes of the transducer used, and the tilted surfaces of the test object. However, the effects described above are not yet fully explained; we are continuing to work on this problem.

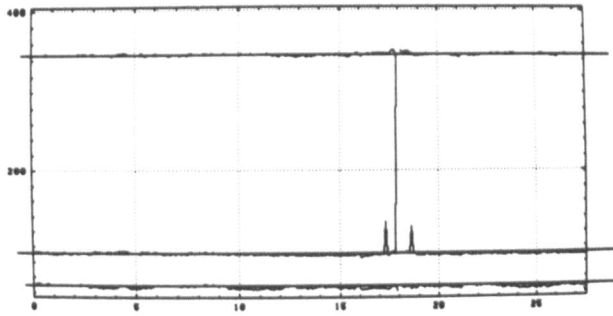

Fig. 4a. Dynamic biometry of the human eye in vivo. Demonstrated are several accommodational changes (distance: 2 m, near: 0.15 m, female, 18 years).
x-axis: measuring time [s]
y-axis: echo transit time [0.1 μs]
y = 0 corresponds to the corneal echo
(y-axis origin suppressed)

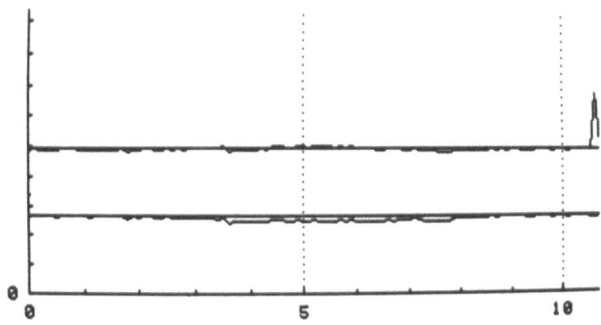

Fig. 4b. Cut-out of a dynamic biometry of the human eye in vivo. Set-up as in Fig. 4a. During accommodation the anterior lens surface moves towards the cornea.

REFERENCES

Coleman, D.J. & Carlin, B. Transducer alignment and electronic measurement of visual axis dimensions in the human eye using time-amplitude ultrasound. In: Proc. Symp. Ultrasonics in Ophthalmology, Münster 1966 (A. Oksala & H. Gernet, eds.) Basel & New York: Karger (1967) p. 207.

Gernet, H., Ostholt, H. & Werner, H. Intraokulare Optik in Klinik und Praxis. München: Rothacker (1978).

Lepper, R.-D., Trier, H.G. & Reuter, R. Neuartige Ultraschallbiometrie Klin. Mbl. Augenheilk. 177: 101 (1980).

Trier, H.G., Hammerla, O. & Reuter, R. Ein hoch auflösendes TAU-System für die Biometrie des Auges. Proc. SIDUO IV, Paris 1971 (M. Massin & J. Poujol, eds.) Paris: Centre National d'Ophtalmologie des Quinze-Vingts (1973) p. 51.

Authors' Address:
Klinisches Institut für experimentelle Ophthalmologie
Bonn (Venusberg)
F.R.G.

INFLUENCE OF EQUIPMENT PARAMETERS ON RESULTS IN OPHTHALMIC ULTRASONOGRAPHY

I. Sensitivity and echo detection capability

W. BUSCHMANN & W. HAIGIS

(Würzburg, F.R.G.)

INTRODUCTION

Equipment parameters may limit the range of useful application of ultrasonic apparatus and transducer probes in ophthalmic ultrasonography. The reliability of ultrasonic diagnosis depends on close-to-optimum parameters and their maintenance. Therefore, the International Electrotechnical Commission, as well as AIUM and other national groups, have developed drafts on measurement of these parameters.

We have performed corresponding measurements in ophthalmic ultrasonography. This paper is devoted to echo detection capability; frequency and spectrum will be dealt with in Part II (poster session). Other parameters like amplifier dynamics, time-gain compensation, lateral and axial resolution and scanning techniques will be discussed at another occasion.

ECHO DETECTION CAPABILITY

1. *Measurement method.* The IEC draft on methods of measuring the performance of ultrasonic pulse-echo diagnostic equipment recommends the use of a working standard plane echo interface in a waterbath. Since the built-in attenuators of many diagnostic apparatus to not allow one to measure the echo of a water/glass interface, we developed another, standardized plane reflector (Fig. 1) which has been described earlier in detail (Buschmann, et al. 1977, Haigis & Buschmann 1979). Its use is discussed in Dr. Haigis' paper at this congress. It is made from 2-hydroxyethylmetacrylate, containing 38% of water. The difference in reflectivity to the ideal plane echo interface (perfect reflector) is -17.4 ± 4.2 dB (W. Haigis & W. Buschmann 1980).

2. *Clinically needed echo detection capability.* The term 'echo detection capability' is now recommended to describe the maximum sensitivity available with distinct diagnostic equipment (apparatus and transducer probe). For more than 15 years we have — in routine diagnostic work — related the sensitivity settings necessary to produce characteristic echo patterns from intraocular lesions to a reference value which described the echo detection capability of the system used. For many years, the measurement of

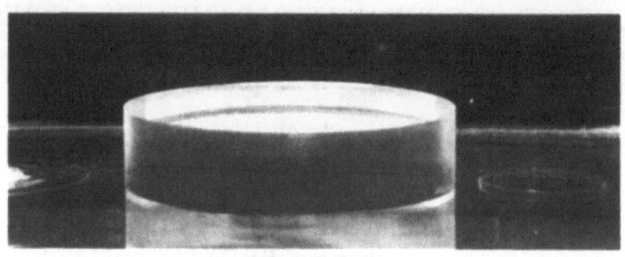

Fig. 1. Test reflector W38 made of soft contact lens material, water content 38%. Plane surface, diameter 30 or 51 mm, thickness 4.0 resp. 11.5 mm. Positioned for use on a plane plexiglass support.

penetration depths in calibrated paraffine oil was successfully used for the calibration of the sensitivity control (Buschmann 1966, Herrmann & Buschmann 1968). Each transducer-apparatus combination could be measured using this method.

Specific relative sensitivity settings were found optimum for the demonstration of 'typical' echogram patterns in numerous diseases of the eye and orbit. The echograms change in a typical manner with the variation of sensitivity. We were able to develope a scheme of typical echograms and their sensitivity-dependent variations, which proved very helpful in differentiation of pathologic echograms (Buschmann 1966).

Now we can refer these results to the standard test reflector W38. They apply for working frequencies between 8.0 and 10.0 MHz. Additional measurement results with the Kretztechnik 7200 MA and transducer probes of 8 MHz and 10 MHz nominal frequency (working frequencies 8.0 MHz resp. 10.0 MHz) are shown in Table 1. Unfortunately we could not yet collect corresponding data with the Ocuscan 400 because of the inaccuracy, which its dB-scale presented until recently. The highest sensitivity is clinically needed to demonstrate echoes from vitreous opacities, vitreous destruction (Fig. 2) and from tissue structures of intraocular tumors (Fig. 3 & 4). According to our measurement results, if the sound beam were directed through the lens, an 8 dB increase in sensitivity would be needed at working frequencies around 10 MHz. This figure is in agreement with the figure of 2 dB $MHz^{-1} cm^{-1}$ given by Lizzi/Feleppa (1979). The echo detection capability of numerous apparatus and transducer probes is not sufficient to provide such high sensitivity. Tumour diagnosis should therefore preferably be done using beam directions with the lens beyond the beam. Similarly, higher echo detection capability is necessary for ultrasonography of the depth of the orbit, if 10 or 15 MHz working frequency is applied. This cannot be provided due to technical limitations. Lower frequencies (5 MHz) must therefore be applied to achieve sufficient penetration.

From Table 1 one can conclude that for work at 8 to 10 MHz working frequencies and unfocussed or weakly focussed probes with 3.5 to 5 mm crystal diameter, the echo detection capability of a specific equipment would be sufficient for intraocular diseases if a dB-reserve of 65–67 dB, above standard 10 mm-echo of test reflector W38, would be available. This

480

Table 1. Minimum echo detection capability necessary to visualize specific lesions in ophthalmic ultrasonography.

Echo producing structure	Minimum echo detection capability in dB with respect to			
	W38 reflector at		Ideal reflector at	
	8 MHz	10 MHz	8 MHz	10 MHz
Ideal plane reflector	−17.4 ± 4.2 (10)	−17.4 ± 4.2 (10)	0	0
Plane glass reflector	−12.3 ± 1.5 (20)	–	5	–
W38 test reflector	0 ± 0.3 (10)	0 ± 0.3 (10)	17	17
W88 test reflector	16.8 ± 0.3 (10)	–	34	–
Sclera (internal surface)	19.9 ± 3.7 (29)	13.5 ± 6.2 (21)	37	31
Detached retina	27.3 ± 5.7 (29)	27.1 ± 6.6 (39)	45	45
Detached choroid	25.4 ± 4.8 (9)	29.6 ± 8.0 (20)	43	47
I.o. melanoblast. surface	26.5 ± 4.4 (8)	25.2 ± 10.2 (21)	44	43
I.o. melanoblast. tissue	–	42 — 59 **	–	68
Fibrin membrane	–	41.3 ± 6.0 (10)	–	59
Vitreous hemorrhage	41.6 ± 9.8 (8)	39.8 ± 5.5 (32)	51	57
Vitreous opacities or destructions	57.7 ± 9.8 (12)	36.2 ± 11.9 (13)	75	54
Tissue sensitivity*	64.8 ± 0.8 (10)	61.4 ± 0.9 (10)	82	79

The figures given in Table 1 relate to the sensitivity settings (formerly refered to as 'overall sensitivity') necessary to produce a 10 mm amplitude of the echo under consideration on the screen of the Kretz 7200 MA with an 8 MHz and a 10 MHz and a 10 MHz flat stalked transducer probe (Kretz 8 MHz 3.5 Fl. and 10 MHz 3.5 Fl.; actual working frequencies 8.0 resp. 10.0 MHz). W38 = working standard plane echo interface, according to IEC SC 29 D4 draft, Nov. 79; made from 2-hydroxyethylmetacrylate (HEMA = material for soft corneal contact lenses) containing 38% of water (Buschmann, Linnert & Eysholdt 1977, Haigis & Buschmann 1979, Haigis & Buschmann 1980). W88 = Co-polymerisate of this material containing 88% of water. Both reflector types as well as the plane glass reflector were measured in saline at a distance equivalent to 30 μsec. time of flight. The figures in brackets give the number of measurements. The last two columns on the right side show rounded values for the echo detection capability with respect to the ideal reflector. Standard deviations have been omitted in these 2 columns for convenience. A value of −17.4 dB was used for the difference in reflectivities between the W38 and the perfect plane reflector (W. Haigis, W. Buschmann, 1980)

*Figures for the 'tissue sensitivities' as measured with a tissue model TM 73 after Till and Ossoinig (1977) are given here relative to W38 and perfect reflector respectively.

**Data from M10/5 F 25 flat stalked transducer probe, nominally 10 MHz, actually working at 10 MHz (Transducer Manufacturing Service, Malmesbury). All values shown in this table were measured carefully adjusting the transducer to get maximum echo amplitude. To evaluate diagnostic echoes the sound beam had been directed past the lens.

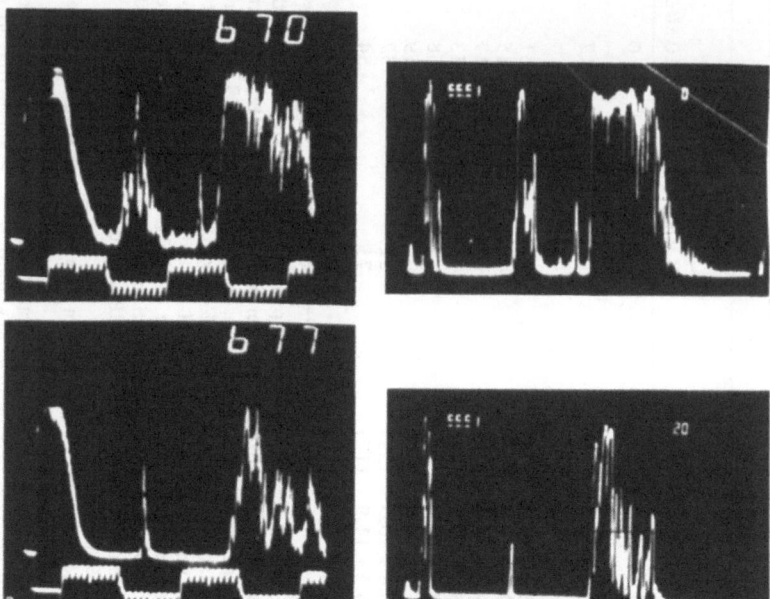

Fig. 2a   Fig. 2b

Fig. 2. Vitreous opacities, examined with two different ultrasonic systems.
Fig. 2a. Kretztechnik 7200 MA, Probe 10 MHz 3.5 Fl (working frequency = 10.0 MHz), position 9c, maximum sensitivity = 68 dB (above) resp. 48 dB (below) above standard echo from W38 test reflector.
Fig. 2b. Ocuscan 400, 10 MHz probe, maximum sensitivity (above) and some 20 dB reduced senstivity.

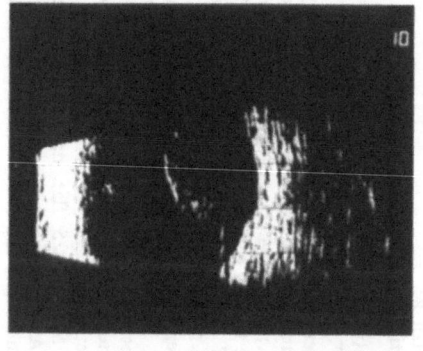 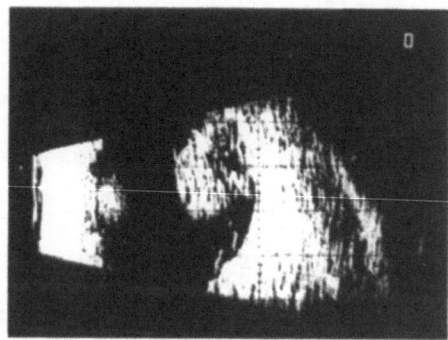

Fig. 3. Intraocular melanoblastoma, Ocuscan 400 contact scan, transducer probe nominal 10 MHz (working frequency = 9.7 MHz)
Fig. 3a. Insufficient sensitivity would suggest a primary retinal detachment.
Fig. 3b. The systems echo detection capability allowed to raise the sensitivity to the level necessary for display of tumour tissue echoes.

482

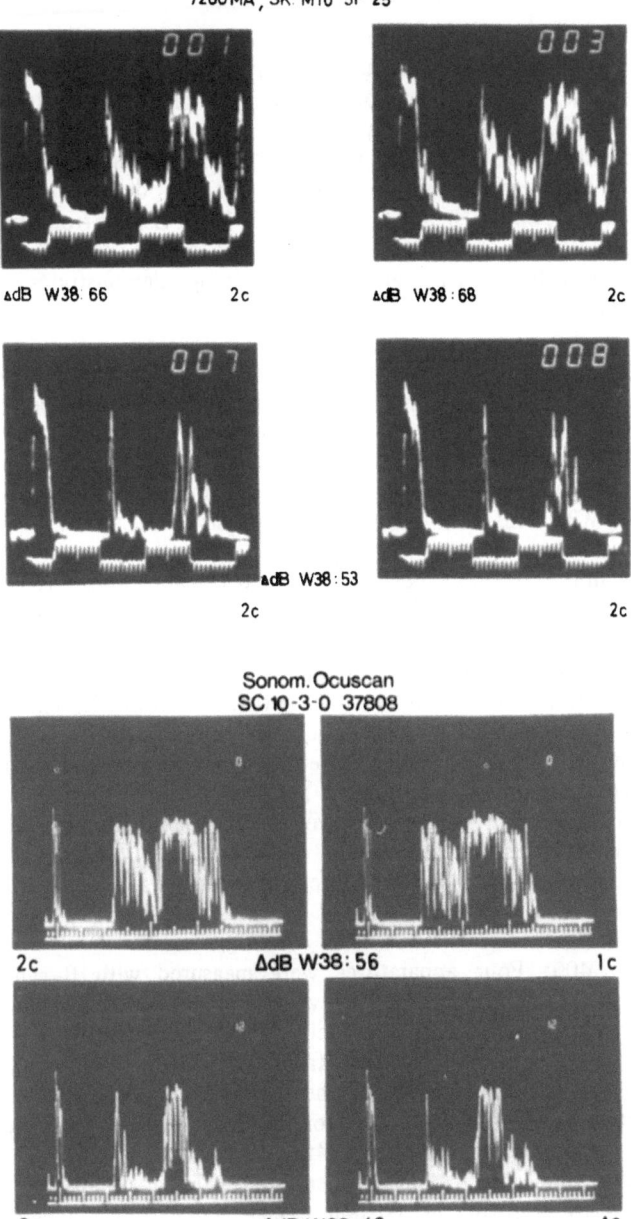

Fig. 4. A-scan of the tumour shown in Fig. 3, taken with two different ultrasonic systems, both used with transducer probes of (or nearby) 10 MHz working frequency. Sensitivity adjustments given (dB values related to 10 mm standard echo of the W38 test reflector) 1c, 2 = probe positions; 1, 2 = clockwise, c = area just before bulbus equator.
Fig. 4a. Kretztechnik 7200 MA
Fig. 4b. Ocuscan 400. The sensitivity and amplitude differences from top to bottom line of echograms demonstrate, compared to Fig. 4a, the error of the dB-scale and the influence of amplifier dynamics.

483

is in agreement with the requirements made by Ossoinig and his group—in as far as their description of 'tissue sensitivity' permits comparison. They use a tissue model instead of a working standard plane echo interface (Till & Ossoinig 1977); thus, frequency spectrum and beam width may well influence their sensitivity measurement. The effect of insufficient echo detection capability on diagnostic criteria of echograms has been described by Baum 1975, Buschmann 1966, 1978, and Coleman, et al. 1977. Echoes from tumour tissue, e.g., would be too weak to be indicated; 'vacuoles' or cyst echograms would be shown on the screen in areas where histology demonstrates solid tumour tissue (Fig. 3 & 4).

3. *Echo detection capability measured in commercially available ophthalmic ultrasonic equipment.* An old Kretz-Technik 7100 MA equipment was measured with an 8 MHz probe (working frequency 8.0 MHz) with 3.5 mm crystal diameter. The echo detection capability (maximum sensitivity) of this combination was 58 dB above the 10 mm standard echo of the test reflector W38. This is too low for safe diagnosis.

Kretztechnik 7200 MA: We have measured ten apparatuses as supplied with 'normal' transducer of 8 MHz *nominal* frequency. Dr. Haigis reported on these measurements. In eight machines, 68 to 75 dB were available in addition to the sensitivity adjustment needed for a 10 mm standard echo from the W38 test reflector. The other two were the noteworthy extremes: 78 dB resp. 57 dB, with the latter being doubtlessly insufficient for diagnostic work. We fully appreciate the manufacturer's attempt to meet some kind of a standard with this type of equipment, but apparently either the standard itself or the checking and maintenance work of the manufacturer (or its numerous service contractors) failed.

The accuracy of the dB-calibrated attenuator was satisfying in all of the ten apparatuses.

Ocuscan 400: Four apparatuses were measured with B-scan transducer probes of 10 MHz *nominal* frequency as supplied with the machines (Table 2). The maximum sensitivities available as conveniently indicated by the crt-readout were found to range from 60–71 dB (2nd row in Table 2). however, the scaling proved to be incorrect in all cases. We therefore calculated – at 10 MHz – figures for the maximum sensitivities with respect to the W38 reflector reference (4th row) which now are seemingly too low. Yet, clinically the echo detection capability of all machines tested appeared to be sufficient. Possible explanations and a detailed description of the above measurements were given by Haigis in his paper. The echo detection capability of the four apparatuses was practically the same, the differences were smaller than in the Kretz 7200 MA machines, which claim to be standardized. At a *working* frequency of 10 MHz the Ocuscan value is somewhat lower than the respective average value for the 7200 MA. For lower frequencies the echo detection capability was higher. Due to the erroneous dB-scale, the figures given in Table 2 had to be derived indirectly. In addition, measurements with the test reflector W38 were also not directly

Table 2. Echo detection capability of four equipments type Ocuscan 400 at nominally 10 MHz.

Ocuscan 400	Nominal attenuation	Actual dB reserve above		Echo detection
Serial No.	Range in dB	W88 reflector	W38 reflector	Capability E in dB
328 124	0–71	38	55	⩾ 72.4
327 990	0–60	35	52	⩾ 69.4
328 025	0–62	38	55	⩾ 72.4
328 094	0–68	43	60	⩾ 77.4

Echo detection capability of Ocuscan 400 at nominally 10 MHz. Third and fourth columns show calculated figures for the echo detection capability with respect to W88 and W38 plane standard reflector 10 mm echoes. Echo detection capability E has been calculated according to IEC 29 D4 draft (Methods for measuring the performance using the value) of -17.4 dB for the difference in reflectivity between the W38 – and the plane ideal reflector.

possible because of insufficient range of attenuation; only the less powerful echoes of W88 test reflectors could adequately be displayed. Thus, Table 2 gives only estimates with some uncertainties still remaining. As a result of our measurements, the manufacturer decided to change the Ocuscan's amplifier design and develop new modules.

Xenotec Ultrascan 500 ABDX: Last year we had opportunity to examine one piece of equipment of this type. It was supplied with a continuous attenuator (dB-scale) and an additional 40 dB attenuation step. We found deviations up to 10 dB between measured actual dB values and dB scale readings. Because of this and other reasons the manufacturer decided for further improvements. We recently received the present version of this apparatus for testing.

CONCLUSION

Our measurement series demonstrate that it is a 'must' to measure the echo detection capability and to check the accuracy of the dB-calibrated attenuator in any equipment before diagnostic use. The measurement technique based on the W38 reflector is applicable to machines of different manufacturers, and the 10 mm standard echo of this reflector is, in addition, a very suitable reference signal for all quantitative echo amplitude evaluation in ultrasonography. The use of at least two test reflectors, providing different reflection factors (just like our test reflectors W38 and W88 do) allows one to check roughly the accuracy of dB-scales; the Echosimulator yields more detailed information (Reuter 1979, Lepper, *et al.* 1979).

Until now, these measurements proved necessary even on so-called 'standardized' apparatus and transducer probes. Without a doubt, good progress has been made in the development of equipment for ophthalmic ultrasonography during the past two decades. However, further improvement is still possible and should be attempted. As a prerequisite to this we should supply the manufacturers with more and better measurement-based information on the influence of technical data on ultrasonic diagnosis.

REFERENCES

Baum, G. Fundamentals of Medical Ultrasonography. New York: Putnam's Sons (1975).

Buschmann, W. Einführung in die ophthalmologische Ultraschalldiagnostik. Leipzig: Georg Thieme (1966).

Buschmann, W., Linnert, D. & Eysholdt, E. Measurement of equipment sensitivity in diagnostic ultrasonography, In: Ultrasound in medicine, Vol. 3B (D. White & R. Brown, eds.) New York: Plenum Publishing Corp. (1977) p. 1925.

Buschmann, W. Tumours of the eye and orbit. In: Ultrasound in Tumour Diagnosis (C.R. Hill, V.R. McCready & D.O. Cosgrove, eds.) Tunbridge Wells: Pitman Medical (1978).

Coleman, J.D., Lizzi, F.L. & Jack, R.L. Ultrasonography of the eye and orbit. Philadelphia: Lea & Febiger (1977).

Haigis, W. & Buschmann, W. Verhandlungsbericht SIDUO VII (H. Gernet, ed.) Münster: R.A. Remy-Verlag (1979) p. 59.

Haigis, W. & Buschmann, W. Die Benutzung von Testreflektoren zur schnellen klinischen Überprüfung von Geräten für die ophthalmologische Ultraschalldiagnostik. Proceedings, Gesellschaft für Biomedizin. Technik Berlin: (Sept. 1980).

Herrmann, G. & Buschmann, W. Kontrolle der Gesamtempfindlichkeit von Ultraschalldiagnostikgeräten und Schallköpfen über lange Zeiträume. v. Graefes Archiv Ophthalmol. 175: 223 (1968).

International Electrotechnical Commission, Technical Comm. 29 Electroacoustics, Subcommittee 29D: Ultrasonics, WG 4: Draft – Methods of measuring the performance of ultrasonic pulse-echo diagnostic equipment (1979).

Lepper, R.D., Trier, H.G. & Reuter, R. Beispiele für die Anwendung des Testprogramms mit Echosimulator an Geräten der Serie 7200 MA Kretztechnik, In: Diagnostica Ultrasonica in Opthalmologia (H. Gernet, ed.) Münster: Remy Verlag (1979) p. 48.

Lizzi, F.L. & Feleppa, E.J. Practical physics and electronics of ultrasound, In: Ophthalmic ultrasonography: Comparative Techniques. Int. Ophthalmol. Clinics 19 (R.L. Dallow, ed.) (1979).

Reuter, R. Der Zusammenhang klinisch relevanter Gerätefunktionen im A- und B-Bild und ihre Überprüfung durch ein differenzierungsfähiges Testprogramm. In: Diagnostica Ultrasonica in Ophthalmologia (H. Gernet, ed.) Münster: Remy-Verlag (1979) p. 44.

Till, P. & Ossoinig, K.C. First experiences with a solid tissue model for the standardization of A- and B-scan instruments in tissue diagnosis. In: Ultrasound in medicine, Vol. 3B (D. White & R.E. Brown, eds.) New York: Plenum Publishing Corp. (1977). p. 2167.

Authors' Address:
University Eye Hospital
Würzburg, F.R.G.

INFLUENCE OF EQUIPMENT PARAMETERS ON RESULTS IN OPHTHALMIC ULTRASONOGRAPHY

II. Frequency and frequency spectrum

W. BUSCHMANN, W. HAIGIS & D. LINNERT

(Würzburg, F.R.G.)

INTRODUCTION

The IEC draft on methods of measuring the performance of ultrasonic pulse-echo diagnostic equipment describes the manufacturer's quotation of frequency as 'nominal frequency'. It may differ considerably from the frequencies actually available for diagnostic work with the equipment, as Haigis has shown in his paper. Frequency affects lateral and axial resolution and — even more important — the rate of attenuation of the beam during its passage through tissue. This rate of attenuation is used as a diagnostic criterion for tissue differentiation (Buschmann 1966, 1972; Ossoinig 1971; Buschmann, Vogel & Herrmann 1972).

1. MEASUREMENT METHODS

The most complete information on the frequencies involved and their relative amplitude would be provided by spectrum analysis. The amplifier's frequency response can be demonstrated on the screen of the ultrasonography apparatus as has been described by Haigis & Buschmann (1980). Also, the so-called Echosimulator (Reuter 1979; Lepper *et al.* 1979; Lepper's paper at this symposium) is a good device to measure — amongst other parameters — this important system characteristic. Spectrum analysis, however, delivers a set of data instead of just one figure.

In diagnostic work the frequencies involved in the emission of an ultrasound pulse are usually well described by the working frequency, i.e. the main frequency component of the sound spectrum which is created by the action of the system pulser on the transducer crystal. The emission spectrum, of course, is strongly influenced by the excitation pulse, mechanical damping as well as all sorts of electrical networks linked to the transducer probe (attenuator, receiver etc.).

To measure the working frequency of a specific transducer the following procedure was adopted, regarding the recommendations given in the IEC draft:

The test reflector W38 (see part I of our contribution to this volume) was used as a working standard plane echo interface in 0.9% buffered NaCl

© *1981. Dr W. Junk Publishers, The Hague*

solution (pH 7.2) at 30 μs distance. Room temperature is appropriate. The transducer probe was oriented to obtain maximum echo amplitude and the radio frequency echo wave form (unrectified echo) was displayed and examined on the screen of the ultrasonic apparatus (if this display mode was provided by the manufacturer). If this facility was lacking, as unfortunately in the 7200 MA Kretztechnik apparatus, a separate oscilloscope had to be used to display the RF waveform of the echo.

The RF oscillations/μs were counted, and the working frequency calculated as the average between maximum amplitude cycle and the last cycle with more than 30% of maximum amplitude.

It is possible to count oscillations also in the video signal, if low filtering would be applied. But the resolution at maximum magnification of the echograms limits this to probes of about 5 MHz at the 7200 MA apparatus. One has to regard half- or full-wave rectification, and Ossoinig's description of frequency calculation (Ossoinig 1971) is incorrect for the machine he uses, because half-wave rectification is applied in the 7200 MA apparatus. It would be correct for the Ocuscan 400 (full-wave rectification), but RF display is available in this machine and this is to be preferred for frequency studies.

The IEC draft mentions our former studies on the rate of attenuation in paraffine oil (more recently: phenyl methyl silicone oil), from which information on frequency and spectrum could be derived (Buschmann 1978). Regarding the influence of the frequency spectrum in present clinical work, the existence of lower frequency components and their relative amplitudes proved to be important. Changes in the rate of attenuation in these oils, which occur with increasing transducer-reflector distance, as well as an apparent frequency decrease in the RF display during distance changes in oil (Fig. 9), demonstrate the existence of powerful low frequency components (Buschman 1972; see also Haigis' paper).

Electronic spectrum analysis was used in addition. We could prove, that the abovementioned simpler methods provide valuable information if spectrum analysis is not available.

2. FREQUENCY AND SPECTRUM REQUIREMENTS IN OPHTHALMIC A- AND B-SCAN ULTRASONOGRAPHY

Controversial recommendations were given and have been realised in diagnostic equipment regarding the frequencies to be used and other frequency related system parameters. A wide frequency range from 5 to 12 or 15 MHz was used by Baum (1975), Oksala (1970), Buschmann (1966, 1972, 1972/73), Holasek, et al. (1975), Coleman, et al. (1977), Decker & Trier (1977), Lizzi et al. (1979).

Contrary to this, Ossoinig (1971) favoured an 8 MHz narrow-bandwidth equipment for all applications in eye and orbit, including restriction to one transducer shape. What is actually necessary for good clinical work? The dependence of ultrasound attenuation in tissue on frequency is documented in the literature (Le Croissette et al. 1979, Parry & Chivers 1979). There is

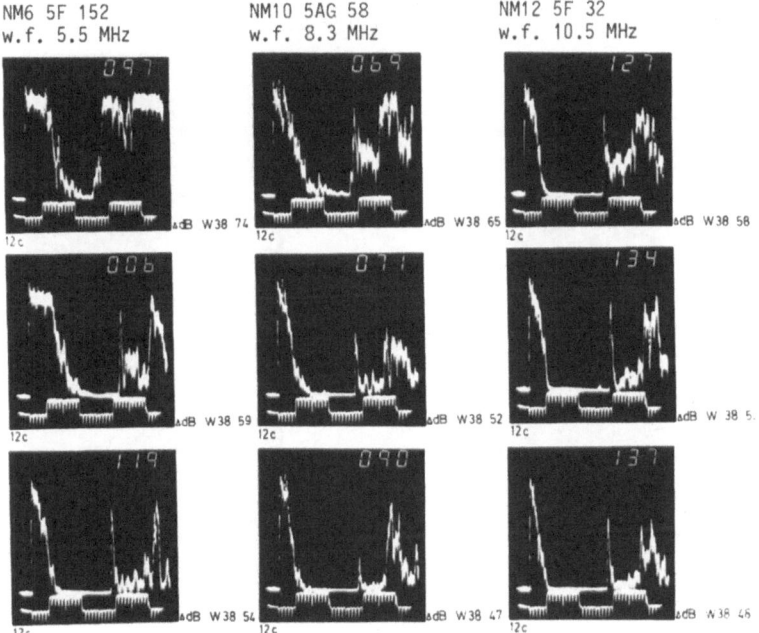

NM6 5F 152   NM10 5AG 58   NM12 5F 32
w.f. 5.5 MHz   w.f. 8.3 MHz   w.f. 10.5 MHz

Fig. 1. Frequency, in the range of 5.5–10.5 MHz, shows no recognizable effect on the A-scans of this i.o melanoblastoma. Very similar echograms were recorded – no matter, whether 5.5 MHz, 8.3 MHz or 10.5 MHz working frequency were used – if the examination direction was the same and if the sensitivity was the same (measured in dB above W38 test reflector standard echo!). Compare echogram No. 006 with No. 127; and No. 119 with No. 071 and No. 134

experimental and clinical evidence according to which the application of different frequencies in the range of 6–15 MHz yields substantially more information.

In routine A-scan echograms, however, no recognizable variations may be seen if different frequencies in the range of 5–10 MHz were applied (Fig. 1). Beam direction affects the tissue echogram much more than frequency (Figs. 2 and 3).

Frequency, nevertheless, matters indeed in tissue differentiation: not only in echo spectrum analysis (Lizzi, *et al.* 1979; Decker & Trier 1977; Holasek *et al.* 1975) but even in the estimation of ultrasound attenuation in a tumour suspected mass with present routine equipment, using the sclera echo as reference signal (comparison of sclera echo amplitude in examination directions through and past the mass lesion, Buschmann 1978). At 5–6 MHz, ultrasound attenuation in most i.o tumour cases was too low; no significant difference was found comparing the directions mentioned. At about 10–12 MHz *working* frequency, averaging repeated measurements, an attenuation of about $1 \, dB \, cm^{-1} \, MHz^{-1}$ was found in i.o. melanoblastomas. This corresponds well to Lizzi *et al.* (1978): $0.9 \, dB \, cm^{-1} \, MHz^{-1}$.

Frequency matters in foreign body diagnosis; the chance to detect a

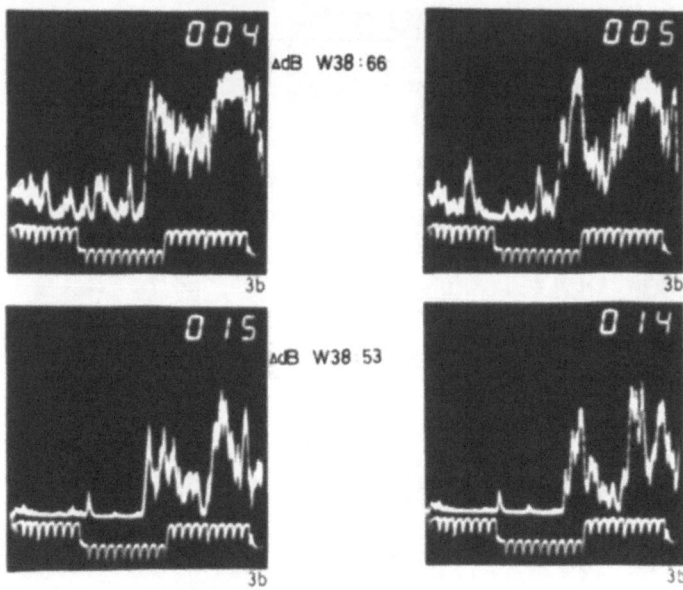

Fig. 2. Beam direction affects the tissue echogram much more than frequency. Intra-ocular melanoblastoma. Transducer position at the globe unchanged. Smallest changes of beam direction result in marked changes of the echo amplitude decrease within the tumour area (compare left and right group of echograms); Kretztechnik 7200 MA; w.f. of the probe: 10 MHz.

a foreign body is about six times better using 10.5 MHz working frequency compared with 5.5 MHz (see Table 1). Safe diagnosis depends on display of an echo with an amplitude well above the sclera echo amplitude range. Such echoes were displayed much more often with probes of higher working frequency, if the same i.o. foreign bodies were subsequently examined with transducer probes of 5.5 MHz, 8.3 MHz and 10.5 MHz working frequency (Linnert & Buschmann 1977).

For the detection of vitreous opacities and vitreous destruction, we prefer, as Oksala (1978) does, a 6 MHz probe. Theoretically, one would expect higher frequencies to be more suitable for the detection of such small reflectors; but the receiver amplifiers of the Kretztechnik 7100 and 7200 apparatus have their highest sensitivity around 6 MHz. With the Ocuscan 400, vitreous opacities could be demonstrated best at 5 MHz. This is also a result of the frequency response of this equipment.

Frequency matters also by partly indirect frequency effects. The differences observed between echograms recorded with probes of lower or higher frequency are partially caused by lower sensitivity of the system at higher frequencies. If corresponding sensitivity adjustments were chosen

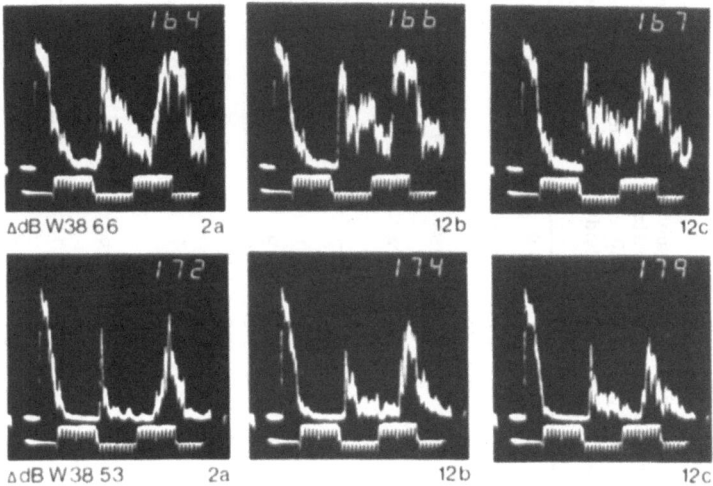

Fig. 3. With change of examination direction, any degree of amplitude decrease within the tumour area (Ossoinig's 'angle kappa') could be achieved in this i.o. melanoblastoma. *Ultrasound attenuation in tissue cannot be evaluated this way.* Electronic averaging of numerous echograms would be necessary for this purpose. Kretztechnik 7200 MA, w.f. of the probe: 10 MHz.

(related to W38 test reflector standard echo), similar echograms, including 'acoustic vacuoles', could be displayed at low and at high frequencies (Fig. 4). For reproducible results, therefore, frequency and sensitivity must be known.

The acoustic shadowing effect behind mass lesions, as well as pronounced orbital fat echoes behind cysts are affected by frequency and usually better demonstrable at higher frequencies (Coleman 1977).

Frequency matters also in orbital diagnosis. Orbital fat tissue can be penetrated better, and the bone walls shown more pronounced, if there is some edema in the orbital tissues (pseudotumor, endocrine ophthalmopathy). A similar effect can be produced by (unexpected) lower working frequency (Figs. 5 & 6). In Fig. 6 two echograms of eye and orbit at the level of the optic nerve are shown. Which one demonstrates an orbital edema? The figures indicate the sensitivity settings of the attenuator. In Fig. 6b, the orbital bone wall is more pronounced, and the orbital fat structure seems to be more inhomogeneous, interrupted by echo-free spaces. One might believe, that this is an orbit with an edema. However it is just the other one, shown in Fig. 6a, which actually has an edema. This makes quite clear that one has to measure the *working* frequency before starting a diagnostic interpretation. Remember, that one commercially available machine supposed to work at 10 MHz (= nominal frequency) was found in our measurements actually to work at 5 MHz as Dr. Haigis reported in his paper. Comparable results depend on the knowledge of the working frequency. Valuable additional diagnostic information becomes available if at least two different frequencies can be applied.

491

Table 1. Frequency dependence of foreign body echo amplitude. 10 i.o. foreign bodies were examined experimentally, using the same series of examination directions and probe positions with three probes subsequently (working frequency 5.5, 8.3 and 10.5 MHz). The figures indicate the number of foreign body echo amplitude measurements performed and the number of high amplitude, typical foreign body echoes found.

The foreign body diagnosis was much safer (and faster) at 10.5 MHz. The chance to detect and to identify a foreign body echo was six times better at 10.5 MHz than with 5.5 MHz. (548 amplitude measurements) Kretztechnik 7200 MA.

Foreign body No.	1	2	3	4	5	6	7	8	9	10	
Transducer probe nom. frequency 6 MHz (w.f. 5.5 MHz NM 6 5F Nr. 152)											
No. of measurements	27	19	17	13	19	19	19	18	19	19	= 189
= 24 dB above W38 echo (= 5 dB above sclera)	1	2	–	2	1	1	1	2	4	–	= 14 (7, 4%)
= 29 dB above W38 echo (= 10 dB above sclera)	–	2	–	–	–	–	–	–	–	–	= 3 (1, 6%)
Transducer probe nom. frequency 10 MHz (w.f. 8.3 MHz) NM 10 5 AG Nr. 58											
No. of measurments	19	19	12	13	19	19	19	16	19	19	= 174
= 24 dB above W38 echo (= 5 dB above sclera)	1	5	–	2	8	4	2	2	13	1	= 38 (21, 8%)
= 29 dB above W38 echo (= 10 dB above sclera)	–	2	–	–	2	2	1	2	7	–	= 16 (9, 2%)
Transducer probe nom. frequency 12 MHz (w.f. 10.5 MHz) NM 12 5F Nr. 32											
No. of measurements	31	19	12	13	19	19	19	18	19	19	= 185
= 24 dB above W38 echo (= 5 dB above sclera)	4	3	3	4	9	4	2	5	7	1	= 42 (22, 7%)
= 29 dB above W38 echo (= 10 dB above sclera)	–	3	–	3	5	2	1	2	2	–	= 18 (9, 7%)

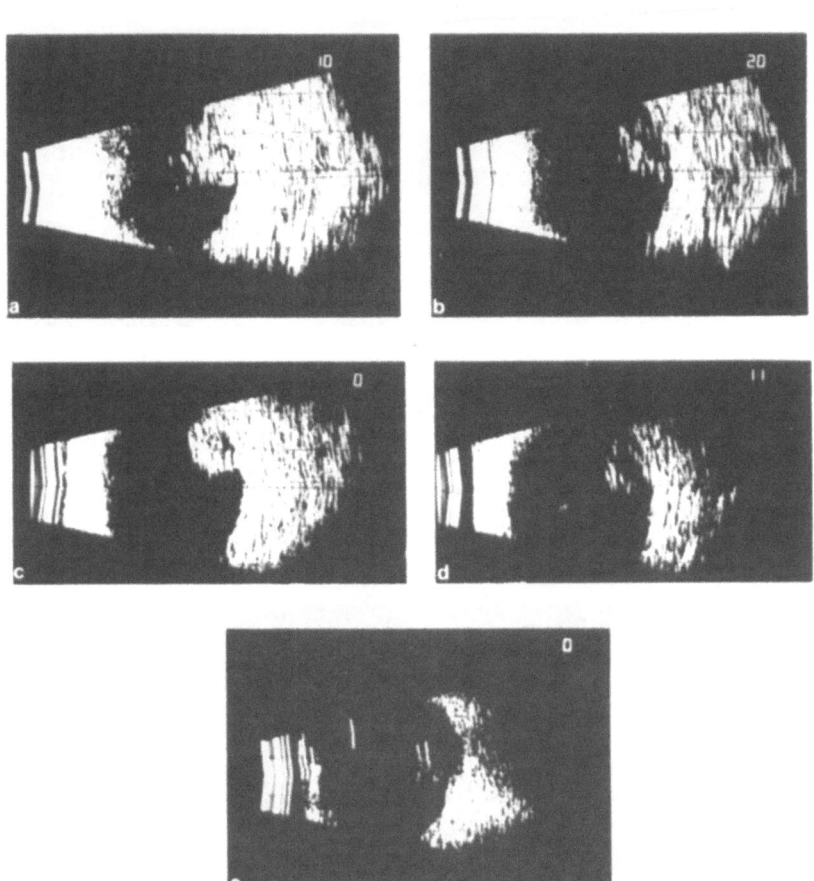

Fig. 4. Partly indirect frequency effects Similar echograms, e.g. 'acoustic vacuoles' in this i.o. melanoblastoma at lower sensitivity and solid tissue echograms (upper line) at higher sensitivity could be displayed with a 5 MHz probe (Fig. 4a, b) as well as with a 10 MHz probe (Fig. 4c, d), if corresponding sensitivity settings were chosen. The system's sensitivity at 15 MHz, however, was insufficient to display tumour tissue echoes in this case (Fig. 4e). The figures within the echograms indicate (roughly) the sensitivity in decibels of receiver attenuation. 0 = no receiver attenuation = maximum sensitivity. Ocuscan 400.

3. WHAT DO WE HAVE? FREQUENCY RESPONSES AND SPECTRA MEASURED IN COMMERCIALLY AVAILABLE OPHTHALMIC ULTRASONIC EQUIPMENT (see W. Haigis's paper for more details)

Measurements proved necessary in all types of commercially available ultrasonic equipment for ophthalmic use; this applies also to the 'standardized' Kretztechnik 7200 MA apparatus and transducers. An example is given in Fig. 7. Nominal frequency: 8 MHz, narrow bandwidth.

Compared to their former model 7100 (with RF signal display facility on the screen, and sufficient scale magnification), in the 7200 MA the

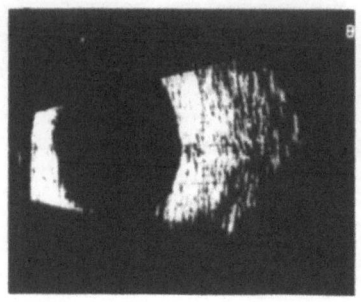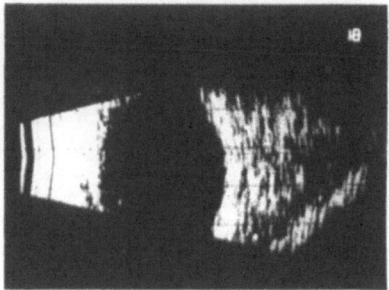

Fig. 5. Endocrine Orbitopathy. Orbital fat edema, lateral rectus muscle slightly swollen, pronounced echoes from the orbital wall. Ocuscan 400, 9.7 MHz (Fig. 5a) resp. 5 MHz (Fig. 5b) transducer probe. The pathologic changes could be displayed with both of the frequencies at corresponding sensitivity levels. Frequency-dependent differences: Smaller echoes (better resolution) in the depth of the orbit at 9.7 MHz (Fig. 5a), but more receiver saturation behind the sclera. In Fig. 5b better penetration at lower frequencies can be seen: less saturation behind the sclera and, nevertheless, more intensive echoes from the orbital wall. Enhancement on.

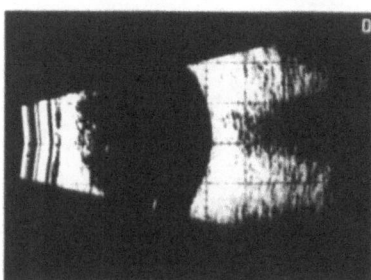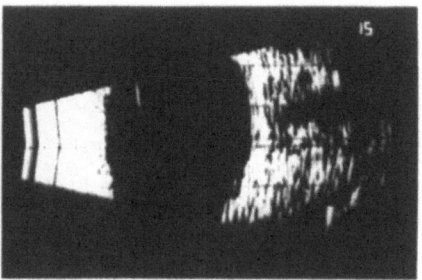

Fig. 6. Which one is the orbit with an edema? Ocuscan 400,
Fig. 6a = 10 MHz (working frequency = 9.7 MHz);
Fig. 6b = 5 MHz (w.f. = 5 MHz).
Without knowledge of the frequencies involved one might easily take figure 6b for an echogram of orbital edema due to the more inhomogeneous appearance of the orbital fat structure and the better penetration of ultrasound (orbital wall partly displayed). However, this is just a normal orbit, examined with a 5 MHz transducer probe at low sensitivity. In Fig. 6a, however, an echogram of an edematous orbit is shown. With regards to the frequency used (9.7 MHz), the penetration into the depth of the orbit is better than normal, and the echoes from this area are too powerful. The rectus muscles are somewhat edematous, too – see concave shape of lateral margin (lower margin in the figure) of orbital fat echogram. Enhancement on.

manufacturers made it difficult for the user to count at least the working frequency: a separate oscilloscope must be applied. Therefore, users may tend to restrict their equipment check to tissue model (Till & Ossoinig 1977) echograms. This would be inadequate (Fig. 8). Considerable differences between nominal and working frequency would be overlooked.

For most applications, the frequency spectrum of diagnostic ultrasound should be narrow; especially lower frequency components of relatively

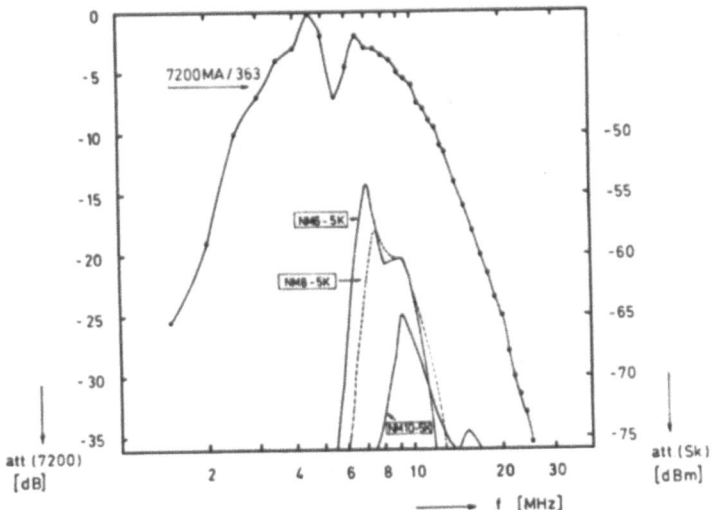

Fig. 7. Frequency response of the 7200 MA No 363 receiver (upper trace), revealing two peaks at 4.5 and 6.5 MHz, *and sound emission spectra* (lower traces) of standard probes, nominal frequencies 6, 8 and 10 MHz, actual peak frequencies 7, 7.5 and 9.1 MHz. Note positions of emission maxima as compared to the receiver response.

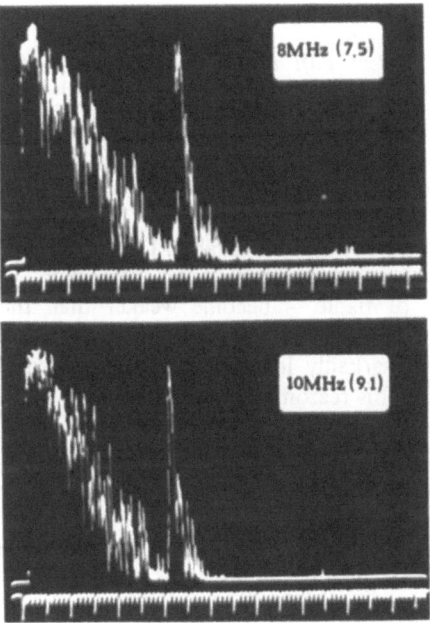

Fig. 8. Tissue model (Till & Ossoinig 1977) echograms taken with (nominal) 8 MHz (Fig. 8a, above) and 10 MHz (below) standard probes (sound emission spectras see Fig. 7) at 'tissue sensitivity' settings. No conclusions as to the actual working frequency can be drawn from these echograms.

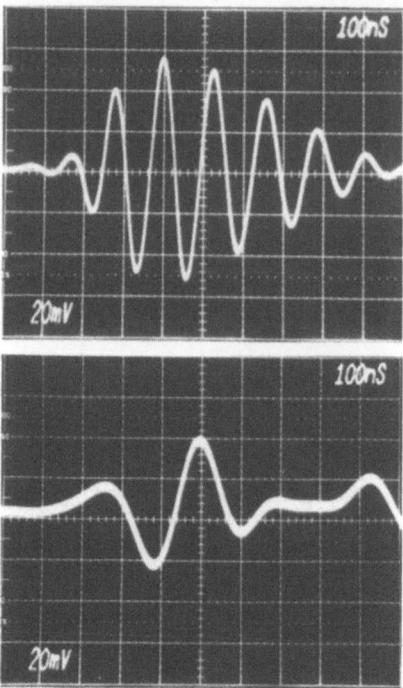

Fig. 9. Absorption-dependent shift in working frequency, revealing low frequency components. RF echogram of W38 test reflector in water bath (distance = focus = 5 mm, Fig. 9a, above) and of plane steel reflector in phenyl methyl silicone oil AP 500 (distance = 33 mm, Fig. 9b, below). Focussed 8 MHz probe. Due to the higher absorption of high frequency spectral components in oil, frequency components become important (see dominant 4 MHz cycle, Fig. 9b, right, compared to 8 MHz in water, Fig. 9a, left echogram).

high amplitude would be very undesirable. Due to the higher attenuation of the higher frequency components in tissue, these may – after penetration of a few millimeters of tissue – become weaker than the lower frequency components. Then, the deeper tissue structures would be examined with an effective frequency markedly lower than the measured working frequency. (See Fig. 9) It is for this reason that we recommend to measure the working frequency not only in a low-attenuation water or saline bath but (if spectrum analysis would not be available) also in a high-attenuation oil. The echoes of a good transducer-apparatus combination would practically maintain their frequency when penetrating increasing distances through oil, as long as echo amplitudes permit frequency evaluation. In case of a wide frequency spectrum, the high frequency components would soon disappear and the echo waveform be determined by the lower frequency components (Fig. 9b). Major changes can easily be detected comparing the RF display of plane interface echoes arising from pulses sent through a waterbath and from pulses having travelled through highly attenuating oil (for details see Dr. Haigis contribution to this volume).

496

CONCLUSION

Summarizing the clinical requirements, for diagnosis of intraocular diseases at least 9–10 and 13–15 MHz working frequency should be applied, and for orbital disorders 5–6 and 9–10 MHz. This can be achieved using a wideband receiver amplifier or several narrow-band channels. On the other hand, the emission spectrum of the transducer connected to the system should preferably be of the narrow-band type, e.g. with a 6 dB bandwidth of not more than 10–20% of the center frequency. Side lobes on the lower frequency side of the spectrum, if present, should have an amplitude 20 dB or more below working frequency amplitude, so that they never can become the prevalent component after tissue penetration.

Frequency response and spectrum in numerous commercially available equipment are not optimum. In addition, nominal frequency is inadequate information. Users need to check frequency response and spectrum to avoid work at unexpected (low) frequencies. Determination of working frequency by counting the RF oscillations, as recommended in the IEC draft, proved to yield adequate information for clinical purposes. For this and other reasons, high-quality apparatus are supplied with a RF display mode and a quartz-calibrated microsecond scale.

As to frequency measurements, especially the check of the frequency response function of the total system, the Echosimulator is a valuable and easy-to-handle instrument, which also can be used to get data on other technical parameters of the diagnostic ultrasonograph. The latter procedures have been dealt with in detail by Dr. Lepper.

The manufacturers of ophthalmic equipment should supply frequency and spectrum information according to the abovementioned IEC draft, as several other manufacturers in the field of ultrasonic pulse-echo techniques already do.

REFERENCES

Baum, G. Fundamentals of Medical Ultrasonography, New York, Putnam's Sons (1975).
Buschmann, W. Einführung in die ophthalmologische Ultraschalldiagnostik. Leipzig: Georg Thieme (1966).
Buschmann, W. Opthalmologische Ultraschalldiagnostik. In: Der Augenarzt, 2nd edition vol. 2, (K. Velhagen, ed.) Leipzig: Georg Thieme (1972) p. 391.
Buschmann, W. Vogel, A. & Herrmann, G. Der Einfluß des Frequenzspektrums auf Gewebsechogramme. Wiss. Zeitschr. der Humboldt-Univ. Berlin, Math.-Nat. R. 21, 45 (1972).
Buschmann, W. Use of the frequency filtering effect of tissues in diagnostic ultrasonography. Ophthalmic Res 4: 122 (1972/73).
Buschmann, W. Tumours of the eye and orbit, In: Ultrasound in Tumour Diagnosis. (C.R. Hill, V.R. McCready & D.O. Cosgrove eds.,) Tunbridge Wells: Pitman Medical (1978).
Buschmann, W. Special techniques. In: Handbook of Clinical Ultrasound. (M. de Vlieger et al., eds.) New York: J. Wiley & Sons (1978).
Coleman, J.D., Lizzi, F.L. & Jack, R.L. Ultrasonography of the eye and orbit. Philadelphia: Lea & Febiger (1977).

Decker, D., & Trier, H.G. Das Projekt 'rechnergestützte Gewebsdifferenzierung' der Arbeitsgemeinschaft Bonn/Stuttgart. In: Diagnostica ultrasonica in ophthalmologia (H. Gernet, ed.) R.A. Remy (1979).

Haigis, W. & Buschmann, W. Klinisch anwendbare Methoden zur Überprüfung von diagnostisch relevanten Geräteparametern von Impuls-Echo-Geräten. Proc. Dreiländertreffen Ultraschall in der Medizin, Böblingen. Stuttgart: Thieme (1980).

Holasek, E., Gans, L.A., Purnell, E.W., & Sokollu, A. A method for spectra-colour B-scan Ultrasonography. J. Clin. Ultrasound, 3, 175, (1975).

International Electrotechnical Commission, Technical Comm. 29 Electroacoustics, Subcommittee 29D: Ultrasonics, WG 4: Draft-Methods of measuring the performance of ultrasonic pulse-echo diagnostic equipment. (1979).

Le Croisette, D.H., Heyser, R.C., Gammell, P.M., & Roseboro, J.A. The attenuation of selected soft tissue as a function of frequency. In: Ultrasonic tissue characterization II, (M. Linzer, ed.), U.S. Department of Commerce, NBS Special Publication 525, (1979), p. 101

Lepper, R.D., Trier, H.G. & Reuter, R. Beispiele für die Anwendung des Testprogramms mit Echosimulator an Geräten der Serie 7200 MA Kretztechnik. In: Diagnostica Ultrasonica in Ophthalmologia. (H. Gernet, ed.) Münster: Remy Verlag (1979), p. 48.

Linnert, D. & Buschmann, W.: Möglichkeiten und Grenzen der echografischen Fremd-körperlokalisation. In: H. Neubauer, Intraokularer Fremdkörper und Metallose. (W. Rüßmann & H. Kilp eds.). München: J.F. Bergmann-Verlag, (1977).

Lizzi, F.L., Coleman, D.J. Franzen, L. & Feleppa, E. Use of spectrum analysis system for characterization of malignant melanoma, In: Ultrasound in Medicine vol. 4. (D. White & E. Lyons eds.) New York: Plenum (1978) p. 559.

Lizzi, F.L., Laviola, M.A. & Coleman, D.J. Tissue signature characterization utilizing frequency domain analysis. In: Collected papers on medical and biological applications. (J. de Klerk & B.R. McAvoy eds.), IEEE Ultrasonic symposium proceedings (1979) p. 410.

Lizzi, F.L. & Feleppa, E.J. Practical physics and electronics of ultrasound, In: Ophthalmic ultrasonography: Comparative Techniques Int Ophthal. Clinics 19. (R.L. Dallow, ed.) (1979).

Oksala, A. Biophysikalische und methodische Fragen in der ophthalmologischen Ultraschalldiagnostik. Klin. Mbl. Augenheilk. 156: 465 (1970).

Oksala, A. Ultrasonic findings in the vitreous body at various ages. A. v. Graefes Arch. klin. exp. Ophthal. 207, 275 (1978).

Ossoinig K. Grundlagen der klinischen Echo-Ophthalmographie. Wien: Verl. Wiener Med. Akad. (1971).

Parry, R.J. & Chivers, R.C. Data of the velocity and attenuation of ultrasound in mammalian tissues – a survey. In: Ultrasonic tissue characterization II, (M. Linzer, ed.), U.S. Dept. of Commerce, NBS Special Publication 525, (1979), p. 343.

Reuter, R. Der Zusammenhang klinisch relevanter Gerätefunktionen im A- und B-Bild und ihre Überprüfung durch ein differenzierungsfähiges Testprogramm. In: Diagnostica Ultrasonica in Ophthalmologia, (H. Gernet, ed.), Münster: Remy Verl. (1979) p. 44.

Till, P. & Ossoinig, K.C. First experience with a solid tissue model for the standardization of A- and B-scan instruments in tissue diagnosis, in: Ultrasound in Medicine, vol. 3B, (D. White & R.E. Brown, eds.) New York: Plenum Publishing Corp. (1977), p. 2167.

Authors' Address:
University Eye Clinic
Würzburg
F.R.G.

498

A NEW OPHTHALMIC ULTRASONOSCOPE

G. BAUM
(Bronx, U.S.A.)

Our experiences in ophthalmic ultrasonography and those of other laboratories have shown that it is extremely difficult to correlate ocular histopathology with ultrasonographic images by visual inspection, despite the use of gray scale, video inversion, color and isometric displays. Julesz (1975) has provided the experimental confirmation of the eye's inability to analyze images of this order of statistical complexity. He has shown that the eye has no difficulty in detecting differences amongst images whose first or second order statistics differ, but has extreme difficulty in arriving at such differentiation when the third or higher order of statistics differ. Thus, in Fig. 1 if one deals with a simple image in which the elements are of equal size and gray scale value, one can readily perceive changes in texture if the spatial distribution amongst the points is altered.

When one goes to more complex images such as shown in Fig. 2, the eye is still able to distinguish between these images when there is a difference in the first or second order statistics. However, when there is a difference in the third order statistics, it is virtually impossible for the eye to detect a difference between these two images. Although it is virtually impossible for the eye to detect differences amongst images which have third or higher order statistical differences, computers do not suffer from the same difficulty that the eye does. For this reason, we have developed the ultrasonographic system shown in Fig. 3. This system employs a digital scan converter and is connected into a high-speed digitizer which has a 20 MHz sampling rate. This system permits us to simultaneously record the RF signal on a disk and to record on film a high resolution-extended gray scale ultrasonogram. Fig. 4.

Digital recording the RF on disks permits us to pre and post process the ultrasound images with the digital scan converter. The disk is played back and the RF data on the disk is rectified and fed into the scan converter. It then becomes possible to carry out pre and post processing studies upon this image, while the stored RF data is unaffected by these routines. The routines in the scan converter enable us to view the image with different levels and different gray scale curves, e.g., log, linear, etc. The digital scan converter also enables us to magnify and study in detail desired portions of the image. These manipulations make it possible to achieve the best image for interpretation.

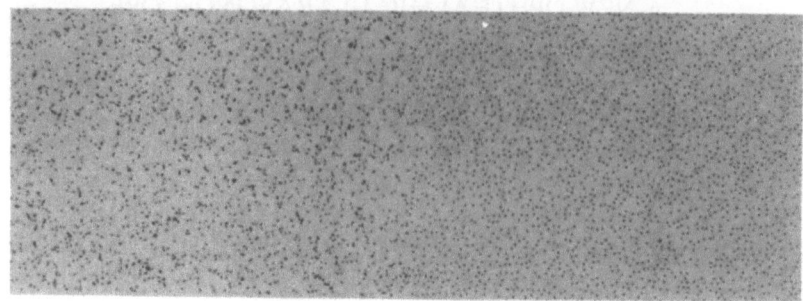

Fig. 1. The difference in second-order statistics, which is readily visible here, and is exemplified by these two textures, which have identical first-order statistics. The first-order statistics of the textures are identical because each texture consists of the same number of black dots, hence there is the same probability in both textures that a given point will have same luminance. In the left field the dots fall at random. In the right field, however, there are at least 10 dot diameters between dots. Thus if a dipole such as a needle were dropped on the two fields, the probability of both ends touching a dot would be different in the two cases. Difference in probabilities signifies a difference in second-order (dipole) statistics.

 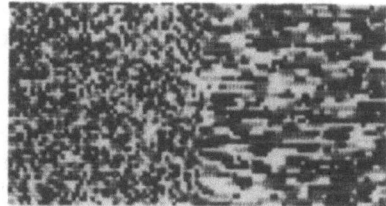

Fig. 2. The difference in third-order statistics, which eludes spontaneous detection is demonstrated in the image at the left. The left and right half-fields in that image have textures that are generated by a Markov process so as to have identical first-order and second-order statistics but to have different third-order statistics based on the sequential arrangement of cells of four different luminance levels: black, dark gray, light gray and white. Only by careful inspection can one see that the left half-field contains a few horizontal stripes of uniform luminance that are formed by three adjacent cells whereas the right half-field contains practically no stripes. In comparison, the two textures in the image at the right can instantly be discriminated because they have different second-order statistics, which appear as a difference in granularity. In both textures cells of three luminance levels (black, gray and white) occur with equal probability; hence first-order statistics are the same. In the texture that largely fills the left side adjacent cells are statistically independent of one another in luminance whereas in the surrounding texture adjacent cells are related mathematically by a Markov process. This gives rise to different second-order statistics.

The keyboard permits us to enter on each ultrasonogram pertinent data about the patient, as well as the operating conditions of the equipment at the time of examination. A dual beam oscilloscope enables us to view one scan line at a time. The upper oscilloscope displays the RF characteristics and the lower the rectified A-mode. The individual frames are automatically numbered. The image can also be monitored as a bistable color-coded and gray scale image. (Fig. 5.)

500

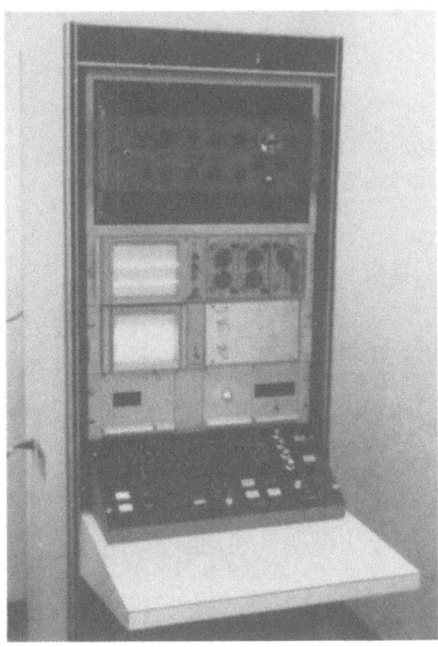

Fig. 3. The new ophthalmic ultrasonographic instrument that we have developed. The digital scan converter is shown at the top most element of the unit. The RF and A-mode displays appear on the upper cathode ray tube and the digitized B-mode image on the lower cathode ray tube. The remaining instrument controls and the keyboard for typing in patient data and equipment operation characteristics can be made from the keyboard shown at the bottom portion of the picture.

The scanner, Fig. 6, is especially advantageous for the studies of the orbit because the geometrical relationships between the transducer and the orbit are held constant by the scanning device. This makes it possible for us to compare virtually identical planes of scan in the two orbits with the eyes in the comparable positions of gaze.

The characteristics of the high-speed digitizer, Fig. 7, are superior to other high-speed digitizers such as the Biomation instrument because the data from the tissues is recorded in real-time in a RAM fast 256 kbyte memory with a scan line to scan line jitter of less than 5 ns. What this means is that we can treat the recorded data as a B-scan and examine it for textural characteristics of pixel size smaller than a wavelength of sound. While this resolution is meaningless in the sense of a classical B-scan, it allows us to process the data without the distortion found when a photograph must be digitized.

For example, we are able to take the raw data and apply published algorithms to smooth it in two dimensions to any degree, alter the gray scale curve and select certain areas for statistical measures. Comparative statistical measures are particularly meaningful here because we are able to work with different areas of an entire B-scan which was recorded in less than 1/2 s, rather than with two separate recordings taken some time apart as would be

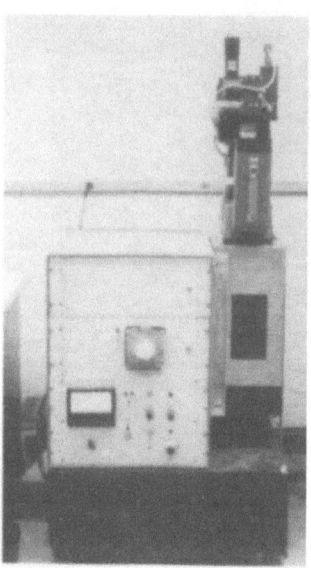

Fig. 4. The high-resolution cathode ray tube and the automatic camera which produces the high resolution, extended gray scale ultrasonogram. The cathode ray tube has an 8.0 mil spot-size. To achieve a stabilized-gray scale, the light output of each scan line is optically monitored and correction made for any drift of the cathode ray tube.

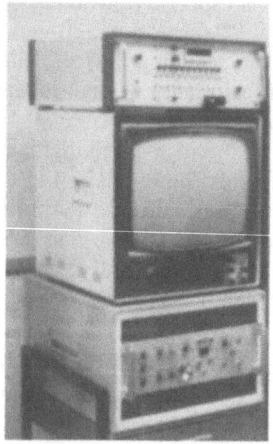

Fig. 5. The colour monitoring portion of the ophthalmic unit. The color monitor is a photodensitometer that is shared with an ultrasound mammographic scanner.

502

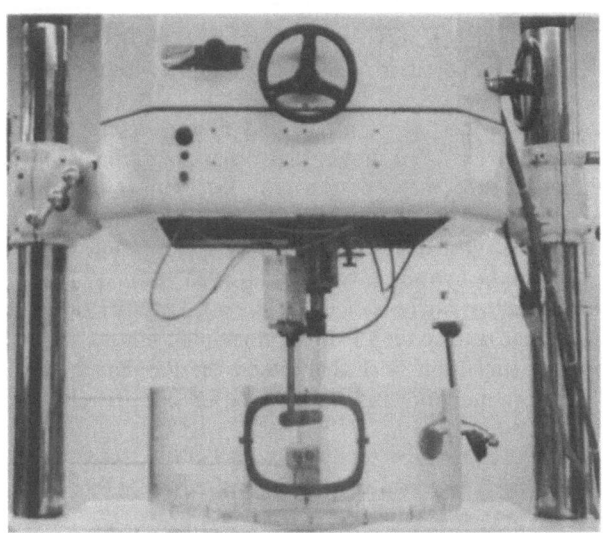

Fig. 6. The eye scanner provides the rigidity required to compare equivalent levels of scan of each eye in comparable levels of gaze. This is essential for examination of the orbits.

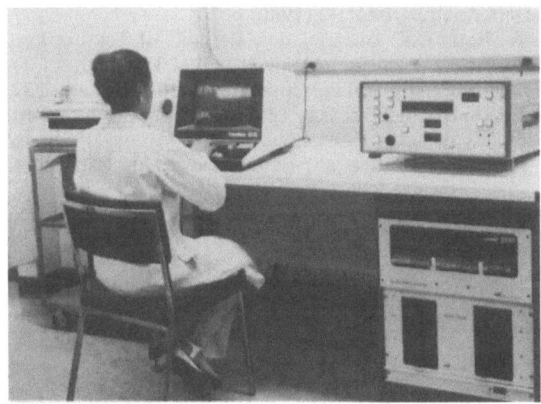

Fig. 7. The high-speed digitizer, printer and microprocessor which is the heart of the system. This system can record an entire plane of scan in real-time with less than 5 nanoseconds of jitter between scan lines. This unit enables us to examine an image for its textural characteristics or pixel size smaller than the wavelength of sound, and allows us to process data without the distortion found when a photograph must be digitized.

required by other commercial digitizers. The system can also be used as a computer to develop and test algorithms which measure the statistical properties of the RF signals.

A number of studies (Conners & Harlow 1980, Faugeras & Pratt 1980, Weszka, *et al.* 1976) have shown that the power spectrum measurement is the least efficacious in discriminating texture. This may be especially true in the

503

study of orbital tumors because Rose, *et al.* (1980) have shown the limitations of spectral analysis in identifying tumors within the fatty tissues of the breast.

The textural properties of ultrasound images resemble those of space satellite images. It has been shown that other algorithms such as the spatial gray level dependence method, the gray level run length method and the gray level difference method are more effective in discriminating such complex textures and may result in improved ultrasonographic classification of tumor type in the eye and orbit. Therefore the primary goal of this system is to carry out texture analysis of the echograms. Studies aimed at identifying the primitives and surrounds of ultrasonographic images are underway. The ability to carry such statistical analysis on the RF data instead of a photograph will result in more precise characterization of different tumor types.

ACKNOWLEDGEMENTS

This work was supported by a grant from the National Eye Institute.

REFERENCES

Conners, R.W. & Harlow, C.A. A Theoretical Comparison of Texture Algorithms, IEEE Trans. on Pattern Analysis, PAM1-2 (1980) p. 204.

Faugeras, O.D. & Pratt, W.K. Decorrelation Methods of Texture Feature Extraction, IEEE Trans. on Pattern Analysis, PAM1-2 (1980) p. 323.

Julesz, B. Experiments in the Visual Perception of Texture, Sci. Am. 232: 34 (1975).

Rose, J.L., Cood, M.S. & Goldberg, B.B. Ultrasonic R-F Waveform Pattern Recognition Analysis of 60 Pathologically Proven Solid Breast Masses, 5th Int. Symp. Untrasonic Imaging & Tissue Characterization, Gaithersburg, Md: Natl. Bureau Stds. (1980) p. 28.

Weszka, J.W. et al. A Comparative Study of Texture Measures for Terrain Classification, IEEE Trans. on Systems, SMC-6 (1976) p. 269.

Author's Address:
Ultrasound Research Laboratory
Albert Einstein College of Medicine
Yeshira University, Dept. of Ophthalmology
Bronx, N.Y.
U.S.A.

IMAGE FREEZING AND GREY SCALE IN OPHTHALMIC ECHOGRAPHY

J. POUJOL, M. MASSIN & N. TOUFIC

(Paris, France)

Since 1979, we have been testing a new echograph for ophthalmology (Triscan E03, Biophysic Medical) with a digital memory (Fig. 1). This device has been used for a long time on instruments for general echography and at last is accessible to ophthalmologists in a commercially available unit. The freeze-frame allowed by the memory can be used in D-mode (isometric display), A-mode and in B-mode where the grey scale of 16 levels is invaluable.

The advantages are numerous. During a dynamic examination, as B-mode allows, it is easy to select cross-sections to be frozen and examined at leisure, without the inconvenience of a continuously moving picture. The grey scale allows the quantitative evaluation of the cross-section, especially in logarithmic amplification. The memory also gives the possibility of analysing all the A-scans of the whole cross-section, whether the latter be in ordinary B-mode or in D-mode (Fig. 2 & 3).

The image freezing also allows the operator to photograph only the most characteristic cross-sections after checking their value and to take several identical photographs if required. It is also possible to use low sensitivity films (Polaroid or other) which reproduce the variations in shades of grey more faithfully than the faster films required for real time. In isometric presentation the advantages of image freezing are the same.

The advantages in A-mode are similar. One of the characteristics of the instrument is that one has the choice between using linear amplification, special (S) amplification and logarithmic amplification. The choice of picture, and especially the time to examine it, are improved and this gives the possibility of a better quantitative evaluation, made over several echograms, without the need to take photographs. The direct reading of amplitudes in logarithmic amplification is of interest here. As in B-mode, the best picture can be chosen for photography thus economising on film. In echometry, even without using the digital values available with the unit, successive measurements can be made leisurely.

The advantages of image freezing and grey scale in ophthalmic echography can, in our opinion, be summarised as follows: speed and precision in the choice of echograms and their interpretation, economy in their recording.

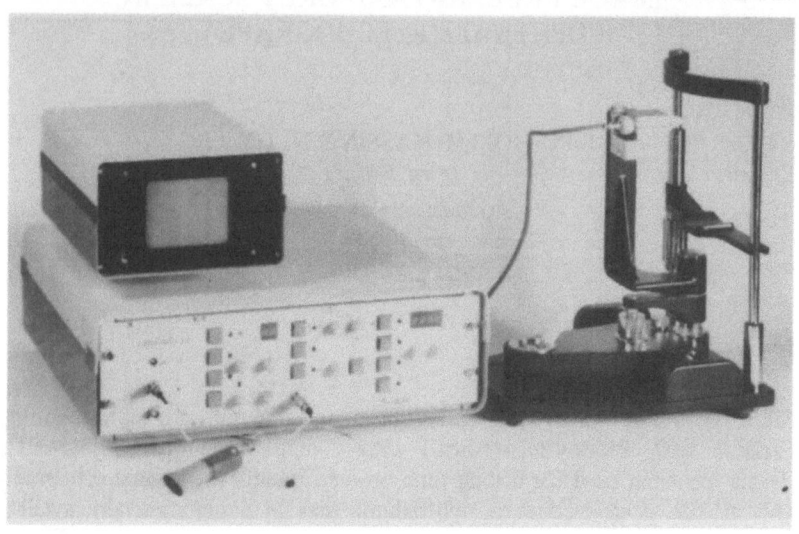

Fig. 1. Biophysic Medical Triscan (E03), with biometry device.

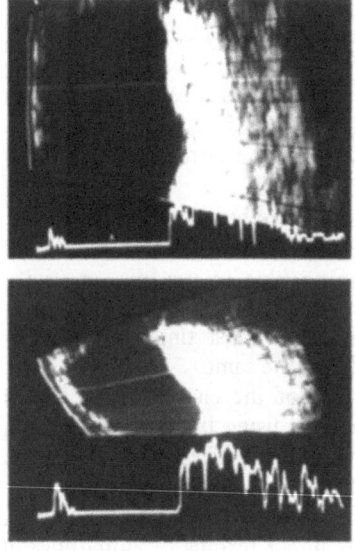

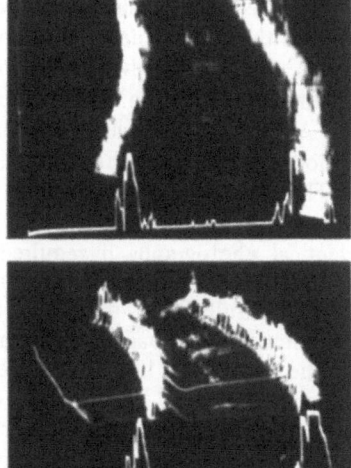

Fig. 2. Choroidal angioma.
Top, B-mode; Bottom, D-mode.

Fig. 3. Orbital hydatic cyst.
B- and D-mode imaging.

Authors' Address:
Centre National d'Ophtalmologie des Quinze-Vingts
Paris
France

506

A NEW CONTACT B-SCAN ULTRASONIC APPARATUS FOR THE OPHTHALMOLOGICAL DIAGNOSIS

A. KANEKO

(*Tokyo, Japan*)

SUMMARY

A new contact B-scan ultrasonic apparatus was developed for the ophthalmo-logical diagnosis. This apparatus can visualize the anterior part of the eye without the use of a waterbath. An improvement was made in the housing of transducer which was mechanically moved in sector from 30° to 90° within paraffin oil. The speed of scanning was adjustable from 1 to 30 cycles/s. This housing head makes contact with the lid through a thin plastic film which has 3.5 cm distance from the transducer. It is made of PZT and has 5 MHz focused crystal of 13 mm diameter. A gray scale and real time image is displayed on CRT. The greatest advantage was gained in diagnosis of leucocoria without general anesthesia. High speed mechanical scanning shortened the time for routine ultrasonic examination. Real time display increased information about mobility of the pathology using dynamic study.

INTRODUCTION

Bronson developed a simple B-scan ultrasonoscope in 1972. This apparatus was one of the revolutionary works in the history of the ultrasonic diagnosis concerning ophthalmology, as B-scan ultrasonography was made possible without the use of a water bath. However, the anterior part of the eye could not be visualized with this apparatus without a water bath. And the images of this ultrasonoscope were relatively poor in resolution and gray scale.

This paper introduces a new contact B-scan apparatus which visualizes the anterior segment of the eye beautifully using no water bath.

METHODS

A 5 MHz focused transducer of 13 mm diameter was put in a container filled with paraffin oil. It was sealed at a depth of 3.5 cm with soft plastic film which neither irritated nor scratched the eyelid. The scanning was mechanical sector whose angle was adjustable from 30° to 90°. The scanning speed could

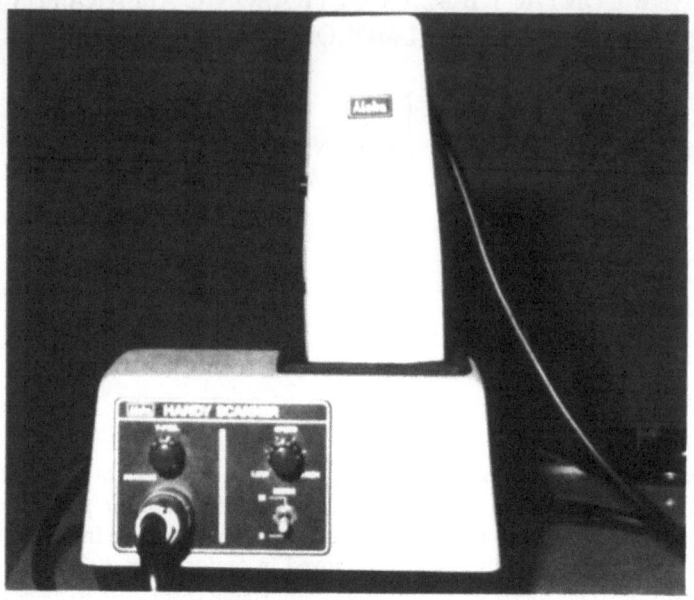

Fig. 1. The scanner and its stand.

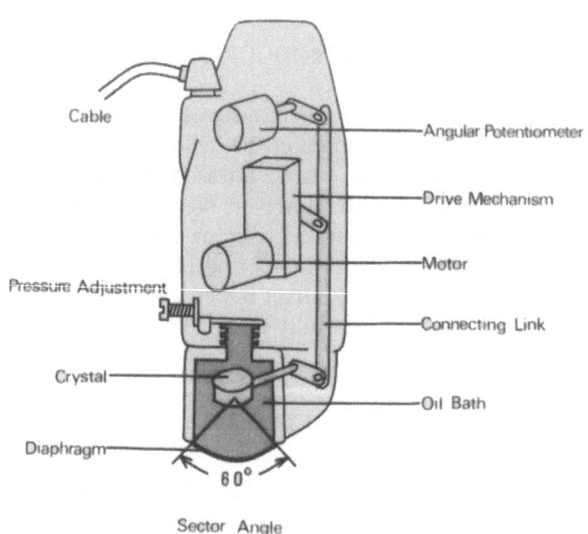

Cable

Angular Potentiometer

Drive Mechanism

Motor

Pressure Adjustment

Connecting Link

Crystal

Oil Bath

Diaphragm

60°

Sector Angle

Fig. 2. The construction of the scanner.

508

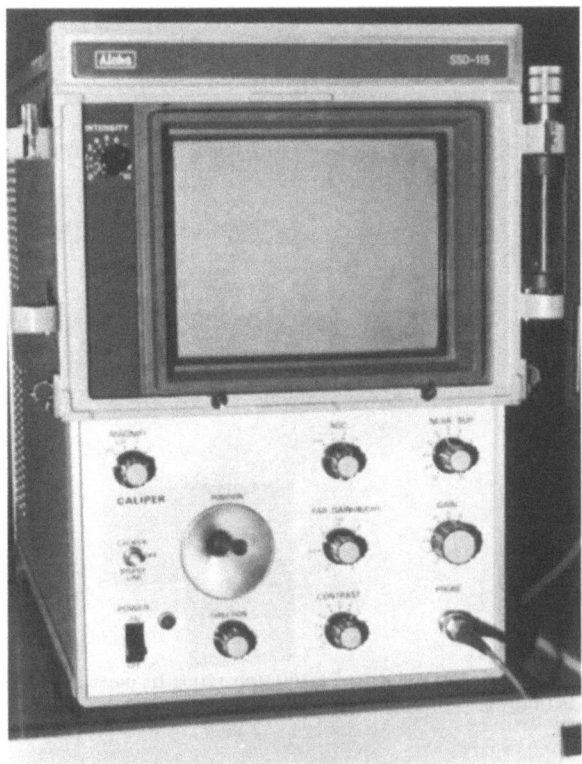

Fig. 3. The cathode ray tube for display with its panel and dials.

be adjusted as high as 30 cycles/s. Ultrasonic images were displayed on a cathode ray tube (CRT) and could be photographied with a Polaroid camera. When the Ultrasonic Image Recorder (Aloka Co. Ltd.) was available, a monochromatic television camera was attached in front of the CRT. A special high quality CRT was used for photography. A large monitor television was used for observation. A videotape recorder could record any real time images during the examination.

During the examination the patients lay on the bed in supine position. If infants were not cooperative for the examination, a nurse restrained them of movements using a bath towel with her arms and hands.

For maximum ultrasonic penetration and accuracy, Scopisol or a similar viscous solution should be used on the eyelid to eliminate the air between the lid and the plastic film of the scanner. It is then possible to manipulate the scanner for optimum diagnostic images on the monitor. Gain and automatic gain control were adjusted to visualize the most suitable images for diagnosis.

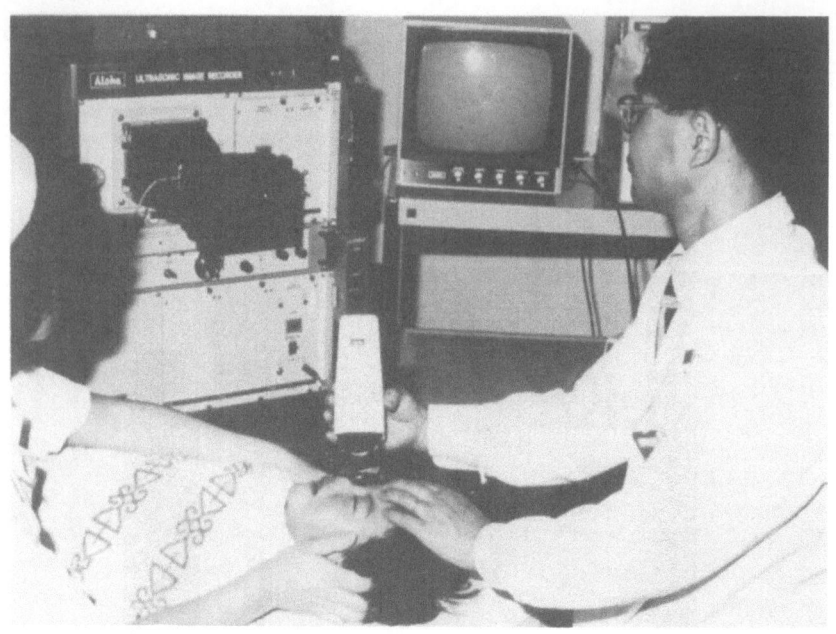

Fig. 4. An infant is being examined with this apparatus. Its movement is restrained by a nurse with a bath towel.

RESULTS

(1) *Normal eye*

The anterior chamber and the lens were distinctly visualized with the sono-lucent vitreous space and the retrobulbar tissue. The movement of the lens and the optic nerve were revealed with that of the eyeball.

(2) *Retinoblastoma*

The solid mass consists of extremely bright spots accompanied by a defect of the retrobulbar tissue directly behind it, because of extensive attenuation of the ultrasound by retinoblastoma. This finding was the same as that of a manual compound scanner reported by the author in 1978.

Although patients were less than two years old, typical findings of retino-blastoma were definitely disclosed without using any anesthesia. It took only 5 min to find the necessary information for the diagnosis because of high speed mechanical scanning.

(3) *Malignant melanoma of the choroid*

A large well circumscribed mass protruded into the vitreous space. It pushed out a part of the posterior capsule of the lens. No spontaneous movements

510

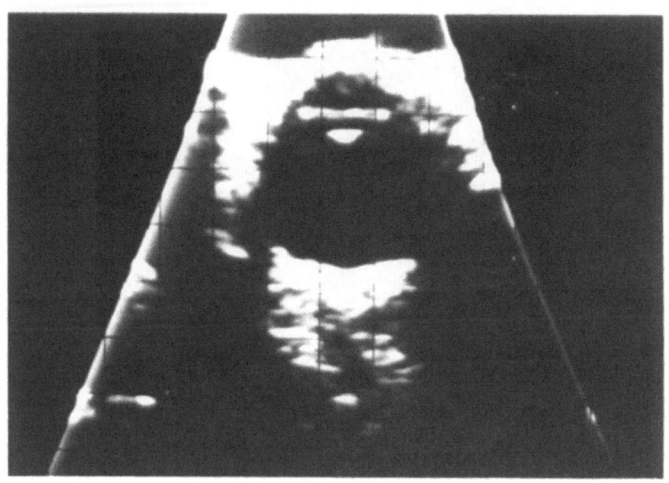

Fig. 5. Ultrasonogram of a normal eye of an infant.

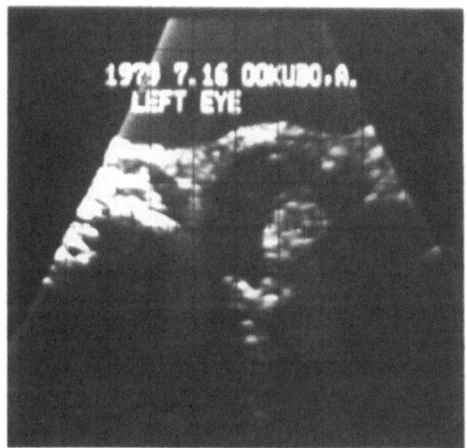

Fig. 6. Ultrasonogram of retinoblastoma.

were visible within the tumor, when the ocular movement was restrained. Retinal detachment was found.

(4) Metallic foreign body on the retina

In this case, a foreign body had been in the eye for 18 years. It caused a traumatic cataract which obstructed direct visualization of the fundus. The X-ray film of the orbit indicated a piece of small foreign body in the orbit. However its relation to the eyeball could not be determined with X-ray examination. The ultrasonic tomography disclosed a small foreign body on

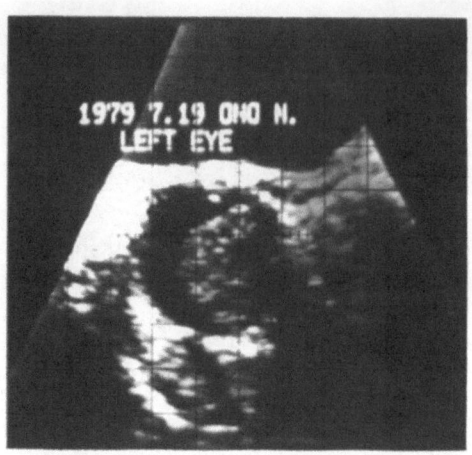

Fig. 7. Ultrasonogram of malignant melanoma of the choroid

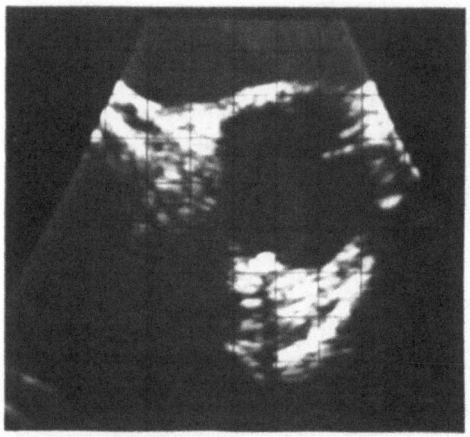

Fig. 8. Ultrasonogram of a metallic foreign body of the retina.

the wall of the eyeball which produced a marked attenuation in the tissue image behind it. The dynamic study revealed that this foreign body was embedded firmly in the retina.

DISCUSSION

B-scan echography is more understandable and reliable than A-scan echography. However, the need for a water bath has made performing ultrasonic tomography of the entire eye a time-consuming process. Infants in particular must be hospitalized and put under general anesthesia. This new contact

B-scan apparatus overcomes these difficulties by means of a built-in water bath and scanner combination.

When the ultrasonic images of this apparatus were compared to those of manual compound scanning combined with a scanconverter, spots of the image of the former method were larger and coarser than the latter. But high speed mechanical scanning enabled the former quickly and easily to detect and visualize the most suitable shape of the pathology for diagnosis. The result of dynamic studies could be recognized reliably only through the real time display of this apparatus. This is a safe, painless, noninvasive and versatile tomographic device that can be used repeatedly. With these advantages, it can improve the prospects of ophthalmic diagnosis and treatment.

ACKNOWLEDGEMENT

I should like to thank the staff of Aloka Co. Ltd. for engineering assistance to develop this new ultrasonic apparatus. This work was supported in part by Grant-in-Aid for Cancer research from the Ministry of Health and Welfare of Japan.

REFERENCES

Bronson, N.R. Development of a simple B-scan ultrasonoscope, Trans. Am. Ophthalmol. Soc. 70: 365 (1972).

Kaneko, A. Diagnosis of leukokoria with ultrasonography and computerized tomography, Proc. 11th Hellenic Ophthalmol. Cong. (1978) p. 239.

Author's Address:
Dept. of Ophthalmology,
National Cancer Center Hospital, 5-1-1, Tsukiji,
Chuwo-ku, Tokyo
Japan 104

FUNCTIONAL REALIZATION OF A SAB-SCANNER

J.M. THIJSSEN

(Nijmegen, The Netherlands)

INTRODUCTION

The SAB (simultaneous A- and B-) scanner was discussed for the first time at the Meeting of the World Federation in San Francisco (Thijssen, *et al.* 1977). We then described many design criteria that seemed clinically or technically important. Here we describe a working model (zero order prototype) that contains many new and valuable features. Recent developments in electronics have been incorporated through which the clinical potentials can be essentially improved. Many graduate and postgraduate students have been working for some time on this project. In the last phase the cooperation of a Dutch firm was formally established. Its employees aided us by decreasing the disadvantages of the working scheme induced by our grant system. We conclude, that the present state of the apparatus is the completion of our developments.

SYSTEM CONCEPT

A block diagram of the system is shown in Fig. 1. The heart of it is the TV-generator which contains a master clock and all other timing is based on it. The motor which rotates a mirror yielding 50 B-mode images/s is slaved by the master oscillator by means of a phase locked loop (P.L.L.) circuit. The transmitter is triggered once every 0.25 msec which corresponds to a 4000 Hz rate necessary for 40 system lines in half a TV-frame.

After transmitting and receiving via the transducer a broadband receiver amplifies the signals and then a threefold parallel processing occurs. The RF processing consists of a buffer amplifier (lx) with a low impedance output. The B-mode signal is logarithmically compressed and filtered by a 4.25 MHz low pass filter (12 dB/octave) after full-wave rectification. The A-mode signal is compressed by a sigmoid gain amplifier and after rectification filtered by a 1 MHz low pass filter (12 dB/octave). The selection of the A-mode trace to be displayed can be made manually and the trace is indicated by a video inversion of the TV-line. If the separate A-mode transducer is being used the motor drive is switched off, and the A-mode triggering is made once every 20 msec, which yields a very low repetition rate (50 Hz) as compared

© *1981. Dr W. Junk Publishers, The Hague*

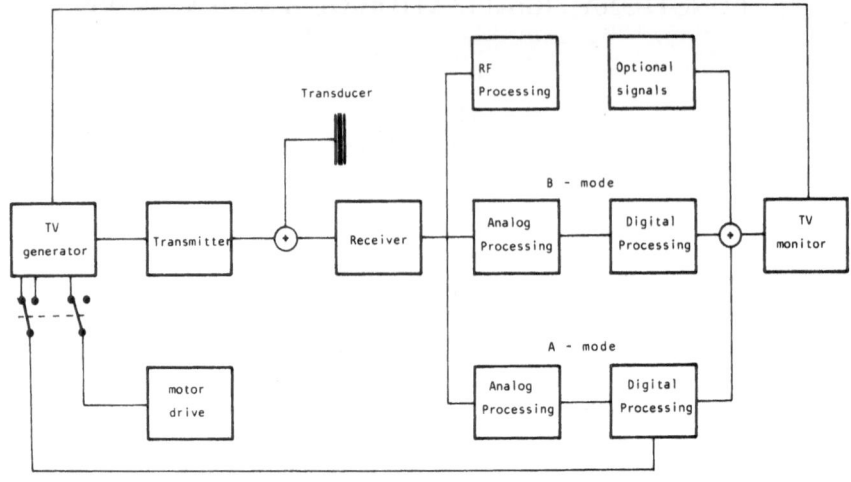

Fig. 1. Block diagram of the SAB-scanner. The master timing circuitry is contained in the TV-generator. The motor is synchronized to it by means of a phase locked loop circuit. Three parallel analog processing routes are present and subsequent digital processing is performed on the A-mode and B-mode signals. Optional signals like the gray level staircase, the microseconds ruler and alpha-numeric symbols are generated and mixed with the A- and B-mode.

to conventional echographic equipment (greater than 500 Hz). The digital processing of the B-mode consists of analog to digital conversion (10 MHz), digital interpolation between consequentive TV-lines and digital to analogue conversion. The A-mode signal is also converted to a digital signal and via a special 'repeating and comparating' circuit it becomes possible to generate an echographic display in A-mode on the TV monitor. Optional signals like ruler, gray wedge etc. are generated and either before, or after digital to analogue conversion they are added to the TV-video signal.

Further details are:

The freeze facility of the complete TV-picture comprises gray wedge, B-mode, µs ruler and text. The biometry can be performed *after* freezing the A-mode echogram with automatic read out on the TV-screen.

Comparison with the original design criteria reveals the following improvements: The A-mode and B-mode displays are integrated with other display facilities in a single TV-frame. Displays of a µs ruler and of alpha-numeric data are added. The latter data may be entered via a keyboard. The axial and the lateral resolution have been improved by almost a factor 2. The number of gray levels has been extended from 8 to 16. The TV-frame rate was increased from 25 Hz to a standard value of 50 Hz. The freeze frame display mode has been added which incorporates the valuable possibility of performing biometrical measurements from the screen and getting an automatic read-out below the A-mode echogram.

Table 1. Technical Specifications.

1. The handpiece		2. The transducer (see Fig. 2)	
Size	150 mm	Center frequency	8 MHz
Diameter	40 mm	Bandwidth	4.25 MHz
Weight	300 gram	Pulse duration	0.25 µs
		Focus at	20 mm
3. The B-scan		Focal diameter (− 6 dB)	1.5 mm
		Focal length	20 mm
Scan mode	linear		
Frame rate	50 Hz	**4. The A-scan**	
Scan width	20 mm		
Scan depth	37 mm	Compression	S-shaped
Shift of depth	10 mm	Bandwidth	1.0 MHz
Compression	logarithmic	Ruler	µs
Video bandwidth	4.25 MHz	Biometry	automatic
			read out µs, mm
Gray levels	16	Keyboard	complete
			Alpha-numeric
Gray wedge	digitally	Separate A-probe	50 Hz trans-
	generated		mission rate

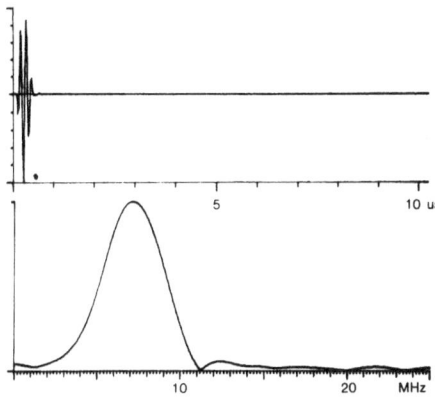

Fig. 2. The radiofrequency echo from a metal plate (upper trace), approximately 8 MHz, and the corresponding amplitude spectrum.

THE FACILITIES OF THE SAB-SCANNER

The display at the screen of the TV monitor is shown in Fig. 3. The gray level staircase can be used to optimally adjust the contrast and intensity levels of the monitor. This facility highly increases the reproducability of the B-mode documentation. The handpiece of the scanner is closed by a milar ® window, so that the B-mode picture begins when this window coincides with the conjunctiva or cornea. The starting point can be shifted by manual control over a 10 mm distance, if for instance deep orbital structures are examined.

The selection of an A-mode trace is made by turning a ten position control switch. The selected TV-line is indicated by video-inversion and is therewith

517

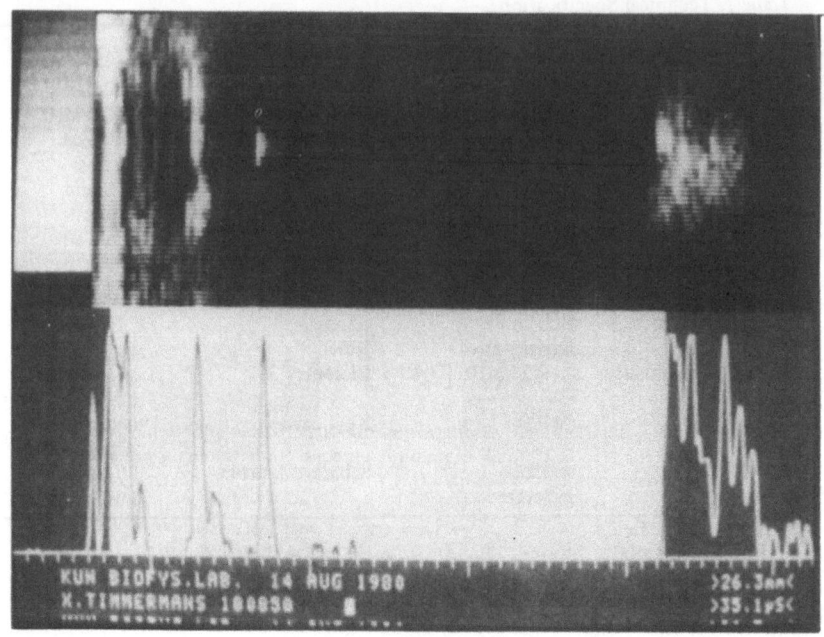

Fig. 3. The SAB-scan picture of a normal eye, polaroid photograph of TV-screen. The white area of the A-mode part is manually controlled and it indicates the region to be measured. The length of it is indicated in microseconds and millimeters in the bottom left characters.

clearly visible. The A-mode echogram is completed with μs ruler with a 0.1 μs accuracy. The biometry facility is illustrated by the black to white and v.v inversion of a part of the A-mode display. This part is manually selected by turning two control knobs either during the scanning, or, which is more attractive, after freezing the complete picture in a digital memory. The most accurate time/distance measurement is obtained by taking the time between the peak values of two echoes. This time is displayed automatically in the bottom left part of the picture, together with the distance in mm (velocity 1550 m/s). Other data can be stored and displayed after typing on the keyboard. Two lines are available and we are developing a device to display some fixed text with intermediate spaces for patient identification data.

Documentation of a complete examination can be made on normal video tape or cassette recorder. Additionally, a small slave monitor is built into the equipment (Fig. 4) and a Polaroid camera is fixed to it. We anticipate that the opportunity of freezing the TV-image during the examination may considerably reduce the need to make photographs, and that the video tape recording may be of value for documentation and educative purposes.

518

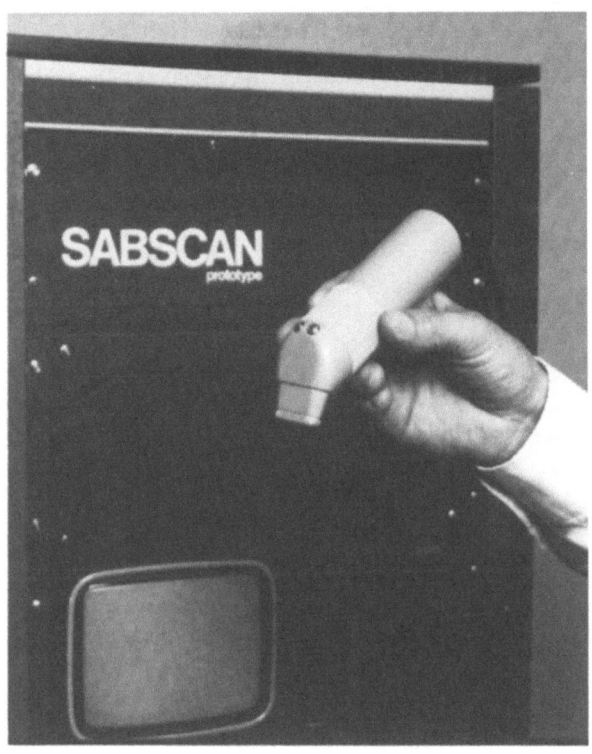

Fig. 4. The front panel of the SAB-scanner with scanner head. The polaroid camera is facing a slave TV-monitor.

ACKNOWLEDGEMENT

This work has been supported by the Health Organization, TNO and Oldelft Inc. The contributions of C. Verhagen, R. Kruizinga, J. van der Wiel, J. van Dullemen, S. Mientky, and X. Timmermans are to be considered of essential importance for the system developments.

REFERENCES

Thijssen, J.M., Kruizinga, R., Verhagen, C., & Koomen, G.J. Design criteria for an ophthalmological B-scan system: simultaneous A- and B-mode equipment (SAB-scan). In: Ultrasound in Medicine, Vol. 3A (D. White & R.E. Brown, eds.) New York: Plenum Press (1977) p. 901.

519

Thijssen, J.M., Kruizinga, R., & Wiel, J.M. van der. A manual scanner for simultaneous A- and B-mode echo-ophthalmography (SAB-scan) In: Diagnostica Ultrasonica in Ophthalmologica (H. Gernet, ed.) Münster: Remy Verlag (1979) p. 5.

Author's Address:
Biophysics Laboratory of the Institute of Ophthalmology
University of Nijmegen
6500 HB Nijmegen
The Netherlands

520

DIGITALIZED ECHO OCULOMETRY

G.W.R.B. VAN MARLE & P.A.M. GOMMERS

(Rotterdam, The Netherlands)

SUMMARY

An ultrasound echograph was expanded with three electronic counters to measure the time intervals between the echoes of cornea and retina, cornea and anterior lens surface, and between both lens surfaces. The thickness of a cataractous lens, often causing multiple echos, can be measured too. The echogram is photographed together with marks indicating which time intervals are measured, furthermore with the numerical values which are obtained. The equipment has already been applied for more than two years, making oculometry more convenient and reliable.

INTRODUCTION

Echooculometry, carried out by means of an A-scan ultrasonograph, is a well-known technique. To prevent deformation of the cornea during the examination, it is preferable to apply the transducer according to the method described by Gernet (1967) as indicated in Fig. 1. Usually, distances between the intraocular structures are measured from a photograph taken from the screen of the echograph.

This procedure is rather inaccurate, furthermore time-consuming and inconvenient for the examiner. An improvement in this aspect was obtained by Coleman (1967) and van der Heijde (1977), using an electronic counter to measure the time difference between two echoes. Though an improvement, their methods have some disadvantages. One disadvantage is that it is only possible to measure one time interval per measurement, while factually three intraocular distances are necessary for calculating the power of an implant lens. These three distances are the depth of the anterior chamber, the thickness of the lens and the axial length of the eye (van der Heijde 1976, Oguchi 1976, Thijssen 1975). The other disadvantage is, that the examiner has to make sure during the measurement that the correct time interval is measured. This is especially obligatory in case phantom echos are present.

To eliminate these disadvantages we have built an instrument with the following features:

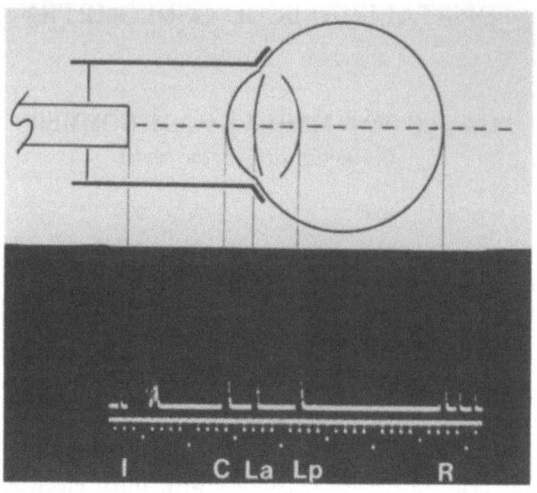

Fig. 1. The fundamental method of measurement.

(1) The three time intervals are measured at the same time by using three counters.
(2) The three intervals are indicated by marks to the echogram.
(3) Both, the marks and the echogram, are documented together with the numerical values of the intervals.

DESCRIPTION OF THE INSTRUMENT

The counters are controlled by the echosignals and by the shutter of the camera. The echosignals are detected and filtered by the echograph itself (see Fig. 2). The echograph we used is a composition of a plug-in module from Sperry Corporation type 10 sdb, together with two Philips oscilloscopes. One scope serves for the registration, the other one is used as a monitor. The transducer is a 10 Mhz type from Kretztechnik.

To reduce the lag in time, caused by the slope of the echosignals, and to separate partly fused echos, the echosignals are firstly differentiated before they are fed to a level comparator. The output of the level comparator determines the time interval according to the leading slope of the echosignals.

A problem occurs in case phantom or artefact echos are present. To solve this problem, two adjustable time delays indicated as t_1 and t_4 in Fig. 3, are introduced. The first echo after t_1 and t_4 is interpreted as to be reflected by the cornea and the retina respectively.

Another problem is met when a cataractous lens is present. Due to the inhomogeneous structure inside such a lens, echos may be expected between the two echos from both lens surfaces. This of course, will hamper the count out of the correct time interval. To circumvent this difficulty, latches (a kind

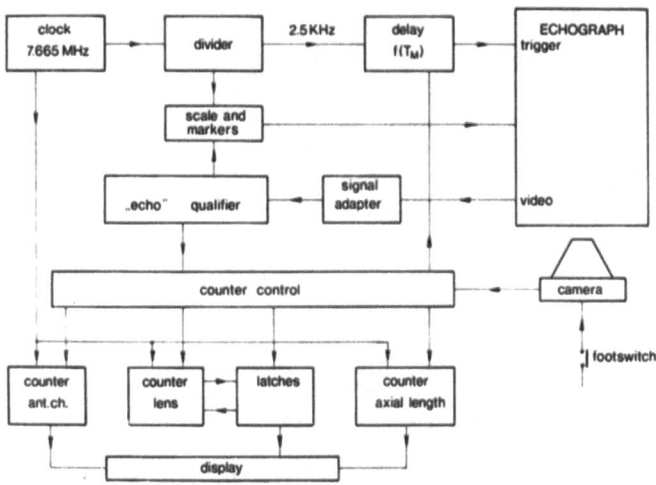

Fig. 2. Block diagram of the instrument.

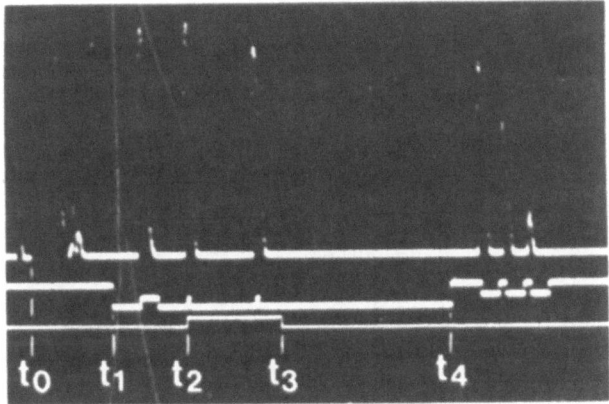

Fig. 3. The time gates to qualify the echosignals.

of memory) are added to the counter (see Fig. 2). Furthermore, a time gate (t_2-t_3 in Fig. 3) is introduced. Within this time gate the last echo is identified as to be from the posterior lens surface. The echo from the anterior lens surface, the second one after t_1, initiates the time gate and starts also the counter. Each echo, which successively arrives, transfers the counter state to the latches. The final value belonging to the last echo is left in the latches. The gate limits the value for the lens thickness to 6.5 mm.

To represent the counted values in mm a clock frequency of 7.665 Mhz is used. This frequency is based on a sound velocity of 1533 m/sec. Since the sound velocity in the crystalline lens is 7% higher, the actual value of the lens thickness and that of the axial length are obtained by adding 7% of the displayed value of the lens.

The resolution of a time measurement with a frequency of 7.665 Mhz equals 130 nsec, which corresponds with 0.1 mm intraocular distance. As this value seems rather inaccurate, the resolution was increased by summing ten successive time intervals. If the ten time intervals are random with respect to the clock, the resolution is improved by $\sqrt{10}$. If, however, they are shifted over 10% of the clock period with respect to the clock, the improvement is ten times. This corresponds in our case with 0.01 mm. This method is realized by delaying 9 of the 10 transmitted sound pulses 10% of the clock period each time again (the delay is $f(T_m)$ in Fig. 2). The fixed relation to the clock is obtaind by triggering the transmitted soundpulse by the clock via a divider. The effect is depicted in Fig. 4. The time interval to be counted is indicated by t_1 and t_2. By shifting the clock each time again, k intervals contain $n + 1$ clockpulses. The remaining ones $(10 - k)$ enclose n pulses. The number of times that $n + 1$ pulses are counted, is proportional to the time fraction Δt. As a result, the final count D impresses as if reached with a ten times higher clock rate. Finally, Fig. 5 represents the timing of the oculometry with the instrument. After pressing the footswitch the whole procedure is finished after 45 msec.

RESULTS

Fig. 6 shows the actual results of an examination of a normal eye (A), an eye with a cataract (B), and of an eye with an implant lens (C). It is clearly seen how the echogram is interpreted by the instrument. With the

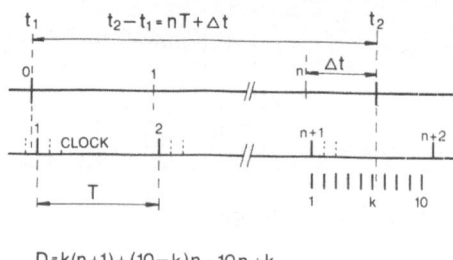

$$D = k(n+1) + (10-k)n = 10n + k$$

Fig. 4. Shifting of the time intervals to improve resolution.

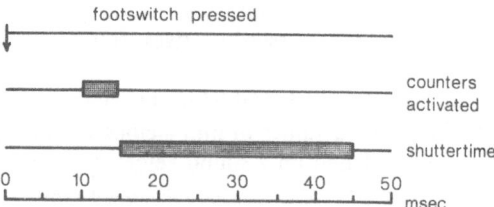

Fig. 5. Time diagram of the measurement.

524

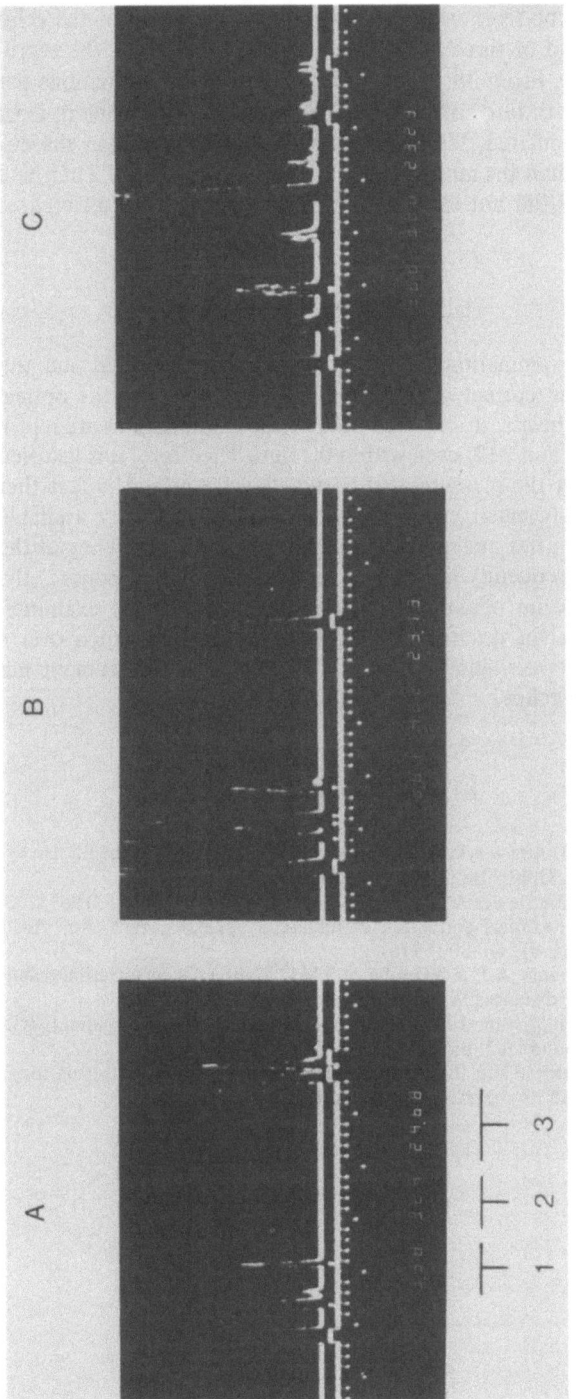

Fig. 6. Results as they are obtained with the instrument.

   A = normal eye.

   B = eye with a cataractous lens.

   C = pseudophakic eye.

   1 = depth of the anterior chamber, indicated by the first broad and the first small mark.

   2 = thickness of the lens, indicated by the first and the last small mark.

   3 = axial length, indicated by the first and the second broad mark.

pseudophakic eye the value for the lens thickness is incorrect due to a phantom echo, as can be seen on the photograph. The method of the echo oculometry requires two or three measurements per eye to check the reproducibility of the result. From 38 patients (75 eyes), three examinations per eye were carried out with our instrument. The maximum difference in axial length per eye was calculated. We found that for 90% of the eyes the differences were smaller than 0.4 mm, for 63% it was smaller than 0.2 mm and for 31% the differences did not exceed 0.1 mm. The mean of the differences was 0.22 mm.

DISCUSSION

The accuracy of the examination depends on the echograph used and the possibility to assure the correct alignment of the transducer to the optical axis of the eye. Nevertheless, in our case 63% of the examinations are reproducible within 0.2 mm and 31% even within 0.1 mm. Therefore, it is justified to have a resolution of the measurement better than 0.1 mm. The fact that the numerical values are electronically measured and are directly available during the examination, has increased the reliability and the efficiency of the echo oculometry, consequently its clinical applicability. Furthermore, the instrument has made echo oculometry more convenient for the examiner. The instrument is now in use for more than two years in which over a thousand patients were examined. Only in a few cases the instrument has failed, due to phantom echos.

REFERENCES

Coleman, D.J. & Carlin, B. A new system for visual axis measurements in the human eye using ultrasound. Arch. Ophthalmol. 77: 124 (1967).
Gernet, H. Ultraschall-Biometrie des Auges. Klin. Mbl. Augenheilk. 151: 853 (1967).
Heijde, G.L. van der. The optical correction of unilateral aphakia. Trans. Am. Acad. Ophthalmol. Otolarying. 81: OP-80 (1976).
Heijde, G.L. van der, Meinema, A.J. & Vlaming, M.S.M.G. Digital A-scan ultrasonography used to measure ocular distances. Am. J. Ophthalmol. 83: 276 (1977).
Oguchi, Y. & Balen, A.Th.M. van. Ultrasonic study of the refraction of patients with pseudophakos. Ultrasound Med. Biol. 1: 267 (1974).
Thijssen, J.M. The emmetropic and the iseikonic implant lens: Computer calculation of the refractive power and its accuracy. Ophthalmologica 171: 467 (1975).

Authors' Address:
Eye Dept.
Eye Hospital
Erasmus University
Rotterdam
The Netherlands

ELECTRONIC TISSUE MODEL (E.T.M.)

J.M. THIJSSEN & S.H.J. VAN KERVEL

(Nijmegen, The Netherlands)

INTRODUCTION

In our clinical and experimental work in echo-ophthalmography we felt the need to have access to the gain characteristic curve of the overall A-mode video system. More specifically, we wanted to decompress the A-mode echogram obtained from our equipment (Kretztechnik 7200 MA), after storage in a digital computer and prior to subsequent quantitative analysis (cf. Thijssen *et al.* 1979, 1980). It also seemed worthwhile to construct a device enabling quick and easy access to the gain characteristic curve for routine check-ups of the equipment. For the latter purpose it should be possible to use a simple gadget like a plexiglass mask to perform the check. Because of the similarity to a solid material 'tissue model' (Till 1976) as regards the latter use of our apparatus we have adopted this name in the title. In this paper the developed apparatus will be shortly outlined and some applications will be discussed. A more extensive description has been presented elsewhere (Kervel & Thijssen 1980).

SYSTEM DESCRIPTION

The dotted part of the block diagram of Fig. 1 contains the electronic system. It will be clear, that the ETM is synchronized to the A-mode apparatus by a trigger signal. This trigger starts a variable delay signal so that it becomes possible to shift the output of the ETM in order to obtain the optimum display positioning at the A-mode oscilloscope. After the delay an exponential decay signal is generated which has a time constant of $14.4\,\mu s$, or correspondingly, an attenuation of $6\,dB/10\,\mu s$. The decay signal is multiplied by a radio frequency (8 MHz) sine wave to produce an exponentially decreasing sine wave voltage. The output signal of the ETM is sketched in Fig. 2. The voltage drop over $100\,\mu s$ is from $100\,mVpp$ to $100\,\mu Vpp$. The actual voltage is displayed on top of Fig. 3 together with the resulting gain characteristic curve that shows up on the screen of our A-mode apparatus. The square wave voltage on the bottom is a 50 kHz calibration trace simultaneously present at the screen.

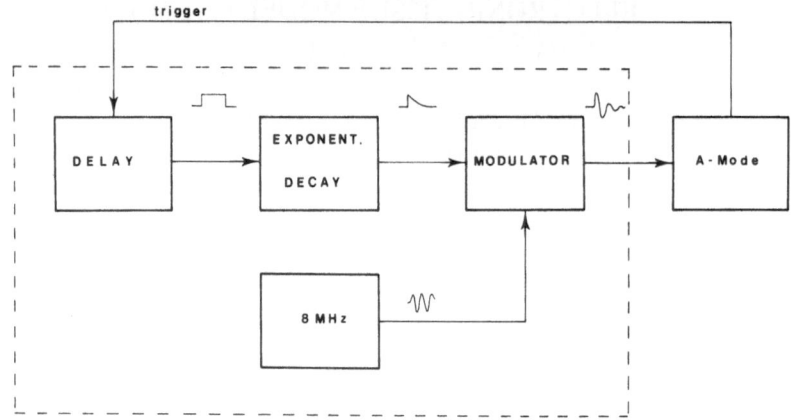

Fig. 1. Block diagram of ETM within dashed lines. For description see text.

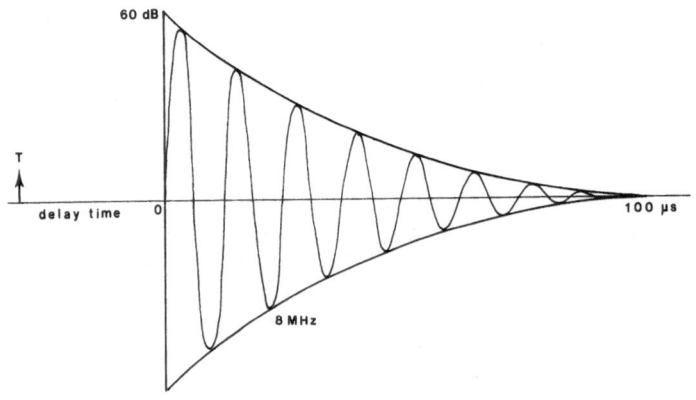

Fig. 2. Time diagram of output signal from ETM.

APPLICATIONS

One application is obvious straight away from Fig. 3. If a standard curve is available on a plexiglass mask the quality of the A-mode equipment can be easily checked at regular intervals. A second characteristic that is available for calibration is the overall amplification of the electronics. This procedure can be performed only if the delay setting of the ETM has been fixed.

If any change has occured in the amplification this will show up in the horizontal position of the gain curve, or alternatively if a mask, as described above, is used the reading of the sensitivity control producing coincidence is indicative.

A further application of the ETM is demonstrated Fig. 4. Here we have decreased the sensitivity of the equipment in 6 dB steps, as read from the

528

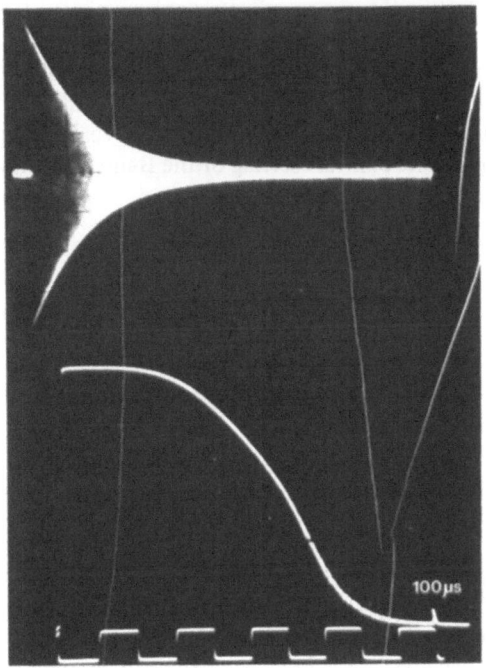

Fig. 3. Top: Oscilloscope picture of output signal of ETM.
Bottom: Sigmoid amplifier gain characteristic curve at screen of A-mode oscilloscope (Kretztechnik 7200 MA).
Square wave: 80 kHz (20 μs period).

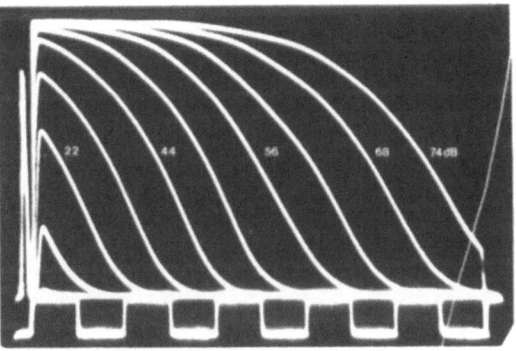

Fig. 4. Amplifier gain curves at 6 dB differing amplification levels.

sensitivity control. Two effects become visible here: the horizontal distances are not equal, i.e. the logarithmic potentiometer used in the equipment is not accurate, and furthermore the slope of the curves changes systematically i.e. the gain characteristic curve is voltage dependent. The latter properties of the echographic equipment stress the need to work with standard settings (threshold, amplification, low-pass filtering) after calibration has been performed. Other applications of the ETM can be found in the calibration of single transducer B-scanners, such as the gray scale setting, the time-gain-compensation and the contrast setting of the B-mode display.

ACKNOWLEDGEMENT

This work was supported by the Health Organization, T.N.O.

REFERENCES

Kervel, S.J.H. van & Thijssen, J.M. A device for the display and adjustment of the non-linear gain curve of ultrasonic A-mode equipment. Ultrasonics 19: 40 (1980).

Thijssen, J.M., Kruizinga, R., Dooren, H.A.F.Q. van & Verbeek, A.M. Computer assisted echographic analysis: In: Diagnostica Ultrasonica in Ophthalmologia. (H. Gernet, ed.) Münster: Remy Verlag (1979) p. 12.

Thijssen, J.M., Bayer, A.L. & Verbeek, A.M. Computer support for ultrasonic diagnosis. Doc. Ophthalmol. 48: 315 (1979).

Thijssen, J.M., Bayer, A.L. & Cloostermans, M. Computer assisted echography: statistical analysis of A-mode video echograms obtained by tissue sampling. In Press: Med. Biol. Engng & Comp.

Till, P. Solid tissue model for the standarization of the echo-ophthalmograph 7200 MA (Kretztechnik). Doc. Ophthalmol. 46: 205 (1976).

Authors' Addresses:
J.M. Thijssen Ph.D.
Biophysics Laboratory of the Institute of Ophthalmology
University of Nijmegen
6500 HB Nijmegen
The Netherlands

Present Address S.H.J. van Kervel
Ultrason, Inc.
P.O. Box 485
Helmond
The Netherlands

ROUND TABLE DISCUSSION ON
TISSUE CHARACTERIZATION

CHAIRMAN: F. LIZZI
PANELISTS: H.G. TRIER, R.D. LEPPER, D. DECKER, J.M. THIJSSEN,
A.L. BAYER, F. LIZZI & S. CHANG

The Tissue Characterization Round Table was conducted as a series of brief presentations by each panel member followed by discussion periods. The Chairman, Dr. Lizzi, introduced the panel members and said that although tissue characterization could, in a certain sense, include A- and B-mode work, the panel would confine itself to newer methods and would discuss points of common interest in terms of general approaches and specific techniques.

Dr. Trier, the first speaker, addressed the topic of clinical conditions for which tissue characterization would be useful. He listed various conditions and corresponding means of obtaining clinically useful information including ultrasound and other diagnostic techniques. He stated that an evaluation of ultrasonography should be based on how well it, by itself, provides diagnostic security. He said that computer-aided A- and B-mode analysis and R.F. analysis would help differential diagnosis of intra-ocular tumors, while better C-mode techniques might help in differentiating vitreous membranes and detached retinas. He alluded to the combined use of ultrasound and magnetic devices to help find small foreign bodies. Improved biometric techniques could be of use in studying intraocular microstructure, choroidal pulsations and, in the orbit, extraocular muscle dimensions. He felt that orbital studies might benefit from vascular assessments using Doppler, TM, and duplex systems.

In the ensuing discussion, Dr. Chang alluded to the importance of human pattern recognition. Dr. Thijssen stated that many traces, not just one, must be evaluated for diagnosis. He said that pulsed Doppler techniques might be beneficial in orbital studies.

Dr. Lepper presented the second talk in which he treated the relation between physical tissue properties and measured ultrasonic signals. He said this relationship is complex. For example, the number of scatterers in a unit volume will influence the received ultrasonic intensity through coherent and incoherent scattering, with unknown fractions of the scatterers acting in each manner. He stated that ultrasonic signals have been studied in a variety of ways. Amplitude variations as functions of time and space are used in clinical instruments. Spectral information from gated tissue segments is affected by internal attenuation. Special features can be studied using deconvolution or correlation techniques. He stated that deconvolution has shortcomings because the impedances and velocities in the examined tissues are unknown. He suggested that it is most useful to store RF signals for subsequent analysis using time- and frequency-domain techniques.

In the discussion Dr. Lizzi agreed with the analytic difficulty in relating physical properties and scattered signals. He stated that internal attenuation in a gated area can sometimes be estimated and compensated for and that it could be kept sufficiently small by using small range gates. Dr. Lepper said that attenuation can vary and that small range gates would limit spectral resolution. Dr. Lizzi responded that there was always a trade-off between spatial and spectral resolution and that computer post-processing permits these parameters to be varied. He also said that deconvolution can be used profitably if correct reference signals were employed. Dr. Lepper said identification of the resolved elements was a problem, and Dr. Lizzi said it's better to present these elements for interpretation than not to.

Dr. Decker presented the third talk and discussed signal processing. He described how he uses a commercial system to find a region of interest; a hand-held transducer is employed with a medium focus and a frequency band from 5- to 22-MHz. Echo signals are digitized and quality control is used to reject unsatisfactory results due to lack of patient cooperation, etc. Average representative echograms are computed for different regions. Signal processing uses a variety of techniques including determination of statistical features such as means, standard deviations, skewness, correlations, etc. Cross-correlation is his preferred method for studying boundary surfaces. For examinations of retinal detachments, thickness is computed and its variation is studied as a function of position. For structures consisting of statistically distributed scatterer elements, (e.g. tumors), a 2-μsec window is used and results from different transducer positions are averaged. A number of features are studied including dominant spectral frequency, spacing between scattering elements, and the number of peaks in a unit distance.

Drs. Lizzi and Decker then discussed spectral techniques for measurement of thin layers. In response to Dr. Thijssen, Dr. Decker stated that scattering element spacing was defined on the basis of A-scan echo peaks.

Dr. Thijssen presented the fourth talk. He started by defining terms for those in the audience who were not familiar with the methods being discussed. He stated that envelope detection used in conventional instruments can suppress information contained in the R.F. waveform. He mentioned that data collection techniques are important; such factors as angle-of-incidence should be considered, and immersion scanners might place constraints on this factor. He stated that intervening tissue factors were also important and that it would be beneficial if one could use internal reference elements in the eye or orbit. He showed experimental data from an *in vitro* liver sample to examine the importance of several factors. He found that spectra can change with stand-off distance in a focused beam and said this must be accounted for. Tissue inhomogeneity is another important factor in such experiments.

In the discussion, Dr. Lizzi agreed with the need for transducer characterization. Dr. Lepper said readings should be taken near the focus where parallel wavefronts are present and said focusing introduces speckling phenomena. Dr. Lizzi said phase cancellation could constitute a problem with unfocused transducers and stated that speckling is a problem in imaging, not in spectrum analysis, and that it is worse for narrow bandwidths.

Dr. Chang posed the question of why tissue characterization stressed the use of focused, broad-band transducers when many clinicians used unfocused, narrow-band systems. Dr. Thijssen said these narrow-band systems might simplify pattern recognition, and Dr. Lepper said high-quality, broad-band amplifiers weren't available when those systems were configured.

Dr. Bayer presented the fifth talk; it dealt with measurements of thin membranes, beyond the resolution of normal systems. He studied inverse filtering approaches, or deconvolution, to compensate for system character-istics, to measure layer thickness and to specify the relative polarity of reflection coefficients. A disadvantage of this method is sensitivity to tilt of the studied membrane. He found spectral resonances were less sensitive to tilting and that scalloping could be used to extract membrane thickness. He showed *in vivo* results from a choroid with an attached pigment epithelium layer. Spectral scalloping suggested two layers; inverse filtering revealed a minor echo between choroid and the pigment epithelium. Corresponding computer simulations were also shown.

In the discussion Dr. Decker asked if cross-correlation techniques had been tried, and Dr. Bayer responded that he had encountered oscillatory corre-lations. Dr. Lizzi agreed that deconvolution should be sensitive to tilt since the reference signal is measured at normal incidence. He said spectral scalloping should be relatively insensitive to tilts which affect both membrane echoes in the same manner.

Dr. Lizzi was the sixth speaker. He showed results obtained with a com-puter system that digitizes R.F. echoes during clinical scans and presents computer generated B-scans that can be used subsequently to retrieve and analyze R.F. echoes from desired tissue regions. As an illustration of a deter-ministic structure, he showed measurements of the surface layer of an *in vitro* kidney sample which yielded spectral scalloping consistent with a membrane thinner than 100 microns. The normalized power spectrum was the same for a large range of chosen analysis sites on the kidney surface. He showed B-scan images where deconvolution was used to image the surfaces of a detached retina. He illustrated returns from a stochastic structure by showing scans of a case of asteroid hyalosis; a normalized power spectrum was computed for the entire volume, treated as an ensemble, and a Rayleigh spectrum was obtained. Probing the volume with inter-actively controlled brackets showed that small regions and line-segments produced spectra with statistical oscillations about the f^4 mean shape. He stated that tissue characterization requires entire tissue volumes to be probed for analysis in a systematic way.

Dr. Chang's presentation followed. He discussed clinical tumor studies that used the computer system described by Dr. Lizzi. He showed a computer-generated B-scan of a tumor obtained prior to surgery and compared it to the post-enucleation histology of the same tumor. Although boundaries were highly correlated, small internal features were not apparent in the B-scan. He then showed computer-generated band-pass images from two scan planes through a different, homogeneous malignant melanoma, showing that band-pass features were the same in both planes and consistent with a slight increase in reflectance at high frequencies. He contrasted this with a larger melanoma that had broken through Bruch's membrane. Here, three scan planes were studied, and high-amplitude, relatively flat spectra were found in the anterior segment of the tumor; he said these were consistent with relatively large scatterers (e.g., vascular 'lakes'). A scan plane through the tumor's base showed the slightly rising, low-amplitude spectra found in homogeneous regions of melanoma; such spectra are associated with melanocyte scattering.

In response to a question, Drs. Chang and Lizzi said that melanoma spectra were being studied by placing analysis gates in anterior segments and plotting scatter diagrams of spectral amplitude and slope as well as attenuation rates (computed from spectral changes with distances).

Dr. Lepper referred to noise evidenced in the high-frequency band-pass images. Dr. Chang replied that this is low-level electronic noise, which is analyzed prior to tissue studies. Dr. Lizzi said that appropriate reject levels could be set to suppress its display. He also said that knowledge of the spectral characteristics of the noise is very important for specifying appropriate filter functions prior to deconvolution.

The session was then concluded with Dr. Thijssen thanking the panel members for their presentations and participation in the discussions.

(Summarized from the taped record by F. Lizzi.)

CLOSING REMARKS BY J.M. THIJSSEN, PRESIDENT OF THE SYMPOSIUM

Ladies and Gentlemen:

Now this Symposium is coming to an end, time has come to try to evaluate how it has been. I would like to invite all of you to send me any positive or negative criticism about the organization of this Congress, and about the functioning and the organization of SIDUO in general so that we can improve upon the future activities of SIDUO. I will distribute your comments to the other members of the Executive Board of SIDUO.

As you may know there is a saying that sounds as follows: 'Not the much is good, but the good is much'. This saying may hold true in general but I am happy that I may say that this Symposium has proved to be a positive exception to this rule. We have had these days many people here and their contribution either as a lecturer in sessions, or as a participant in the discussions has been of a high level in all respects. Therefore, we have had very much of the very good, which is exceptional indeed. Thank you very much for this because it makes us, the members of the organization committee, feel extremely satisfied.

I would like to thank all of you, the Board of SIDUO in particular, for the confidence you have had to give the organization in my hands. It has been an exciting experience and I have done it with great pleasure. I have to thank Prof. Deutman and the other members of the staff of the Department of Ophthalmology who allowed us to do this organization work. I may express my gratitude to the Board of our Faculty of Medicine and in particular to the people of the domestic service of this preclinical building and to the people of the garden service who prepared for us these splendid flowers. I would like to thank also the people of the Restaurant of the Hospital who prepared for us very good meals during this week and the Public Relations Department of both our Hospital and the University who helped us a lot in our work.

You will have noticed that I needed much assistance in the organization. My way of working is that after the decisions are made and the tasks made clear I expect everybody to do his very best until the end and personal signs of satisfaction or gratitude may be rare. You therefore will understand that now the time has come to make very clear to everyone who is present here how grateful I really am to the other members of the organization committee who all did an extremely good job. And to be more specific, I can assure you that whithout the work of Marion van Tongerloo and José Koot this Congress might not have been possible at all. They have continuously devoted their energy to the benefit of this Symposium for almost a whole year. Like I said, I myself, but all the participants as well, would like to express our gratefulness to you both so please would you come here and take these flowers as a symbol of this gratitude. I would also like to thank Anja Derks, Jolanda Hennink and Jeanette van Namen who, as you all have noticed, have had their part in keeping things running smoothly during the Symposium.

I am of course also very grateful to my colleagues in the Committee, Ad Verbeek, Ton der Weyer, and René van den Broek. Please be so kind and accept my little present which shows my gratitude. I would like to thank also my coworkers and students Joop Kerkhof, Johan Taks, Marco Timmer, Marius Cloostermans, and Ton Bayer for helping us a lot during this time. You will also agree that the projectionists Cornelius and Maurits, who, together with Marco, did a splendid job in preventing any problem with the slides, are to be thanked for their excellent work.

Last but not least I would like to thank my wife, Loes, who not only took the responsibility for the Ladies Program, but who together with my children had to endure my retraction from family life in much of the week-ends and evenings of the past year.

Ladies and Gentlemen, I have the honour and the pleasure to officially close this SIDUO VIII Symposium. Thank you for coming and I would like to see you again in Leeds, 1982, at the SIDUO IX Symposium.

LIST OF CONTRIBUTORS

537